Prevention in Mental Health

Prevention in Mental Health

Marco Colizzi · Mirella Ruggeri
Editors

Prevention in Mental Health

From Risk Management to Early Intervention

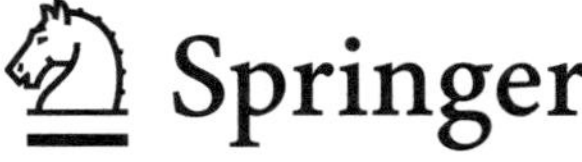 Springer

Editors
Marco Colizzi
Department of Medicine (DAME)
University of Udine
Udine, Italy

Mirella Ruggeri
Department of Neurosciences,
Biomedicine and Movement Sciences
University of Verona
Verona, Italy

ISBN 978-3-030-97908-9   ISBN 978-3-030-97906-5   (eBook)
https://doi.org/10.1007/978-3-030-97906-5

This Springer imprint is published by the registered company Springer Nature Switzerland AG
The registered company address is: Gewerbestrasse 11, 6330 Cham, Switzerland

An ounce of prevention is worth a pound of cure

Benjamin Franklin, 1736

To new beginnings, harbingers of change

Preface

When I received the proposal to edit a book for Springer Nature, I had recently come back to Italy after having spent over 5 years at my *scientific mecca*, the King's College London. After completing a PhD in Neuroscience, I had gained insight, and possibly experience, into the implementation of clinical and research services for mental health. The opportunity to discuss the book proposal with the Springer Editor would have been the Congress of the Italian Society of Psychopathology, held in Rome, where I had to deliver a presentation about the modulatory effects of cannabis on neurotransmitter systems involved in the pathophysiology of psychosis, my *workhorse*. Having both commitments, we did not manage to meet, and the COVID-19 pandemic did not give us a second chance.

However, never let yourselves be discouraged by circumstances. We still did not know, but the entire project, from its initial phases to the chapter collection to the production, would have been accomplished remotely while the pandemic is still raging in most of the world. For all these reasons, I am doubly grateful to all the people who have contributed to this work, namely the publisher's staff and the authors. They have done a tremendous effort to keep the book on top of their priorities while the research commitments were rapidly shifting in response to the pandemic outbreak; indeed, the global health research agenda has dramatically changed to pool resources in the fight against COVID-19.

In a certain way, the book was supposed to build on my research interests into the effects of cannabis on mental health. Such book would have certainly pleased several colleagues, some of whom I know personally, working in the field. Also, it would have been easier to rely on a list of experts, already in my possession, and my chance of success would have been substantially greater. Please, do not misunderstand me. I still wanted—and want—to explore the connections between cannabinoids and mental health. However, along with my co-editor, professor Mirella Ruggeri, we had the ambition to write a book which could possibly catch the interest of a wider audience of physicians, nurse practitioners, physician assistants, nurses, and students in different disciplines relevant to mental health. Most importantly, our aim was to fuel the ongoing paradigm shift in treatment and research of mental disorders which highlights the crucial contribution of preventive approaches. Also incorporating evidence about the endocannabinoid system and its potential implications, of course!

For a long time, we have been used to recognize and diagnose mental disorders based on late-stage symptoms, with schizophrenia being probably the most paradigmatic example. However, if we consider mental disorders as conditions at risk of chronicity, with roots in neurodevelopment, then we should be able to detect subtle changes in brain and behavioral functioning many years before the frank manifestation of the disorder in its most disabling form. The preventing approach promises to improve outcome by intervening early, before the full and severe symptomatic presentation of the disorder, possibly re-aligning the neurodevelopmental trajectory of the individual. Consistently, as for instance cardiology has been able to *rewind the tape* from myocardial infarction to atherosclerotic cardiovascular disease, and similar paths can be found in oncologic practice, also psychiatrists have, at least in part, linked the diagnosis of mental disorders to their pathophysiology and associated risk factors rather than to symptoms, thus redefining mental disorders as historically known.

Over the last few years, I have had the terrific opportunity of putting theory into practice. By working on the *border* between child and adolescent mental health services on one hand and adult services on the other, I was able to give a closer look at neurodevelopmental trajectories and their implications for diagnosis, treatment, and longer-term outcome. Aware of skimming just the surface of an ocean, I felt that I was heading in the right direction.

However, epidemiological data indicate that we need to do more. What would that mean for mental health? A much more socially embedded structural prevention, accompanied by a reduction of major determinants, is required for diagnosable mental health conditions to subside. There are signs of this pivot beginning to happen, calling for more research and for its more rapid translation into practice.

We hope that this book will offer some help, providing some of the most advanced knowledge, from risk management to early intervention. We tried to provide a holistic approach, encompassing biological, psychological, and environmental contributions to mental health prevention in most mental disorders. Whenever possible and supported by evidence, preventive strategies were discussed in a trans-diagnostic approach, with the goal to benefit the wider possible stakeholders.

No disease has been eradicated without a universal, multi-level, and comprehensive intervention. There is a compelling reason to inform all healthcare professionals, policy makers, and the general public about the presence and the need for mental health preventive strategies, even in healthy or subclinical populations. In parallel, efforts need to be made to implement preventive approaches in the wider possible context, to sustain individuals' ability to reach satisfactory outcomes in life.

It is time.

Udine, Italy   Marco Colizzi

Introduction

Mental Health Prevention: What Is New and What Should Be Done

This volume is a report on the current state of prevention and early intervention in mental health. It offers a representative and critical survey of general aspects and paradigms of mental health preventive strategies, deeply informed transdisciplinary evidence of the literature in specific areas for intervention and improvement, and a reappraisal of what to expect in the near future. Experts in the field from different European universities, university hospitals, and research facilities, and with different clinical and research backgrounds including humanities and social sciences, psychiatry, and neuroscience, have contributed to the realization of this project.

In alternating sections presenting psychosocial, environmental, and neurobiological arguments for the present and the future of mental health prevention from the perinatal period to adulthood, the book concludes with a call for renewal in mental health prevention. In particular, neglected areas for intervention as well as neurobiological pathways worthy of intensifying research into the development of novel preventive therapeutic options are discussed. The volume is richly documented, supported by capsule summaries of chapters' key points as well as figures, tables, and cartoons, helping the reader navigating through the contents.

Readers may be surprised how many major determinants on which to act have been identified by clinical research evidence summarized in this book. There is more as the list is certainly not exhaustive. That simply reflects the vastness of arguments for mental health prevention, most of which with unfulfilled potential, and the need for healthcare services providing primary, social, and mental care to be implemented and integrated hand in hand for preventive strategies to succeed.

Personally, editing this book was an experience that will shape our future years of dedicated work on implementing a multidisciplinary and trans-diagnostic model for care in mental health prevention. We hope that evidence-based mental health prevention inputs presented here by experienced and talented clinical researchers will orient readers' clinical and research practice too. Thanking them in advance for their critical attention to this material, we hope they will enjoy their reading.

Department of Medicine (DAME),   Marco Colizzi
University of Udine, Udine, Italy

Department of Neurosciences,   Mirella Ruggeri
Biomedicine and Movement Sciences
University of Verona,
Verona, Italy

Part I

General Aspects and Paradigms

Gender and Mental Health Prevention: When Differences Matter

Carla Comacchio

1.1 Introduction

This chapter focuses on gender-specific mental health prevention strategies. There have been many studies investigating the impact of gender on mental health, but few studies have taken into account gender differences in mental health prevention. The chapter aims to provide a comprehensive overview of mental health preventive strategies that have been developed for men and women with mental health problems. Additionally, gaps in the existing literature will be highlighted with the purpose of increasing the awareness of the importance of gender differences in mental health prevention. The chapter is divided into four main sections, each one focusing on a specific area of prevention in mental health. A fifth section represents the conclusion. The first section is named "individual factors": it provides a summary of gender differences in neurodevelopment and of the impact of gender and childhood traumatic experiences on mental health. Preventive strategies for mental health consequences of childhood abuse are discussed. The second section is called "familiar factors" and addresses the impact of maternity on mental health. Mental health promotion strategies during pregnancy and postpartum are discussed, with a specific focus on intimate partner violence prevention. The third section is "social factors": it focuses on the impact of gender and education, employment, discrimination, relationships, and nutrition on mental health. Studies on gender and mental health prevention that included these variables are presented. The fourth section is "healthcare factors" and explores the provision of gender-specific mental health prevention programs by mental health services.

C. Comacchio (✉)
Aulss 9 Scaligera and Università degli Studi di Verona, Verona, Italy
e-mail: carla.comacchio@univr.it; carla.comacchio@aulss9.veneto.it

© The Author(s), under exclusive license to Springer Nature Switzerland AG 2022
M. Colizzi, M. Ruggeri (eds.), *Prevention in Mental Health*,
https://doi.org/10.1007/978-3-030-97906-5_1

1.2 Individual Factors

There are many gender differences in developmental patterns of brain morphology, and they are due to global and local maturational changes [1]. Sex differences in the brain are organized during a critical period of neural development and have an instrumental role in determining the physiology and behavior of an individual throughout the lifespan. Understanding the impact of sex differences in neurodevelopment can advance our understanding of the potential risk for a number of neurodevelopmental, neurological, and mental health disorders that exhibit sex biases. Sex determination occurs at the moment of conception, when a female's egg is fertilized by a male's sperm. Sexual differentiation is the process by which the developing embryo becomes male or female after sex determination. It is the process by which primary sex characteristics develop, including the development of the gonads and sex organs, and it is also the process by which many sex differences in the brain are established. The organization of sexually dimorphic brain regions relies on gonadal sex hormones and involves sex differences in gene expression [2]. Among sex differences in the size of brain nuclei, it is important to cite the spinal nucleus of the bulbocavernosus; the bed nucleus of the stria terminalis, which shows a higher numbers of neurons in males compared to females [3]; and the anteroventral periventricular nucleus of the hypothalamus, which is significantly larger in females compared with males [4]. These differences can be explained by different functions of these brain regions: neurons of the spinal nucleus of the bulbocavernosus are motoneurons that are more represented in males than females [5]; the bed nucleus of the stria terminalis is involved in the vasopressin system which shows higher immunoreactivity in males compared to females [6]; and the anteroventral periventricular nucleus of the hypothalamus is involved in the surge of luteinizing hormone (LH) [7]. During postnatal brain development, the male hippocampus is only slightly larger than the female hippocampus [8], and this is thought to be the result of more neurons and glia in the male compared to the female hippocampus [9]. In males, there is an increased cell proliferation that occurs prenatally, and it is driven by androgen exposure [10]. Even the amygdala has an overall larger size in males compared to females [11]; however, the female amygdala has significantly more cell proliferation than males during early postnatal brain development, and these cells differentiate into astrocytes as opposed to neurons [12]. It is likely that these sex differences in cell number in both hippocampus and amygdala have an important role in generating sex differences in social and perhaps also cognitive behaviors; however, that remains to be fully determined. Gonadal hormones can also impact on epigenetic modifications to the DNA [13]. Therefore, given the sexually dimorphic nature of gonadal hormone secretion, epigenetic processes are likely contributors in the process of sexual differentiation, thereby determining in which sex and under what circumstances certain genes are expressed in the body and the brain.

1.2.1   Neuroimmune Impact of Childhood Adversities

Early-life experiences—both positive and negative—can have profound effects on brain development. While good parental care can offer resilience to insults later in life such as psychological stressors [14], childhood adversities can yield a myriad of deleterious deviations in brain circuitry, stress responsivity, cognitive function, and general health [15]. Many significant childhood stressors differentially disadvantage women compared with men. Childhood discrimination, violence, and physical, sexual, and emotional abuse remain problems that differentially affect women worldwide [16]. The impact of childhood adversities shows a "dose-response" effect, with a graded relationship between the number of adverse childhood events (such as abuse, neglect, or household dysfunction) and the number of adult psychiatric and inflammatory disorders [17]. Excess psychological stress has been shown to cause unhealthy sensitization of the immune response [18] that persists in later life. It causes subsequent oxidative stress damage [19] that can lead to excitotoxicity [20] or can alter typical developmental patterns of neural innervation and receptor activity [21]. Moreover, childhood adversities have been hypothesized to impact males and females differently depending on when exposure takes places, since microglial maturation also follows sexually dimorphic trajectories, such that phagocytic activity [22], transcriptomic changes [23], and responses to sensitizing stimuli [24] appear different between males and females at specific developmental time points. Immunological disturbances have been implicated as being part of the pathophysiology of mental disorders including major depressive disorder (MDD) [25], bipolar disorder [26], and schizophrenia [27]. It has been proposed that childhood adversities may generate a population with increased vulnerability to mental illness through a pipeline of amplified signaling between the brain and immune system. Lastly, it has been found that women who are homozygous for the 5HTTLPR "s" allele produce higher and more prolonged levels of cortisol in response to a stressful laboratory test than women with at least one 5HTTLPR "l" allele, indicating that women with this genetic predisposition may be more biologically reactive to stressors [28].

1.2.2   Preventing Childhood Trauma

Child maltreatment is a serious public health problem [29], affecting up to 80% of children worldwide [30]. The definition of childhood trauma is broad and comprises eight main dimensions: physical abuse, sexual abuse, psychological abuse, witnessing interpersonal violence, physical neglect, emotional neglect, significant separations from caregivers, and loss of caregiver [31]. Childhood abuse rates are two to three times higher in women compared to men [32], and it is associated with a number of negative sequelae, such as depression [33], post-traumatic stress disorder [34], suicidality [35], eating disorders [36], and drug abuse [37]. Victims of childhood abuse are also at risk for revictimization as adults, when they go on to experience high rates of intimate partner violence [38], and their offspring are at increased risk for being abused [39]. However, childhood abuse prevention is challenging to achieve in public health programming, in part due to the level of support needed to overcome risk factors and bolster protective factors for families and communities [40]. Most interventions designed to prevent childhood abuse are based on home visits [41]. At-risk parents are usually identified among low-income families, focusing on those families with parental young age, maternal depression and substance abuse, family stress, lack of social support, and intimate partner violence [41]. Most home-visiting interventions are delivered by trained paraprofessionals or nurses [41]. One study compared nurses and lay visitors and found that while lay visitors were more successful in helping mothers to feel a sense of mastery and self-empowerment, nurse visitors were more effective in supporting depressed mothers with limited psychological resources as well as improving cognitive outcomes for their children [42]. Most home-visiting interventions start during pregnancy [43], in order to establish a sense of trust between the mother and the visitor that allows the mother to rely on the visitor immediately after birth, and continues up to 2 years after childbirth [44]. Home visit frequency is weekly or biweekly in the immediate postpartum period, gradually decreasing to monthly or bimonthly [41]. Intervention targets usually include accessing prenatal care and pediatric care, understanding infant development, enhancing parent-infant interaction, mobilizing psychosocial support, delaying repeat pregnancy, and improving maternal life trajectory [41]. Cognitive behavioral therapy (CBT) has been used in one study to increase parental problem-solving skills [45]. These interventions have found to positively impact on reducing child abuse rates as well as increasing mother-infant interaction, maternal depression, repeat pregnancy, maternal employment, cognitive development, and externalizing behaviors of children [41]. Moreover, they have shown long-term protective effects on children, who display lower rates of substance use, better academic achievement, and fewer arrests and convictions [46]. Evidence on interventions other than home visitation is limited. Two studies have assessed the efficacy and cost differential of postpartum groups as compared to home visits. The studies suggest that groups can improve parenting knowledge [47] and maternal mental health [48] at a lower cost. However, these studies did not measure the impact upon child abuse events [41].

However, not all traumatic experiences occur during the first years postpartum. Research shows that different children having essentially the same upsetting experience may be impacted in different ways [49]. Some will have few or no symptoms of traumatic stress; some will have symptoms that diminish over several weeks; and some others may have long-lasting emotional, behavioral, and cognitive difficulties that affect multiple domains of life as a result of the experience(s). Thus, screening for traumatic stress symptoms among children with a history of potentially traumatic experiences can identify those who may benefit from evidence-based trauma treatment. There are several useful screening tools to identify and more effectively care for children and adolescents who have been exposed to violence. The Trauma Symptom Checklist for Children/Trauma Symptom Checklist for Young Children (TSCC/TSCYC) short form is a 20-item parent report measure for the assessment of trauma-related symptoms in children ages 3–12. The clinical scales include PTS-Intrusion, PTS-Avoidance, PTS-Arousal, Sexual Concerns, Anxiety, Depression, Dissociation, and Anger/Aggression [50]. The UCLA PTSD Reaction Index (UCLA PTSD-RI) is a tool that assesses trauma exposure and PTSD symptoms in children and adolescents [51]. It includes parent-report and self-report versions. Informants are asked to indicate whether the child has been exposed to 12 different traumatic events, and an option is also provided to describe additional traumatic events not already queried. It subsequently asks individuals to identify the current most impairing event and asks questions about the child's reactions during or directly after exposure to that event. Finally, it assesses PTSD symptom frequency on a five-point Likert scale within the past month. The Child PTSD Symptom Scale (CPSS) is a 26-item child (ages 8–18) self-report measure which parallels DSM-IV diagnostic criteria for PTSD. Respondents indicate how often they experienced each symptom in the past month on a four-point Likert scale from 0 (not at all) to 3 (five or more times a week). Higher total scores indicate greater PTSS [52]. Once traumatic experiences are disclosed, trauma-focused cognitive behavioral therapy (TFCBT) for children and adolescents should be offered. It is a structured, short-term psychotherapeutic treatment model that effectively improves trauma-related outcomes for children/teens and their caregivers. TFCBT is intended to address affective, cognitive, and behavioral problems, to promote optimal support at home; to strengthen parenting skills, and to reduce child and caregiver distress about the child's traumatic experiences. This form of CBT has shown to have superior outcomes to other methods in different settings and with diverse populations and varied life circumstances [53, 54]. However, to our knowledge, no study has focused on gender-specific intervention to prevent childhood abuse. Available intervention research largely focuses on response to traumatic experiences rather than prevention [55]. Nevertheless, the differential susceptibility of girls and boys to various forms of maltreatment should be addressed in dedicated preventive programs. Childhood abuse preventive programs for boys should be more focused on preventing harsh physical punishment and its consequences, since being victim of physical violence in childhood increases the likeliness of becoming perpetrators of physical violence in later life [56]. On the other side, preventive programs for childhood abuse in girls should have different features and involve sexual abuse prevention, female genital mutilation prevention, and neglect and infanticide prevention that arise from child's gender prevention. They could be helpful in reducing the incidence of adult revictimization [41], HIV and other sexually transmitted disease infections [57], and selective abortion practices [58]. Moreover, interventions specifically designed for preventing childhood abuse in boys and girls are likely to decrease the incidence and the impact of such events and, in the long run, to decrease gender inequalities in the community.

1.3   Familiar Factors

Among familial factors, maternity is considered the most important period for promoting mental health. Maternity is a major life transition and the perinatal period is characterized by several biological and psychosocial changes [59]. During pregnancy, maternal attitude toward their developing child is predictive of the quality of maternal behavior both during and after birth [60, 61] and of infant's later attachment style [62]. During the first weeks after birth, women start to know their infant and manage childcare tasks, developing a mother-infant relationship. A positive mother-infant relationship is described as the mothers' ability of understanding their child's expression of emotions and respond to the child's need in a timely and appropriate manner [63]. It is influenced by maternal well-being [64], mentalization [65], self-efficacy [66], and breastfeeding [67], and it is crucial for the development of infant's secure attachment [68]. Secure attachment is associated with several positive outcomes for the child in terms of emotional, social, and behavioral development and adjustment, as well as school performance [69]. While most women gradually develop confidence and satisfaction with their new roles [70], a significant proportion of mothers do experience distress. Maternal distress occurs when the infant's demands are perceived as exceeding the available resources for coping [71], and it is a risk factor for the development of mental health problems.

Mental health problems are common during the perinatal period, affecting around 16% of women during pregnancy and 20% postpartum [72]. Despite one in five women would experience a perinatal mental health disorder, many of them do not receive a correct diagnosis [73]. Moreover, it has been calculated that among women who are identified as having a mental health problem, only 15% receive adequate treatment [74]. Perinatal mental health problems are associated with poor mother-infant relationship, insecure attachment, and increased risk for child's emotional, behavioral, and cognitive problems in later life [75–78]. Since preventive interventions during early childhood are more effective than those that occur later in a child's life [79], the perinatal period constitutes a window of opportunity for preventing mental health problems.

An important issue related to maternal mental health is intimate partner violence (IPV), since it is estimated that one in three women is victim of physical, sexual, or emotional abuse by their partner [80]. Although IPV can occur at any time of life, the highest prevalence is during a woman's reproductive years [81], and more than 25% of women are pregnant when violence occurs [82]. As previously stated, maternity presents new challenges to each parent and their relationship, which, in some cases, can lead to the initiation, continuation, or increased frequency or severity of aggression [81], making IPV one of the most common health risks in the perinatal period [83]. Perinatal IPV is associated with several psychiatric disorders, especially postpartum depression [84] and child adverse outcomes [85]. Risk factors for IPV in pregnancy include abuse before pregnancy, lower educational level, low socioeconomic status, being single or living apart, alcohol abuse, unintended/unwanted pregnancy, and lifetime adversity/exposure to violence [86]. Perinatal mental health problems are a major public issue [87], and studies indicate that they can be minimized if women and families engage with dedicated services [88]. There are three key elements in promoting mental health during the perinatal period: (1) detection of at-risk mothers, (2) availability of effective perinatal interventions, and (3) availability of an organizational framework for the interdisciplinary work [63].

1.3.1   Detection of at-Risk Mothers

Detection of at-risk mothers involves assessment of preexisting mental health or substance abuse disorders, screening for domestic and intimate partner violence, and evaluation of familial, social, and economic support [89]. There are six assessment tools to screen risk factors for perinatal mental health problems. The Antenatal Psychosocial Health Assessment (ALPHA) tool uses 35 questions to identify antenatal psychosocial risk factors that would lead to poor postnatal psychosocial outcomes. These risk factors are associated with woman abuse, child abuse, postpartum depression, and couple dysfunction, and the risk factors are further grouped into four categories: family factors, maternal factors, substance use, and family violence. Questions are scored using a three-point tick-box system of "low," "some," and "high" [90]. The Antenatal Risk Questionnaire (ANRQ) consists of 12 items. This tool assesses the following psychosocial risk domains: emotional support from subject's own mother in childhood, past history of depressed mood or mental illness and treatment received, perceived level of support available following the birth of the baby, partner emotional support, life stresses in the previous 12 months, personality style (anxious or perfectionistic traits), and history of abuse (emotional, physical, and sexual). It is scored using a combination of categorical and continuous data, with a possible maximum score of 62 and minimum score of 5 [91]. The Australian Routine Psychosocial Assessment (ARPA) includes 12 questions (support, stressors, personality, mental health, childhood abuse, family violence, and current mood) [92]. The Camberwell Assessment of Need—Mothers (CAN-M) covers the 26 domains of accommodation, food, looking after the home, self-care, daytime activities, general physical health, pregnancy care, sleep, psychotic symptoms, psychological distress, information, safety to self, safety to child and others, substance misuse, company, intimate relationships, sexual health, violence and abuse, practical demands of childcare, emotional demands of childcare, basic education, telephone, transport, budgeting, benefits, language, culture, and religion. Domains were assessed on a five-point Likert scale of importance (ranging from "not at all" to "essential") [93]. The Contextual Assessment of Maternity Experience (CAME) explores recent life adversity or stressors, the quality of social support and key relationships including partner relationship, and maternal feelings toward pregnancy, motherhood, and the baby [94]. The Pregnancy Risk Questionnaire (PRQ) assesses the mother's attitude to her pregnancy, mother's experience of parenting in childhood, history of physical or sexual abuse, history of depression, impact of depression on psychosocial function, whether treatment was sought or recommended, presence of emotional support from partner and mother, presence of other supports, presence of stressors during pregnancy, trait anxiety, obsessional traits, and self-esteem. A five-point Likert scale is used, from 1 "not at all" to 5 "very much" [95]. However, none of these tools has been considered reliable in adequately detecting antenatal mental health problems due to low positive predictive values, insufficient information regarding clinical performance, or insufficient sample size [96]. Despite their limitations, these tools can be used to determine the need for further intervention or to refer women to mental health services.

The most common psychiatric disorder in the perinatal period is postnatal depression, which affects up to 15% of pregnant women [97]. Approximately 40% of women will experience their first depressive episode postpartum [98] and when left untreated, are more likely to experience further episodes of depression later in life (10 in Pettman). There are seven commonly used screening tools for perinatal depression [99]. The Postpartum Depression Screening Scale (PDSS) is divided into seven dimensions with each dimension composed of five items. The seven dimensions are Sleeping/Eating Disturbances, Anxiety/Insecurity, Emotional Lability, Cognitive Impairment, Loss of Self, Guilt/Shame, and Contemplating Harming Oneself. On completing the scale, a mother is asked to select a label from (1) to (5) to reflect her degree of disagreement or agreement, where (1) means strongly disagree and (5) means strongly agree [100]. The Edinburgh Postnatal Depression Scale (EPDS) is the most widely tested screening tool for postnatal depression, but its sensitivity varies from 22% to 96% [101, 102]. The EPDS is a ten-item self-report questionnaire used by healthcare providers to assess perinatal depression. Possible scores range from 0 to 30, with 11 and 13 being the most commonly used cutoffs to detect "probable" depression [103]. However, EPDS limits questions to feelings of sadness or anxiety, without screening for physical symptoms [99], which are a common presentation of depression. In addition, the EPDS reference period is narrow, since it allows patients to report symptoms felt during the week before the assessment. Lastly, there are differences in the cutoff scores that allow for disparities in depressive level detection [104]. Despite this, EPDS is routinely used to screen for depressive levels in the postpartum. Beck's Depression Inventory-II (BDI-II) is a 21-item self-report instrument for measuring the severity of depression with four response options ranging from 0 to 3 for each item, with a total maximum score for all items being 63. A score of 0–13 is considered minimal, 14–19 mild, 20–28 moderate, and 29–63 severe depression [105]. The General Health Questionnaire-12 (GHQ-12) is a scale of 12 items, with four response options and an overall rating from 0 to 12 used to assess mental health and psychological adjustment [106]. The Center for Epidemiological Studies Depression Scale (CES-D) is a 20-item Likert-format screening tool that asks respondents how often they experienced a particular symptom in the past week, where 0 represents "rarely or none of the time" and 3 represents "most or all of the time" (range 0–60). Higher scores indicate greater depressive symptoms [107]. The Patient Health Questionnaire (PHQ) is the preferred screening tool for depressive symptoms in most primary care settings. The PHQ-9 is a multipurpose self-rating nine-item, depression-screening scale, which assesses the experiencing of depressive symptoms over the last 14 days. Scores on the PHQ-9 range from 0 to 27 and are calculated by assigning scores of 0, 1, 2, or 3 to response categories of "not at all," "several days," "more than half the days," or "nearly every day," respectively, and then summing up the scores. Greater scores on the PHQ-9 indicate more severe depressive symptoms [108]. The Pregnancy Risk Questionnaire has been previously described. However, a recent review concluded that none of these could be deemed best at detecting perinatal depression on the basis of sensitivity and specificity. Moreover, there was no agreement on time duration in which screening tools should be administered [99].

Concerning IPV, since pregnancy involves repeated contact with healthcare providers, it offers a unique opportunity to develop trust between women and healthcare team, which can increase the possibility of disclosure of abusive situations. Moreover, women may be motivated by the desire to protect their children from possible abuse by intimate partner. Most pregnant women are accepting of inquiry regarding IPV, provided there is enough privacy and confidentiality and the inquiry and disclosure lead to positive consequences [109]. For these reasons, checking any relationship stress during each antenatal and postpartum visit may be helpful. There are three commonly used screening tools for detecting IPV in pregnancy. The RADAR is an acronym-mnemonic that helps summarize key action steps that physicians should take in recognizing and treating patients affected by IPV. The tool includes (1) routinely screen adult patients, (2) ask direct questions, (3) document your findings, (4) assess patient safety, and (5) review options and referrals [110]. The HIITS tool asks a patient the following questions: How often does your partner physically hurt you, insult or talk down to you, threaten you with harm, and scream or curse at you? Each category is graded on a scale of 1 (never) to 5 (frequently) and a sum of all the categories is generated. A total score of 10 or above is suggestive of IPV [111]. Abuse Assessment Screen (AAS) tool is perhaps one of the most widely used IPV screening tools in the pregnant population. It is a short, five-question screen that involves the following open-ended questions: (1) Have you ever been emotionally or physically abused by your partner or someone important to you? (2) Since I saw you last, have you been hit, slapped, kicked, or otherwise physically hurt by someone? If *yes*, by whom? Number of times? Nature of injury? (3) Since you have been pregnant, have you been hit, slapped, kicked, or otherwise physically hurt by someone? If *yes*, by whom? Number of times? Nature of injury? (4) Within the past year, has anyone made you do something sexual that you did not want to do? If *yes*, then who? (5) Are you afraid of your partner or anyone else? [112]. Once IPV is disclosed, it is essential to determine whether the woman is in immediate danger, whether there are weapons at home, if violence has recently escalated, if substance abuse is involved, and if there is an alternate environment where the woman can ensure her safety and protection [113]. It is important to note that effective protocols for immediate access or referral to adequate support are most successful in increasing IPV identification [114]. In no case, women should be blamed or pressed to leave their partner [84]. Despite this, fewer than half of pregnant women with mental health problems are identified in clinical settings [74]. Reasons for that include inadequate training in detecting mental health issues by maternity healthcare staff, insufficient interventions for women with psychiatric problems in the peripartum, and barriers in accessing psychiatric services due to stigma, fear of child welfare consequences, and lack of adequate childcare [74].

1.3.2 Availability of Effective Perinatal Interventions

There are several interventions available for preventing perinatal mental health disorders, including medication, health promotion interventions, and psychological interventions. Nearly all studies have focused on preventing perinatal depression, since it is the most common mental health problem in the peripartum and it can lead to severe consequences, both for the mother and the offspring. Concerning medication, it has been estimated that the risk of subsequent incidence of postpartum depression following a first episode of postpartum depression is 1 in 4 [115]. Prophylactic medication in the postpartum with nortriptyline, a tricyclic antidepressant, has been tested in two small trials [116, 117] with conflicting results. In one study prophylactic nortriptyline appeared to be effective in reducing postpartum depression relapse at 12 weeks postpartum [116], whereas the other study found no difference in depressive levels at 20 weeks postpartum between women taking antidepressant and controls [117]. It is not clear whether these inconsistencies are due to methodological limitations, inadequate drug mechanism, or intervention or approach ineffectiveness. At present, there is thus no indication for prophylactic antidepressant therapy in postpartum women who already had suffered from postpartum depression. It has been hypothesized that postpartum depression may be related to the rapidly decreasing levels of sex hormones following delivery, and four small trials have tested the prophylactic effect of estrogen and progesterone therapy in preventing postpartum depression [118–121]. Results were promising for prophylactic estrogen therapy [118], but highly inconsistent for prophylactic progesterone therapy, with two small studies showing a reduction in the postpartum depression recurrence rate [119, 120], and another larger trial showing an increased risk of developing depressing symptoms in women taking progesterone therapy compared to controls [121]. Postpartum depression has been linked to thyroid antibodies in pregnancy [122], but a small trial failed to show an effect in the occurrence of depression in women taking thyroxine postpartum [123]. The effect of docosahexaenoic acid (DHA) administration in postpartum women at risk for postpartum depression has been tested in a small trial [124], under the observation that populations with high intakes of omega-3 fatty acids have lower rates of depression than do populations with low consumption of omega-3 fatty acids [125], without showing a significant effect on postpartum depression rates. Lastly, calcium supplementation in women at risk for postpartum depression has showed a promising effect in preventing postpartum depression in a small trial [126], since calcium metabolism is influenced by fluctuations in gonadal hormones that are exacerbated in the postpartum period [127]. Concluding, given the current evidence, there is no specific biological approach recommended for preventing postpartum depression in clinical practice. However, women with perinatal mental health problems indicate a preference for health promotion and psychological interventions over medications [128].

Regarding psychological interventions, preventive treatments for perinatal depression have focused on interpersonal therapy, cognitive behavioral therapy (CBT), and psychological debriefing. In two trials, interpersonal therapy appeared to be effective in preventing depression compared to controls at 4 weeks postpartum

[129, 130], but this prophylactic effect was not maintained at 24 weeks postpartum [130]. Preventive CBT for postpartum depression has been tested in two trials: one study showed no difference in depressive levels at 12 weeks postpartum between intervention and control groups [131], whereas in the other study, women in the CBT group showed lower levels of depressive symptoms at 6 weeks postpartum compared to controls [132]. Psychological debriefing midwife-led for preventing postpartum depression has been analyzed in four studies with inconsistent results: in one study, women in the psychological debriefing group presented with less depressive symptoms at 3 weeks postpartum compared to controls [133]; in another study, women in the experimental group showed higher levels of depressive symptoms at 24 weeks postpartum compared to controls; and in two studies, no difference in depressive levels was found between treated women and controls [134, 135].

Among psychosocial interventions for preventing postpartum depression, we can list antenatal and postnatal classes, intrapartum support, and supportive interaction strategies. Antenatal classes showed to be effective in preventing postpartum depression only in two trials [136, 137], whereas in four studies, no differences were found in depressive levels between experimental and control groups [138–140]. Intrapartum support showed to be effective in preventing postpartum depression at 6 weeks but not at 1 year postpartum [141, 142], but the positive result at 6 weeks postpartum was not replicated in other studies [143, 144]. Interaction strategies for preventing postpartum depression include extensive nursing home visits [145, 146] or additional support provided by trained postpartum workers [147, 148]. They showed a reduction in depressive levels at 6 weeks postpartum compared to controls, but these results were not maintained at follow-up assessments [145–148]. Despite home visits and home-based psychological interventions (interpersonal therapy, CBT, and counseling) appearing to be promising for the treatment of postpartum depression [149], there is insufficient evidence to recommend them for preventing postpartum depression.

1.3.3 Availability of an Organizational Framework for the Interdisciplinary Work

It has been advised that continuity of care may increase woman's satisfaction, and three trials have been conducted to compare midwife-managed care with shared care (care divided among midwives, hospital physicians, and general practitioners) in preventing postnatal depression. Midwives have been identified as case managers because typically obstetricians and gynecologists are not trained to identify psychiatric disorders, and even when mental health problems are identified, perinatal mental health providers are frequently insufficient [74]. Moreover, the waiting lists for psychiatric appointments are often too long to be of use during pregnancy, and, in addition, women often refuse to seek mental healthcare in psychiatric settings due to stigma, fear of child welfare consequences, cost, inconvenience, and lack of adequate childcare [74]. In a large trial, women in the midwife-managed group showed lower depressive levels compared to women in the shared care group [150], whereas the other two trials showed no differences in depressive levels between experimental and control groups [151, 152]. Interestingly, while continuous midwifery care did not prevent postpartum depression, it appeared to be highly successful at engaging women in treatment [152].

Antenatal classes have been claimed to be a good opportunity for delivering preventive interventions for postpartum depression, but a randomized controlled trial showed no differences in depression levels between experimental and control groups at 16 weeks postpartum [153]. Neither early postpartum appointments delivered 2–6 weeks postpartum in order to prevent postpartum depression appeared to be effective in reducing depressive levels compared to controls [154, 155]. On the other side, educational strategies focusing on postpartum depression, which were delivered during antenatal classes and early postpartum appointments, appeared to be successful in decreasing the severity of postpartum depression and the time between onset of depressive symptoms and seeking professional help [156, 157]. However, a larger trial failed to replicate the result [158]. To date, despite a good number of available trials, there is insufficient evidence to unequivocally recommend any particular intervention for preventing postpartum depression.

1.4 Social Factors

Many social factors contribute to mental well-being and should be involved in mental health preventive strategies. Unfortunately, there are a few studies on social factors and mental health preventive interventions, and for most of them, the impact of gender has not been taken into consideration. These social factors are analyzed in the next paragraphs.

1.4.1 Education

Several studies have suggested that formal education offers benefits for mental health and may be protective specifically against depression [159]. High education may be protective against mental health problems because it can lead to more fulfilling careers and higher socioeconomic position. It may also sustain healthy lifestyle behaviors and provide better access to healthcare. Moreover, higher education may help developing qualities that increase the ability to cope with stress, such as self-efficacy and cognitive and socio-emotional skills. It has been found that high education levels are a protective factor for the perceived quality of life in women but not in men, whereas low levels of education are associated with higher use of health services in women compared with men [160]. Globally, women have fewer socioeconomic resources such as power, authority, and earnings compared with men [161]. They face more economic dependency; restricted opportunities for paid employment, routine, being poorly paid, and unfulfilling work; and less authority at work [162] than men. The "theory of resource substitutions" suggests that higher education is more positively impactful for individuals with previous disadvantages [161]. On this basis, three studies have shown that the protective effects of education on depressive symptoms are larger for women compared with men [161, 163, 164]. This larger beneficial effect has been attributed to the greater effect of education-related work creativity and sense of control on depressive symptoms in women than men [161]. However, these results have not been replicated by recent trials [165]. While the differential impact of gender and education on depression has not been completely disentangled, it is known that school difficulties may be, in some cases, a consequence of a mental disorder [166]. School difficulties in both genders and academic failure for men are associated with an increased risk for suicide before the age of 35 [167]. Given this, schools and universities could be a good place to deliver mental health prevention interventions. Even though a few mental health preventive interventions in schools have been developed [168], no study has been made on the impact of gender on mental health preventive interventions in schools and universities.

1.4.2   Employment

The effect of employment on mental health can be both positive, by providing regular activity, time structure, social contact, a sense of collective effort, and social identity [169], and negative, as a source of psychological stress related to job demands and lack of social support in the workplace. Statistically speaking, women are less occupationally active than men. In 2017, among people aged 20–64, the share of working women in Europe was 66.5% and the share of working men was 78% [170]. For people aged >50, these differences were even larger. The activity rate for women aged 50–64 was 51.1%, and for men 67.2%. Taking into account only people aged 60–64, this rate was 22.1% of working women, compared to almost 50% of working men [171]. Mental health is negatively affected by economic recession [172], and mental distress and depression are more common among unemployed than employed people [173]. Studies conducted in the 1960s and the 1970s reported worse health consequences in unemployed men compared to unemployed women. At least two explanations were offered for such finding: first, as masculine identity has been historically linked to having a job in Western countries, unemployment was suggested to threaten it [174]; second, women have been suggested to compensate for the negative effect of unemployment by returning to their position as housewives [175]. However, with the increasing participation of women in the labor market, these results have been overturned by more recent studies indicating that unemployment has a stronger association with negative health outcomes in women than men [176–178]. Nowadays, poor mental health seems to have a stronger association with unemployment in men compared to women only in conservative countries [179]. Conservative countries are those that tend to display lower levels of social welfare, using the principle of subsidiarity where the state only intervenes when, for example, citizens are unable to find gainful employment or source financial means from family members (i.e., Belgium, Germany, France, the Netherlands) [180]. A possible explanation for this is that the breadwinner role in the traditional family model could contribute to a stigmatization of unemployed men [181]. By contrast, in liberal countries, defined as countries in which the principle of the free market is the bedrock and welfare state provides minimal support and aims to intervene as little as possible (i.e., United Kingdom, Ireland) [180], unemployed women seem to show lower levels of mental well-being compared with men [179], possibly because of lower social insurance benefits and salaries compared to men [181]. Instead, in Southern-European countries, characterized by the prominent role of families in providing welfare and generally high levels of inequality [180] (i.e., Portugal, Greece, Italy), there seem to be no gender difference in mental well-being among unemployed people [179]. This may be due to the increased women participation in labor market during economic crisis in order to set the drop in earnings of their partners [179]. Moreover, women tend to report lower health status, more somatic and psychological symptoms [182], and higher levels of smoking and alcohol consumption during recession periods compared with men [178]. Lastly, women with low socioeconomic status appear to be particularly hit by the consequences of recession [183], possibly because of the detrimental effect of financial strain and social isolation [184].

A number of male-dominated industries (i.e., industries in which more than 70% of workers are men) [185] have higher than average rates of anxiety and mood disorders. These industries include agriculture, construction, mining, and utilities [186]. Generally speaking, men are more reticent to access professional mental health services and seek help for psychological problems [187]. This may be due to "traditional masculine behavior" (emphasis on being rational, stoical, and not showing weakness) [188], perceived stigma around mental health [189], and employment status [190]. Therefore, workers in male-dominated industries are at higher risk of mental health disorders but are less likely to access treatment than the general population [191]. As such, interventions delivered in settings where men gather, including the workplace, hold promise for promoting mental health among men [192]. The available evidence suggests that key elements to promote mental health among workers in male-dominated industries include distribution of information to workers about mental health issues, provision of additional social support, access to treatment and advice for workers, education for managers about mental health in the workplace, addressing excessive workloads, and providing relief periods from heavy workloads [193]. Additional elements that can improve mental health in male-dominated industries are team environment, job demand, job variety, and control [191]. Moreover, structural factors such as economic climate, labor market conditions, employment policies, and job security can contribute to workers' psychological well-being [194]. Lastly, it has been proved that interventions that target the whole workplace, utilize team-based approaches, and use multiple strategies are the most effective [195]. However, most studies on promoting mental health among men in workplaces have examined a wide range of psychological outcomes and used a variety of different measures, making it difficult to compare results [196]. The most commonly investigated outcome measure was stress reduction [197–201]. Studies involving both sexes tend to support a more effective role of mental health promotion in female as opposed to male workers [199, 202], possibly because men are less likely to participate in planning workshops compared to women.

Another life status transition with implications for workforce participation, lifestyle, and social roles among older adults is retirement. Retirement has been associated with poor mental health, particularly with higher levels of depression, in men but not in women [203]. This has been attributed to decreased financial stability [204], loss in work role and social networks [205], or loss of eligibility for receipt of social security benefits [206]. Moreover, men tend to consider work to have a central role in their lives and have a much more continuous employment career compared with women [203].

1.4.3   Discrimination

Discrimination is defined as being treated unfairly in any field of public life based on one's personal characteristics, such as race, gender, or religion [207]. Perceived discrimination is strongly associated with poor indicators of both physical [208] and mental health, particularly with anxiety [209], depression [210], and PTSD [211]. Gender discrimination in the workplace includes harassment, unequal pay, and implementation of rules that puts one gender at a disadvantage [212]. Although gender discrimination is illegal in many countries, it is still far from being eradicated. For instance, statistics from Europe show that women earn on average 20% less than men [213]. In addition, more than 50% of employed women report being victims of sexual harassment in the workplace [214]. Lastly, evidence shows gender-biased hiring preferences with men being favored over women, even though qualifications and experience are identical [215]. Despite political efforts to reduce gender gap in the labor market, different conditions for men and women in this field still persist. The horizontal segregation of the labor market means that men mainly work in male-dominated sectors, while women work in female-dominated sectors [216]. Vertical segregation means that men are overrepresented at the highest levels with regard to status, power, and income. As a consequence, women have lower wages than men, even in the same job [217]. These gender differences in labor market are posited to be associated with differences in mental health problems reported by men and women [218]. However, to date few studies have focused on workplace-related gender discrimination [210]. One large cohort study [219] has focused on the effect of age discrimination on mental health in the workplace and found that perceived age discrimination is a significant predictor of women's depressive symptoms and life satisfaction over the life course.

One important risk factor for mental health problems in the workplace is burnout. Burnout is a psychological syndrome that encompasses symptoms of emotional exhaustion, cynicism, and self-inefficacy in work role performance and results from chronic exposure to excessive demands from the work environment [220]. It affects 4–13% of the workforce [221] and women tend to report higher levels of burnout compared with men [222]. This has been attributed to lower levels of decision latitude in women compared with men [223]. In several working environments, women are overqualified in greater proportion than men [224]. Overqualification may express a glass ceiling effect where women are less likely to be promoted to higher-level positions characterized by greater levels of decision latitude. On the other side, burnout in men appears to be related to their longer working hours and irregular shifts compared to women. Burnout is a risk factor for sickness absence, and the length of sickness absence is increased by physical violence, bullying, and shift work in women only [225]. Few studies have focused on preventing burnout in workplaces, and have showed that high levels of job support, workplace justice, and job controls are protective against burnout. Moreover, job control has found to be protective also against depression [226]. However, none of these studies has adopted a gendered perspective. Although there is a large increase in the proportion of women in managerial jobs, they still tend to be overrepresented in the helping professions such as teaching, nursing, and social work. In contrast, men are still the majority within physics, engineering, and chemistry [227]. People having jobs in which they are in a cultural and numerical minority may be especially vulnerable to stress-related problems, regardless of gender [228]. Gender differences in burnout rates appear to be largely dependent on profession, with women in medicine being at particular risk. Burnout appears to be 20 to 60% higher among women physicians than men physicians [229], because of the high levels of gender-based discrimination in this field [230]. Maternal discrimination is a risk factor for burnout, and it is also very frequent among female physicians. It is most frequently manifested as disrespectful treatment by colleagues, exclusion from administrative decision-making, and inequitable pay and benefits [231], which can contribute to burnout. In addition, motherhood has other implications for women in medicine, predisposing them to life stressors such as delays in childbirth and/or adoption, fertility struggles [232], infertility, and pregnancy-related complications or risk exposure during pregnancy (e.g., radiation or chemical exposure) [233]. Other gender differences in burnout rates have been found in teachers, with women reporting higher levels of emotional exhaustion [234] and psychological fatigue compared with men [235]. A possible explanation for this can be found in the emotional labor which characterizes these professions. Teachers are often required to hide or suppress one's own (negative) emotions which have been related to burnout [236]. As a consequence, women in education tend to retire earlier than men [237], increasing pressure on the teacher labor market and leading to increasing teacher shortages [238]. Interventions specific to prevent burnout in female physicians should thus include addressing barriers to career satisfaction, work-life integration, and mental health, identification and reduction of gender and maternal bias, mentorship and sponsorship opportunities, and family leave, lactation, and childcare policies and support [239].

1.4.4 Relationships

Marriage impacts on both physical and mental health, and married individuals of both sexes show better physical health than unmarried ones [240]. However, the impact of marriage on mental health is controversial, with some early studies showing that married women exhibit higher rates of mental disorders compared with men, and others reporting that the mental health benefits of being married extend equally to men and women [241]. It has been hypothesized that marriage may confer benefits to mental health because it provides an intimate, emotionally fulfilling relationship that satisfies individuals' needs for social integration and support [242]. Spouses also monitor one another, encouraging healthy behaviors that promote emotional well-being, i.e., responsible drinking [243]. Lastly, marriage can also create an important sense of identity and purpose for many people, which may contribute to mental well-being [244]. Generally speaking, entry into marriage is associated with lower levels of distress, whereas a transition out of marriage increases psychological distress in both sexes [245]. However, women report significantly greater increases in psychological distress than men when their marriages break down [246]. Moreover, increased vulnerability to distress may also occur for women who become widowed or remarried [241]. In addition, there is evidence that the costs of loss and separation or divorce fall more heavily on women than men, exerting a strong and often permanent downward pull on the economic well-being of widowed and divorced women [247]. Given the physical and mental health benefits of marriage, some countries have developed programs to promote healthy marriages via relationship education as a strategy to improve public health. Key elements of these programs are couples and marriage education and support for adults, relationships and marriage education for high school students, and fatherhood programs with co-parenting or marriage components [248]. Couples and marriage education programs aim to change attitudes and dispel myths about marriage and to teach relationship skills—especially related to communication and conflict resolution—to adults at various life stages: single, dating, engaged, newly married, marriages in crisis, and those who are remarried [248]. Relationship education for students focuses on teaching middle and high school students about skills for building successful relationships and marriages [248]. Fatherhood programs aim to promote the importance of fatherhood and to help fathers to become more involved with their children. They encompass job training and placement, child support payment assistance, peer support groups, parenting classes, legal assistance, and individual counseling [248]. All these programs include capacity building activities and public education, community awareness, and outreach components of service programs, and they have shown to be effective in increasing longevity of marriages [248].

Early studies on mental health, work, and gender revealed that there has been no significant change in the housework division following the increased participation of women in the workforce [249]. In Western countries, employed women spend on average 4 h per day on housework, compared to the 2 h spent by men [250]. On the contrary, employed men watch television an hour longer, sleep half an hour longer [251], and spend longer time eating meals [252] compared to their wives. A large body of literature identifies work-family conflicts as a factor for adverse health outcomes among employed women [253]. Husbands' participation in housework is associated with wives' satisfaction with housework division and perception of fairness [254]. Conversely, the unequal division of domestic work and family responsibility is associated with less life satisfaction, poor self-rated health [255], and perceived physical/psychosomatic symptoms in women [256]. Specifically, inequity in the division of housework has been associated with depressive symptoms [257] and increased risk for suicidal ideation [258]. Moreover, a higher domestic workload has reported to be associated with increased psychological distress [256] and suboptimal self-rated health [259]. Possible strategies to decrease domestic job stress include removal of traditional gender roles at home and discussing the social norms for domestic work and their redefinition in the light of social, cultural, emotional, and environmental contexts [260].

1.4.5 Nutrition

In the last years, there has been growing attention on the impact of nutrition on mental health. In the beginning, most studies have focused on the association of depression with specific nutrients or foods [261], whereas recent research has shifted toward the relationship between depression and dietary patterns [262]. Generally speaking, healthy dietary patterns are associated with reduced odds of depression [263]. A healthy diet is characterized by high intakes of fruit, vegetables, whole grains, poultry, fish, and reduced fat dairy products [264]. Several potential mechanisms underlying this association have been proposed: the anti-inflammatory properties of foods in the healthy diet have been shown to influence concentrations of monoamines, which are thought to play a role in the regulation of emotions and cognition [265]. The antioxidant compounds in fruit and vegetables could reduce oxidative stress-induced neuronal damage, particularly neurons in the hippocampus [266]. Evidence also suggests that a high consumption of long-chain omega-3 (n23) and PUFAs [267] reduces the risk of depression. There could also be a cumulative effect of all these nutrients and their biochemical properties on the risk of depression [268]. However, it is not clear whether a poor dietary pattern precedes the development of depression or if depression causes poor dietary intake. Indeed, some studies have shown that depressed individuals seek to self-medicate with high-fat and high-sugar food [269, 270]. Fast-food consumption has been found to be associated with symptoms of depression [271], and depressed women have increased odds of reporting high fast-food consumption compared with nondepressed ones [272]. On the contrary, high fruit and vegetable consumption has been associated with decreased odds of depression in women but not in men [273]. Therefore, given that women are at greater risk of depression than men [274], fruit and vegetable consumption may be helpful to reduce depression in women. Despite this, nutritional education has not been included in any mental health prevention program yet.

1.5 Healthcare Factors

Gender differences in mental health service use are widely known, with men being less likely to seek services for mental health than women [275]. There is a variety of possible explanations for gender differences in mental health service use, with studies emphasizing the role of education [276], socioeconomic factors [277], and relationship status [276]. Moreover, service use has been claimed to be related to willingness to disclose depressive symptoms [276], and perceived stigma around mental health, such as internalized stigma [278]. Lastly, the adherence to the "traditional masculine behavior" could prevent men from attending mental health services when needed [188]. When striving for equitable access to services, it is important to consider both horizontal and vertical equity. Horizontal equity is the provision of equal care for equal needs, whereas vertical equity is the provision of different treatments for people with different needs [279]. Many solutions have been proposed to increase access to mental health services, including integrating behavioral health services into primary or community-based care, augmenting the workforce through task-shifting (e.g., utilizing community health workers or peer navigators to provide some services), imparting training and supervision to novel providers via the Internet, or delivering services to people where they live (e.g., via minute clinics, medical vans, or telemental health services) rather than expecting people to travel long distances to access services [280]. Unfortunately, none of these solutions has involved a gendered perspective.

1.6   Conclusion

Despite the acknowledged gender differences in mental health, there is limited availability of mental health preventive strategies specifically targeted for men and women. Mental health preventive strategies during childhood are mainly focused on childhood abuse and do not take into account gender differences in childhood abuse rates. Most sex-specific preventive strategies are focused on pregnancy and postpartum and mainly address depressive symptoms. Regarding employment, despite persisting gender differences and discrimination in the workplace, limited sex-specific mental health preventive programs have been developed. Some mental health preventive strategies have been developed specifically for men in male-dominated industries and are focused on stress reduction. Concerning relationships, given the greater negative impact of marriage disruption in women compared with men, there is a certain amount of gendered mental health preventive strategies available. Other factors that impact on mental health in a gender-specific manner are education and nutrition, and they should be implemented in mental health prevention strategies. In this context, even though it is well known that men are more reluctant than women to access mental health services, mental health services appear to be slow in developing strategies that guarantee equal access to care for men and women with mental health problems (refer to Fig. 1.1).

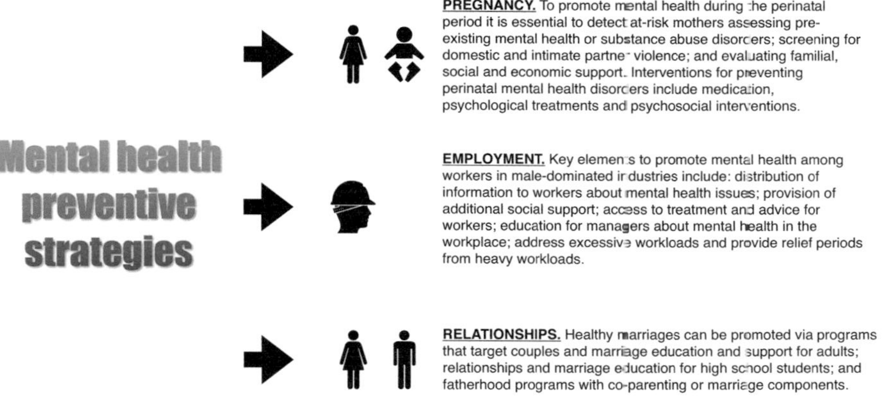

Fig. 1.1   Summary of available mental health preventive strategies

References

1. Narvacan K, Treit S, Camicioli R, Martin W, Beaulieu C. Evolution of deep gray matter volume across the human lifespan. Hum Brain Mapp. 2017;38(8):3771–90.
2. Arnold AP, Chen X. What does the "four core genotypes" mouse model tell us about sex differences in the brain and other tissues? Front Neuroendocrinol. 2009;30:1–9.
3. Sengelaub DR, Forger NG. The spinal nucleus of the bulbocavernosus: firsts in androgen dependent neural sex differences. Horm Behav. 2008;53(5):596–612. https://doi.org/10.1016/j.yhbeh.007.11.008.
4. Bleier R, Byne W, Siggelkow I. Cytoarchitectonic sexual dimorphisms of the medial preoptic and anterior hypothalamic areas in Guinea pig, rat, hamster, and mouse. J Comp Neurol. 1982;212(2):118–30.
5. Lubischer JL, Arnold AP. Evidence for target regulation of the development of androgen sensitivity in rat spinal motoneurons. Dev Neurosci. 1995;17(2):106–17.
6. Bales KL, Kramer KM, Lewis-Reese AD, Carter CS. Effects of stress on parental care are sexually dimorphic in prairie voles. Physiol Behav. 2006;87:424–9.
7. Hu MH, Li XF, McCausland B, Li SY, Gresham R, Kinsey-Jones JS, et al. Relative importance of the arcuate and anteroventral periventricular kisspeptin neurons in control of puberty and reproductive function in female rats. Endocrinology. 2015;156(7):2619–31. https://doi.org/10.1210/en.2014-1655.
8. McCarthy MM, Konkle AT. When is a sex difference not a sex difference? Front Neuroendocrinol. 2005;26(2):85–102.
9. Conejo NM, Gonzalez-Pardo H, Pedraza C, Navarro FF, Vallejo G, Arias JL. Evidence for sexual difference in astrocytes of adult rat hippocampus. Neurosci Lett. 2003;339(2):119–22.
10. Zhang JM, Konkle AT, Zup SL, McCarthy MM. Impact of sex and hormones on new cells in the developing rat hippocampus: a novel source of sex dimorphism? Eur J Neurosci. 2008;27(4):791–800. https://doi.org/10.1111/j.1460-9568.2008.06073.x.
11. Cooke BM. Steroid-dependent plasticity in the medial amygdala. Neuroscience. 2006;138(3):997–1005.
12. Krebs-Kraft DL, Hill MN, Hillard CJ, McCarthy MM. Sex difference in cell proliferation in developing rat amygdala mediated by endocannabinoids has implications for social behavior. Proc Natl Acad Sci U S A. 2010;107(47):20535–40. https://doi.org/10.1073/pnas.1005003107.
13. Auger AP, Auger CJ. Epigenetic turn ons and turn offs: chromatin reorganization and brain differentiation. Endocrinology. 2011;152(2):349–53. https://doi.org/10.1210/en.2010-0793.
14. Francis DD, Diorio J, Plotsky PM, Meaney MJ. Environmental enrichment reverses the effects of maternal separation on stress reactivity. J Neurosci. 2002;22(18):7840–3.
15. Brown DW, Anda RF, Felitti VJ, Edwards VJ, Malarcher AM, Croft JB, Giles WH. Adverse childhood experiences are associated with the risk of lung cancer: a prospective cohort study. BMC Public Health. 2010;10:20. https://doi.org/10.1186/1471-2458-10-20.
16. Vigod SN, Stewart DE. Emergent research in the cause of mental illness in women across the lifespan. Curr Opin Psychiatry. 2009;22(4):396–400. https://doi.org/10.1097/YCO.0b013e3283297127.
17. Edwards VJ, Holden GW, Felitti VJ, Anda RF. Relationship between multiple forms of childhood maltreatment and adult mental health in community respondents: results from the adverse childhood experiences study. Am J Psychiatry. 2003;160(8):1453–60.
18. Hennessy MB, Paik KD, Caraway JD, Schiml PA, Deak T. Proinflammatory activity and the sensitization of depressive-like behavior during maternal separation. Behav Neurosci. 2011;125(3):426–33. https://doi.org/10.1037/a0023559.
19. Spiers JG, Chen HJ, Bradley AJ, Anderson ST, Sernia C, Lavidis NA. Acute restraint stress induces rapid and prolonged changes in erythrocyte and hippocampal redox status. Psychoneuroendocrinology. 2013;38(11):2511–9. https://doi.org/10.1016/j.psyneuen.2013.05.011.

20. Moghaddam B. Stress preferentially increases extraneuronal levels of excitatory amino acids in the prefrontal cortex: comparison to hippocampus and basal ganglia. J Neurochem. 1993;60(5):1650–7.
21. Tottenham N, Sheridan MA. A review of adversity, the amygdala and the hippocampus: a consideration of developmental timing. Front Hum Neurosci. 2009;3:68. https://doi.org/10.3389/neuro.09.068.2009.
22. Nelson LH, Warden S, Lenz KM. Sex differences in microglial phagocytosis in the neonatal hippocampus. Brain Behav Immun. 2017;64:11–22.
23. Hanamsagar R, Alter MD, Block CS, Sullivan H, Bolton JL, Bilbo SD. Generation of a microglial developmental index in mice and in humans reveals a sex difference in maturation and immune reactivity. Glia. 2017;65(9):1504–20.
24. Ganguly P, Thompson V, Gildawie K, Brenhouse HC. Adolescent food restriction in rats alters prefrontal cortex microglia in an experience-dependent manner. Stress. 2018;21(2):162–8.
25. Raison CL, Miller AH. Is depression an inflammatory disorder? Curr Psychiatry Rep. 2011;13(6):467–75. https://doi.org/10.1007/s11920-011-0232-0.
26. Hamdani N, Tamouza R, Leboyer M. Immuno-inflammatory markers of bipolar disorder: a review of evidence. Front Biosci (Elite Ed). 2012;4:2170–82.
27. Mansur RB, Zugman A, de Miranda Asevedo E, da Cunha GR, Bressan RA, Brietzke E. Cytokines in schizophrenia: possible role of anti-inflammatory medications in clinical and preclinical stages. Psychiatry Clin Neurosci. 2012;66(4):247–60. https://doi.org/10.1111/j.1440-1819.2012.02354.x.
28. Gotlib IH, Joormann J, Minor KL, Hallmayer J. HPA axis reactivity: a mechanism underlying the associations among 5-HTTLPR, stress, and depression. Biol Psychiatry. 2008;63:847–51.
29. Children's Bureau. Child maltreatment 2015. Washington, DC: Administration on Children Youth and Families.
30. Sege RD, Amaya-Jackson L, AMERICAN ACADEMY OF PEDIATRICS Committee on Child Abuse and Neglect, Council on Foster Care, Adoption, and Kinship Care, AMERICAN ACADEMY OF CHILD AND ADOLESCENT PSYCHIATRY Committee on Child Maltreatment and Violence, NATIONAL CENTER FOR CHILD TRAUMATIC STRESS. Clinical considerations related to the behavioral manifestations of child maltreatment. Pediatrics. 2017;139(4):e20170100. https://doi.org/10.1542/peds.2017-0100.
31. Roy CA, Perry JC. Instruments for the assessment of childhood trauma in adults. J Nerv Ment Dis. 2004;192(5):343–51.
32. Afifi TO, MacMillan HL, Boyle M, Taillieu T, Cheung K, Sareen J. Child abuse and mental disorders in Canada. CMAJ. 2014;186(9):E324–32.
33. Li XB, Li QY, Liu JT, Zhang L, Tang YL, Wang CY. Childhood trauma associates with clinical features of schizophrenia in a sample of Chinese inpatients. Psychiatry Res. 2015;228(3):702–7.
34. Carey PD, Walker JL, Rossouw W, Seedat S, SteinRisk DJ. Indicators and psychopathology in traumatised children and adolescents with a history of sexual abuse. Eur Child Adolesc Psychiatry. 2008;17(2):93–8.
35. Devries KM, Mak JYT, Child JC, Falder G, Bacchus LJ, Astbury A, et al. Childhood sexual abuse and suicidal behavior: a meta-analysis. Pediatrics. 2014;133(5):1331–44.
36. Monteleone AM, Ruzzi V, Patriciello G, Pellegrino F, Cascino G, Castellini G, et al. Parental bonding, childhood maltreatment and eating disorder psychopathology: an investigation of their interactions. Eat Weight Disord. 2019; https://doi.org/10.1007/s40519-019-00649-0.
37. Meshesha LZ, Abrantes AM, Anderson BJ, Blevins CE, Caviness CM, Stein MD. Marijuana use motives mediate the association between experiences of childhood abuse and marijuana use outcomes among emerging adults. Addict Behav. 2019;93:166–72. https://doi.org/10.1016/j.addbeh.2019.01.040.
38. Bensley L, Van Eenwyk J, Wynkoop Simmons K. Childhood family violence history and women's risk for intimate partner violence and poor health. Am J Prev Med. 2003;25(1):38–44.
39. Madigan S, Wade M, Plamondon A, Vaillancourt K, Jenkins JM, Shouldice M, Benoit D. Course of depression and anxiety symptoms during the transition to parenthood for female

adolescents with histories of victimization. Child Abuse Negl. 2014;38(7):1160–70. https://doi.org/10.1016/j.chiabu.2014.04.002.
40. Frioux S, Wood JN, Fakeye O, Luan X, Localio R, Rubin DM. Longitudinal association of county-level economic indicators and child maltreatment incidents. Matern Child Health J. 2014;18(9):2202–8. https://doi.org/10.1007/s10995-014-1469-0.
41. Levey EJ, Gelaye B, Bain P, Rondon MB, Borba CPC, et al. 1A systematic review of randomized controlled trials of interventions designed to decrease child abuse in high-risk families. Child Abuse Negl. 2017;65:48–57. https://doi.org/10.1016/j.chiabu.2017.01.004.
42. Olds DL, Robinson J, Pettitt L, Luckey DW, Holmberg J, Ng RK, et al. Effects of home visits by paraprofessionals and by nurses: age 4 follow-up results of a randomized trial. Pediatrics. 2004;114(6):1560–8. https://doi.org/10.1542/peds.2004-0961.
43. Barlow J, Davis H, McIntosh E, Jarrett P, Mockford C, Stewart-Brown S. Role of home visiting in improving parenting and health in families at risk of abuse and neglect: results of a multicentre randomised controlled trial and economic evaluation. Arch Dis Child. 2007;92(3):229–33. https://doi.org/10.1136/adc.2006.095117.
44. DuMont K, Mitchell-Herzfeld S, Greene R, Lee E, Lowenfels A, Rodriguez M, Dorabawila V. Healthy Families New York (HFNY) randomized trial: effects on early child abuse and neglect. Child Abuse Negl. 2008;32(3):295–315. https://doi.org/10.1016/j.chiabu.2007.07.007.
45. Bugental DB, Ellerson PC, Lin EK, Rainey B, Kokotovic A, O'Hara N. A cognitive approach to child abuse prevention. J Fam Psychol. 2002;16(3):243–58.
46. Centers for Disease Control and Prevention. Preventing adverse childhood experiences (ACEs): leveraging the best available evidence. Atlanta, GA: National Center for Injury Prevention and Control, Centers for Disease Control and Prevention. https://www.cdc.gov/violenceprevention/pdf/preventingACES-508.pdf.
47. McNeil HJ, Holland SS. A comparative study of public health nurse teaching in groups and in home visits. Am J Public Health. 1972;62(12):1629–37.
48. de Camps Meschino D, Philipp D, Israel A, Vigod S. Maternal-infant mental health: postpartum group intervention. Arch Womens Ment Health. 2016;19(2):243–51. https://doi.org/10.1007/s00737-0150551-y.
49. Copeland WE, Keeler G, Angold A, Costello EJ. Traumatic events and posttraumatic stress in childhood. Arch Gen Psychiatry. 2007;64(5):577–84. https://doi.org/10.1001/archpsyc.64.5.577.
50. Wherry JN, Huffhines LP, Walisky DN. A short form of the trauma symptom checklist for children. Child Maltreat. 2016;21(1):37–46. https://doi.org/10.1177/1077559515619487.
51. Steinberg AM, Brymer MJ, Kim S, Briggs EC, Ippen CG, Ostrowski SA, et al. Psychometric properties of the UCLA PTSD reaction index: part I. J Trauma Stress. 2013;26(1):1–9. https://doi.org/10.1002/jts.21780.
52. Foa EB, Johnson KM, Feeny NC, Treadwell KR. The child PTSD Symptom Scale: a preliminary examination of its psychometric properties. J Clin Child Psychol. 2001;30(3):376–84. https://doi.org/10.1207/S15374424JCCP3003_9.
53. Murray LA, Skavenski S, Kane J, Mayeya J, Dorsey S, Cohen JA, et al. Effectiveness of trauma-focused cognitive behavioral therapy among trauma-affected children in Lusaka, Zambia: a randomized clinical trial. JAMA Pediatr. 2015;169:761–9. https://doi.org/10.1001/jamapediatrics.2015.0580.
54. Cohen JA, Mannarino AP, Perel JM, Staron V. A pilot randomized controlled trial of combined trauma-focused CBT and sertraline for childhood PTSD symptoms. J Am Acad Child Adolesc Psychiatry. 2007;46(7):811–9. https://doi.org/10.1097/chi/0b013e3180547105.
55. Ellsberg M, Arango DJ, Morton M, Gennari F, Kiplesund S, et al. Prevention of violence against women and girls: what does the evidence say? Lancet. 2015;385(9977):1555–66. https://doi.org/10.1016/S0140-6736(14)61703-7.
56. MacMillan HL, Jamieson E, Wathen C, Boyle M, Walsh C, Omura J, et al. Development of a policy-relevant child maltreatment research strategy. Milbank Q. 2007;85:337–74. https://doi.org/10.1111/j.1468-0009.2007.00490.x.

57. Wagman JA, Gray RH, Campbell J, Thoma M, Ndyanabo A, Ssekasanvu J, et al. Impact of an integrated intimate partner violence and HIV prevention intervention: a cluster randomised trial in Rakai, Uganda. Lancet Glob Health. 2014;3(1):e23–33. https://doi.org/10.1016/S2214-109X(14)70344-4.
58. Roberts LR, Montgomery SB. India's distorted sex ratio: dire consequences for girls. J Christ Nurs. 2016;33(1):E7–E15. https://doi.org/10.1097/CNJ.0000000000000244.
59. O'Hara MW, Mc Cabe JE. Postpartum depression: current status and future directions. Annu Rev Clin Psychol. 2013;9:379–407. https://doi.org/10.1146/annurev-clinpsy-050212-185612.
60. Lindgren K. Relationships among maternal-fetal attachment, prenatal depression, and health practices in pregnancy. Res Nurs Health. 2001;24:203–17.
61. Foley S, Hughes C. Great expectations? Do mothers' and fathers' prenatal thoughts and feelings about the infant predict parent-infant interaction quality? A meta-analytic review. Dev Rev. 2018;48:40–54.
62. Crawford A, Benoit D. Caregivers' disrupted representations of the unborn child predict later infant-caregiver disorganized attachment and disrupted interactions. Infant Ment Health J. 2009;30:124–44.
63. Aarestrup AK, Væver MS, Petersen J, Røhder K, Schiøtz M. An early intervention to promote maternal sensitivity in the perinatal period for women with psychosocial vulnerabilities: study protocol of a randomized controlled trial. BMC Psychol. 2020;8(1):41. https://doi.org/10.1186/s40359-020-00407-3.
64. Jones TL, Prinz RJ. Potential roles of parental self-efficacy in parent and child adjustment: a review. Clin Psychol Rev. 2005;25(3):341–63.
65. Fonagy P, Target M. Bridging the transmission gap: an end to an important mystery of attachment research? Attach Hum Dev. 2005;7(3):333–43.
66. Teti DM, O'Connell MA, Reiner CD. Parenting sensitivity, parental depression and child health: the mediational role of parental self-efficacy. Early Dev Parent. 1996;5(4):237–50.
67. Papp LM. Longitudinal associations between breastfeeding and observed mother-child interaction qualities in early childhood. Child Care Health Dev. 2014;40:740–6.
68. Fish M, Stifter CA. Patterns of mother-infant interaction and attachment: a cluster-analytic approach. Infant Behav Dev. 1995;18(4):435–46.
69. Sroufe LA. Attachment and development: a prospective, longitudinal study from birth to adulthood. Attach Hum Dev. 2005;7:349–67.
70. Carvalho JMN, Gaspar MFRF, Cardoso AMR. Challenges of motherhood in the voice of primiparous mothers: initial difficulties. Investigacion y Educacion en Enfermeria. 2017;35(3):285–94.
71. Deater-Deckard K. Parenting stress and child adjustment: some old hypotheses and new questions. Clin Psychol Sci Pract. 1998;5(3):314–32.
72. Howard LM, Molyneaux E, Dennis C-L, Rochat T, Stein A, Milgrom J. Nonpsychotic mental disorders in the perinatal period. Lancet. 2014;364:1775–88.
73. Dennis C-L, Chung-Lee L. Postpartum depression help-seeking barriers and maternal treatment preferences: a qualitative systematic review. Birth. 2006;33(4):323–31.
74. Guille C, Newman RB. Treatment of peripartum mental health disorders: an essential element of prenatal care. Obstet Gynecol Clin N Am. 2018;45(3):xv–xvi. https://doi.org/10.1016/j.ogc.2018.06.001.
75. Bernard K, Nissim G, Vaccaro S, Harris JL, Lindhiem O. Association between maternal depression and maternal sensitivity from birth to 12 months: a meta-analysis. Attach Hum Dev. 2018;20(6):578–99. https://doi.org/10.1080/14616734.2018.1430839.
76. Martins C, Gaffan E. Effects of early maternal deprivation on patterns of infant-mother attachment: a meta-analytic investigation. J Child Psychol Psychiatry. 2000;41:737–46.
77. Bauer A, Pawlby S, Plant DT, King D, Pariante CM, Knapp M. Perinatal depression and child development: exploring the economic consequences from a South London cohort. Psychol Med. 2015;45:51–61.
78. Yarcheski A, Mahon NE, Yarcheski TJ, Hanks MM, Cannella BL. A metaanalytic study of predictors of maternal-fetal attachment. Int J Nurs Stud. 2009;46:708–15.

79. Heckman JJ. Giving kids a fair chance. Cambridge: The MIT Press; 2013.
80. Belay S, Astatkie A, Emmelin M, Hinderaker SG. Intimate partner violence and maternal depression during pregnancy: a community-based cross-sectional study in Ethiopia. PLoS One. 2019;14(7):e0220003. https://doi.org/10.1371/journal.pone.0220003.
81. Van Parys A-S, Verhamme A, Temmerman M, Verstraelen H. Intimate partner violence and pregnancy: a systematic review of interventions. PLoS One. 2014;9:e85084.
82. Gazmararian JA, Petersen R, Spitz AM, Goodwin MM, Saltzman LE, Marks JS. Violence and reproductive health: current knowledge and future research directions. Mat Child Health J. 2000;4:79–84.
83. Devries KM, Kishor S, Johnson H, Stöckl H, Bacchus LJ, Garcia-Moreno C, et al. Intimate partner violence during pregnancy: analysis of prevalence data from 19 countries. Reprod Health Matters. 2010;18:158–70.
84. Stewart DE, MacMillan H, Wathen N. Intimate partner violence. Can J Psychiatr. 2013;58:1–15.
85. Campbell JC. Health consequences of intimate partner violence. Lancet. 2002;359:1331–6.
86. James L, Brody D, Hamilton Z. Risk factors for domestic violence during pregnancy: a meta-analytic review. Violence Vict. 2013;28:359–80.
87. Buist A, Bilszta J, Barnett B, Milgrom J, Ericksen J, Condon J, et al. Recognition and management of perinatal depression in general practice: a survey of GPs and postnatal women. Aust Fam Physician. 2005;34(9):787–90.
88. Shaw E, Levitt C, Wong S, Kaczorowski J. Systematic review of the literature on postpartum care: effectiveness of postpartum support to improve maternal parenting, mental health, quality of life, and physical health. Birth. 2006;33(3):210–20.
89. Choi KR, Records K, Low LK, Alhusen JL, Kenner C, Bloch JR, et al. Promotion of maternal-infant mental health and trauma-informed care during the COVID-19 pandemic. J Obstet Gynecol Neonatal Nurs. 2020;49(5):409–15. https://doi.org/10.1016/j.jogn.2020.07.004.
90. Reid AJ, Biringer A, Carroll JD, Midmer D, Wilson LM, Chalmers B. Stewart DE using the ALPHA form in practice to assess antenatal psychosocial health. CMAJ. 1998;159(6):667–84.
91. Austin M-P, Colton J, Priest S, Reilly N, Hadzi-Pavlovic D. The Antenatal Risk Questionnaire (ANRQ): acceptability and use for psychosocial risk assessment in the maternity setting. Women Birth. 2013;26(1):17–25. https://doi.org/10.1016/j.wombi.2011.06.002.
92. Matthey S, Phillips J, White T, Glossop P, Hopper U, Panasetis P. Routine psychosocial assessment of women in the antenatal period: frequency of risk factors and implications for clinical services. Arch Womens Ment Health. 2004;7:223–9.
93. Howard L, Hunt K, Slade M, O'Keane V, Senevirante T, Leese M, Thornicroft G. Assessing the needs of pregnant women and mothers with severe mental illness: the psychometric properties of the Camberwell Assessment of Need—Mothers (CAN-M). Int J Methods Psychiatr Res. 2007;16(4):177–85.
94. Bernazzani O, Marks MN, Bifulco A, Siddle K, Asten P, Conroy S. Assessing psychosocial risk in pregnant/postpartum women using the Contextual Assessment of Maternity Experience (CAME): recent life adversity, social support and maternal feelings. Soc Psychiatry Psychiat Epidemiol. 2005;40(6):497–508.
95. Austin M-P, Hadzi-Pavlovic D, Saint K, Parker G. Antenatal screening for the prediction of postnatal depression: validation of a psychosocial Pregnancy Risk Questionnaire. Acta Psychiatr Scand. 2005;112:310–7.
96. Johnson M, Schmeid V, Lupton S, Austin MP, Matthey SM, Kemp L, et al. Measuring perinatal mental health risk. Arch Womens Ment Health. 2012;15(5):375–86. https://doi.org/10.1007/s00737-012-0297-8.
97. Howard LM, Molyneaux E, Dennis C-L, Rochat T, Stein A, Milgrom J. Nonpsychotic mental disorders in the perinatal period. Lancet. 2014;384(9956):1775–88.
98. Woolhouse H, Gartland D, Mensah F, Brown SJ. Maternal depression from early pregnancy to 4 years postpartum in a prospective pregnancy cohort study: implications for primary health care. BJOG. 2015;122:312–21.

99. Ukatu N, Clare CA, Brulja M. Postpartum depression screening tools: a review. Psychosomatics. 2018;59(3):211–9. https://doi.org/10.1016/j.psym.2017.11.005.
100. Beck CT, Gable RK. Further validation of the postpartum depression screening scale. Nurs Res. 2001;50(3):155–64. https://doi.org/10.1097/00006199-200105000-00005.
101. Chae S, Chae M, Tyndall A, Ramirez M, Winter R. Can we effectively use the two-item PHQ-2 to screen for postpartum depression? Fam Med. 2012;44(10):698–703.
102. Yawn B, Pace W, Wollan P, Bertram S, Kurland M, Graham D, Dietrich A. Concordance of Edinburgh postnatal depression scale (EPDS) and patient health questionnaire (PHQ-9) to assess increased risk of depression among postpartum women. J Am Board Fam Med. 2009;22(5):483–91.
103. Cox JL, Holden JM, Sagovsky R. Detection of postnatal depression. Development of the 10-item Edinburgh Postnatal Depression Scale. Br J Psychiatry. 1987;150:782–6. https://doi.org/10.1192/bjp.150.6.782.
104. Venkatesh K, Zlotnick C, Triche E, Ware C, Phipps M. Accuracy of brief screening tools for identifying postpartum depression among adolescent mothers. Pediatrics. 2013;133(1):e45–53.
105. Beck AT, Ward CH, Mendelson M, Mock J, Erbaugh J. An inventory for measuring depression. Arch Gen Psychiatry. 1961;4:53–63.
106. Navarro P, Ascaso C, Garcia-Esteve L, Aguado J, Torres A, Martín-Santos R. Postnatal psychiatric morbidity: a validation study of the GHQ-12 and the EPDS as screening tools. Gen Hosp Psychiatry. 2007;29(1):1–7.
107. Radloff LS. The CES-D scale: a self-report depression scale for research in the general population. Appl Psychol Meas. 1977;1:385–401.
108. Kroenke K, Spitzer RL, Williams JB. The PHQ-9: validity of a brief depression severity measure. J Gen Intern Med. 2001;16(9):606–13. https://doi.org/10.1046/j.1525-1497.2001.016009606.x.
109. Stöckl H, Hertlein L, Himsl I, Ditsch N, Blume C, Hasbargen U, et al. Acceptance of routine or case-based inquiry for intimate partner violence: a mixed method study. BMC Pregnancy Childbirth. 2013;13:77.
110. Basile KC, Hertz MF, Back SE. Intimate partner violence and sexual violence victimization assessment instruments for use in healthcare settings: version 1. Atlanta, GA: Centers for Disease Control and Prevention, National Center for Injury Prevention and Control; 2007.
111. Sherin KM, Sinacore JM, Li XQ, Zitter RE, Shakil A. HITS: a short domestic screening tool for use in a family practice setting. Fam Med. 1998;30:508–12.
112. Soeken KL, McFarlane J, Parker B, Lominack MC. The abuse assessment screen: a clinical instrument to measure frequency, severity, and perpetrator of abuse against women. In: Campbell JC, editor. Empowering survivors of abuse: health care for battered women and their children. Thousand Oaks, CA: Sage; 1998. p. 195–203.
113. Deshpande NA, Lewis-O'Connor A. Screening for intimate partner violence during pregnancy. Rev Obstet Gynecol. 2013;6(3–4):141–8.
114. Renker PR, Tonkin P. Women's views of prenatal violence screening: acceptability and confidentiality issues. Obstet Gynecol. 2006;107:348–54.
115. Davidson J, Robertson E. A follow-up study of postpartum illness, 1946–1978. Acta Psychiatr Scand. 1985;71:451–7.
116. Wisner KL, Wheeler SB. Prevention of recurrent postpartum major depression. Hosp Community Psychiatry. 1994;45:1191–6.
117. Wisner KL, Perel JM, Peindl KS, Hanusa BH, Findling RL, Rapport D. Prevention of recurrent postpartum depression: a randomized clinical trial. J Clin Psychiatry. 2001;62(2):82–6.
118. Sichel DA, Cohen LS, Robertson LM, Ruttenberg A, Rosenbaum JF. Prophylactic estrogen in recurrent postpartum affective disorder. Biol Psychiatry. 1995;38:814–8.
119. Dalton K. Postnatal depression and prophylactic progesterone. Br J Fam Plann. 1994;19(Suppl):10–2.
120. Dalton K. Progesterone or progestogens? Br Med J. 1976;2(6046):1257.

121. Lawrie TA, Hofmeyr GJ, De Jager M, Berk M, Paiker J, Viljoen E. A double-blind randomised placebo controlled trial of postnatal norethisterone enanthate: the effect on postnatal depression and serum hormones. Br J Obstet Gynecol. 1998;105:1082–90.
122. Harris B, Fung H, Johns S, Kologlu M, Bhatti R, McGregor AM, et al. Transient post-partum thyroid dysfunction and postnatal depression. J Affect Disord. 1989;17:243–9.
123. Harris B, Oretti R, Lazarus J, Parkes A, John R, Richards C, et al. Randomised trial of thyroxine to prevent postnatal depression in thyroid-antibody-positive women. Br J Psychiatry. 2002;180:327–30.
124. Llorente AM, Jensen CL, Voigt RG, Fraley JK, Berretta MC, Heird WC. Effect of maternal docosahexaenoic acid supplementation on postpartum depression and information processing. Am J Obstet Gynecol. 2003;188:1348–53.
125. Hibbeln JR. Fish consumption and major depression. Lancet. 1998;351:1213.
126. Harrison-Hohner J, Coste S, Dorato V, Curet LB, McCarron D, Hatton D. Prenatal calcium supplementation and postpartum depression: an ancillary study to a randomized trial of calcium for prevention of preeclampsia. Arch Women Ment Health. 2001;3:141–6.
127. Thys-Jacobs S, Alvir MJ. Calcium-regulating hormones across the menstrual cycle: evidence of a secondary hyperparathyroidism in women with PMS. J Clin Endocrinol Metab. 1995;80:2227–32.
128. Battle CL, Salisbury AL, Schofield CA, Ortiz-Hernandez S. Perinatal antidepressant use: understanding women's preferences and concerns. J Psychiatr Pract. 2013;19:443–53.
129. Zlotnick C, Johnson SL, Miller IW, Pearlstein T, Howard M. Postpartum depression in women receiving public assistance: pilot study of an interpersonal-therapy-oriented group intervention. Am J Psychiatry. 2001;158:638–40.
130. Gorman LL. Prevention of postpartum depression in a high risk sample. Iowa City, IA: Department of Psychology, University of Iowa; 2001.
131. Saisto T, Salmela-Aro K, Nurmi JE, Kononen T, Halmesmaki E. A randomized controlled trial of intervention in fear of childbirth. Obstet Gynecol. 2001;98:820–6.
132. Chabrol H, Teissedre F, Saint-Jean M, Teisseyre N, Roge B, Mullet E. Prevention and treatment of post-partum depression: a controlled randomized study on women at risk. Psychol Med. 2002;32:1039–47.
133. Lavender T, Walkinshaw SA. Can midwives reduce postpartum psychological morbidity? A randomized trial. Birth. 1998;25:215–9.
134. Small R, Lumley J, Donohue L, Potter A, Waldenstrom U. Randomised controlled trial of midwife led debriefing to reduce maternal depression after operative childbirth. BMJ. 2000;321:1043–7.
135. Priest SR, Henderson J, Evans SF, Hagan R. Stress debriefing after childbirth: a randomised controlled trial. Med J Aust. 2003;178:542–5.
136. Gordon R, Gordon K. Social factors in prevention of postpartum emotional problems. Obstet Gynecol. 1960;15:433–8.
137. Elliott SA, Leverton TJ, Sanjack M, Turner H, Cowmeadow P, Hopkins J, et al. Promoting mental health after childbirth: a controlled trial of primary prevention of postnatal depression. Br J Clin Psychol. 2000;39:223–41.
138. Stamp GE, Williams AS, Crowther CA. Evaluation of antenatal and postnatal support to overcome postnatal depression: a randomized, controlled trial. Birth. 1995;22:138–43.
139. Brugha TS, Wheatley S, Taub NA, Culverwell A, Friedman T, Kirwan P, et al. Pragmatic randomized trial of antenatal intervention to prevent post-natal depression by reducing psychosocial risk factors. Psychol Med. 2000;30:1273–81.
140. Buist A, Westley D, Hill C. Antenatal prevention of postnatal depression. Arch Women Ment Health. 1999;1:167–73.
141. Wolman WL, Chalmers BE, Hofmeyr J, Nikodem VC. Postpartum depression and companionship in the clinical birth environment: a randomized, controlled study. Am J Obstet Gynecol. 1993;168:1388–93.

142. Nikodem VC, Nolte AG, Wolman W, Gulmezoglu AM, Hofmeyr GJ. Companionship by a lay labour supporter to modify the clinical birth environment: long-term effects on mother and child. Curationis. 1998;21(1):8–12.
143. Gordon NP, Walton D, McAdam E, Derman J, Gallitero G, Garrett L. Effects of providing hospital-based doulas in health maintenance organization hospitals. Obstet Gynecol. 1999;93:422–6.
144. Hodnett ED, Lowe NK, Hannah ME, Willan AR, Stevens B, Weston JA, et al. Effectiveness of nurses as providers of birth labor support in North American hospitals: a randomized controlled trial. JAMA. 2002;288:1373–81.
145. Armstrong KL, Fraser JA, Dadds MR, Morris J. A randomized, controlled trial of nurse home visiting to vulnerable families with newborns. J Paediatr Child Health. 1999;35:237–44.
146. Armstrong KL, Fraser JA, Dadds MR, Morris J. Promoting secure attachment, maternal mood and child health in a vulnerable population: a randomized controlled trial [comments]. J Paediatr Child Health. 2000;36:555–62.
147. Morrell CJ, Spiby H, Stewart P, Walters S, Morgan A. Costs and effectiveness of community postnatal support workers: randomised controlled trial. BMJ. 2000;321:593–8.
148. Reid M, Glazener C, Murray GD, Taylor GS. A two-centred pragmatic randomised controlled trial of two interventions of postnatal support. BJOG. 2002;109:1164–70.
149. Leis JA, Mendelson T, Tandon SD, Perry DF. A systematic review of home-based interventions to prevent and treat postpartum depression. Arch Womens Ment Health. 2009;12(1):3–13. https://doi.org/10.1007/s00737-008-0039-0.
150. Shields N, Reid M, Cheyne H, Holmes A. Impact of midwife-managed care in the postnatal period: an exploration of psychosocial outcomes. J Reprod Infant Psychol. 1997;15(2):91–108.
151. Waldenstrom U, Brown S, McLachlan H, Forster D, Brennecke S. Does team midwife care increase satisfaction with antenatal, intrapartum, and postpartum care? A randomized controlled trial. Birth. 2000;27:156–67.
152. Marks MN, Siddle K, Warwick C. Can we prevent postnatal depression? A randomized controlled trial to assess the effect of continuity of midwifery care on rates of postnatal depression in high-risk women. J Matern Fetal Neonatal Med. 2003;13:119–27.
153. Webster J, Linnane J, Roberts J, Starrenburg S, Hinson J, Dibley L. IDentify, Educate and Alert (IDEA) trial: an intervention to reduce postnatal depression. BJOG. 2003;110:842–6.
154. Serwint JR, Wilson MH, Duggan AK, Mellits ED, Baumgardner RA, DeAngelis C. Do postpartum nursery visits by the primary care provider make a difference? Pediatrics. 1991;88:444–9.
155. Gunn J, Lumley J, Chondros P, Young D. Does an early postnatal check-up improve maternal health: results from a randomised trial in Australian general practice. BJOG. 1998;105:991–7.
156. Okano T, Nagata S, Hasegawa M, Nomura J, Kumar R. Effectiveness of antenatal education about postnatal depression: a comparison of two groups of Japanese mothers. J Ment Health. 1998;7:191–8.
157. Heh SS, Fu YY. Effectiveness of informational support in reducing the severity of postnatal depression in Taiwan. J Adv Nurs. 2003;42:255–67.
158. Hayes BA, Muller R, Bradley BS. Perinatal depression: a randomized controlled trial of an antenatal education intervention for primiparas. Birth. 2001;28(1):28–35.
159. Lorant V, Deliege D, Eaton W, Philippot P, Ansseau M. Socioeconomic inequalities in depression: a meta-analysis. Am J Epidemiol. 2003;157:98–112.
160. Gil-Lacruz M, Gil-Lacruz AI, Gracia-Pérez ML. Health-related quality of life in young people: the importance of education. Health Qual Life Outcomes. 2020;18(1):187. https://doi.org/10.1186/s12955-020-01446-5.
161. Ross CE, Mirowsky J. Sex differences in the effect of education on depression: resource multiplication or resource substitution? Soc Sci Med. 2006;63(5):1400–13. https://doi.org/10.1016/j.socscimed.2006.03.013.
162. Ross CE, Mirowsky J. Age and the gender gap in the sense of personal control. Soc Psychol Q. 2002;65:125–45.

163. Ross CE, Mirowsky J. The interaction of personal and parental education on health. Soc Sci Med. 2011;72(4):591–9. https://doi.org/10.1016/j.socscimed.2010.11.028.

164. Schaan B. The interaction of family background and personal education on depressive symptoms in later life. Soc Sci Med. 2014;102:94–102. https://doi.org/10.1016/j.socscimed.2013.11.049.

165. Cermakova P, Pikhart H, Kubinova R, Bobak M. Education as inefficient resource against depressive symptoms in the Czech Republic: cross-sectional analysis of the HAPIEE study. Eur J Pub Health. 2020;30(5):948–52. https://doi.org/10.1093/eurpub/ckaa059.

166. Thompson EA, Connelly CD, Thomas-Jones D, Eggert LL. School difficulties and co-occurring health risk factors: substance use, aggression, depression, and suicidal behaviors. Child Adolesc Psychiatr Nurs. 2013;26(1):74–84. https://doi.org/10.1111/jcap.12026.

167. Ligier F, Giguère CE, Notredame CE, Lesage A, Renaud J, Séguin M. Are school difficulties an early sign for mental disorder diagnosis and suicide prevention? A comparative study of individuals who died by suicide and control group. Child Adolesc Psychiatry Ment Health. 2020;14:1. https://doi.org/10.1186/s13034-019-0308-x.

168. Waddell C, Wong W, Hua J, Godderis R. Preventing and treating conduct disorder in children and youth. 2004. http://childhealthpolicy.ca/wpcontent/themes/chpc/pdf/RR-4-04-full-report.pdf.

169. Cercarelli R, Allsop S, Evans M, Velander F. Reducing alcohol-related harm in the workplace: an evidence review: full report. Melbourne: Victorian Health Promotion Foundation; 2012.

170. Eurostat [Internet]. Brussels: Eurostat; 2018 [Employment statistics]. Available from: https://ec.europa.eu/eurostat/statistics-explained/index.php?title=Employment_statistics.

171. Eurostat [Internet]. Activity rates by sex, age and educational attainment level (%)]. Brussels: Eurostat; 2018. Available from: https://ec.europa.eu/eurostat/web/products-datasets/product?code=lfsq_argaed.

172. Katikireddi SV, Niedzwiedz CL, Popham F. Trends in population mental health before and after the 2008 recession: a repeat cross-sectional analysis of the 1991–2010 health surveys of England. BMJ Open. 2012;2:e001790. https://doi.org/10.1136/bmjopen-2012-001790.

173. Wadell G, Burton KA. Is work good for your health and well-being? London Government of the Stationery Office; 2006.

174. Paul KI, Moser K. Unemployment impairs mental health. Meta-analyses. J Vocational Behav. 2009;74:264–82.

175. Jahoda M. Employment and unemployment. A social psychological analysis. Cambridge: Cambridge University Press; 1982.

176. Blomqvist S, Burström B, Backhans MC. Increasing health inequalities between women in and out of work--the impact of recession or policy change? A repeated cross-sectional study in Stockholm county, 2006 and 2010. Int J Equity Health. 2014;13:51. https://doi.org/10.1186/1475-9276-13-51.

177. Brydsten A, Hammarström A, San Sebastian M. Health inequalities between employed and unemployed in northern Sweden: a decomposition analysis of social determinants for mental health. Int J Equity Health. 2018;17(1):59. https://doi.org/10.1186/s12939-018-0773-5.

178. Hammarström A, Gustafsson PE, Strandh M, Virtanen P, Janlert U. It's no surprise! Men are not hit more than women by the health consequences of unemployment in the Northern Swedish Cohort. Scand J Public Health. 2011;39(2):187–93. https://doi.org/10.1177/1403494810394906.

179. Cortès-Franch I, Puig-Barrachina V, Vargas-Leguás H, Arcas MM, Artazcoz L. Is being employed always better for mental wellbeing than being unemployed? Exploring the role of gender and welfare state regimes during the economic crisis. Int J Environ Res Public Health. 2019;16(23):4799. https://doi.org/10.3390/ijerph16234799.

180. Esping-Andersen G. Social foundations of postindustrial economies. Oxford: Oxford University Press; 1999.

181. Bambra C, Eikemo TA. Welfare state regimes, unemployment and health: a comparative study of the relationship between unemployment and self-reported health in 23 European countries. J Epidemiol Community Health. 2009;63:92–8.

182. Novo M, Hammarström A, Janlert U. Do high levels of unemployment influence those who are not unemployed? A gendered comparison of young men and women during boom and recession. Soc Sci Med. 2001;53:293–303.
183. Burström B, Nylén L, Barr B, Clayton S, Holland P, Whitehead M. Delayed and differential effects of the economic crisis in Sweden in the 1990s on health-related exclusion from the labour market: a health equity assessment. Soc Sci Med. 2012;75:2431–6.
184. Hetzler A, Melén D, Bjerstedt D. Sjuk-Sverige: försäkringskassan, rehabilitering och utslagning från arbetsmarknaden. Eslöv: B. Östlings bokförlag Symposion; 2005.
185. Australian Bureau of Statistics. Australian and New Zealand standard industrial classification. Canberra: Commonwealth of Australia and Crown Copyright New Zealand; 2008.
186. Australian Bureau of Statistics. 4326.0 – National survey of mental health and wellbeing: summary of results, 2007. Sydney: Australian Bureau of Statistics; 2008a. Available at: www.abs.gov.au/ausstats/abs@.nsf/mf/4326.0%3E.
187. Tynan RJ, Considine R, Rich JL, Skehan J, Wiggers J, Lewin TJ, et al. Help-seeking for mental health problems by employees in the Australian Mining Industry. BMC Health Serv Res. 2016;16:498.
188. Seidler ZE, Dawes AJ, Rice SM, Oliffe JL, Dhillon HM. The role of masculinity in men's help-seeking for depression: a systematic review. Clin Psychol Rev. 2016;49:106–18.
189. Addis ME, Mahalik JR. Men, masculinity, and the contexts of help seeking. Am Psychol. 2003;58:5–14.
190. Ahs A, Burell G, Westerling R. Care or not care – that is the question: predictors of healthcare utilisation in relation to employment status. Int J Behav Med. 2012;19:29–38.
191. Battams S, Roche AM, Fischer J, Lee NK, Cameron J, Kostadinov V. Workplace risk factors for anxiety and depression in male-dominated industries: a systematic review. Health Psychol Behav Med. 2014;2(1):983–1008.
192. Robertson S, White A, Gough B, Robinson M, Seims A, Raine G, Hanna E. Promoting mental health and wellbeing in men and boys: what works? Leeds: Leeds Beckett University; 2015.
193. Lee NK, Roche A, Duraisingam V, Fischer JA, Cameron J. Effective interventions for mental health in male-dominated workplaces. MHRJ. 2014;19(4):1361–9322.
194. Meltzer H, Bebbington P, Brugha T, Jenkins R, McManus S, Stansfeld S. Job insecurity, socio-economic circumstances and depression. Psychol Med. 2010;40(8):1401–7.
195. Lamontagne AD, Keegel T, Louie AM, Ostry A, Landsbergis PA. A systematic review of the job-stress intervention evaluation literature, 1990–2005. Int J Occup Env Heal. 2007;13(3):268–80.
196. Seaton CL, Bottorff JL, Jones-Bricker M, Oliffe JL, DeLeenheer D, Medhurst K. Men's mental health promotion interventions: a scoping review. Am J Mens Health. 2017;11(6):1823–37. https://doi.org/10.1177/1557988317728353.
197. Bilderbeck AC, Farias M, Brazil IA, Jakobowitz S, Wikholm C. Participation in a 10-week course of yoga improves behavioural control and decreases psychological distress in a prison population. J Psychiatr Res. 2013;47(10):1438–45. https://doi.org/10.1016/j.jpsychires.2013.06.014.
198. Hirokawa K, Taniguchi T, Tsuchiya M, Kawakami N. Effects of a stress management program for hospital staffs on their coping strategies and interpersonal behaviors. Ind Health. 2012;50(6):487–98.
199. Jarman L, Martin A, Venn A, Otahal P, Sanderson K. Does workplace health promotion contribute to job stress reduction? Three-year findings from partnering Healthy@Work. BMC Public Health. 2015;15(1):1293. https://doi.org/10.1186/s12889-015-2625-1.
200. Kim S, Lee H, Kim H, Noh D, Lee H. Effects of an integrated stress management program (ISMP) for psychologically distressed students: a randomized controlled trial. Perspect Psychiatr Care. 2016;52(3):178–85. https://doi.org/10.1111/ppc.12114.
201. Weltman G, Lamon J, Freedy E, Chartrand D. Police department personnel stress resilience training: an institutional case study. Glob Adv Health Med. 2014;3(2):72–9. https://doi.org/10.7453/gahmj.2014.015.

202. Kobayashi Y, Kaneyoshi A, Yokota A, Kawakami N. Effects of a worker participatory program for improving work environments on job stressors and mental health among workers. J Occup Health. 2008;50(6):455–70.
203. Noh JW, Kwon YD, Lee LJ, Oh IH, Kim J. Gender differences in the impact of retirement on depressive symptoms among middle-aged and older adults: a propensity score matching approach. PLoS One. 2019;14(3):e0212607. https://doi.org/10.1371/journal.pone.0212607.
204. Kim JE, Moen P. Retirement transitions, gender, and psychological Well-being: a life-course, ecological model. J Gerontol B Psychol Sci Soc Sci. 2002;57:212–22.
205. van Solinge H, Henkens K. Adjustment to and satisfaction with retirement: two of a kind? Psychol Aging. 2008;23:422–34. https://doi.org/10.1037/0882-7974.23.2.422.
206. Clarke P, Marshall V, House J, Lantz P. The social structuring of mental health over the adult life course: advancing theory in the sociology of aging. Soc Forces. 2011;29:1287–313. https://doi.org/10.1353/sof.2011.0036.
207. Bayer PB. Mutable characteristics and the definition of discrimination under title VII. UC Davis L Rev. 1986;20:769.
208. Pascoe EA, Smart Richman L. Perceived discrimination and health: a meta-analytic review. Psychol Bull. 2009;135(4):531. https://doi.org/10.1037/a0016059.
209. Mickelson KD, Williams DR. The prevalence, distribution, and mental health correlates of perceived discrimination in the United States. J Health Soc Behav. 1999;40:208–30.
210. Kim G, Kim J, Lee SK, Sim J, Kim Y, Yun BY, Yoon JA. Multidimensional gender discrimination in workplace and depressive symptoms. PLoS One. 2020;15(7):e0234415. https://doi.org/10.1371/journal.pone.0234415.
211. McLaughlin KA, Hatzenbuehler ML, Keyes KM. Responses to discrimination and psychiatric disorders among black, hispanic, female, and lesbian, gay, and bisexual individuals. Am J Public Health. 2010;100:1477–84.
212. Hosang GM, Bhui K. Gender discrimination, victimisation and women's mental health. Br J Psychiatry. 2018;213(6):682–4. https://doi.org/10.1192/bjp.2018.244.
213. EIGE. Gender Equality Index 2015. Measuring gender equality in the European Union 2005–2012. 2015. https://doi.org/10.2839/763764.
214. TUC and everyday sexism project. Still just a bit of banter? 2016.
215. Moss-Racusin CA, Dovidio JF, Brescoll VL, Graham MJ, Handelsman J. Science faculty's subtle gender biases favor male students. Proc Natl Acad Sci. 2012;109:16474–9.
216. Lagerlöf, E. Women, work and health. National report Sweden, Ds 1993:98. Stockholm: Ministry of Health and Social Affairs; 1993.
217. Asplund R, Barth E, Smith N, Wadensjö E. The male–female wage gap in the Nordic counties. In: Wadensjö E, editor. The Nordic labour markets in the 1990's. Part 1. Amsterdam: Elsevier; 1996. p. 55–82.
218. Springer KW, Hankivsky O, Bates LM. Gender and health: relational, intersectional, and biosocial approaches. Soc Sci Med. 2012;74:1661–6.
219. Shippee TP, Wilkinson LR, Schafer MH, Shippee ND. Long-term effects of age discrimination on mental health: the role of perceived financial strain. J Gerontol B Psychol Sci Soc Sci. 2019;74(4):664–74. https://doi.org/10.1093/geronb/gbx017.
220. Maslach C, Schaufeli WB, Leiter MP. Job burnout. Ann Rev Psychol. 2001;52:397–422.
221. Maske UE, Riedel-Heller SG, Seiffert I, Jacobi F, Hapke U. Prevalence and comorbidity of self-reported diagnosis of burnout syndrome in the general population—results of the German health interview and examination survey for adults (DEGS1). Psychiatr Prax. 2016;43:e1.
222. Purvanova RK, Muros JP. Gender differences in burnout: a meta-analysis. J Vocat Behav. 2010;77:168–85.
223. Beauregard N, Marchand A, Bilodeau J, Durand P, Demers A, Haines VV. Gendered pathways to burnout: results from the SALVEO study. Ann Work Expo Health. 2018;62(4):426–37. https://doi.org/10.1093/annweh/wxx114.
224. Gagnon S. La surqualification: Qui la vit? Où s'observet-elle? Travail et remuneration. 2008;9:1–5.

225. Niedhammer I, Chastang JF, Sultan-Taïeb H, Vermeylen G, Parent-Thirion A. Psychosocial work factors and sickness absence in 31 countries in Europe. Eur J Pub Health. 2013;23(4):622–9. https://doi.org/10.1093/eurpub/cks124.
226. Stepanikova I, Baker EH, Simoni ZR, Zhu A, Rutland SB, Sims M, et al. The role of perceived discrimination in obesity among African Americans. Am J Prev Med. 2017;52(1S1):S77–85.
227. Halpern DF, Murphy SE. From balance to interaction: why the metaphor is important. In: Halpern DF, Murphy SE, editors. From work-family balance to work-family interaction: changing the metaphor. Mahwah: Lawrence Erlbaum Associates, Inc. Publishers; 2004. p. 3–11.
228. Evans O, Steptoe A. The contribution of gender-role orientation, work factors and home stressors to psychological wellbeing and sickness absence in male- and female-dominated occupational groups. Soc Sci Med. 2002;54:481–92.
229. Dyrbye LN, Sinsky T, Cipriano C, Bhatt P, Ommaya J, West A, Meyers CD. Burnout among health care professionals: a call to explore and address this underrecognized threat to safe, high-quality care. NAM Perspect. 2017;7 https://doi.org/10.31478/201707b.
230. Wang C, Sweetman A. Gender, family status and physician labour supply. Soc Sci Med. 2013;94:17–25.
231. Adesoye T, Mangurian C, Choo EK, Girgis C, Sabry-Elnaggar H, Linos E. Perceived discrimination experienced by physician mothers and desired workplace changes: a cross-sectional survey (in Eng). JAMA Intern Med. 2017;177(7):1033–6.
232. Stentz NC, Griffith KA, Perkins E, Jones RD, Jagsi R. Fertility and childbearing among American female physicians (in eng). J Women's Health. 2016;25(10):1059–65.
233. Sarma AA, Nkonde-Price C, Gulati M, Duvernoy CS, Lewis SJ, Wood MJ. Cardiovascular medicine and society: the pregnant cardiologist. J Am Coll Cardiol. 2017;69(1):92–101.
234. Grayson JL, Alvarez HK, Grayson JLAHK. School climate factors relating to teacher burnout: a mediator model. Teach Teach Education. 2008;24(5):1349–63.
235. Van Droogenbroeck F, Spruyt B. I ain't gonna make it. Comparing Job Demands-Resources and attrition intention between senior teachers and senior employees of six other occupational categories in Flanders. Int J Aging Hum Dev. 2016;83(2):128–55. https://doi.org/10.1177/0091415016647729.
236. Hochschild AR. The managed heart: commercialization of human feeling. Berkeley, CA: University of California Press; 2012.
237. Borman GD, Dowling NM. Teacher attrition and retention: a metaanalytic and narrative review of the research. Rev Educ Res. 2008;78(3):367–409.
238. Organisation for Economic Co-operation and Development [OECD]. Education at a glance 2012: OECD indicators. Paris.
239. Shanafelt TD, Noseworthy JH. Executive leadership and physician Well-being: nine organizational strategies to promote engagement and reduce burnout. Mayo Clin Proc. 2017;92(1):129–46.
240. Cotten S. Marital status and mental health revisited: examining the importance of risk factors and resources. Fam Relat. 1999;48:225–33.
241. Williams K. Has the future of marriage arrived? A contemporary examination of gender, marriage and psychological Well-being. J Health Soc Behav. 2003;44(4):470–87.
242. House JS, Umberson D, LandisKR. Structures and processes of social support. Ann. Rev Sociol. 1988;14:293–318.
243. Lewis MA, Butterfield RM. Social control in marital relationships: effect of one's partner on health behaviors. J Appl Soc Psychol. 2007;37:298–319. https://doi.org/10.1111/j.0021-902 9.2007.00161.x.
244. Gove WR, Style CB, Hughes M. The effect of marriage on the Well-being of adults. J Fam Issues. 1990;11:4–35.
245. Strohschein L, McDonough P, Monette G, Shao Q. Marital transitions and mental health: are there gender differences in the short-term effects of marital status change? Soc Sci Med. 2005 Dec;61(11):2293–303. https://doi.org/10.1016/j.socscimed.2005.07.020.

246. Simon R. Revisiting the relationships among gender, marital status and mental health. Am J Sociol. 2002;107(4):1065–96.
247. Bianchi SM, Subaiya L, Kahn JR. The gender gap in the economic Well-being of nonresident fathers and custodial mothers. Demography. 1999;36(2):195–203.
248. Ooms T, Bouchet S, Parke M. Beyond marriage licenses: efforts to strengthen marriage and two-parent families. Washington, DC: Center for Law and Social Policy; 2004.
249. Dennerstein L. Mental health, work, and gender. Int J Health Serv. 1995;25(3):503–9. https://doi.org/10.2190/QJRA-8NMB-KR1R-QH4Q.
250. Organisation for Economic Cooperation and Development. OECD. Stat. 2019. https://stats.oecd.org/index.aspx?queryid=54757
251. Szalai A, editor. The use of time: daily activities of urban and suburban populations in twelve countries. The Hague: Mouton; 1972.
252. Coveman S. Gender, domestic labor time and wage inequality. Am Sociol Rev. 1983;48(626):1983.
253. Kobayashi T, Honjo K, Eshak ES, Iso H, Sawada N, Tsugane S, et al. Work family conflict and self-rated health among Japanese workers: how household income modifies associations. PLoS One. 2017;12:e0169903.
254. Himsel AJ, Goldberg WA. Social comparisons and satisfaction with the division of housework: implications for men's and women's role strain. J Fam Issues. 2003;24(7):843–66.
255. Wagman P, Nordin M, Alfredsson L, Westerholm PJ, Fransson EI. Domestic work division and satisfaction in cohabiting adults: associations with life satisfaction and self-rated health. Scand J Occup Ther. 2017;24:24–31.
256. Eek F, Axmon A. Gender inequality at home is associated with poorer health for women. Scand J Public Health. 2015;43:176–82.
257. Jung JW, Cho SY. Factors influencing household work sharing and perceptions of equitable and unequitable household work sharing in dual-earner households. Korean J Commun Living Sci. 2015;26(4):717–29.
258. Lee SA, Park EC, Ju YJ, Han KT, Yoon JG, Kim TH. The association between satisfaction with husband's participation in housework and suicidal ideation among married working women in Korea. Psychiatry Res. 2018;261:541–6. https://doi.org/10.1016/j.psychres.2018.01.039.
259. Molarius A, Granstrom F, Linden-Bostrom M, Elo S. Domestic work and self-rated health among women and men aged 25-64 years: results from a population-based survey in Sweden. Scand J Public Health. 2014;42:52–9.
260. Maeda E, Nomura K, Hiraike O, Sugimori H, Kinoshita A, Osuga Y. Domestic work stress and self-rated psychological health among women: a cross-sectional study in Japan. Environ Health Prev Med. 2019;24(1):75. https://doi.org/10.1186/s12199-019-0833-5.
261. Murakami K, Sasaki S. Dietary intake and depressive symptoms: a systematic review of observational studies. Mol Nutr Food Res. 2010;54:471–88.
262. McNaughton S. Dietary patterns and diet quality: approaches to assessing complex exposures in nutrition. Aust Epidemiol. 2010;17:35–7.
263. Lai JS, Hiles S, Bisquera A, Hure AJ, McEvoy M, Attia J. A systematic review and meta-analysis of dietary patterns and depression in community-dwelling adults. Am J Clin Nutr. 2014;99(1):181–97. https://doi.org/10.3945/ajcn.113.069880.
264. National Health and Medical Research Council. Australian dietary guidelines. Canberra: National Health and Medical Research Council; 2013.
265. Kiecolt-Glaser JK. Stress, food, and inflammation: psychoneuroimmunology and nutrition at the cutting edge. Psychosom Med. 2010;72:365–9.
266. Calder PC, Albers R, Antoine J-M, Blum S, Bourdet-Sicard R, Ferns GA, et al. Inflammatory disease processes and interactions with nutrition. Br J Nutr. 2009;101(Suppl 1):1–45.
267. Appleton KM, Rogers PJ, Ness AR. Updated systematic review and meta-analysis of the effects of n23 long-chain polyunsaturated fatty acids on depressed mood. Am J Clin Nutr. 2010;91:757–70.
268. Jacka F, Berk M. Food for thought. Acta Neuropsychiatr. 2007;19:321–3.
269. Christensen L. The effect of food intake on mood. Clin Nutr. 2001;20(Suppl 1):161–6.

270. Wurtman RJ, Wurtman J. Carbohydrates and depression. Sci Am. 1989;260:68–75.
271. Irigoyen Camacho ME, Lazarevich I, Velazquez-Alva MC, Najera Medina O, Flores NL, Zepeda MA. Depression and food consumption in Mexican college students. Nutricion Hospitalaria. 2018;35(3):620–6. https://doi.org/10.20960/nh.1500.
272. Crawford GB, Khedkar A, Flaws JA, Sorkin JD, Gallicchio L. Depressive symptoms and self-reported fast-food intake in midlife women. Prev Med. 2011;52(3–4):254–7. https://doi.org/10.1016/j.ypmed.2011.01.006.
273. Lee J, Allen J. Gender differences in healthy and unhealthy food consumption and its relationship with depression in young adulthood. Community Ment Health J. 2020;57(5):898–909. https://doi.org/10.1007/s10597-020-00672-x.
274. Hasin DS, Sarvet AL, Meyers JL, Saha TD, Ruan J, Stohl M, Grant BF. Epidemiology of adult DSM-5 major depressive disorder and its specifiers in the United States. JAMA Psychiat. 2018;75(4):336–46. https://doi.org/10.1001/jamapsychiatry.2017.4602.
275. Hauge LJ, Stene-Larsen K, Grimholt TK, Oien-Odegaard C, Reneflot A. Use of primary health care services prior to suicide in the Norwegian population 2006–2015. BMC Health Serv Res. 2018;18(1):619. https://doi.org/10.1186/s12913-018-3419-9.
276. Doherty DT, Kartalova-O'Doherty Y. Gender and self-reported mental health problems: predictors of help seeking from a general practitioner. Br J Health Psychol. 2010;15(1):213–28.
277. Milner A, Scovelle A, King T. Treatment-seeking differences for mental health problems in male-and non-male-dominated occupations: evidence from the HILDA cohort. Epidemiol Psychiatr Sci. 2018;28(6):630–7.
278. Schnyder N, Panczak R, Groth N, Schultze-Lutter F. Association between mental health-related stigma and active helpseeking: systematic review and meta-analysis. Br J Psychiatry. 2017;210(4):261–8. https://doi.org/10.1192/bjp.bp.116.189464.
279. Alegría A, Nakash O, NeMoyer A. Increasing equity in access to mental health care: a critical first step in improving service quality. World Psychiatry. 2018;17(1):43–4. https://doi.org/10.1002/wps.20486.
280. Fairburn CG, Patel V. The global dissemination of psychological treatments: a road map for research and practice. Am J Psychiatry. 2014;171(5):495–8. https://doi.org/10.1176/appi.ajp.2013.13111546.

Clinical Staging of Psychiatric Disorders: Its Utility in Mental Health Prevention

Grazia Rutigliano and Claudia Del Grande

2.1 Diagnostic Process in Psychiatry: Shortcomings of Current Diagnostic Classifications and Future Directions

In clinical medicine, "diagnosis" is defined as the application to an individual case of a given category or "type" from a classification. The purpose of diagnosis should be that of guiding treatment and predicting outcome or prognosis [1]. Despite the value of diagnosis being clearly established in clinical medicine, in psychiatry it has been repeatedly questioned; particularly, the most concerns regard the clinical utility and predictive validity of diagnostic processes [2].

Diagnostic categories traditionally described in the official diagnostic systems (DSM/ICD) are artificial divisions based on cross-sectional symptom sets mainly observed in entrenched or chronic mental illness [2]. This categorical approach has been criticized for its intrinsically limited clinical utility: first, it failed to identify discrete disease entities corresponding to specific etiology and/or pathogenesis; second, diagnostic categories demonstrated to have relative, limited implications in terms of guiding treatment choice and predicting outcomes, namely, the two key elements of "clinical utility"; finally, they only embody the "end-state" of illness trajectories, failing to represent the progressive and dynamic nature of emerging psychopathology [3, 4]. Despite the efforts made to improve the clinical utility of psychiatric diagnosis in both the DSM-5 and the ICD-11, current diagnostic

G. Rutigliano (✉)
Institute of Clinical Sciences, Faculty of Medicine, Imperial College London, London, UK
e-mail: grutigli@ic.ac.uk

C. Del Grande
Azienda USL Toscana Nord Ovest, UFSMA Zona Pisana, Pisa, Italy
e-mail: claudia.delgrande@uslnordovest.toscana.it

M. Colizzi, M. Ruggeri (eds.), *Prevention in Mental Health*,
https://doi.org/10.1007/978-3-030-97906-5_2

systems are still inadequate to provide satisfactory characterization of patients in the complexity of the clinical realm. It has been observed that patients sharing the same psychiatric diagnosis may respond differently to a specific treatment, as well as patients with different diagnostic framework may respond similarly to a given treatment; clinical trajectories and outcomes of patients receiving the same diagnosis are dynamic and extremely variable; and a large extent of comorbidity and psychopathological phenomena (i.e., psychomotor retardation or agitation, anhedonia, delusions) are present across different diagnostic entities, especially in earlier phases of illness trajectories, thus supporting the need for a different operationalization of psychopathology [3, 4]. Moreover, subthreshold conditions are frequently observed to precede full-threshold disorders, aligning with the dimensional models of mental disorders that conceptualize psychopathology on a continuum of severity [5, 6].

Many experts worldwide have converged on the need of focusing on a better characterization of the individual case with respect to the relevant psychopathological dimensions and to the current stage of development of the diagnosed disorder. The characterization of the individual case should include the exploration of a series of antecedent (i.e., family history of mental illness, other parental factors, perinatal factors, early environmental exposure, psychomotor development, premorbid social adjustment, psychopathological antecedents, polygenic risk scores) and concomitant variables (personality traits, cognitive functions, social functioning, soft neurological signs, substance abuse, recent environmental exposure, biological markers), as well as careful assessment of the severity of the clinical picture. Alternative approaches are expected to improve illness management and outcome prediction, with special emphasis on social functioning and personal recovery.

2.2 Clinical Staging Model: Principles and Criteria for Staging

Clinical staging is a proven strategy in general medicine, where it is used routinely for potentially serious or chronic physical disorders, mainly cancer, but also diabetes, autoimmune diseases, arthritis, and cardiovascular diseases. The staging model meets the purpose of (a) characterizing a disorder by describing the link between clinical phenotypes, the degree of disease extent, and progression and biomarkers and (b) promoting a personalized or stratified medicine approach to treatment planning. Its value and utility is most notably recognized in clinical oncology, where quality of life and survival largely depend on the earliest possible delivery of effective interventions. A prototype of staging is the tumor-node-metastasis staging model applied to breast cancer, where the extent of disease progression is defined by the size of primary tumor, its spread to other locations within the body, and involvement of other systems [2].

Clinical staging defines the extent of disease progression at a particular point in time, thus placing an individual's current state along a continuum from stage 0 (at-risk or latency stage) to stage 4 (chronicity) [2].

The clinical staging framework incorporates some fundamental assumptions:

1. The disease does not inevitably progress.
2. Treatment during earlier stages of illness may arrest disease progression and achieve better response and prognosis (i.e., arrests progression).
3. Treatments during earlier stages have a more favorable risk-benefit ratio.
4. Early interventions modify stage distribution of the disease over time (toward less severe stages).
5. Clinical stages are associated with stage-specific biological, social, and environmental factors.

2.3   Clinical Staging Model in Psychiatry

Initial support for the concept of staging in psychiatry became over three decades ago from Fava and Kellner [7]. These authors realized that official diagnostic classifications neglected the longitudinal perspective of mental disorders, including the prodromes. Since then, a prototypical clinical staging model was elaborated [2], initially for psychotic disorders and later adapted to bipolar disorder (BD), depression, eating disorders, and anxiety disorders. The clinical staging model spans from stage 0 to stage 4. Stage 0 identifies a premorbid asymptomatic at-risk state (usually defined by genetic vulnerability). Stage 1 corresponds to the emergence of subthreshold symptoms and functional decline. It can be further distinguished in stage 1a, characterized by mild symptoms, cognitive changes, and functional changes, and stage 1b, which represents the so-called "clinical high-risk" or "ultrahigh-risk" state, i.e., moderate subthreshold symptoms and disability. Stage 2 represents full-threshold first episode of illness (i.e., psychotic or severe mood disorder) associated with further functional drop. This may fully remit, or further evolve, toward stage 3, "late/incomplete recovery." Stage 3 encompasses 3a, incomplete recovery from the first episode; 3b, single relapse which stabilizes with treatment at a level of symptoms, cognition, and functioning below the best level achieved following remission from first episode; and 3c, multiple relapses, related to worsening of clinical extent. Finally, stage 4 identifies severe, persistent, or unremitting mental health disorders characterized by chronicity [2].

In contrast with staging in clinical medicine, where anatomic extent and impact of the disease determine stage, it appears evident that the concept of staging in psychiatry is closely related to that of illness course. This course-based definition of stages utilizes duration and relapse criteria and key social variables (i.e., social isolation or vocational failure) as indicators of illness extent and progression [2]. This model assumes that clear syndromic specificity and stability progressively increases from early to advanced stages that are associated with severe symptom burden, significant functional impairment, and persistent/recurrent pattern. Remission and recovery are an integral part of the staging process, and are possible to occur at every stage, although the chances of remission and recovery decrease with progression and a return to previous stages is not possible. Then, identifying young people at enhanced risk for developing serious mental illness and prevention of progression to more advanced stages through early successful treatments are the primary goals of this prevention-oriented framework [2, 4]. This is of particular relevance, if we consider that three quarters of major mental disorders emerge between childhood and young adulthood, with a peak onset during adolescence. This can have a significant impact on the psychosocial trajectories of affected individuals and contributes considerably to the global economic burden of mental diseases [4, 8].

An old dilemma and ongoing debate in the proposed clinical staging model concerns the "splitting" versus "lumping" issue. The splitting approach proposes distinct staging models for different disorders (eating disorders, unipolar depression, psychotic, and BDs), and conceptualizes stages 2–4 as identifying clinical subtypes within those diagnostic categories, rather than focusing on disease progression [9–11]. Conversely, the lumping approach favors a transdiagnostic view, based on the observation that early stages of several of major psychiatric disorders are nonspecific and substantially overlap [2, 12]. The relative concentration of specific diagnosis in families and the differences in course and treatment outcomes across different disorders support the splitting approach, while the lumping one is supported by the evidence for shared genetic risk factors and biomarkers, common childhood precursors, shared environmental risk factors (e.g., traumatic experiences, substance misuse), extensive comorbidity between disorders, and similar response to common psychological and pharmacological treatments across currently defined diagnostic categories. Transdiagnostic staging models may probably be optimal for the study of at-risk and prodromal phases, while disorder-specific models can contribute to the understanding of the later more clearly defined syndromic phenotypes [10].

2.3.1 Application of the Clinical Staging Model to Psychotic Disorders

The first attempts to systematically operationalize the clinical staging model were made for psychotic disorders. About 25 years ago, the Melbourne Group of the Personal Assessment and Crisis Evaluation (PACE) Clinic pioneered the at-risk mental state (ARMS) train of research, which coincides with stage 1, help-seeking clinical high-risk individuals. They prospectively developed a set of high-risk diagnostic criteria, named "ultrahigh-risk" (UHR) criteria, and conceived the first UHR psychometric tool, the Comprehensive Assessment of At-Risk Mental States (CAARMS) [13]. A few years later, the Prevention through Risk Identification, Management and Education (PRIME) Clinic in New Haven (USA) introduced another UHR diagnostic instrument, the Structured Interview for Psychosis-Risk

Syndrome (SIPS) [14]. Albeit slightly different operationalization, the two instruments address the same constructs, as follows:

- Genetic risk and deterioration syndrome (GRD), including a combination of vulnerability trait (first-degree family history of psychosis or schizotypal personality disorder) and significant decrease in functioning or chronic low functioning.
- Attenuated psychotic symptoms (APS), including young people who experience psychotic symptoms at subthreshold intensity or frequency.
- Brief Limited Intermittent Psychotic Symptoms (BLIPS), defined by the presence of a full-blown psychotic episode lasting less than a week and spontaneously remitting without drug therapy or hospitalization.

According to the staging framework, individuals meeting these criteria already present some decline in functioning and quality of life [15]. UHR individuals are at increased risk of transitioning to stage 2, full-threshold first episode psychosis (about 20% risk after 2 years) [16], while there is no evidence of an increased risk of developing nonpsychotic disorders [17]. However, substantial heterogeneity exists in the possible outcomes of the ARMS (see below, *Transdiagnostic Approach to Clinical Staging*). Furthermore, stage 1 was further subdivided into different clinical stages, based on a gradient of risk at 2-year follow-up. Individuals showing negative and cognitive symptoms (i.e., stage 1a) have about 3% risk; risk increases to 19% for those complaining of APS (i.e., stage 1b), and peaks to 39% in BLIPS (i.e., stage 1c) [16]. Of note, stage 1 is preceded by an asymptomatic stage 0, including individuals at genetic risk exposed to environmental factors before symptoms and help-seeking behavior manifest. At present, there are no known preventive strategies to arrest progression from stage 0. In addition, it is not recommended to use UHR criteria in stage 0, or even worse, in the general population for screening purposes, because, due to the meta-analytically demonstrated poor positive predictive value of UHR criteria, this would lead to risk dilution [18]. On the other hand, every effort should be put to further enrich risk in stage 1 through sequential testing methods [19], to identify those more in need of indicated preventive treatments. Stage 2 encompasses the acute phase or crisis that is characterized by sustained psychotic symptoms, lasting at least 4 weeks and followed by an early recovery phase or post-acute phase observed within 6–12 months. The individual who manifested a first episode of psychosis might recover completely (stage 2), achieve recovery but relapse (stage 3a), undergo multiple relapses (stage 3b), and not respond to treatment (stage 3c). Adequate secondary preventive interventions in stage 2 are therefore fundamental to avoid incomplete recovery (i.e., stage 3). Multiple recurrences or a severe, persistent illness finally qualifies as stage 4. Unfortunately, despite much research being conducted, there is no conclusive evidence about the clinical utility of discrete stages in psychotic disorders, also because of lack of consensus on interventions able to alter long-term course.

2.3.2 Application of the Clinical Staging Model to Bipolar Disorders

The stages of BD are described in terms of severity of symptoms (subthreshold phenomena or full-blown episodes), quality of remissions (full remission and recovery, episodic course with inter-episode full or partial remission, or recurrent/persistent illness), as well as associated cognitive and functional impairment. These latter are often related to one another and to severity of mood disorders and prognosis [20]. All staging models of BD involve a latent or preclinical stage of enhanced vulnerability (stage 0). The asymptomatic stage can follow dynamic and variable trajectories that may or may not lead to subthreshold clinical phenomena (stage 1) incorporating some aspects of current diagnostic categories (e.g., brief or recurrent hypomania, mild depressive symptoms which do not satisfy criteria for a major depressive episode for intensity or duration, disrupted sleep-wake cycle, increased or decreased energy). This can evolve to the first sustained full-threshold episode of mania, severe depression, or affective psychosis (stage 2). Stage 3 may be characterized by single or multiple relapses or recurrent/persistent illness course, and, finally, stage 4 is characterized by unremitted illness associated with poor outcome, treatment-refractory symptoms, severely impaired functioning, and heavy medical comorbidity. Obesity, insulin resistance, type II diabetes, and cardiovascular diseases are all viewed as correlates of poor outcome and appear to be related to BD in a complex, bidirectional way [20]. It is now established that physical comorbidities, especially cardiovascular diseases, account for the majority of premature mortality observed in these patients that show a reduction in life expectancy of 10–17.5 years compared to the general population [21]. Psychiatric comorbid conditions are also common in BD, particularly anxiety and substance use disorders, and contribute to poor outcome and less favorable treatment response.

Despite the staging model capturing the aggregate course and evolution of BD, linear stepwise progression through more severe phases may not be applicable to illness course in all patients: in fact, some individuals may have a more severe and deteriorating presentation from the onset of illness, while others may have a favorable episodic course characterized by full inter-episode recovery [10]. Shah and Scott (2016) highlighted the pluripotential, heterotypic, and dynamic course of early-stage, subthreshold syndromes that may potentially evolve in recurrent depression, BD, or psychosis but, in some cases, represent just time-limited adjustment problems with no transition to more severe mental disorders [22].

Evidence supporting staging in BD was initially derived from observational studies of the course and natural history of illness, which consistently highlighted how the periods of euthymia become shorter with an increasing number of successive episodes of illness [10]. In addition, the Systematic Treatment Enhancement Program for Bipolar Disorders (STEP-BD) study recently showed that the number of episodes was positively associated with severity of manic and depressive symptoms, as well as poorer functioning and quality of life [23]. Moreover, lithium treatment, the gold standard for BD prophylaxis, is observed to be more effective if used earlier in the illness course; conversely, its efficacy declines when administered to patients with multiple prior illness episodes [24].

There is evidence for a positive association between illness progression and cognitive dysfunction and, to some extent, brain structural changes [25, 26]. Cognitive dysfunction is widely recognized as a major driver of functional disability and patients' psychosocial outcomes; it often persists in remission periods and may emphasize affective components [27]. Therefore, addressing cognitive deficits is a major challenge of new therapeutic approaches to BD.

2.3.3   Application of the Clinical Staging Model to Major Depressive Disorder

The elements for a clinical staging model are present in major depressive disorder (MDD) as well. The onset of MDD is anticipated by risk factors (stage 0), such as family history of depression, low maternal care, parental divorce in early childhood, somatic health concerns, substance use, poor diet, and physical inactivity [28]. In particular, it has been reported that having a depressed parent is associated with a three- to five-fold increase of MDD or other mental disorders [29, 30]. A MDD prodrome (stage 1) has been tentatively described: besides family history of affective disorders, it consists of subthreshold depressive and anxiety symptoms and substance use. However, the formal operationalization of such prodrome is still in its infancy. In 2015, Verduijn et al. [11] demonstrated the predictive validity of a staging model, in which they distinguished stage 1a and 1b. As far as we are aware, this approach has not been adopted and followed up by other groups. Among people with good social support, the highest transition rates to a first depressive episode (stage 2) are related to multiple stress events in the past year. On the other hand, stressful events seem to have less of a role in those with poor social support [31]. Stage 2 does not inevitably progress to later stages. In fact, in a 23-year longitudinal study, one third of participants with a first MDD episode did not develop a second episode during the follow-up, and one third of those with a second episode did not develop a third episode [32]. However, in many patients, MDD shows a progressive course, as Kraepelin already noted at the beginning of the twentieth century. The risk of relapses increases with the number and duration of previous depressive episodes [33, 34]. Furthermore, as MDD progresses, illness severity increases, the interval between episodes shortens, and the disease grows "autonomous" from stressful events (stage 3) [35]. Discussion of the pathophysiological mechanisms underlying this type of progression, i.e., the sensitization and the kindling models, is beyond the scope of this chapter (please refer to [36]). Nonetheless, some evidence suggests that antidepressant treatment does not lose efficacy for recurrent depressive episodes [28]. If inadequately addressed, stage 3 may accelerate the progressive cognitive and functional decline characteristic of stage 4. The higher the duration of MDD, the less the chance of recovery [37]. Furthermore, each depressive episode is associated with 2–3% memory decline and 13% increased dementia risk [35]. In conclusion, clinical observations support the progressive nature of MDD, hence the applicability of a staging model. However, formal operationalization and research are needed.

2.3.4 Transdiagnostic Approach to Clinical Staging

A quarter of a century after the formulation of the ARMS concept, it has become evident that transition to psychosis is only one of the possible clinical outcomes in UHR individuals. A large proportion of them complain of persistent subthreshold psychotic symptoms and achieve poor functional adjustment [38]. Moreover, incident/recurrent nonpsychotic "comorbid" disorders are not uncommon, including mood, anxiety, personality, and/or substance use disorders [38]. Besides its pluripotency, the ARMS construct is also characterized by substantial heterotypy, meaning that symptoms progress from one category to the other. It was reported that subjects deemed at risk for nonpsychotic disorders evolved toward a psychotic outcome with a 77-fold higher rate than the general population (4% in 3 years vs 25% in UHR) [39]. Another criticism of the ARMS model comes with the so-called prevention paradox, referring to the observation that only a small proportion of people presenting with a first episode of psychosis (range: 4–13%) are previously under the care of UHR services, where they exist. While some authors make the case for insufficient cost-effectiveness of prodromal services in public health [40], it is possible that these data indicate that UHR services are not well suited to intercept the early—mostly undifferentiated—stages of psychopathology [41]. Accordingly, the retrospective analysis of a first episode psychosis sample showed that, in most cases, psychosis onset was preceded by depressive and anxiety symptoms and poor functioning, rather than subthreshold psychotic symptoms [22]. The earliest stages of mental disorders are characterized by waxing and waning states of anxiety and depression, possibly combining with psychotic-like experiences, emotional dysregulation, and basic symptoms, in a "kaleidoscopic series of microphenotypes" [41]. This laid the foundations for a broader transdiagnostic approach to risk detection, under the name of Clinical High At Risk Mental State (CHARMS). Operationally, the CHARMS framework expands UHR criteria, to include, in stage 1b, psychotic symptoms, bipolar states, depression, and borderline personality features, all at intensity and frequency under the diagnostic threshold. Stage 2 is also broadened to any "exit syndrome," rather than specific evolution to psychosis onset. Adopting this approach in the next generation of preventive interventions may allow to better capture at-risk individuals and to offer psychosocial or biological treatments tailored to the presenting symptomatology, rather than targeting attenuated psychotic experiences to prevent transition to full-blown psychosis.

2.4 Toward a Clinicopathological Staging Model

An important advantage of the clinical staging model is that it allows gathering data on biological, social, and environmental factors linked to stage-specific clinical features. To date, much of the search for neurobiological correlates of major psychiatric disorders has been conducted on patients with stable diagnostic features, meaning in an advanced stage of the disease course. This methodological approach affects the ability to discriminate between markers of vulnerability and sequelae of disease

[2]. This is, for instance, the case of hippocampal atrophy that has been detected in depressed patients: it is unclear whether this alteration may reflect etiological processes or is simply a correlate of untreated illness [42, 43]. We hope that a clearer knowledge of the pathophysiological changes underlying illness onset and progression, i.e., integrated clinicopathological staging model, may more accurately guide clinicians in treatment selection and prognostic evaluations. Some of the biological markers are thought to represent etio-pathogenetic mechanisms (e.g., neuroinflammation, oxidative stress, hypothalamic-pituitary-adrenal (HPA) axis hyperactivity), while others may be pathogenic consequences (e.g., cognitive and brain structure abnormalities). As illustrated in our proposal for a clinicopathological staging model (Fig. 2.1), biomarkers seem to have a gradient of appearance across clinical stages, with earlier biomarkers being shared by different mental disorders (reminiscent of shared early experiences in undifferentiated subthreshold illness stages), and later biomarkers acquiring more and more illness specificity. It should be noted, though, that further research is needed and no definitive clinicopathological model of staging can be used yet. In this paragraph, we will describe two of the most investigated and best-replicated biological markers, neuroinflammation/oxidative and nitrosative (O&NS) stress and brain structural changes, in the context of schizophrenia, BD, and MDD. The reader is invited to refer to [35, 45, 46] for a more comprehensive overview.

2.4.1 Neuroinflammation and O&NS Markers

A large body of evidence supports chronic inflammation as a pathophysiological mechanism in schizophrenia, BD, and MDD. Cytokines were consistently found elevated in multiple psychiatric states [45]. In detail, anti-inflammatory cytokines, such as interleukin-10 (IL-10), were increased only during the early stages, while levels of pro-inflammatory cytokines, such as the tumor necrosis factor-alpha (TNF-α) and IL-6, progressively increased across stages, possibly in relation to neurodegeneration [47]. A similar pattern has been described for O&NS. Mental disorders, especially in later stages, are characterized by a decompensation of antioxidant mechanisms, such as coenzyme Q10, vitamin E, zinc, glutathione, and glutathione peroxidase. Thus, oxidative stress leads to lipid and DNA damage, as shown by increased peripheral levels of by-products of lipid peroxidation and DNA lesions, respectively [35]. Furthermore, O&NS processes modify protein chemical structure, thus inducing autoimmune responses, shown by increased immunoglobulin M, that amplify inflammation and interfere with cell signaling pathways [35].

2.4.2 Brain Structural Changes

Progressive brain changes were shown in schizophrenia, starting from early stages, i.e., UHR individuals. Subtle gray matter reductions are even observed in non-affected relatives, especially in those who present schizotypal features and cognitive

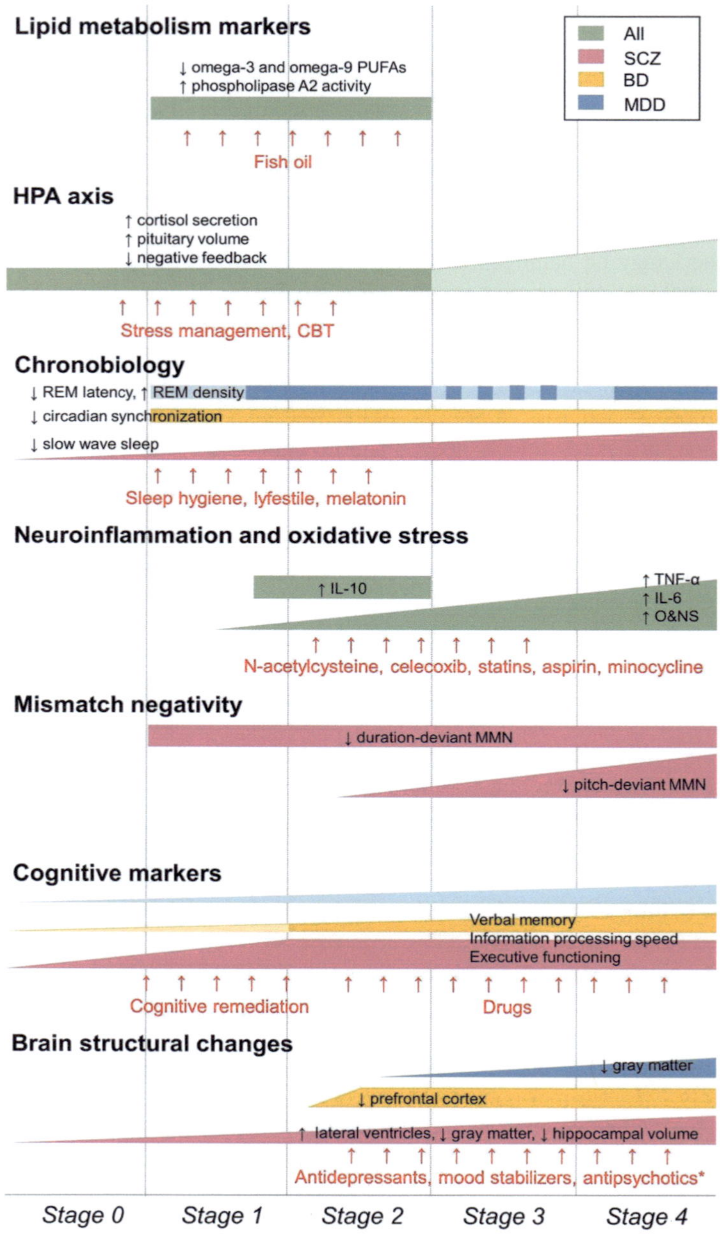

Fig. 2.1 Proposal for a clinicopathological staging model. *BD* bipolar disorder, *CBT* cognitive behavioral therapy, *HPA* hypothalamic-pituitary-adrenal axis, *IL* interleukin, *MDD* major depressive disorder, *MMN* mismatch negativity, *O&NS* oxidative and nitrosative stress, *PUFA*, polyunsaturated fatty acids, *REM* rapid eye movement sleep, *SCZ* schizophrenia, *TNF-α* tumor necrosis factor-alpha. *Antipsychotic treatment intensity was associated to brain tissue loss. It is recommended to use the lowest possible antipsychotic dose to prevent relapse [44]

deficits, possibly reflecting vulnerability [48]. Progressive gray matter loss occurs throughout illness stages, mostly affecting the frontal cortex, the superior temporal gyri, and insular cortex [49–51]. Hippocampal structural changes are found in late stages, while evidence in first episode psychosis (stage 2) or earlier is less clear-cut [52]. The most consistent neuroimaging finding in chronic schizophrenia is the enlargement of lateral ventricles, which could represent a marker of neuroprogression and poor outcome [53]. Structural changes were also described in bipolar disorder and MDD. To simplify, evidence gathered so far seems to indicate that brain loss in affective disorders is a consequence of the pathogenic process. In fact, there is no sufficient data to support the presence of structural changes during the first mood episode. Focal changes in ventral and rostral prefrontal cortex, brain areas involved in affect regulation, rapidly emerge in young adults who develop bipolar disorder [54]. In MDD, significant correlations were described between hippocampal volume and clinical features, such as illness duration, number of episodes, duration of untreated depression, and memory [55].

2.5 Staging Treatment in the Clinicopathological Staging Framework

The clinical staging model implies a hypothetical "step function." Progression from one stage to the next is thought to be preventable through adequate intervention. In this context, "adequate" means that interventions should balance benefits versus risks, in keeping with the maxim "primum non nocere." In early stages, safety should be put first. Interventions with higher risk for side effects should be reserved for severe and chronic disorders. The great promise of the clinicopathological framework is to make treatment optimization, stratification, and personalization possible. Most of the biological factors underlying clinicopathological progression are indeed modifiable, hence amenable to treatment (Fig. 2.1). Although there is no definite consensus, several interventions have been proposed as benign neuroprotective options to be used transdiagnostically during early stages. These include antioxidants and anti-inflammatory agents (e.g., omega-3 polyunsaturated fatty acids, N-acetylcysteine, statins, aspirin, celecoxib). Preliminary evidence supports psychotherapeutic interventions targeting symptoms of psychological distress (i.e., family-focused treatment, cognitive behavioral therapy, stress management) for young at clinical high-risk people, including children and adolescents with mild symptoms of depression, cyclothymia, and other specified and unspecified bipolar and psychotic disorders [56]. Treatments suited for clear full-blown clinical phenotypes, such as antipsychotic drugs and mood stabilizers, are less justifiable in the earlier stages, and the evidence for their utility and efficacy is poor [57]. The aspiration that appropriate therapy can both prevent neuroprogression and have neuroprotective effects is supported by observational studies indicating that lithium treatment reduces brain tissue loss in the cortex, especially in the anterior cingulate and paralimbic cortices, as well as in the hippocampus; increases the length of telomeres; exerts neuroprotective effects by preventing apoptosis, increasing neurotrophins and cell survival molecules, and stimulating hippocampal neurogenesis; exerts anti-inflammatory properties; and prevents the accumulation of medical comorbidities and progression to dementia [58]. Notably, while exposure to antidepressants and mood stabilizers seems to mitigate gray matter loss, antipsychotic treatment intensity, particularly with first-generation antipsychotics, has been shown to predict brain tissue loss. Notwithstanding this, antipsychotic treatment remains a key strategy to prevent relapse, since relapse is itself associated with brain structural changes, but an effort should be made to use the lowest possible doses [44, 59].

In conclusion, the adoption of the clinical staging model holds the potential to transform psychiatry into a more modern medical discipline better grounded on the knowledge of neurobiological pathogenetic processes. The integration of such knowledge in mental health care will allow offering stratified and personalized preventive interventions, with the ultimate goal to arrest neuroprogression and improve personal outcomes.

References

1. Jablensky A. Psychiatric classifications: validity and utility. World Psychiatry. 2016;15(1):26–31.
2. McGorry PD, Hickie IB, Yung AR, Pantelis C, Jackson HJ. Clinical staging of psychiatric disorders: a heuristic framework for choosing earlier, safer and more effective interventions. Aust N Z J Psychiatry. 2006;40(8):616–22.
3. Maj M. Why the clinical utility of diagnostic categories in psychiatry is intrinsically limited and how we can use new approaches to complement them. World Psychiatry. 2018;17(2):121–2.
4. Hartmann JA, McGorry PD, Destree L, Amminger GP, Chanen AM, Davey CG, et al. Pluripotential risk and clinical staging: theoretical considerations and preliminary data from a transdiagnostic risk identification approach. Front Psych. 2020;11:553578.
5. van Os J, Linscott RJ, Myin-Germeys I, Delespaul P, Krabbendam L. A systematic review and meta-analysis of the psychosis continuum: evidence for a psychosis proneness-persistence-impairment model of psychotic disorder. Psychol Med. 2009;39(2):179–95.
6. Krueger RF, Markon KE. A dimensional-spectrum model of psychopathology: progress and opportunities. Arch Gen Psychiatry. 2011;68(1):10–1.
7. Fava GA, Kellner R. Staging: a neglected dimension in psychiatric classification. Acta Psychiatr Scand. 1993;87(4):225–30.
8. Patel V, Flisher AJ, Hetrick S, McGorry P. Mental health of young people: a global public-health challenge. Lancet. 2007;369(9569):1302–13.
9. Treasure J, Stein D, Maguire S. Has the time come for a staging model to map the course of eating disorders from high risk to severe enduring illness? An examination of the evidence. Early Interv Psychiatry. 2015;9(3):173–84.
10. Berk M, Post R, Ratheesh A, Gliddon E, Singh A, Vieta E, et al. Staging in bipolar disorder: from theoretical framework to clinical utility. World Psychiatry. 2017;16(3):236–44.
11. Verduijn J, Milaneschi Y, van Hemert AM, Schoevers RA, Hickie IB, Penninx BW, et al. Clinical staging of major depressive disorder: an empirical exploration. J Clin Psychiatry. 2015;76(9):1200–8.
12. McGorry P, Nelson B. Why we need a transdiagnostic staging approach to emerging psychopathology, early diagnosis, and treatment. JAMA Psychiat. 2016;73(3):191–2.
13. Yung AR, Yuen HP, McGorry PD, Phillips LJ, Kelly D, Dell'Olio M, et al. Mapping the onset of psychosis: the comprehensive assessment of at-risk mental states. Aust N Z J Psychiatry. 2005;39(11–12):964–71.

14. McGlashan T, Walsh B, Woods S. The psychosis-risk syndrome: handbook for diagnosis and follow-up. Oxford: Oxford University Press; 2010.
15. Fusar-Poli P, Rocchetti M, Sardella A, Avila A, Brandizzi M, Caverzasi E, et al. Disorder, not just state of risk: meta-analysis of functioning and quality of life in people at high risk of psychosis. Br J Psychiatry. 2015;207(3):198–206.
16. Fusar-Poli P, Cappucciati M, Borgwardt S, Woods SW, Addington J, Nelson B, et al. Heterogeneity of psychosis risk within individuals at clinical high risk: a meta-analytical stratification. JAMA Psychiat. 2016;73(2):113–20.
17. Fusar-Poli P, Rutigliano G, Stahl D, Davies C, De Micheli A, Ramella-Cravaro V, et al. Long-term validity of the At Risk Mental State (ARMS) for predicting psychotic and non-psychotic mental disorders. Eur Psychiatry. 2017;42:49–54.
18. Fusar-Poli P, Cappucciati M, Rutigliano G, Schultze-Lutter F, Bonoldi I, Borgwardt S, et al. At risk or not at risk? A meta-analysis of the prognostic accuracy of psychometric interviews for psychosis prediction. World Psychiatry. 2015;14(3):322–32.
19. Schmidt A, Cappucciati M, Radua J, Rutigliano G, Rocchetti M, Dell'Osso L, et al. Improving prognostic accuracy in subjects at clinical high risk for psychosis: systematic review of predictive models and meta-analytical sequential testing simulation. Schizophr Bull. 2017;43(2):375–88.
20. Alda M, Kapczinski F. Staging model raises fundamental questions about the nature of bipolar disorder. J Psychiatry Neurosci. 2016;41(5):291–3.
21. Correll CU, Solmi M, Veronese N, Bortolato B, Rosson S, Santonastaso P, et al. Prevalence, incidence and mortality from cardiovascular disease in patients with pooled and specific severe mental illness: a large-scale meta-analysis of 3,211,768 patients and 113,383,368 controls. World Psychiatry. 2017;16(2):163–80.
22. Shah J, Scott J. Concepts and misconceptions regarding clinical staging models. J Psychiatry Neurosci. 2016;41(6):E83–E4.
23. Magalhaes PV, Dodd S, Nierenberg AA, Berk M. Cumulative morbidity and prognostic staging of illness in the Systematic Treatment Enhancement Program for Bipolar Disorder (STEP-BD). Aust N Z J Psychiatry. 2012;46(11):1058–67.
24. Hui TP, Kandola A, Shen L, Lewis G, Osborn DPJ, Geddes JR, et al. A systematic review and meta-analysis of clinical predictors of lithium response in bipolar disorder. Acta Psychiatr Scand. 2019;140(2):94–115.
25. Robinson LJ, Ferrier IN. Evolution of cognitive impairment in bipolar disorder: a systematic review of cross-sectional evidence. Bipolar Disord. 2006;8(2):103–16.
26. Bora E, Yucel M, Pantelis C. Cognitive endophenotypes of bipolar disorder: a meta-analysis of neuropsychological deficits in euthymic patients and their first-degree relatives. J Affect Disord. 2009;113(1–2):1–20.
27. Sole B, Jimenez E, Torrent C, Reinares M, Bonnin CDM, Torres I, et al. Cognitive impairment in bipolar disorder: treatment and prevention strategies. Int J Neuropsychopharmacol. 2017;20(8):670–80.
28. Dodd S, Berk M, Kelin K, Mancini M, Schacht A. Treatment response for acute depression is not associated with number of previous episodes: lack of evidence for a clinical staging model for major depressive disorder. J Affect Disord. 2013;150(2):344–9.
29. Weissman MM, Wickramaratne P, Nomura Y, Warner V, Pilowsky D, Verdeli H. Offspring of depressed parents: 20 years later. Am J Psychiatry. 2006;163(6):1001–8.
30. Hartmann JA, Nelson B, Ratheesh A, Treen D, McGorry PD. At-risk studies and clinical antecedents of psychosis, bipolar disorder and depression: a scoping review in the context of clinical staging. Psychol Med. 2019;49(2):177–89.
31. Hill RM, Pettit JW, Lewinsohn PM, Seeley JR, Klein DN. Escalation to Major Depressive Disorder among adolescents with subthreshold depressive symptoms: evidence of distinct subgroups at risk. J Affect Disord. 2014;158:133–8.
32. Eaton WW, Shao H, Nestadt G, Lee HB, Bienvenu OJ, Zandi P. Population-based study of first onset and chronicity in major depressive disorder. Arch Gen Psychiatry. 2008;65(5):513–20.

33. Kendler KS, Thornton LM, Gardner CO. Stressful life events and previous episodes in the etiology of major depression in women: an evaluation of the "kindling" hypothesis. Am J Psychiatry. 2000;157(8):1243–51.
34. Solomon DA, Keller MB, Leon AC, Mueller TI, Lavori PW, Shea MT, et al. Multiple recurrences of major depressive disorder. Am J Psychiatry. 2000;157(2):229–33.
35. Moylan S, Maes M, Wray NR, Berk M. The neuroprogressive nature of major depressive disorder: pathways to disease evolution and resistance, and therapeutic implications. Mol Psychiatry. 2013;18(5):595–606.
36. Post RM. Transduction of psychosocial stress into the neurobiology of recurrent affective disorder. Am J Psychiatry. 1992;149(8):999–1010.
37. Keller MB, Lavori PW, Mueller TI, Endicott J, Coryell W, Hirschfeld RM, et al. Time to recovery, chronicity, and levels of psychopathology in major depression. A 5-year prospective follow-up of 431 subjects. Arch Gen Psychiatry. 1992;49(10):809–16.
38. Rutigliano G, Valmaggia L, Landi P, Frascarelli M, Cappucciati M, Sear V, et al. Persistence or recurrence of non-psychotic comorbid mental disorders associated with 6-year poor functional outcomes in patients at ultra high risk for psychosis. J Affect Disord. 2016;203:101–10.
39. Lee TY, Lee J, Kim M, Choe E, Kwon JS. Can we predict psychosis outside the clinical high-risk state? A systematic review of non-psychotic risk syndromes for mental disorders. Schizophr Bull. 2018;44(2):276–85.
40. van Os J, Guloksuz S. A critique of the "ultra-high risk" and "transition" paradigm. World Psychiatry. 2017;16(2):200–6.
41. McGorry PD, Hartmann JA, Spooner R, Nelson B. Beyond the "at risk mental state" concept: transitioning to transdiagnostic psychiatry. World Psychiatry. 2018;17(2):133–42.
42. Hickie I, Naismith S, Ward PB, Turner K, Scott E, Mitchell P, et al. Reduced hippocampal volumes and memory loss in patients with early- and late-onset depression. Br J Psychiatry. 2005;186:197–202.
43. Sheline YI, Gado MH, Kraemer HC. Untreated depression and hippocampal volume loss. Am J Psychiatry. 2003;160(8):1516–8.
44. Andreasen NC, Liu D, Ziebell S, Vora A, Ho BC. Relapse duration, treatment intensity, and brain tissue loss in schizophrenia: a prospective longitudinal MRI study. Am J Psychiatry. 2013;170(6):609–15.
45. McGorry P, Keshavan M, Goldstone S, Amminger P, Allott K, Berk M, et al. Biomarkers and clinical staging in psychiatry. World Psychiatry. 2014;13(3):211–23.
46. Wood SJ, Yung AR, McGorry PD, Pantelis C. Neuroimaging and treatment evidence for clinical staging in psychotic disorders: from the at-risk mental state to chronic schizophrenia. Biol Psychiatry. 2011;70(7):619–25.
47. Kauer-Sant'Anna M, Kapczinski F, Andreazza AC, Bond DJ, Lam RW, Young LT, et al. Brain-derived neurotrophic factor and inflammatory markers in patients with early- vs. late-stage bipolar disorder. Int J Neuropsychopharmacol. 2009;12(4):447–58.
48. Boos HB, Aleman A, Cahn W, Hulshoff Pol H, Kahn RS. Brain volumes in relatives of patients with schizophrenia: a meta-analysis. Arch Gen Psychiatry. 2007;64(3):297–304.
49. Sun D, Phillips L, Velakoulis D, Yung A, McGorry PD, Wood SJ, et al. Progressive brain structural changes mapped as psychosis develops in 'at risk' individuals. Schizophr Res. 2009;108(1–3):85–92.
50. Takahashi T, Wood SJ, Yung AR, Soulsby B, McGorry PD, Suzuki M, et al. Progressive gray matter reduction of the superior temporal gyrus during transition to psychosis. Arch Gen Psychiatry. 2009;66(4):366–76.
51. Takahashi T, Wood SJ, Soulsby B, McGorry PD, Tanino R, Suzuki M, et al. Follow-up MRI study of the insular cortex in first-episode psychosis and chronic schizophrenia. Schizophr Res. 2009;108(1–3):49–56.
52. Velakoulis D, Wood SJ, Wong MT, McGorry PD, Yung A, Phillips L, et al. Hippocampal and amygdala volumes according to psychosis stage and diagnosis: a magnetic resonance imaging study of chronic schizophrenia, first-episode psychosis, and ultra-high-risk individuals. Arch Gen Psychiatry. 2006;63(2):139–49.

53. Olabi B, Ellison-Wright I, McIntosh AM, Wood SJ, Bullmore E, Lawrie SM. Are there progressive brain changes in schizophrenia? A meta-analysis of structural magnetic resonance imaging studies. Biol Psychiatry. 2011;70(1):88–96.
54. Kalmar JH, Wang F, Spencer L, Edmiston E, Lacadie CM, Martin A, et al. Preliminary evidence for progressive prefrontal abnormalities in adolescents and young adults with bipolar disorder. J Int Neuropsychol Soc. 2009;15(3):476–81.
55. Schmaal L, Veltman DJ, van Erp TG, Samann PG, Frodl T, Jahanshad N, et al. Subcortical brain alterations in major depressive disorder: findings from the ENIGMA Major Depressive Disorder working group. Mol Psychiatry. 2016;21(6):806–12.
56. Colizzi M, Lasalvia A, Ruggeri M. Prevention and early intervention in youth mental health: is it time for a multidisciplinary and trans-diagnostic model for care? Int J Ment Health Syst. 2020;14:23.
57. Francey SM, Nelson B, Thompson A, Parker AG, Kerr M, Macneil C, et al. Who needs antipsychotic medication in the earliest stages of psychosis? A reconsideration of benefits, risks, neurobiology and ethics in the era of early intervention. Schizophr Res. 2010;119(1–3):1–10.
58. Dell'Osso L, Del Grande C, Gesi C, Carmassi C, Musetti L. A new look at an old drug: neuroprotective effects and therapeutic potentials of lithium salts. Neuropsychiatr Dis Treat. 2016;12:1687–703.
59. Ho BC, Andreasen NC, Ziebell S, Pierson R, Magnotta V. Long-term antipsychotic treatment and brain volumes: a longitudinal study of first-episode schizophrenia. Arch Gen Psychiatry. 2011;68(2):128–37.

The Role of Psychopharmacology in Mental Health Prevention

3

Christopher Lemon and Andrew Thompson

3.1 Introduction

The chronicity and debilitating impact of inadequately treated mental illnesses makes any form of prevention attractive for consumers, families, carers and communities. The task of prevention at any level in mental health is complex and must consider a range of interconnected biological, social and psychological factors across the lifespan [1, 2]. In clinical practice, prevention often involves firstly, treatment of a full-threshold mental disorder, followed by strategies for avoiding relapse. In this chapter, however, we explore research on prevention using psychopharmacology alone or in combination with other treatments before the emergence of full-threshold disorders.

Prevention strategies can be distinguished into categories: primary, secondary, tertiary and quaternary, as well as universal, selective and indicated. Primary prevention strategies describe strategies for avoiding the development of disease and target those who are considered 'at risk' but have not yet developed a disorder. Primary prevention strategies have been studied in mental health, such as using phosphatidylcholine to improve foetal brain development, early childhood

C. Lemon
NorthWestern Mental Health, Melbourne Health, Royal Melbourne Hospital, Parkville, VIC, Australia
e-mail: Christopher.lemon@mh.org.au

A. Thompson (✉)
Orygen, Centre for Youth Mental Health, The University of Melbourne, Parkville, VIC, Australia

Centre for Youth Mental Health, The University of Melbourne, Parkville, VIC, Australia

Unit of Mental Health and Wellbeing, Warwick Medical School, University of Warwick, Coventry, UK
e-mail: Andrew.thompson@orygen.org.au

behaviour and reduce risk of major mental illnesses later in life [3] as well as vitamin and mineral supplementation to prevent dementia [4]. However, overall studies are few, effect sizes generally small and many potential confounders are hard to exclude. Secondary prevention involves intervention at a latent phase of illness where some initial evidence of disease has emerged. Many examples exist in physical medicine, such as implementing lifestyle programmes for those with 'prediabetes' or 'prehypertension' [1]. Screening tools in psychiatry have been of significant interest in recent decades, especially for young people with characteristics that may place them 'at-risk' of developing mental disorders, but have also attracted considerable controversy [5]. It should be recognized that this is an ongoing, active area of research with a need to more clearly define such characteristics that drive the focus of prevention. Tertiary prevention refers to strategies designed to limit disability and impact after a disease has been established, and includes relapse prevention [1, 6]. Quaternary prevention, seeking to limit iatrogenic harm from 'overmedicalization', is an emerging concept [7], but has been of limited focus in mental health research to date. Universal prevention targets entire populations irrespective of their risk of developing a particular illness. Selective prevention targets populations with a higher risk than the general population. Indicated prevention is for those at high risk who may already have some early, evidence of developing illness, but at a level below the threshold for diagnosis [6]. In this chapter, we focus on using pharmacological interventions in those with evidence of being at-risk of developing a major mental disorder as a form of secondary indicated prevention.

Medication is one aspect of psychiatric care that often receives significant attention from consumers, their families and carers, as well as society more broadly. Although non-pharmacological treatments, such as psychotherapy, remain more popular, attitudes towards psychiatric medications have become increasingly positive in recent decades, particularly in the United States and Europe [8]. The specific role of medications in primary prevention of mental illness in several populations is a developing but controversial area of research. Substantial attention has been given to primary prevention of mental disorders in young people, and there has been significant interest in determining whether there is a role for pharmacotherapies. Most mental disorders have their onset during the ages of late teens to mid-20s [9]. This finding has led to changes in clinical practice, particularly the emergence of mental health services specifically for young people in this age range, with a strong focus on all forms of prevention. Medications are used in these services, though often not as a first-line intervention and only when symptoms or functioning worsens despite use of alternative treatments [10–12].

In line with the increasing focus on youth mental health in psychiatric research, prescribing of psychotropic medications has increased substantially in recent decades [13–15]. This has included increases in prescribing antipsychotics, antidepressants, stimulants and mood stabilizing agents [16–19]. Some treatments have been recognized as generally beneficial, such as fluoxetine in moderate-to-severe depression, but not in the absence of other therapies, including psychotherapy [20]. Changing trends in prescribing amongst young people may reflect improved access and awareness of potential roles of psychotropics, but this change in practice has also attracted significant controversy. Debates have emerged around several aspects of prescribing psychotropic medications in young people. These include the risk-benefit ratios of antipsychotics with focus on the emergence of adverse metabolic side effects in children and adolescents [21], as well as debates on the efficacy of selective serotonin reuptake inhibitors (SSRIs) and possible associations with increased risk of suicidal ideation [22–27]. In addition, many children taking anti-depressants and antipsychotics have had them prescribed "off-label" for management of challenging behaviours, most commonly for conduct or disruptive behaviour disorder, attention deficit hyperactivity disorder (ADHD) and pervasive developmental disorder (which has also included intellectual disabilities) [28–30]. In many cases, once given a medication, many stop receiving concomitant psychological treatment, particularly those diagnosed with ADHD and autism spectrum disorder [30, 31].

In this chapter, we aim to provide an overview of important research to date on the use of psychotropic medications in young people who fall into the category of being at-risk of developing a major mental disorder. Importantly, in other approaches to prevention, including psychological and social strategies, as covered elsewhere in this book, there is an impasse where further investment into evidence generation and implementation trials is needed, but investment requires good evidence in the first place [2]. This problem extends to research on biological therapies for mental disorder prevention. Nonetheless, the starting point is to consider what evidence we have available now and how we can use it to examine whether there is any potential for medications to help in preventing the suffering of mental disorders. We provide an overview of the concept of clinical staging and current research into at-risk mental states. We then summarize current evidence on using medications for secondary indicated prevention that are otherwise used for treatment of full-threshold disorders, as well as discuss emerging novel pharmacotherapies. We also explore relevant research, clinical and ethical challenges and consider how they shape the future work on defining the potential role of pharmacotherapy in this area. The focus of this chapter is limited to prescribing for prevention of mental disorders in young people. It is beyond the scope to review all the evidence regarding all established psychotropic treatments, recognizing the literature continues to rapidly grow (see reviews, e.g. [31–35] and Cochrane collaboration reviews, e.g. [25, 36–38]). In addition, studies on herbal medicines in young people with mental disorders are also recognized as an emerging area, but will not be reviewed in detail here (see [39] for relevant background). We also limit our focus to secondary indicated prevention and will not fully explore primary and tertiary prevention.

3.2   Preventative Psychopharmacology in Young People

3.2.1   The Staging Model and Prevention of Mental Disorders

The approach of identifying and treating psychiatric disorders early in young people has been influenced by the findings and growth of early intervention/detection paradigms, which have been described elsewhere (see [40, 41]). Early intervention approaches initially focused on psychotic disorders but have more recently expanded to include other major mental disorders, such as bipolar affective disorder (BPAD) and depression. More recently, the concept of 'clinical staging' has been introduced, which seeks to define a framework for early, prodromal symptoms or syndromes more broadly. This concept has been successfully applied in several areas of medicine, most notably in the treatment of cancer where earlier 'precancerous' stages are recognized and treated, with interventions tailored according to clinical stage of illness. The proposed staging model of psychiatric disorders by McGorry and colleagues [42] claims the majority of mental disorders will progress through a number of distinct clinical stages, like in cancer, where more diffuse, less severe pathology presents early on during the development of a disorder and may respond to less intensive interventions to alter its overall course. With respect to psychopharmacological interventions, this suggests that medications with a greater number or more potent side effects would be reserved for the later stages of a disorder, as in the use of clozapine for schizophrenia. It also suggests a need for less intensive therapies that may alter or at least delay the course of the disorder. This still could include pharmacotherapies, but with better side effect profiles alongside comparable clinical efficacy to alternatives.

Several potential examples of the staging approach are worth mentioning. First, for the illness schizophrenia, the first stage of an illness might be a diffuse 'prodromal' stage, which consists of non-specific symptoms such as sleep disturbance, mood disturbance and more specific low-grade psychotic-like experiences, such as fleeting hallucinations or paranoid thoughts [43]. This has led to the development of clinical criteria based on such 'prodromal' symptoms and other risk factors, including family history and lower functioning; those who appear to be at-risk of developing schizophrenia and meet these criteria have been termed 'ultra high risk' (UHR) for psychosis or 'clinical high risk' (CHR) [44–46]. For clarity, for the remainder of this chapter, we will refer to this cohort as UHR. The potential to prevent or delay the development of a psychotic disorder in the UHR group continues to receive considerable research attention [47].

BPAD also has a proposed at-risk mental state involving a unique set of 'prodromal' symptoms, which again may respond to a different treatment approach than a full-threshold BPAD [48, 49]. Whilst the immediate predictive validity for these criteria is lower than for psychotic disorders, there remains optimism that such criteria may prove clinically useful. The predictive validity for these criteria has been calculated in a review paper suggesting relatively high specificity but poor sensitivity [48], indicating instruments for detection still require further refining [50]. In one study [51], the clinical value of Bechdolf et al.'s (2010) bipolar disorder at-risk (BAR) criteria was demonstrated in a small convenience sample, showing that that cyclothymia has good clinical utility for case finding and screening, as well as subthreshold mania. Other clinical features, such as family history, probable antidepressant-emergent elation and atypical depression, were found to be useful for screening-out non-cases rather than case finding [49, 51].

Staging models have also been considered for depressive disorders with the aim of early detection and prevention of poor outcome, including recurrent depression in adulthood. Hetrick et al. (2008) have outlined an early potential risk stage or set of risk factors that might respond to more benign interventions [52]. An at-risk state and 'prodrome' for diagnosis and early intervention in depressive disorders has also been proposed [53, 54]. There appear to be significant psychosocial and functional deficits associated with sub-syndrome depression and the associated burden to society of these symptoms [55]. This remains an area of ongoing research.

There are significant biological dimensions to the idea of at-risk states. Staging models imply a less severe form of disorder is present in the early stages of a psychiatric illness. For instance, in consumers meeting the UHR criteria, longitudinal magnetic resonance imaging findings demonstrate excessive neuroanatomical changes in those who do convert to psychosis, most notably in the medial temporal and prefrontal cortical regions [56]. Some evidence indicates that changes are specific to the type of psychotic disorder experienced, with anatomical changes differing in those who develop schizophrenia compared to an affective psychosis [57]. This supports the view that there may be biological targets for treatment in at-risk states, and a role for pharmacotherapy as an indicated form of secondary prevention in this cohort.

However, the discriminative validity of signs and symptoms in at-risk states has challenged efforts to identify clear biological targets for preventative pharmacotherapies. This is especially evident in the overlap between the prodromal stage of depressive disorders, bipolar disorders [58, 59] and other psychotic disorders [60] with diagnosis only becoming clear over differing time frames of illness, or at a point where the disorder has progressed to meet the diagnostic threshold of a fullblown disorder. Furthermore, the categorical distinctiveness of disorders is also unclear, highlighted by recent work showing overlap between BPAD with hypomanic symptoms and major depressive disorder [61].

3.2.2 Pharmacological Treatments for Emerging Psychiatric Disorders/'At-Risk' States

There have been several approaches to the treatment of at-risk states in young people. These approaches have included both the use of medications known to be efficacious in full-blown disorders and the use of new or novel medications aimed at arresting or preventing the onset of the illness. In the youth population, the focus on at-risk states has often been with respect to the major psychiatric disorders of schizophrenia, BPAD and major depression.

3.2.3 Using Medications Known to be Effective in Full-Threshold Mental Disorders

3.2.3.1 At Risk for Psychosis

There have been several small randomized controlled trials using antipsychotic medications in the UHR for psychosis group in youth populations. The first of these trials reported that the number of individuals developing a psychotic disorder was significantly lower after 6 months in those receiving a low dose of risperidone. Participants also received cognitive behavioural therapy (CBT) [62]. However, the effect was lost at 12-month follow-up [63]. Another similar trial suggested an emerging difference in 'transition' to a full-threshold psychotic disorder at 12 months amongst UHR consumers treated with olanzapine, but findings did not reach statistical significance. The prevalence of side effects (especially weight gain and extrapyramidal symptoms) was much greater in those on active medication in both trials [64]. Ruhrmann and colleagues reported a non-placebo-controlled randomized trial of the antipsychotic amisulpride with or without a 'needs-focused' intervention in an UHR group [65]. They reported that the amisulpride plus needs-focused group ($n = 56$) produced superior effects on attenuated and full-blown psychotic symptoms; basic, depressive and negative symptoms, and global functioning. They reported that the main side effects were prolactin-related. However, they concluded that the 'effects require confirmation by a placebo-controlled study' [65]. A more recent antipsychotic medication randomized trial failed to find a difference between those receiving low-dose risperidone, CBT and befriending [66, 67] with all groups having lower than expected rates of onset of, or transition to, a frank psychotic illness. This, and the positive reports of psychological interventions in this group [68, 69], has led to caution regarding the use of antipsychotics in this at-risk population. Other considerations include the relatively high number of individuals in the recent trials (nearly 90% in some trials) who do not go on to develop a psychotic disorder even if not receiving antipsychotic medication (false positives) [67, 70] and the concern over the stigma of a relatively aggressive treatment for what still remains an at-risk state rather than a full-threshold disorder [71].

3.2.3.2 Bipolar At-Risk Populations

There has been less research into 'traditional' or mood stabilizing treatments in this population, primarily because the at-risk state is much less well defined and at present does not have strong short-term positive predictive value. This markedly weakens any argument for using traditional psychopharmacological agents in this group. One placebo-controlled trial [72] investigated the use of divalproex sodium in a sample of young people deemed at risk of developing a bipolar illness. Importantly, this was not based on the population being defined as at risk, but rather either having a diagnosis of bipolar illness 'not otherwise specified', cyclothymia or a family history of bipolar disorder. The population ($n = 56$) was young (mean age of 10) although it included consumers up to the age of 17. The primary outcome was time to discontinuation for any reason. Neither time to discontinuation due to a mood event nor mood symptoms were significantly different in the divalproex group, and the authors concluded that it did not produce 'clinically meaningful improvements in the treatment of this potential at-risk group'. Another placebo-controlled single-site trial by the same researchers examined the use of aripiprazole in young people with one parent and another first- or second-degree relative with bipolar disorder and had limited benefit from psychotherapeutic treatment. Participants were outpatients between the ages of 5 and 17 years old with either bipolar 'not otherwise specified' ($n = 23$) or 'cyclotaxia' ($n = 7$). The primary outcome was mean change from baseline on Young Mania Rating Scale (YMRS) total score. At the 12-week endpoint, there were greater changes from baseline in the YMRS in those given aripiprazole compared with placebo, with acute treatment response generally noted around week 5–6. Overall, aripiprazole was well-tolerated, but in those who took the medication, weight gain was higher (2.3 kg vs. 0.7 kg), and those given aripiprazole were more likely to report emesis, increased appetite and coughing compared with placebo [73]. However, the small sample sizes and short duration of these studies limit their clinical utility. It is also worth recognizing that bipolar disorder not otherwise specified remains a controversial diagnosis in children [74].

3.2.3.3 Emerging Depressive Disorders or At-Risk States

There are no trials to our knowledge of traditional antidepressant agents in those deemed at risk for depression. The at-risk state for depression is less well developed than previously discussed disorders. Early features are likely to be less discriminative for later depression as previously discussed. In addition, there is the questionable efficacy of antidepressants in mild depressive disorder, as well as efficacy in youth populations [75]. There are also ongoing concerns about increases in suicidal ideation and behaviour related to use of SSRIs in young people [22]. These concerns make the rationale and ethics for such trials much less robust.

3.2.4   Current Clinical Guidelines

Guidelines exist for consumers considered at-risk of developing psychosis, but not other disorders. In general, there is consensus that all consumers at-risk of developing psychosis should be offered psychological therapy, particularly CBT. Some recommendations are made about using pharmacotherapy, but with caution and in acknowledgement of the limitations of current evidence. Guidelines differ on the relationship between psychological and pharmacological interventions.

The British Association for Psychopharmacology guidelines from 2020 indicate most consumers prefer and should be offered psychological interventions, but for those with attenuated psychotic symptoms, "off-label" low-dose antipsychotics can be considered for short-term symptom relief whilst acknowledging evidence for guidance on specific practices has significant limitations [76]. Other guidelines, such as the European Psychiatric Association guidelines [77] and the Australian Clinical Guidelines for Early Psychosis [78], suggest considering antipsychotics if CBT has failed or there is sustained attenuated or rapidly progressing frank psychotic symptoms.

In contrast, National Institute for Health and Care Excellence (NICE) guidelines, last updated in 2014, advise all consumers considered at-risk of psychosis should have CBT with or without family intervention, as well as targeted treatment of comorbidities. There is specific guidance against using antipsychotic medications in consumers considered at-risk or for the purpose of decreasing risk of developing a psychotic disorder [79].

Whilst a full analysis of the efficacy of treatments for at-risk mental states and full-threshold disorders is beyond the scope of this chapter, it is worth noting that CBT has a relatively good evidence base for UHR consumers. Although antipsychotics have shown overall similar efficacy, across current guidelines, side effects seem to drive low tolerance and limit recommendations for use [80].

3.3 New Frontiers: Novel Agents for Secondary Indicated Prevention

Supplementation and agents for protecting the brain are an exciting area of new research for at-risk mental states. Although the literature is still developing, existing studies indicate such agents may have significant clinical utility as well as being more ethically justifiable than existing pharmacotherapies known to be effective in full-threshold disorders but with significant side effects. Here, we discuss the concept of neuroprotection as a form of indicated secondary prevention in at-risk mental states and current areas of research on agents that may protect the brain from developing major psychiatric pathology. Most of the research in this field relates to young people.

3.3.1 Neuroprotective Agents and Nutraceuticals

Researchers have proposed that disruptions in the normal neuroprotective pathways are important in the development of psychotic and bipolar disorders, making them potential targets for preventative pharmacological interventions [81, 82]. The concept of neuroprotective interventions is established in neurological disorders [83]. The concept appears theoretically attractive to those who are displaying some signs of a disorder but not a full-threshold disorder. Several theoretical explanations have been offered with the dominant one being that psychiatric disorders are partly underpinned by an alteration in apoptosis leading to altered synaptic pruning during critical developmental periods [81, 84]. Neuroprotective strategies may arrest or delay progression of such pathological processes.

Some existing psychiatric treatments are associated with neuroprotective properties. These include atypical antipsychotic medication, mood stabilizers (lithium, anticonvulsants) and antidepressants [85–90]. In particular, monoamine oxidase inhibitors, tetracyclic antidepressants, tricyclic antidepressants, SSRIs and serotonin and noradrenaline reuptake inhibitors have all been associated with neuroprotection of hippocampal neurons through modulation of brain-derived neuroprotective factor (BDNF), with some effects possibly mediated by dose [89, 91, 92].

More novel agents proposed to be neuroprotective have been termed 'nutraceuticals', a concept combining 'nutrition' and 'pharmaceutical', as they are often also dietary supplements. These agents function like food or food products associated with health and medical benefits, such as prevention and treatment of disease. One with the most research interest is long-chain omega-3 polyunsaturated fatty acids or 'fish oil'. Importantly, many trials of nutraceuticals are dissimilar to other psychopharmacological trials in that they rarely have pharmaceutical industry sponsorship, given such compounds tend not to be novel and are widely available for other uses.

3.3.2   Neuroprotective Properties of Established Treatments for Mental Disorders in At-Risk Mental States

A research group from New York reported a possible beneficial effect of antidepressant medication on progression to a full-threshold psychotic disorder in an UHR group, arguing that antidepressants have neuroprotective properties [93]. The study was a prospective naturalistic treatment study of 48 participants, where 20 were prescribed antidepressants and 28 were prescribed second-generation antipsychotics. The rate of developing a psychotic disorder was 25% in the group treated primarily with antipsychotics, and there were no 'conversions' to a psychotic disorder in the primarily antidepressant-treated group. However, there were differences between the two groups at baseline, with the antipsychotic group having more disorganized thinking and over the follow-up period they were more likely to be noncompliant with medications. Despite these methodological shortcomings, the study does suggest that this is likely an area worth further research in this population. However, as the rates of lifetime depressive disorders in UHR individuals can be as high as 60% [94, 95], the possibility of a randomized controlled trial to further investigate this treatment approach on its own (which would mean randomizing to placebo) is ethically challenging [96]. Another trial is underway that uses a stepped approach to treatment in UHR that has the use of antidepressants as a later step in the pathway when more 'benign' treatments have not been effective. The results are awaited [97]. Lithium is also thought to have neuroprotective properties, and its efficacy in reducing risk of psychosis in the UHR population has been investigated. Preliminary results from one study suggest that lithium may have some neuroprotective effects but does not delay psychosis onset. However, the trial was a small, single-site study [81, 98, 99].

Whilst these therapies are established in the treatment of psychiatric disorders in general, they are not without well-documented and significant side effects, which in a population who are not necessarily guaranteed to develop full-threshold disorders raises several questions about the balance between risk and potential benefit. Attention has therefore turned to even more benign pharmacological interventions.

3.3.3   Supplementation Agents in At-Risk Mental States

3.3.3.1 Supplementation in Ultra High Risk

Supplementation with long-chain omega-3 polyunsaturated fatty acids (PUFAs) (fish oil) has received considerable research interest in psychotic disorders. Research into the beneficial effects of omega-3 PUFAs as an adjunctive treatment or supplement in individuals with established schizophrenia and first-episode psychosis has yielded some positive results [100]. In the UHR population, 12 weeks of omega-3 PUFAs reduced risk of development of psychotic disorder at 12-month follow-up [101], and even at a later 7-year follow-up [102]. A significant reduction in positive and negative symptoms and improved functioning was also found in the omega-3-treated group compared to placebo. Adverse effects did not differ between the two groups. However, two subsequent replication studies failed to find a benefit of omega-3 PUFAs in transition rate or reduction in symptoms [103, 104]. There is some data to suggest those whose omega-3 levels increase with supplementation or have higher baseline levels may have more improvement in symptoms and functioning [105]. There is ongoing research in this area.

Another treatment of interest is the hypothalamic neuropeptide, oxytocin. Oxytocin has been recognized as playing a role in social and emotional functioning with mixed findings on its potential role in mediating social cognition in consumers with established psychosis [10]. Interest in the use of oxytocin in UHR especially in relation to hippocampal function has increased recently. In one study [106], intranasal oxytocin was associated with increased cerebral perfusion in the left hippocampal region in UHR consumers. However, the clinical significance of these findings remains largely speculative [106].

More recently, interest has emerged in using cannabidiol (CBD) in consumers at-risk of developing a major psychotic disorder [107]. CBD has been examined as an adjunctive treatment in psychosis, and has been shown alongside regular antipsychotic treatment to modestly improve positive psychotic symptoms and illness severity, with mild side effects, most of which resolved spontaneously [108]. In UHR consumers, a single dose of CBD has been associated with attenuation of abnormal insular cortex function [109] as well as normalization of medial temporal lobe, mid-brain and striatal dysfunction [110]. UHR consumers with lower levels of anandamide have been found to have a higher risk of transition to full-threshold psychotic disorders compared to those with higher levels [111]. A three-arm randomized controlled trial with placebo and two different doses of CBD has commenced in 2021, and will assess the effects of CBD on positive psychotic symptoms in UHR individuals after 12 weeks of daily dosing [112].

There has also been a short pilot study demonstrating glycine supplementation may improve symptoms and cognition in young people at-risk of psychosis [113]. However, a small sample size was used, and the study duration was short, highlighting the need for more comprehensive studies to confirm findings.

3.3.3.2 Bipolar 'At Risk' and Emerging Depressive Disorders

Several nutraceuticals have been investigated in depression and BPAD. Despite there being no trials of indicated secondary prevention in at-risk groups, it is worth briefly mentioning some of these compounds used either on their own or as adjunct in established disorders. The use of omega-3 PUFAs as an adjunct in the treatment of depression and bipolar depression has some evidence of efficacy [100, 114, 115]. The evidence for the efficacy of omega-3 PUFAs as a treatment alone is less robust. There has been one trial on the efficacy of omega-3 treatment alone in childhood depression (aged 6–12) [116] but nothing specifically about older or youth populations. Again, there is encouraging evidence to support the notion that supplementation may be beneficial. Epidemiological studies indicate an association between depression and low dietary intake of omega-3 fatty acids, and biochemical studies have shown reduced levels of omega-3 fatty acids in red blood cell membranes in depressed consumers. Animal studies of fatty acid supplementation have also shown reduced 'depression-like' behaviours in rats, though applying these findings to humans is complex [117].

Another nutraceutical of interest in depression is folate. This is based on the findings of low levels of plasma and red cell folate in depression, especially in those with poor response to treatment [118, 119]. There is no convincing evidence to recommend the use of folate in adults yet [120], although some small studies have suggested folate as an adjunct to treatment in established depression is associated with reduced symptomatology [121], with similar findings in schizophrenia [122], though more data is needed.

In one trial on established depression in adolescents aged 12–17 who had also previously attracted a diagnosis of BPAD, the nutraceutical ginseng (*Acanthopanax senticosus*) was added to lithium and compared to fluoxetine [123]. There was no difference in response rate, remission or depressive symptoms. There is evidence that N-acetylcysteine may be an effective adjunct in bipolar depression in adults [124], but there are currently no trials in the youth population.

3.4   Issues in Research, Clinical Practice and Ethics Relevant to Preventative Prescribing in At-Risk Mental States

The concept of at-risk states in mental illness remains contentious in research and clinical practice. Debates have included suggestions ranging from reframing early intervention services [125] abandoning the concept entirely [126], as well as responses pointing out misunderstandings of the evidence and calls for more research [127].

Fusar-Poli et al. [10] point to the 'Gartner Hype Cycle' in UHR research. The hype cycle includes (1) innovative trigger, (2) peak of inflated expectations, (3) trough of disillusionment, (4) slope of enlightenment and (5) plateau of productivity or knowledge. Fusar-Poli et al. indicate after several negative early intervention trials, current research efforts align with the trough of disillusionment. In their umbrella review of the evidence for preventative interventions in UHR consumers [10], they found no pooled effect sizes across pharmacological, psychological or other treatments for the prevention of psychosis onset, nor favour for any particular preventative treatment over another. Outcomes included risk of developing first-episode psychosis, acceptability of treatments, severity of attenuated positive or negative psychotic symptoms, symptom-related distress, level of social functioning, level of general functioning and quality of life [10]. Equally, systematic reviews in this area have reported that for reducing transition from UHR to full-threshold psychotic disorder, the best evidence is for omega-3 fatty acids, but the quality of evidence is low and most other pharmacotherapy interventions seem to have poor support, overall. In other reviews, psychological treatments seem to have more promising results, with some data indicating a number needed to treat of 13 over 12 months for CBT in UHR consumers [128, 129].

However, as Fusar-Poli et al. [10] also suggest, the 'uncertain stage of knowledge' is often the precipitant to productive generation of knowledge, growing from the limitations of current evidence, and occurring after the 'peak of inflated expectations'. This has occurred in other areas of medicine, such as cancer prevention, where contemporary preventative practices are well-established [10]. In addition, there are significant methodological challenges in conducting research in this area, including difficulty blinding therapists, high attrition and non-adherence rates in youth. Furthermore, a large number of studies are underpowered, and it is difficult to determine the degree of symptom reduction needed to conclusively determine clinical improvement [129].

3.4.1　Prescribing for Prevention in At-Risk Mental States

The use of pharmacotherapies to prevent illness poses a set of unique challenges for clinicians, consumers and their families and carers. This is certainly not limited to mental health. An example in physical medicine is the treatment of hypertension in young adults. Elevated blood pressure or stage 1 or stage 2 hypertension in adults under the age of 40 is associated with a significantly higher risk of cardiovascular disease, compared with those who are normotensive [130]. However, treatment of hypertension in young adults remains controversial. Although the presence of cardiovascular and brain changes in young adults with hypertension indicates a need to initiate treatment, there are conflicting thresholds for diagnosis, inappropriate or invalid use of risk-based models derived from literature about older age groups and an overall lack of data on the benefits and drawbacks of using pharmacotherapy in young people [131].

Another example is the use of pharmacotherapies as an early intervention for multiple sclerosis (MS). Optic neuritis (ON) results from acute, demyelinating inflammation of the optic nerve and is one of the most common initial presentations of MS. However, the predictive value of ON has been the subject of debates that resemble discourse around at-risk mental states [132]. One key study by the Optic Neuritis Study Group in 2008 [133] demonstrated that the aggregate probability of developing MS 15 years after the onset of ON was 50%, while the risk was 25% for those with no lesions on MRI compared with 72% for those with one or more lesions on MRI at initial screen. Some demographic variables have also been associated with development of MS in consumers presenting with ON, such as low body mass index [134]. Like treatment of first-episode psychosis, however, the use of ongoing disease modifying pharmacotherapies beyond treatment of the initial attack remains contested [135]. Equally, like guidelines for those considered at-risk of developing psychosis, guidelines from advisory groups about ON and MS are complex and reflect the unknowns of working with an at-risk condition. Based on observational studies, the American Academy of Neurology recommends initiation of disease modifying agents for consumers with an isolated demyelinating event such as ON with two or more MRI-detected neurological lesions, but also advises ongoing screening only in those with an isolated clinical syndrome. Similar to the area of focus in this chapter, these guidelines highlight the need for further evidence regarding clinical benefit, adverse effects and burden of taking long-term medication [136].

These examples provide evidence that prescribing for secondary prevention in mental health is as complex as in other areas of medicine. In addition, societal and self-stigma related to most if not all diagnoses, as well as maintaining adherence can be particularly challenging in mental health care.

3.4.2   Aspects of the Therapeutic Alliance in Preventative Psychopharmacology

Given a large proportion of the research on preventative psychopharmacology relates to young people with at-risk mental states, it is worth mentioning some unique dimensions of working with young people taking pharmacotherapy. Young people living with chronic illnesses face several ongoing challenges in addition to the usual stressors of adolescence and early adulthood. Use of any therapy requires regular involvement of health professionals in a young person's life, which may be a novel experience compared to healthy peers, and can be difficult to accept. Healthcare providers promoting a young person's independence and control around decisions about their care and managing both positive and negative consequences are important for maintaining compliance and achieving good longitudinal outcomes [137, 138]. Technology-based approaches, such as text-messaging and mobile apps, may also be useful in giving a sense of control and maintaining adherence [139].

The significance of possible adverse effects in preventative psychopharmacology should be considered with respect to the unique experience of working with young people. Unintended harms of pharmacotherapies, including side effects, the burden of consistently monitoring a chronic illness and adhering to a treatment regimen can have a major impact on the effectiveness of pharmacotherapies [140]. A diverse range of side effects from psychotropic medications are described in the literature from young people's perspectives, and there is recognition that they can lead to dislike of pharmacotherapies. Concerns include discontinuation syndromes, becoming dependent on medications and in some cases, needing to use illicit substances to cope with adverse effects [138]. Sexual dysfunction and weight gain, which are likely to be considered significant for young people with at-risk mental states, should be given particular consideration.

3.4.3   Ethical Challenges

There are several ethical dimensions worth briefly considering in relation to developing research on preventative psychopharmacology in young people. Most have been considered in relation to studies on the UHR mental state, though many apply to research on other at-risk mental states. More broadly, they highlight the difficulty in researching and establishing any practice designed to prevent illness.

One of the most significant challenges in this area is working with the possibility that treatments, including pharmacotherapies and others, can challenge the principle of nonmaleficence when they are given to people who do not ever developing a mental disorder but do suffer adverse effects. The probability of developing a full-threshold psychotic disorder from its putative at-risk state has been recognized as being less than 50% [127]. It currently remains challenging to identify which UHR consumers are in the group who do not convert to full-threshold disorders once medication has been commenced, and distinguish them from *false*-false positives (people who would have developed psychosis, were it not for the treatment they received before the condition's onset) [141, 142]. In addition, others also argue symptoms associated with at-risk states are often mild positive symptoms occurring alongside largely non-psychotic symptoms, such as concentration difficulties, motivational impairment, low mood, sleep changes and anxiety, leading to the view that treatments designed for more severe positive symptoms, such as antipsychotics, are not justified in this population [143]. This may be the case, and is well-recognized by proponents of research in this area. This has also been one factor leading to increasing focus on exploring the potential benefits of more benign alternatives, such as nutraceuticals. In addition, it partly explains the conservative approach of some current guidelines, as described previously, which recommend treatments such as CBT over antipsychotic medications, largely due to the potential impact of pharmacological side effects [76, 78].

In addition, there have been concerns around young people being stigmatized by being 'labelled' as UHR, with this being considered another threat to nonmaleficence. In a similar vein, there are concerns around at-risk states being used instead of diagnostic terms such as 'psychosis', and initiating treatment in this setting with terms like 'at-risk' posing a threat to fully informed consent [142]. Some argue these concerns gain increased magnitude in the setting of the high false positive rate of the UHR diagnosis and the likely prospect of adverse effects of some medications considered for prevention [144]. However, stigma is a complex issue in this area, and several aspects continue to be debated. Evidence is mixed, with some findings indicating young people with an UHR diagnosis feel increased internalized stigma and perceived discrimination compared with those with non-psychotic disorders, but others report feelings of relief, validation and improved help-seeking behaviours [145]. Regarding pharmacotherapies, taking medication has been reported as stigmatizing for young people with chronic physical illnesses due to concerns that it may make it obvious to others that they have a chronic health problem [140]. Alternative evidence indicates young people who self-label as 'mentally ill' tend to have greater willingness to seek help and take psychiatric medications [146].

The complexity of the ethical aspects of this area of research, considered alongside some of the promising findings in the empirical literature highlights the need for more data on at-risk prediction models, more benign treatments for at-risk states such as nutraceuticals and the qualitative experience of those considered at-risk of developing major mental disorders. There is no area of research without ethical dilemmas, and in real-world practice, the absence of research is likely to facilitate more unpredictable, "off-label" prescribing in clinical practice.

3.5   Conclusions and Future Directions

We have discussed pharmacological prevention in mental disorders focusing primarily on secondary indicated prevention for at-risk mental states in young people. The emergence of early intervention paradigms and the clinical staging model for major mental illnesses has encouraged investigation into the role of pharmacological treatments in very early treatment and prevention of mental disorders in young people. To date, the literature and current guidelines suggest pharmacotherapy in the absence of psychological and psychosocial treatments is not indicated, although more research is needed to define their role as adjunctive treatments. The most promising area of interest seems to be in defining the potential role of more benign pharmacological treatments including nutraceuticals or putative neuroprotective compounds. Although the area of indicated prevention in psychopharmacology is in its infancy and subject to ethical dilemmas, there are some promising signs that some of these agents may have a useful preventative role or potentially a neuroprotective effect in these disabling disorders and therefore a wider public health benefit.

Glossary

'At-risk' mental state Mental states with cognitive, perceptual and functional signs and symptoms suggesting, though not confirming, the emergence of a major mental disorder

Nutraceuticals Compounds that can be derived from foods and naturally occurring products with properties that may mitigate the emergence or severity of disease

Prodrome Early clinical evidence of illness preceding the development of an acute, fully developed recognizable disorder

Psychotropic medications Pharmacological compounds known to mitigate the signs and symptoms of major mental disorders through biological mechanisms in the brain

Ultra high risk state Individuals suffering cognitive, perceptual and functional symptoms with individual, genetic and functional risk factors, suggestive of very high likelihood of developing a first-episode psychosis and meeting a set of predefined criteria

References

1. Compton MT, Shim RS. Mental illness prevention and mental health promotion: when, who, and how. Psychiatr Serv. 2020;71:981–3.
2. Ormel J, VonKorff M. Reducing common mental disorder prevalence in populations. JAMA Psychiatry. 78(4):359–60. https://doi.org/10.1001/jamapsychiatry.2020.3443.
3. Freedman R, Hunter SK, Hoffman MC. Prenatal primary prevention of mental illness by micronutrient supplements in pregnancy. Am J Psychiatry. 2018;175:607–19.

4. Rutjes AW, Denton DA, Di Nisio M, et al. Vitamin and mineral supplementation for maintaining cognitive function in cognitively healthy people in mid and late life. Cochrane Database Syst Rev. 2018;12:CD011906. https://doi.org/10.1002/14651858.CD011906.pub2.

5. Mrazek PJ, Haggerty RJ. Reducing risks for mental disorders: frontiers for preventive intervention research. Washington, DC: National Academies Press; 1994.

6. Soneson E, Perez J, Jones PB. Principles of risk, screening, and prevention in psychiatry. In: Thompson A, Broome M, editors. Risk factors psychosis: paradigms, mechanisms and prevention. London: Academic Press; 2020. p. 11–43.

7. Pandve HT. Quaternary prevention: need of the hour. J Family Med Prim Care. 2014;3:309–10.

8. Angermeyer MC, van der Auwera S, Carta MG, Schomerus G. Public attitudes towards psychiatry and psychiatric treatment at the beginning of the 21st century: a systematic review and meta-analysis of population surveys. World Psychiatry. 2017;16:50–61.

9. Kessler RC, Amminger GP, Aguilar-Gaxiola S, Alonso J, Lee S, Üstün TB. Age of onset of mental disorders: a review of recent literature. Curr Opin Psychiatry. 2007;20:359–64.

10. Fusar-Poli P, Davies C, Solmi M, Brondino N, De Micheli A, Kotlicka-Antczak M, Shin JI, Radua J. Preventive treatments for psychosis: umbrella review (just the evidence). Front Psychiatry. 2019;10:764. https://doi.org/10.3389/fpsyt.2019.00764.

11. Hickie IB, Scott EM, Cross SP, et al. Right care, first time: a highly personalised and measurement-based care model to manage youth mental health. Med J Aust. 2019;211:S3–S46.

12. Salazar de Pablo G, Estradé A, Cutroni M, Andlauer O, Fusar-Poli P. Establishing a clinical service to prevent psychosis: what, how and when? Systematic review. Transl Psychiatry. 2021;11:43.

13. Zuvekas SH. Prescription drugs and the changing patterns of treatment for mental disorders. Health Aff. 2005;24:195–205.

14. Zito JM, Safer DJ, DosReis S, Gardner JF, Magder L, Soeken K, Boles M, Lynch F, Riddle MA. Psychotropic practice patterns for youth: a 10-year perspective. Arch Pediatr Adolesc Med. 2003;157:17–25.

15. Wong ICK, Murray ML, Camilleri-Novak D, Stephens P. Increased prescribing trends of paediatric psychotropic medications. Arch Dis Child. 2004;89:1131–2.

16. Olfson M, Marcus SC. National patterns in antidepressant medication treatment. Arch Gen Psychiatry. 2009;66:848–56.

17. Wong ICK, Asherson P, Bilbow A, et al. Cessation of attention deficit hyperactivity disorder drugs in the young (CADDY)—a pharmacoepidemiological and qualitative study. Health Technol Assess. 2009;13:1–120.

18. Moreno C, Laje G, Blanco C, Jiang H, Schmidt AB, Olfson M. National trends in the outpatient diagnosis and treatment of bipolar disorder in youth. Arch Gen Psychiatry. 2007;64:1032–9.

19. Olfson M, Blanco C, Liu L, Moreno C, Laje G. National trends in the outpatient treatment of children and adolescents with antipsychotic drugs. Arch Gen Psychiatry. 2006;63:679–85.

20. Zhou X, Teng T, Zhang Y, et al. Comparative efficacy and acceptability of antidepressants, psychotherapies, and their combination for acute treatment of children and adolescents with depressive disorder: a systematic review and network meta-analysis. Lancet Psychiatry. 2020;7:581–601.

21. Fraguas D, Correll CU, Merchán-Naranjo J, Rapado-Castro M, Parellada M, Moreno C, Arango C. Efficacy and safety of second-generation antipsychotics in children and adolescents with psychotic and bipolar spectrum disorders: comprehensive review of prospective head-to-head and placebo-controlled comparisons. Eur Neuropsychopharmacol. 2011;21:621–45.

22. Hammad TA, Laughren T, Racoosin J. Suicidality in pediatric patients treated with antidepressant drugs. Arch Gen Psychiatry. 2006;63:332–9.

23. Hebebrand J. Commentary on "Forum: Use of antidepressants in children and adolescents". Curr Opin Psychiatry. 2010;23:62–3.

24. Hetrick SE, McKenzie JE, Merry SN. The use of SSRIs in children and adolescents. Curr Opin Psychiatry. 2010;23:53–7.

25. Hetrick S, Merry S, McKenzie J, Sindahl P, Proctor M. Selective serotonin reuptake inhibitors (SSRIs) for depressive disorders in children and adolescents. Cochrane Database Syst Rev. 2007;3:CD004851.

26. Goodyer IM, Wilkinson P, Dubicka B, Kelvin R. Forum: the use of selective serotonin reuptake inhibitors in depressed children and adolescents: commentary on the meta-analysis by Hetrick et al. Curr Opin Psychiatry. 2010;23:58–61.
27. Dubicka B, Hadley S, Roberts C. Suicidal behaviour in youths with depression treated with new-generation antidepressants: meta-analysis. Br J Psychiatry. 2006;189:393–8.
28. Pillay J, Boylan K, Newton A, Hartling L, Vandermeer B, Nuspl M, MacGregor T, Featherstone R, Carrey N. Harms of antipsychotics in children and young adults: a systematic review update. Can J Psychiatry. 2018;63:661–78.
29. Hoon D, Taylor MT, Kapadia P, Gerhard T, Strom BL, Horton DB. Trends in off-label drug use in ambulatory settings: 2006–2015. Pediatrics. 2019;144:e20190896.
30. Bushnell GA, Crystal S, Olfson M. Trends in antipsychotic medication use in young privately insured children. J Am Acad Child Adolesc Psychiatry. 2021;60:877–86.
31. Dinnissen M, Dietrich A, van der Molen JH, Verhallen AM, Buiteveld Y, Jongejan S, Troost PW, Buitelaar JK, Hoekstra PJ, van den Hoofdakker BJ. Prescribing antipsychotics in child and adolescent psychiatry: guideline adherence. Eur Child Adolesc Psychiatry. 2020;29:1717–27.
32. Carlisle LL, McClellan J. Psychopharmacology of schizophrenia in children and adolescents. Pediatr Clin North Am. 2011;58:205–18.
33. Kaplan G, Ivanov I. Pharmacotherapy for substance abuse disorders in adolescence. Pediatr Clin North Am. 2011;58:243–58.
34. Kodish I, Rockhill C, Ryan S, Varley C. Pharmacotherapy for anxiety disorders in children and adolescents. Pediatr Clin North Am. 2011;58:55–72.
35. Smiga SM, Elliott GR. Psychopharmacology of depression in children and adolescents. Pediatr Clin North Am. 2011;58:155–71.
36. Kennedy E, Kumar A, Datta SS. Antipsychotic medication for childhood-onset schizophrenia. Cochrane Database Syst Rev. 2007;3:CD004027. https://doi.org/10.1002/14651858. CD004027.pub2.
37. Ipser JC, Stein DJ, Hawkridge S, Hoppe L. Pharmacotherapy for anxiety disorders in children and adolescents. Cochrane Database Syst Rev. 2009;3:CD004027.
38. Hazell P, Mirzaie M. Tricyclic drugs for depression in children and adolescents. Cochrane Database Syst Rev. 2013;6:CD002317. https://doi.org/10.1002/14651858.CD002317.pub2.
39. Feucht C, Patel DR. Herbal medicines in pediatric neuropsychiatry. Pediatr Clin North Am. 2011;58:33–54.
40. Yung AR, McGorry PD. The prodromal phase of first-episode psychosis: past and current conceptualizations. Schizophr Bull. 1996;22:353–70.
41. McGorry PD, Hartmann JA, Spooner R, Nelson B. Beyond the "at risk mental state" concept: transitioning to transdiagnostic psychiatry. World Psychiatry. 2018;17:133–42.
42. McGorry PD, Hickie IB, Yung AR, Pantelis C, Jackson HJ. Clinical staging of psychiatric disorders: a heuristic framework for choosing earlier, safer and more effective interventions. Aust N Z J Psychiatry. 2006;40:616–22.
43. Yung AR, McGorry PD. The initial prodrome in psychosis: descriptive and qualitative aspects. Aust N Z J Psychiatry. 1996;30:587–99.
44. Yung A, Phillips L, PD MG. Treating schizophrenia in the prodromal phase. London: Taylor & Francis; 2004.
45. Miller TJ, McGlashan TH, Rosen JL, Cadenhead K, Cannon T, Ventura J, McFarlane W, Perkins DO, Pearlson GD, Woods SW. Prodromal assessment with the structured interview for prodromal syndromes and the scale of prodromal symptoms: predictive validity, interrater reliability, and training to reliability. Schizophr Bull. 2003;29:703–15.
46. Yung AR, McGorry PD, McFarlane CA, Jackson HJ, Patton GC, Rakkar A. Monitoring and care of young people at incipient risk of psychosis. Schizophr Bull. 1996;22:283–303.
47. Fusar-Poli P, Borgwardt S, Bechdolf A, et al. The psychosis high-risk state: a comprehensive state-of-the-art review. JAMA Psychiat. 2013;70:107–20.
48. Howes OD, Lim S, Theologos G, Yung A, Goodwin GM, McGuire P. A comprehensive review and model of putative prodromal features of bipolar affective disorder. Psychol Med. 2011;41:1567–77.

49. Bechdolf A, Nelson B, Cotton SM, et al. A preliminary evaluation of the validity of at-risk criteria for bipolar disorders in help-seeking adolescents and young adults. J Affect Disord. 2010;127:316–20.
50. Waugh MJ, Meyer TD, Youngstrom EA, Scott J. A review of self-rating instruments to identify young people at risk of bipolar spectrum disorders. J Affect Disord. 2014;160:113–21.
51. Scott J, Marwaha S, Ratheesh A, Macmillan I, Yung AR, Morriss R, Hickie IB, Bechdolf A. Bipolar at-risk criteria: an examination of which clinical features have optimal utility for identifying youth at risk of early transition from depression to bipolar disorders. Schizophr Bull. 2017;43:737–44.
52. Hetrick SE, Parker AG, Hickie IB, Purcell R, Yung AR, McGorry PD. Early identification and intervention in depressive disorders: towards a clinical staging model. Psychother Psychosom. 2008;77:263–70.
53. Fava GA, Grandi S, Canestrari R, Molnar G. Prodromal symptoms in primary major depressive disorder. J Affect Disord. 1990;19:149–52.
54. Fava GA, Tossani E. Prodromal stage of major depression. Early Interv Psychiatry. 2007;1:9–18.
55. Sadek N, Bona J. Subsyndromal symptomatic depression: a new concept. Depress Anxiety. 2000;12:30–9.
56. Wood SJ, Pantelis C, Velakoulis D, Yücel M, Fornito A, McGorry PD. Progressive changes in the development toward schizophrenia: studies in subjects at increased symptomatic risk. Schizophr Bull. 2008;34:322–9.
57. Dazzan P, Soulsby B, Mechelli A, et al. Volumetric abnormalities predating the onset of schizophrenia and affective psychoses: an MRI study in subjects at ultrahigh risk of psychosis. Schizophr Bull. 2012;38:1083–91.
58. Biederman J, Mick E, Faraone SV, Spencer T, Wilens TE, Wozniak J. Pediatric mania: a developmental subtype of bipolar disorder? Biol Psychiatry. 2000;48:458–66.
59. Hillegers MHJ, Reichart CG, Wals M, Verhulst FC, Ormel J, Nolen WA. Five-year prospective outcome of psychopathology in the adolescent offspring of bipolar parents. Bipolar Disord. 2005;7:344–50.
60. Häfner H, Maurer K, Trendler G, An Der Heiden W, Schmidt M, Könnecke R. Schizophrenia and depression: challenging the paradigm of two separate diseases—a controlled study of schizophrenia, depression and healthy controls. Schizophr Res. 2005;77:11–24.
61. O'Donovan C, Alda M. Depression preceding diagnosis of bipolar disorder. Front Psychiatry. 2020;11:500. https://doi.org/10.3389/fpsyt.2020.00500.
62. McGorry PD, Yung AR, Phillips LJ, et al. Randomized controlled trial of interventions designed to reduce the risk of progression to first-episode psychosis in a clinical sample with subthreshold symptoms. Arch Gen Psychiatry. 2002;59:921–8.
63. Phillips LJ, McGorry PD, Yuen HP, Ward J, Donovan K, Kelly D, Francey SM, Yung AR. Medium term follow-up of a randomized controlled trial of interventions for young people at ultra high risk of psychosis. Schizophr Res. 2007;96:25–33.
64. McGlashan T, Zipursky RB, Perkins D, et al. Randomized, double-blind trial of olanzapine versus placebo in patients prodromally symptomatic for psychosis. Am J Psychiatry. 2006;163:790–9.
65. Ruhrmann S, Bechdolf A, Kühn KU, et al. Acute effects of treatment for prodromal symptoms for people putatively in a late initial prodromal state of psychosis. Br J Psychiatry. 2007;191:88–95.
66. McGorry PD, Nelson B, Phillips LJ, et al. Randomized controlled trial of interventions for young people at ultra-high risk of psychosis: twelve-month outcome. J Clin Psychiatry. 2013;7:349–56.
67. Yung AR, Phillips LJ, Nelson B, et al. Randomized controlled trial of interventions for young people at ultra high risk for psychosis: 6-month analysis. J Clin Psychiatry. 2011;4:430–40.
68. Morrison AP, French P, Walford L, Lewis SW, Kilcommons A, Green J, Parker S, Bentall RP. Cognitive therapy for the prevention of psychosis in people at ultra-high risk: randomised controlled trial. Br J Psychiatry. 2004;185:291–7.

69. Van Der Gaag M, Smit F, Bechdolf A, French P, Linszen DH, Yung AR, McGorry P, Cuijpers P. Preventing a first episode of psychosis: meta-analysis of randomized controlled prevention trials of 12 month and longer-term follow-ups. Schizophr Res. 2013;149:56–62.

70. Yung AR, Yuen HP, Berger G, Francey S, Hung TC, Nelson B, Phillips L, McGorry P. Declining transition rate in ultra high risk (prodromal) services: dilution or reduction of risk? Schizophr Bull. 2007;33:673–81.

71. Corcoran C, Malaspina D, Hercher L. Prodromal interventions for schizophrenia vulnerability: the risks of being "at risk". Schizophr Res. 2005;73:173–84.

72. Findling RL, Frazier TW, Youngstrom EA, McNamara NK, Stansbrey RJ, Gracious BL, Reed MD, Demeter CA, Calabrese JR. Double-blind, placebo-controlled trial of divalproex monotherapy in the treatment of symptomatic youth at high risk for developing bipolar disorder. J Clin Psychiatry. 2007;65:781–8.

73. Findling RL, Youngstrom EA, Rowles BM, Deyling E, Lingler J, Stansbrey RJ, McVoy M, Lytle S, Calabrese JR, McNamara NK. A double-blind and placebo-controlled trial of aripiprazole in symptomatic youths at genetic high risk for bipolar disorder. J Child Adolesc Psychopharmacol. 2017;27:864–74.

74. Duffy A, Carlson G, Dubicka B, Hillegers MHJ. Pre-pubertal bipolar disorder: origins and current status of the controversy. Int J Bipolar Disord. 2020;8(1):18. https://doi.org/10.1186/s40345-020-00185-2.

75. Jureidini JN, Doecke CJ, Mansfield PR, Haby MM, Menkes DB, Tonkin AL. Efficacy and safety of antidepressants for children and adolescents. Br Med J. 2004;328:879–83.

76. Barnes TRE, Drake R, Paton C, et al. Evidence-based guidelines for the pharmacological treatment of schizophrenia: updated recommendations from the British Association for Psychopharmacology. J Psychopharmacol. 2020;34:3–78.

77. Schmidt SJ, Schultze-Lutter F, Schimmelmann BG, et al. EPA guidance on the early intervention in clinical high risk states of psychoses. Eur Psychiatry. 2015;30:388–404.

78. Early Psychosis Guidelines Writing Group and EPPIC National Support Program. Australian clinical guidelines for early psychosis. 2nd ed. Melbourne: The National Centre of Excellence in Youth Mental Health; 2016.

79. National Institute of Health Care and Excellence. Psychosis and schizophrenia in adults: Prevention and management. 2014. https://www.nice.org.uk/guidance/cg178/chapter/Update-information

80. van der Gaag M, van den Berg D, Ising H. CBT in the prevention of psychosis and other severe mental disorders in patients with an at risk mental state: a review and proposed next steps. Schizophr Res. 2019;203:88–93.

81. Berger G, Dell'Olio M, Amminger P, Cornblatt B, Phillips L, Yung A, Yan Y, Berk M, McGorry P. Neuroprotection in emerging psychotic disorders. Early Interv Psychiatry. 2007;1:114–27.

82. Berk M, Conus P, Kapczinski F, et al. From neuroprogression to neuroprotection: implications for clinical care. Med J Aust. 2010;193:36–40.

83. Meldrum BS. Implications for neuroprotective treatments. Prog Brain Res. 2002;135:487–95.

84. Berger GE, Wood S, McGorry PD. Incipient neurovulnerability and neuroprotection in early psychosis. Psychopharmacol Bull. 2003;37:79–101.

85. Bai O, Wei Z, Lu W, Bowen R, Keegan D, Li XM. Protective effects of atypical antipsychotic drugs on PC12 cells after serum withdrawal. J Neurosci Res. 2002;69:278–83.

86. Wei Z, Mousseau DD, Richardson JS, Dyck LE, Li XM. Atypical antipsychotics attenuate neurotoxicity of β-Amyloid(25-35) by modulating Bax and Bcl-XL/S expression and localization. J Neurosci Res. 2003;74:942–7.

87. Manji HK, Moore GJ, Chen G. Clinical and preclinical evidence for the neurotrophic effects of mood stabilizers: implications for the pathophysiology and treatment of manic-depressive illness. Biol Psychiatry. 2000;48:740–54.

88. Manji HK, Moore GJ, Chen G. Bipolar disorder: leads from the molecular and cellular mechanisms of action of mood stabilisers. Br J Psychiatry. 2001;178:s107–19.

89. Xu H, Richardson JS, Li XM. Dose-related effects of chronic antidepressants on neuroprotective proteins BDNF, Bcl-2 and Cu/Zn-SOD inrat hippocampus. Neuropsychopharmacology. 2003;28:53–62.
90. Seymour CB, Mothersill C, Mooney R, Moriarty M, Tipton KF. Monoamine oxidase inhibitors I-deprenyl and clorgyline protect nonmalignant human cells from ionising radiation and chemotherapy toxicity. Br J Cancer. 2003;89:1979–86.
91. Nibuya M, Morinobu S, Duman S. Regulation of BDNF and trkB mRNA in rat brain by chronic electroconvulsive seizure and antidepressant drug treatments. J Neurosci. 1995;15:7539–47.
92. Nibuya M, Nestler EJ, Duman RS. Chronic antidepressant administration increases the expression of cAMP response element binding protein (CREB) in rat hippocampus. J Neurosci. 1996;16:2365–72.
93. Cornblatt BA, Lencz T, Smith CW, et al. Can antidepressants be used to treat the schizophrenia prodrome? Results of a prospective, naturalistic treatment study of adolescents. J Clin Psychiatry. 2007;68:546–57.
94. Rosen JL, Miller TJ, D'Andrea JT, McGlashan TH, Woods SW. Comorbid diagnoses in patients meeting criteria for the schizophrenia prodrome. Schizophr Res. 2006;85:124–31.
95. Lin A, Wood SJ, Nelson B, Beavan A, McGorry P, Yung AR. Outcomes of nontransitioned cases in a sample at ultra-high risk for psychosis. Am J Psychiatry. 2015;172:249–58.
96. Fusar-Poli P, Valmaggia L, McGuire P. Can antidepressants prevent psychosis? Lancet. 2007;370:1746–8.
97. Nelson B, Amminger GP, Yuen HP, et al. Staged treatment in early psychosis: a sequential multiple assignment randomised trial of interventions for ultra high risk of psychosis patients. Early Interv Psychiatry. 2018;12:292–306.
98. Berk M, Hallam K, Lucas N, Hasty M, Mcneil CA, Conus P, Kader L, Mcgorry PD. Early intervention in bipolar disorders: opportunities and pitfalls. Med J Aust. 2007;187:S11–4.
99. Berger GE, Wood SJ, Ross M, et al. Neuroprotective effects of low-dose lithium in individuals at ultra-high risk for psychosis: a longitudinal MRI/MRS study. Curr Pharm Des. 2012;18:1381–6128.
100. Peet M, Stokes C. Omega-3 fatty acids in the treatment of psychiatric disorders. Drugs. 2005;65:1051–9.
101. Amminger GP, Schäfer MR, Papageorgiou K, Klier CM, Cotton SM, Harrigan MSM, Mackinnon A, McGorry PD, Berger GE. Long-chain ω-3 fatty acids for indicated prevention of psychotic disorders: a randomized, placebo-controlled trial. Arch Gen Psychiatry. 2010;67:146–54.
102. Amminger GP, Schäfer MR, Schlögelhofer M, Klier CM, McGorry PD. Longer-term outcome in the prevention of psychotic disorders by the Vienna omega-3 study. Nat Commun. 2015;6:7934. https://doi.org/10.1038/ncomms8934.
103. McGorry PD, Nelson B, Markulev C, et al. Effect of ω-3 polyunsaturated fatty acids in young people at ultrahigh risk for psychotic disorders: the NEURAPRO randomized clinical trial. JAMA Psychiat. 2017;74:19–27.
104. Cadenhead K, Addington J, Cannon T, et al. Omega-3 fatty acid versus placebo in a clinical high-risk sample from the North American Prodrome Longitudinal Studies (NAPLS) consortium. Schizophr Bull. 2017;43:S16.
105. Amminger GP, Nelson B, Markulev C, et al. The NEURAPRO biomarker analysis: long-chain Omega-3 fatty acids improve 6-month and 12-month outcomes in youths at ultra-high risk for psychosis. Biol Psychiatry. 2020;87:243–52.
106. Davies C, Paloyelis Y, Rutigliano G, et al. Oxytocin modulates hippocampal perfusion in people at clinical high risk for psychosis. Neuropsychopharmacology. 2019;44:1300–9.
107. Davies C, Bhattacharyya S. Cannabidiol as a potential treatment for psychosis. Ther Adv Psychopharmacol. 2019;9:1–16.
108. McGuire P, Robson P, Cubala WJ, Vasile D, Morrison PD, Barron R, Taylor A, Wright S. Cannabidiol (CBD) as an adjunctive therapy in schizophrenia: a multicenter randomized controlled trial. Am J Psychiatry. 2018;175:225–31.

109. Wilson R, Bossong MG, Appiah-Kusi E, Petros N, Brammer M, Perez J, Allen P, McGuire P, Bhattacharyya S. Cannabidiol attenuates insular dysfunction during motivational salience processing in subjects at clinical high risk for psychosis. Transl Psychiatry. 2019;9:203. https://doi.org/10.1038/s41398-019-0534-2.
110. Bhattacharyya S, Wilson R, Appiah-Kusi E, O'Neill A, Brammer M, Perez J, Murray R, Allen P, Bossong MG, McGuire P. Effect of Cannabidiol on medial temporal, midbrain, and striatal dysfunction in people at clinical high risk of psychosis: a randomized clinical trial. JAMA Psychiat. 2018;75:1107–17.
111. Koethe D, Giuffrida A, Schreiber D, Hellmich M, Schultze-Lutter F, Ruhrmann S, Klosterkotter J, Piomelli D, Leweke FM. Anandamide elevation in cerebrospinal fluid in initial prodromal states of psychosis. Br J Psychiatry. 2009;194:371–2.
112. Amminger GP, Lin A, Kerr M, et al. Cannabidiol for at risk for psychosis youth: a randomised controlled trial. Early Interv Psychiatry. 2021; https://doi.org/10.1111/eip.13182.
113. Woods SW, Walsh BC, Hawkins KA, Miller TJ, Saksa JR, D'Souza DC, Pearlson GD, Javitt DC, McGlashan TH, Krystal JH. Glycine treatment of the risk syndrome for psychosis: report of two pilot studies. Eur Neuropsychopharmacol. 2013;23:931–40.
114. Williams A-l, Katz D, Ali A, Girard C, Goodman J, Bell I. Do essential fatty acids have a role in the treatment of depression? J Affect Disord. 2006;93:117–23
115. Osher Y, Belmaker RH. Omega-3 fatty acids in depression: a review of three studies. CNS Neurosci Ther. 2009;15:128–33.
116. Nemets H. Omega-3 treatment of childhood depression: a controlled, double-blind pilot study. Am J Psychiatry. 2006;163:1098.
117. Ferraz AC, Kiss Á, Araújo RLF, Salles HMR, Naliwaiko K, Pamplona J, Matheussi F. The antidepressant role of dietary long-chain polyunsaturated n-3 fatty acids in two phases in the developing brain. Prostaglandins Leukot Essent Fatty Acids. 2008;78:183–8.
118. Fava M, Borus J, Alpert JE, Nierenberg AA, Rosenbaum JF, Bottiglieri T. Folate, vitamin B12, and homocysteine in major depressive disorder. Am J Psychiatry. 1997;154:426–8.
119. Beydoun MA, Shroff MR, Beydoun HA, Zonderman AB. Serum folate, vitamin b-12, and homocysteine and their association with depressive symptoms among U.S. adults. Psychosom Med. 2010;72:862–73.
120. Taylor MJ, Carney SM, Geddes J, Goodwin G. Folate for depressive disorders. Cochrane Database Syst Rev. 2003;2:CD003390.
121. Coppen A, Bailey J. Enhancement of the antidepressant action of fluoxetine by folic acid: a randomised, placebo controlled trial. J Affect Disord. 2000;60:121–30.
122. Godfrey PSA, Toone BK, Carney MWP, Flynn TG, Bottiglieri T, Laundy M, Chanarin I, Reynolds EH. Enhancement of recovery from psychiatric illness by methylfolate. Lancet. 1990;336:392–5.
123. Weng S, Tang J, Wang G, Wang X, Wang H. Comparison of the addition of Siberian ginseng (Acanthopanax senticosus) versus fluoxetine to lithium for the treatment of bipolar disorder in adolescents: a randomized, double-blind trial. Curr Ther Res. 2007;68:280–90.
124. Berk M, Dean O, Cotton SM, et al. The efficacy of N-acetylcysteine as an adjunctive treatment in bipolar depression: an open label trial. J Affect Disord. 2011;135:389–94.
125. Moritz S, Gaweęda Ł, Heinz A, Gallinat J. Four reasons why early detection centers for psychosis should be renamed and their treatment targets reconsidered: we should not catastrophize a future we can neither reliably predict nor change. Psychol Med. 2019;49:2134–40.
126. Ajnakina O, David AS, Murray RM. "At risk mental state" clinics for psychosis—an idea whose time has come—and gone! Psychol Med. 2019;49:529–34.
127. Yung AR, Wood SJ, Malla A, Nelson B, McGorry P, Shah J. The reality of at risk mental state services: a response to recent criticisms. Psychol Med. 2021;51:212–8.
128. Bosnjak Kuharic D, Kekin I, Hew J, Rojnic Kuzman M, Puljak L. Interventions for prodromal stage of psychosis. Cochrane Database Syst Rev. 2019,11:CD012236. https://doi.org/10.1002/14651858.CD012236.pub2.

129. Nelson B, Amminger GP, Bechdolf A, et al. Evidence for preventive treatments in young patients at clinical high risk of psychosis: the need for context. Lancet Psychiatry. 2020;7:378–80.
130. Yano Y, Reis JP, Colangelo LA, et al. Association of Blood Pressure Classification in Young Adults using the 2017 American College of Cardiology/American Heart Association Blood pressure guideline with cardiovascular events later in life. JAMA. 2018;320:1774–82.
131. Hinton TC, Adams ZH, Baker RP, Hope KA, Paton JFR, Hart EC, Nightingale AK. Investigation and treatment of high blood pressure in young people: too much medicine or appropriate risk reduction? Hypertension. 2020;75:16–22.
132. Kale N. Optic neuritis as an early sign of multiple sclerosis. Eye Brain. 2016;8:195–202.
133. The Optic Neuritis Study Group. Multiple sclerosis risk after optic neuritis. Arch Neurol. 2008;65:727–32.
134. Ro LS, Yang CC, Lyu RK, Lin KP, Tsai TC, Lu SR, Chang KH, Huang LC, Tsai CP. A prospective, observational study on conversion of clinically isolated syndrome to multiple sclerosis during 4-year period (MS NEO study) in Taiwan. PLoS One. 2019;14:1–15.
135. Filippini G, Del Giovane C, Clerico M, Beiki O, Mattoscio M, Piazza F, Fredrikson S, Tramacere I, Scalfari A, Salanti G. Treatment with disease-modifying drugs for people with a first clinical attack suggestive of multiple sclerosis. Cochrane Database Syst Rev. 2017;4:CD012200. https://doi.org/10.1002/14651858.CD012200.pub2.
136. Rae-Grant A, Day GS, Marrie RA, et al. Practice guideline recommendations summary: disease-modifying therapies for adults with multiple sclerosis. Neurology. 2018;90:777–88.
137. Wilson EV. Engaging young people with a chronic illness. Aust Fam Physician. 2017;46:572–6.
138. McMillan SS, Wilson B, Stapleton H, Wheeler AJ. Young people's experiences with mental health medication: a narrative review of the qualitative literature. J Ment Health. 2020; https://doi.org/10.1080/09638237.2020.1714000.
139. Badawy SM, Thompson AA, Kuhns LM. Medication adherence and technology-based interventions for adolescents with chronic health conditions: a few key considerations. JMIR Mhealth Uhealth. 2017;5:e202.
140. Hanghøj S, Boisen KA. Self-reported barriers to medication adherence among chronically ill adolescents: a systematic review. J Adolesc Health. 2014;54:121–38.
141. Yung AR. Antipsychotic treatment of UHR ('prodromal') individuals. Early Interv Psychiatry. 2010;4:197–9.
142. Corcoran CM. Ethical and epidemiological dimensions of labeling psychosis risk. AMA J Ethics. 2016;18:633–42.
143. Van Os J, Guloksuz S. A critique of the "ultra-high risk" and "transition" paradigm. World Psychiatry. 2017;16:200–6.
144. Raven M, Stuart GW, Jureidini J. "Prodromal" diagnosis of psychosis: ethical problems in research and clinical practice. Aust N Z J Psychiatry. 2012;46:64–5.
145. Colizzi M, Ruggeri M, Lasalvia A. Should we be concerned about stigma and discrimination in people at risk for psychosis? A systematic review. Psychol Med. 2020;50:705–26.
146. Xu Z, Müller M, Heekeren K, et al. Self-labelling and stigma as predictors of attitudes towards help-seeking among people at risk of psychosis: 1-year follow-up. Eur Arch Psychiatry Clin Neurosci. 2016;266:79–82.
147. Thomas T, Stansifer L, Findling RL. Psychopharmacology of pediatric bipolar disorders in children and adolescents. Pediatr Clin North Am. 2011;58:173–87.

Part II

Areas for Intervention and Improvement

Postpartum (Puerperal) Psychosis: Risk Factors, Diagnosis, Management and Treatment

4

Paola Dazzan, Alessandra Biaggi, Katie Hazelgrove, Carmine M. Pariante, Chaitra Jairaj, and Gertrude Seneviratne

4.1 What Is Postpartum (or Puerperal) Psychosis

Whilst extensive research has been conducted on the aetiology, pathophysiology and optimal management of psychoses unrelated to the puerperium, as seen throughout this book, not much has been done on postpartum psychosis. This chapter aims to provide an overview on the main risk factors, clinical characteristics and possibilities for prevention and management of this rare but very severe psychosis.

Postpartum psychosis (PP) is the most severe perinatal mental health problem and a psychiatric and obstetric emergency. PP is rare and usually presents with a sudden onset following childbirth, occurring in approximately 1–2 per 1000 live births [1]. It is most commonly associated with a personal or family history of bipolar disorder, and women with a history of bipolar disorder have a

P. Dazzan (✉) · C. M. Pariante
Department of Psychological Medicine, Institute of Psychiatry, Psychology and Neuroscience, King's College London, London, UK

National Institute for Health Research (NIHR) Mental Health Biomedical Research Centre at South London and Maudsley NHS Foundation Trust and King's College London, London, UK
e-mail: paola.dazzan@kcl.ac.uk; carmine.pariante@kcl.ac.uk

A. Biaggi · K. Hazelgrove · C. Jairaj
Department of Psychological Medicine, Institute of Psychiatry, Psychology and Neuroscience, King's College London, London, UK
e-mail: alessandra.biaggi@kcl.ac.uk; katie.1.hazelgrove@kcl.ac.uk; chaitra.1.jairaj@kcl.ac.uk

G. Seneviratne
Channi Kumar Mother and Baby Unit, Bethlem Royal Hospital, South London and Maudsley NHS Foundation Trust, London, UK
e-mail: gertrude.seneviratne@slam.nhs.uk

M. Colizzi, M. Ruggeri (eds.), *Prevention in Mental Health*, https://doi.org/10.1007/978-3-030-97906-5_4

significantly higher risk of suffering an episode after delivery, estimated at between 30 and 50% [2–4]. The risk is also significantly higher in women who suffered from PP following a previous birth. The fact that the risk of PP is particularly high in these groups of women makes it highly predictable and thus provides ample opportunities for the prevention and early management of this severe type of psychosis.

The onset of PP is usually rapid (within hours) and symptoms most often appear within 72 h to 4 weeks after delivery [5], although they may still present up to 12 weeks after childbirth [6], and even up to 6 months after delivery, although with a significantly reduced risk. Vigilance and monitoring are therefore important given the potentially devastating impact of psychosis during this period.

Symptoms of PP typically include mood swings, confusion, disorganised behaviour, delusions and hallucinations that may involve the baby, creating additional risk for his/her safety, and in rare cases may lead to suicide and/or infanticide [7–9]. There can be significant fluctuations in mental state, with women at times appearing to be well, and yet within a few hours appearing confused, with a labile mood and at times paranoia. Whilst some of these symptoms, like hypomania or anxiety, are similar to those that precede a relapse of bipolar disorder, others such as feeling confused or unreal appear to be more specific to PP. Other common symptoms include agitation, fearfulness, tearfulness, lack of sleep and grossly disorganised behaviour. A disturbance of consciousness characterised by confusion, catatonia or perplexity is also a common presentation [10]. In fact, a study conducted in India found that 20% of 200 women with PP experienced catatonia during that episode, most commonly in the form of mutism, withdrawal and negativism [11]. These symptoms represent a dramatic change from the previous level of functioning in these women [5, 9], who usually have little insight into the seriousness of their condition. An episode can last at least 1 day and usually resolves in 1–2.5 months, although an episode of postpartum depression with psychotic features often has a longer duration compared to postpartum mania [12, 13]. Thus, PP can result in considerable distress, and may have long-term consequences for women's well-being, as well as that of their baby and their family, together with implications for wider society [14]. Women usually eventually return to their previous levels of functioning, with a more favourable prognosis for women with shorter episodes [13, 15].

Due to its severity, PP requires rapid and intensive psychiatric treatment and hospitalisation (sometimes requiring involuntary hospital admission) for mother and baby safety, and for treatment to be initiated as soon as possible, as discussed later in this chapter.

4.2 Risk Factors for the Onset of PP

The strongest risk factor for the onset of PP is a personal history of bipolar disorder, schizoaffective disorder [4] or a history of previous PP [13]. More specifically, about 26% of women with bipolar disorder I and schizoaffective disorder bipolar type can develop an episode of PP after giving birth [4]. Women who have experienced an episode of PP following a previous pregnancy are also at increased risk of a new episode after a subsequent delivery, with rates ranging between 54.4 and 57% [13, 16].

A thorough review and meta-analysis has confirmed the higher risk in women with a history of bipolar disorder or PP, although this study found relapse rates to be lower than those reported in previous studies [17]. In particular, these authors found that 17% of women with a diagnosis of bipolar disorder and 29% of women with a history of PP experienced a severe postpartum relapse, defined as having a psychotic, manic or mixed episode and/or a psychiatric hospitalisation [17].

In addition to a personal history, having a family history of PP in a first-degree relative has also been found to increase the risk of PP [4], with the risk reported as being as high as 57% in women with both a diagnosis of bipolar disorder and a family history of PP [4]. Importantly, evidence shows that diagnoses of schizophrenia or major depressive disorder are not associated with a higher risk of psychosis in the postnatal period. For example, Kendell found that only 3% of women with schizophrenia and 2% of women with a history of depression developed a severe postpartum relapse requiring hospital admission in the postpartum [18].

4.2.1 Obstetric, Psychosocial and Sleep-Related Risk Factors

Although a number of obstetric factors for the development of PP have been investigated, including pregnancy and delivery complications, caesarean section, primiparity, length of gestation, neonatal complications, infant gender and inter-pregnancy interval, results across studies have not always been consistent. The obstetric factor that has been most consistently associated with an increased risk of PP is primiparity [14], particularly in women with a first episode of PP [19] but also in those with a previous history of bipolar or schizoaffective disorder [20]. Although the higher risk related to primiparity has been suggested to reflect the fact that women who develop PP may be less likely to have other children, studies that have controlled for this factor do not provide support for this suggestion [20]. An alternative hypothesis is that the higher risk for PP in primiparae women could be related to greater psychological stress, as a first pregnancy is an unknown quantity for the women and every aspect, including transition to parenthood, may increase stress levels. On the other hand, specific biological changes occur in first pregnancies, similar to those occurring in other disorders, like pregnancy-induced hypertension and pre-eclampsia, which also occur more frequently in first pregnancies. Some studies have also reported an increased risk of PP in women with long inter-pregnancy intervals [19], possibly because the biological differences between first and subsequent pregnancies become fewer when the interval between pregnancies increases, thus resulting in higher rates of PP [19].

Some evidence also suggests that delivery—but not pregnancy-related complications—could increase the risk of developing PP, and also of being admitted to hospital after delivery [20, 21]. Perhaps not surprisingly, considering its role in mania, sleep loss has been found to increase the risk of PP. Sleep disruption is thought to be a trigger in the development of mania and psychosis unrelated to childbirth, and is also a common symptom in women with PP [22, 23]. Sleep disruption in the perinatal period can result from the physiological changes of pregnancy and the postpartum, and the need to care for the newborn after giving birth [22, 23]. Despite this evidence, little research has been conducted in this area. A study has found that women with PP were more likely to give birth during the night and to have longer labours compared to control women [24], whilst another study found that women with a history of bipolar disorder and/or a history of psychosis did not differ from healthy women in their sleep behaviour in pregnancy and in the first 6 months of the postpartum. Interestingly, a recent study [25] found that women with bipolar I disorder who reported sleep loss as a trigger to their manic episodes were twice as likely to have experienced an episode of PP during their lifetime. On the contrary, women with bipolar I disorder reporting a history of sleep loss triggering an episode of depression were not more likely to experience an episode of PP following childbirth. This suggests that the presence of a specific vulnerability to the development of mania induced by sleep loss also increases the risk of developing PP [25].

With regard to demographic factors, research is limited and results have been inconsistent. Whilst one study [26] found an increased risk for PP in single and older women, another study [18] found that single women had an increased risk for admission to hospital, although this was not specific to psychosis and maternal age was not associated with PP. Level of education was not found to be associated with an increased risk of PP [26].

Stressful life events and childhood adversity have been consistently associated with an increased risk of developing psychosis and psychotic relapses unrelated to the puerperium, but their role has been much less frequently investigated in the occurrence of PP. Whilst some studies have not found an association between stressors and the onset of PP [14], our recent work has found that women with current PP actually report more frequent recent stressful life events, as well as higher perceived stress than healthy women in the same postpartum period [27]. Those women also show an activation of the stress and immune response, with higher levels of cortisol, the main stress hormone, during the day and of C-reactive protein, an indicator of inflammation, than control women. In a more recent and larger sample of women at risk of PP evaluated since pregnancy, we replicated evidence for a role of stress and its biological response, and found that severe childhood maltreatment and higher daily cortisol levels in the third trimester of pregnancy (with odds ratios of 4.9 and 3.7, respectively) predicted a psychiatric relapse in the first 4 weeks' postpartum in women at risk of PP, after adjusting for clinical and sociodemographic covariates [28]. Together, these data provide support for the role of psychosocial stress and the biological stress system in increasing the risk of postpartum relapse in women at risk of this disorder [28].

4.2.2 Biological, Genetic and Brain-Related Risk Factors

The clear temporal relationship between childbirth and PP suggests that biological factors are involved in the onset of the illness [29]. For example, the rapid decline of reproductive hormones (oestrogen and progesterone) that occurs after delivery has been long thought to play a role in the development of this disorder. In fact, oestrogen has a modulatory effect on dopaminergic function, which is involved in the development of psychosis [30].

However, absolute levels of reproductive hormones have not been found to differ between women who develop PP and unaffected women, and the administration of oestrogen to women at risk of PP has not been found to prevent the onset of an episode [31, 32]. It is possible that women who develop PP have an altered response to the normal hormonal fluctuations associated with the perinatal period and that hormonal changes interact with an underlying vulnerability of biological systems involved in the origin of psychosis [30, 33].

Similarly to reproductive hormones, cortisol also undergoes dramatic changes during pregnancy and the early postpartum, and rapidly declines after delivery [30]. Alterations in the hypothalamic-pituitary-adrenal axis and in cortisol levels have also been observed in depression and psychosis unrelated to gestation [30], and as mentioned above, are now also emerging in relation to the onset of PP, thus providing important pointers to the role of stress as a potential area for intervention.

Another biological system possibly involved in the origin of PP, as mentioned earlier, is the immune system. In fact, the perinatal period is characterised by changes in the maternal immune system, and pregnancy is a time of immunosuppression, necessary to promote tolerance towards the genetically different foetal tissue. However, after delivery, there is usually a "rebound" phenomenon, with an over-activation of the immune system [34]. An increase in inflammatory markers has been observed in both affective and non-affective psychoses unrelated to gestation [30], and evidence has built over the last decade to support a role for immune dysregulation also in the onset of PP. In addition to the findings mentioned above from our group [27], Bergink and colleagues [34] found evidence of an immune system dysregulation in women with a first episode of PP, suggesting the presence of an inflammatory state in these women similar to that reported in individuals with non-puerperal psychosis.

Finally, evidence of a familial component in the risk of PP suggests an important role for genetic factors [4]. Evidence points to the involvement of one or more susceptibility genes on the long arm of chromosome 16, as well as of others involved in serotoninergic, hormonal and inflammatory pathways. However, studies are still in progress and until now no genetic variants have been consistently observed [14, 33].

Other potential risk factors include alterations in brain structure and function. Although a considerable body of research has shown that individuals who develop affective and non-affective psychosis unrelated to gestation present alterations in brain structure and function at their first episode of the illness or even prior to psychosis onset, very little has been done in women with, or at risk of, PP [30]. In the last few years, our group has provided evidence for both structural and functional alterations in women at risk who develop an episode of PP and in women at risk who remain well. For example, we found that women with PP show smaller volumes of the anterior cingulate gyrus, superior temporal gyrus and parahippocampal gyrus compared to women who were at risk but remain well following the index pregnancy [35]. On the other hand, women who remain well postnatally were observed to have larger superior and inferior frontal gyrus compared to healthy women. More recently, in another sample of women at risk of PP followed up since pregnancy, we found that these women, and specifically those who developed a psychiatric relapse in the postpartum, showed increased resting connectivity within an executive network compared to women not at risk [36]. Women at risk also showed decreased connectivity in the executive network, and altered emotional load-dependent connectivity between executive, salience and default-mode networks during the execution of an emotional task. Those women at risk who became unwell particularly showed increased salience network-dependent modulation of the default-mode and executive network relative to those at risk who remained well, who showed greater executive network-dependent modulation of the salience network. These findings point to an important role for the executive network and its interplay with other brain networks implicated in goal-directed behaviour, which could be considered neural phenotypes for PP and help advance our understanding of the pathophysiology of this disorder.

4.3 Differential Diagnosis

The prodromal symptoms of PP can be easily confused with those of postpartum blues, as these both develop soon after delivery, and usually in the first week postpartum. However, contrary to the baby blues, symptoms of PP do not recover spontaneously but worsen rapidly [37]. Although PP can also present with a predominant depressive affect, it should be differentiated from postpartum depression. PP develops very quickly after childbirth, most often within 2 weeks, with symptoms escalating rapidly, whilst postpartum depression symptoms usually do not start before 2 weeks after delivery [38].

Also, it is important to differentiate the delusional thought content about harming the infant that can occur in PP from that of obsessions and compulsions. Obsessions are characterised by intrusive images and thoughts which are ego-dystonic, which occur in the context of an obsessive compulsive disorder and sometimes in postnatal depression. In these, women recognise them as being intrusive images and thoughts, and are able to maintain rational judgement and reality testing. These women are not typically at increased risk of harming their infants, although they may avoid them to reduce anxiety and fear of causing them harm. On the contrary, delusional thoughts about harming the infant are ego-syntonic, and women who experience them are unable to distinguish them from reality, and to understand the potential consequences of their behaviour, and may in some occasions feel forced to act on them [5, 9, 39].

As well as a detailed mental state assessment, the differential diagnosis of PP requires a thorough evaluation of the patient's history, a physical and neurologic examination and basic medical workup. This should include a complete blood count, metabolic profile and urine toxicology screen and thyroid function tests and thyroid autoantibodies, serum calcium levels, B12, thiamine and folate levels and erythrocyte sedimentation rate [5]. Investigation should also include C-reactive protein, autoantibodies like NMDA and voltage-gated k channels (VGKC) complex and glutamic acid decarboxylase (GAD).

The differential diagnosis should also exclude the possibility of delirium (with a screen to include HIV and hepatitis), acute infections, anaemia due to peripartum blood loss, endocrine and autoimmune disorders and eclampsia [5, 40]. Other conditions that should be considered include metabolic or nutritional deficiencies, as well as primary hypoparathyroidism, uremic encephalopathy, hepatic failure, vitamin deficiencies, stroke and drug or medication-induced psychosis [12]. Neuroimaging investigations and EEG should be routinely performed, particularly in women presenting with neurological symptoms such as seizures, impaired consciousness or dyskinesia.

It is also important to observe women for substance-related disorders, as substance use and psychotic disorders may coexist and/or substance use may cause psychotic symptoms in the absence of a psychotic disorder.

Finally, it is important to distinguish between women who have a pre-existing psychotic disorder and those who develop a first-onset psychotic disorder, as both the course of the disorder and treatment option would vary significantly in these two populations.

4.4 Prevention and Prophylaxis

4.4.1 Screening for Postpartum Psychosis

There are currently no easily implemented self-report screening tools for PP. Some authors have advocated the use of the Mood Disorder Questionnaire (MDQ) [5], a brief self-report screen of 13 symptoms and their timing and degree of impairment, completed in approximately 5 min that detects bipolar disorder.

At present, appropriate preconception counselling represents the best approach to reduce the risks and impact of PP, together with careful management and support. Any woman at risk, or who experiences an episode of PP, should also receive psychoeducation about the risk in current as well as subsequent pregnancies, and be informed that the highest risk of recurrent episodes is conferred by a pre-existing bipolar disorder or previous episodes of PP. Advice should include education about sleep hygiene and prevention of sleep loss near delivery, as discussed earlier in this chapter. Clinicians and mothers should also develop, with specialist services, an integrated treatment plan involving the woman, her family support and all healthcare (and social care if present) professionals involved.

4.4.2 The Role of Medications

Postpartum relapse rates seem to be higher in unmedicated than in medicated women with a diagnosis of bipolar disorder or a history of PP. As such, in the above-mentioned meta-analysis, Wesseloo and colleagues found that 66% of the women with bipolar disorder who had not taken prophylactic medication in pregnancy had a postpartum relapse, in contrast with 23% of those who had taken medication in pregnancy [17]. Similarly, these authors also found higher relapse rates (65%) in women who did not take medication in the postpartum period compared to those who took medication (29%).

Experiencing an episode of illness in pregnancy has been described as another significant risk factor for a relapse in the postpartum in women with a previous diagnosis of bipolar disorder with or without a history of puerperal episodes, a finding that we have also recently replicated [28, 41]. Relapse rates have been reported to be high (around 24%) in pregnancy in women with bipolar disorder, and 60% of the women who had an episode during pregnancy have been found to also experience a postpartum relapse, despite being on medication after the episode suffered in pregnancy. On the contrary, those women with a history of PP, even when medication-free, have not been reported to be at risk of relapse in pregnancy but only in the postpartum [42]. It is therefore important to make women aware that those with a history of isolated PP are not at increased risk for episodes *during* pregnancy.

Still, to date it remains unclear whether starting prophylaxis following delivery is sufficient to prevent an episode in women at risk, or whether medications should also be taken during pregnancy. Some evidence suggests that for women with a history of bipolar disorder, the rates of postpartum relapses are significantly lower in those who are maintained on medications during pregnancy [17].

Prophylactic medications such as lithium or antipsychotics given immediately after delivery may reduce the risk of developing PP, and some advocate that these medications should start already in the second or third trimester, although this remains controversial [5]. There is a body of evidence that particularly supports the use of lithium for the postpartum prophylaxis of PP, in those women at high risk because of a previous history of bipolar disorder or PP [42–44]. Use of lithium at this time has however important implications, considering the shifts in fluids that occur around childbirth, and the passage of lithium in breast milk. For these reasons, atypical antipsychotics are often preferred to lithium, although there is no sufficient evidence to support their use in the prophylaxis of PP.

The risks and benefits of treatment with any of these medications, and the desire to breastfeed, should all be discussed prior to delivery. It is important to closely monitor mental state and to have a plan to identify any early sign of relapse as soon as they emerge in those women with bipolar disorder who prefer to discontinue medications in pregnancy and not to recommence medications immediately after childbirth.

For women who do already take medications in pregnancy, the discussion should focus on costs and benefits of treatment and of not receiving treatment, and on considering which medications have been effective in treating previous illness episodes. The conversation should consider continuing the current regime, stopping some or all medications or switching to other medications if there are options with greater evidence of safety in pregnancy.

In women with bipolar disorder, lithium prophylaxis in pregnancy is often a recommended option, in view of its established efficacy, although this drug carries known maternal and infant risks [45]. A study by Viguera and colleagues [46] compared relapse rates in women with bipolar disorder who discontinued lithium during pregnancy with rates in non-pregnant women with bipolar disorder who discontinued lithium, over an equivalent period of time. These authors found that, whilst relapse rates were similar in the first 40 weeks after lithium discontinuation, they were 2.9 more frequent in the postpartum period in pregnant compared with non-pregnant women (70% compared with 24%).

Whilst second-generation antipsychotics are often considered in alternative to lithium, there are no data available at present to support the superiority of one antipsychotic over another in terms of safety, although second-generation antipsychotics may have greater efficacy and fewer short-term side effects [47]. Furthermore, existing data suggest that first- and second-generation antipsychotics are not major teratogens [48–50]. The choice should therefore be informed by a discussion with the patient, based on personal preference and expectation for efficacy, and information from both personal and family history. Even in the context of a cost/benefit discussion, it should still be considered that women who take antipsychotic medications are also at higher risk for adverse maternal and perinatal outcomes compared to the general population and should therefore be monitored for their occurrence [49].

4.5 Treatment and Management of Postpartum Psychosis

Once it occurs, PP is primarily managed with specialist treatment and medications, which may be complemented by non-pharmacological therapies, particularly in the post-acute phase, and hospitalisation is usually required.

There have been very few studies on the specific treatment of PP, mostly case reports and retrospective studies. The pharmacological approach is therefore based on information derived from the treatment of mood disorders and psychoses not related to the puerperium. Treatment choices are often based on factors such as the individual symptoms experienced and previous treatments, the level of disturbance and the side effect profile. Excessive sedation, for example, may be problematic in the mother's ability to care for her newborn child.

In general, the first-line treatment of PP is represented by antipsychotic medications. Mood stabilisers and benzodiazepines are also used in the acute stages, with benzodiazepines specifically used as short-term treatment to help control the symptoms until antipsychotic medications take effect, and also to treat insomnia [51]. Antidepressants are usually best avoided because of the risk of inducing rapid cycling or mixed states, although they may be required if the presentation is more that of a depressive psychosis. Of note, brexanolone, a progesterone agonist also acting on GABA receptors and causing sedation, has been shown to improve symptoms of depression in the immediate postpartum [52], and there may be value in exploring whether this compound could also be beneficial in the treatment of PP. Electroconvulsive therapy (ECT) is also an option to consider in women with severe postpartum episodes, particularly in the presence of significant suicidal risk or in women with severe psychomotor retardation of catatoria [53].

An interesting study conducted in the last few years implemented an algorithm involving four sequential interventions in 64 women with first-onset psychosis or mania in the postpartum period: benzodiazepines, antipsychotics, lithium and ECT [12]. The authors found that nearly all women (98.4%) achieved complete remission within the first three steps and that none required ECT. However, only 3.7% of the women responded to benzodiazepines alone. Furthermore, remission at 9 months postpartum was sustained in 79.7%, and women treated with lithium showed a significantly lower rate of relapse than those treated with antipsychotic monotherapy. Then again, the number maintained on antipsychotics alone was too small (eight women) to conduct a significant comparison [54].

Women who have experienced PP should be supported in planning for more intensive postnatal support (midwife/maternal and child health nurse visits): education about maintaining regular sleep patterns and about the possible consequences of sleep deprivation against the benefits of breastfeeding. Additionally, they should be offered support for mother-infant interaction. Childcare support should also be in place prior to discharge from hospital.

Family psychoeducation and psychological therapies are important components of the treatment plan, and women and carers should receive information about PP, its risk factors and its treatment. Useful resources can be found in websites such as that of Action on Postpartum Psychosis, the UK Postpartum Psychosis Network, which produces several helpful insider guides for patients and carers, and the Royal College of Psychiatrists.

4.5.1 Treatment Continuation

There are no formal recommendations for the duration of treatment of PP after resolution of the most acute phase. Consideration should thus be given to the risk of recurrent illness. Women that are maintained on lithium monotherapy could have a lower rate of relapse than those maintained on antipsychotic monotherapy, according to the study mentioned above, which has however several caveats [12]. It is recommended that women who do not have a history of episodes outside of the postpartum period are treated for at least 6–9 months and that if they remain stable, any medication is tapered slowly with close clinical monitoring [40].

4.6 Prognosis of Postpartum Psychosis

Despite its severity, PP commonly carries a favourable prognosis, and with treatment, women can recover within 2–6 months. However, for many women, particularly those with a manic type of illness, the psychotic symptoms are often followed by a lengthy period of depression before full recovery is achieved [37, 55]. Nevertheless, most women will achieve full recovery, particularly women who developed symptoms within a month postpartum, compared to those with later onset [5].

Still, as mentioned earlier in this chapter, after a first episode of PP, women have 50–80% chance of developing a later psychiatric episode [56]. Some studies have shown that between 62 and 69% of women who suffer from PP develop a subsequent affective episode outside the perinatal period, and between 54.4 and 57% of women will experience a new episode of PP after a new delivery [13, 16]. Moreover, some women with a history of PP will develop non-psychotic depression after a new delivery [13]. The risk of psychiatric relapses after a new delivery is considerably higher in women who have suffered from PP compared to those with episodes of bipolar disorder unrelated to the perinatal period [16]. Interestingly, a retrospective study of 116 women who experienced PP showed that a longer duration of the index episode and a longer latency between the index PP and next pregnancy predicted a higher risk of PP in a subsequent pregnancy [13].

4.7   Conclusions

PP is a very severe disorder with a clearly identifiable time of onset. Despite this, very little research has been done to understand the aetiological factors associated with its occurrence, particularly in women known to carry a high risk. We are particularly lacking prospective studies that follow women at risk from pregnancy to the postpartum, to understand which biological, psychological and environmental factors are associated with an increased risk of developing the illness, and to understand if PP has a long-term impact on child development and on mother-infant relationship [57]. This lack of evidence has significantly limited advances in the prevention and management of this disorder, for which data on new targets for intervention are urgently needed.

Acknowledgements   This work was partly supported by the UK Medical Research Foundation, by the UK Medical Research Council and the UK National Institute for Health Research (NIHR) Biomedical Research Centre at South London and Maudsley NHS Foundation Trust and King's College London. CMP is a NIHR Senior Investigator.

References

1. Jones I. Perinatal psychiatry. Medicine (Baltimore). 2012;40:654–7. https://doi.org/10.1016/j.mpmed.2012.09.001.
2. Di Florio A, Forty L, Gordon-Smith K, Heron J, Jones L, Craddock N, Jones I. Perinatal episodes across the mood disorder spectrum. JAMA Psychiat. 2013;70:168–75. https://doi.org/10.1001/jamapsychiatry.2013.279.
3. Doyle K, Heron J, Berrisford G, Whitmore J, Jones L, Wainscott G, Oyebode F. The management of bipolar disorder in the perinatal period and risk factors for postpartum relapse. Eur Psychiatry. 2012;27:563–9. https://doi.org/10.1016/j.eurpsy.2011.06.011.
4. Jones I, Craddock N. Familiality of the puerperal trigger in bipolar disorder: results of a family study. Am J Psychiatry. 2001;158:913–7. https://doi.org/10.1176/appi.ajp.158.6.913.
5. Sit D, Rothschild AJ, Wisner KL. A review of postpartum psychosis. J Womens Health. 2006;6(4):421–34. https://doi.org/10.1089/jwh.2006.15.352.

6. Munk-Olsen T, Laursen TM, Pedersen CB, Mors O, Mortensen PB. New parents and mental disorders: a population-based register study. JAMA. 2006;296(21):2582–9. https://doi.org/10.1001/jama.296.21.2582.
7. Knight M, Bunch K, Tuffnell D, Jayakody H, Shakespeare J, Kotnis R, Kenyon S, Kurinczuk JJ. MBRRACE—UK report: saving lives, improving mothers' care, 2014–16. Oxford: National Perinatal Epidemiology Unit; 2018.
8. Rai S, Pathak A, Sharma I. Postpartum psychiatric disorders: early diagnosis and management. Indian J Psychiatry. 2015;57:216–21. https://doi.org/10.4103/0019-5545.161481.
9. Spinelli MG. Postpartum psychosis: detection of risk and management. Am J Psychiatry. 2009;166:405–8. https://doi.org/10.1176/appi.ajp.2008.08121899.
10. Brockington I. Puerperal psychosis. In: Brockington I, editor. Motherhood and mental health. Oxford: Oxford University Press; 1996.
11. Nahar A, Kondapuram N, Desai G, Chandra PS. Catatonia among women with postpartum psychosis in a mother-baby inpatient psychiatry unit. Gen Hosp Psychiatry. 2017;45:40–3. https://doi.org/10.1016/j.genhosppsych.2016.12.010.
12. Berghink V, Burgerhout KM, Koorengevel KM, Kamperman AM, Hoogendijk WJ, Lambregtse-Van Den Berg MP, Kushner SA. Treatment of psychosis and mania in the postpartum period. Am J Psychiatry. 2015;172(2):115–23. https://doi.org/10.1176/appi.ajp.2014.13121652.
13. Blackmore ER, Rubinow DR, O'Connor TG, Liu X, Tang W, Craddock N, Jones I. Reproductive outcomes and risk of subsequent illness in women diagnosed with postpartum psychosis. Bipolar Disord. 2013;15(4):394–404. https://doi.org/10.1111/bdi.12071.
14. Jones I, Chandra PS, Dazzan P, Howard LM. Bipolar disorder, affective psychosis, and schizophrenia in pregnancy and the post-partum period. Lancet. 2014;384:1789–99. https://doi.org/10.1016/S0140-6736(14)61278-2.
15. Burgerhout KM, Kamperman AM, Roza SJ, Lambregtse-Van Den Berg MP, Koorengevel KM, Hoogendijk WJG, Kushner SA, Berghink V. Functional recovery after postpartum psychosis: a prospective longitudinal study. J Clin Psychiatry. 2017;78(1):122–8. https://doi.org/10.4088/JCP.15m10204.
16. Robertson E, Jones I, Haque S, Holder R, Craddock N. Risk of puerperal and non-puerperal recurrence of illness following bipolar affective puerperal (post-partum) psychosis. Br J Psychiatry. 2005;186:258–9. https://doi.org/10.1192/bjp.186.3.258.
17. Wesseloo R, Kamperman AM, Munk-Olsen T, Pop VJM, Kushner SA, Berghink V. Risk of postpartum relapse in bipolar disorder and postpartum psychosis: a systematic review and meta-analysis. Am J Psychiatry. 2016;173:117–27. https://doi.org/10.1176/appi.ajp.2015.15010124.
18. Kendell RE, Chalmers JC, Platz C. Epidemiology of puerperal psychoses. Br J Psychiatry. 1987;150:662–73. https://doi.org/10.1192/bjp.150.5.662.
19. Munk-Olsen T, Jones I, Laursen TM. Birth order and postpartum psychiatric disorders. Bipolar Disord. 2014;16(3):300–7. https://doi.org/10.1111/bdi.12145.
20. Blackmore ER, Jones I, Doshi M, Haque S, Holder R, Brockington I, Craddock N. Obstetric variables associated with bipolar affective puerperal psychosis. Br J Psychiatry. 2006;188:32–6. https://doi.org/10.1192/bjp.188.1.32.
21. Hellerstedt WL, Phelan SM, Cnattingius S, Hultman CM, Harlow BL. Are prenatal, obstetric, and infant complications associated with postpartum psychosis among women with pre-conception psychiatric hospitalisations? BJOG. 2013;120(4):446–55. https://doi.org/10.1111/1471-0528.12073.
22. Bilszta JLC, Meyer D, Buist AE. Bipolar affective disorder in the postnatal period: investigating the role of sleep. Bipolar Disord. 2010;12(5):568–78. https://doi.org/10.1111/j.1399-5618.2010.00845.x.
23. Sharma V. Role of sleep loss in the causation of puerperal psychosis. Med Hypotheses. 2003;61(4):477–81. https://doi.org/10.1016/S0306-9877(03)00200-7.
24. Sharma V, Smith A, Khan M. The relationship between duration of labour, time of delivery, and puerperal psychosis. J Affect Disord. 2004;83(2-3):215–20. https://doi.org/10.1016/j.jad.2004.04.014.

25. Lewis KJS, Di Florio A, Forty L, Gordon-Smith K, Perry A, Craddock N, Jones L, Jones I. Mania triggered by sleep loss and risk of postpartum psychosis in women with bipolar disorder. J Affect Disord. 2018;225:624–9. https://doi.org/10.1016/j.jad.2017.08.054.
26. Nager A, Johansson LM, Sundquist K. Are sociodemographic factors and year of delivery associated with hospital admission for postpartum psychosis? A study of 500,000 first-time mothers. Acta Psychiatr Scand. 2005;112(1):47–53. https://doi.org/10.1111/j.1600-0447.2005.00525.x.
27. Aas M, Vecchio C, Pauls A, Mehta M, Williams S, Hazelgrove K, Biaggi A, Pawlby S, Conroy S, Seneviratne G, Mondelli V, Pariante CM, Dazzan P. Biological stress response in women at risk of postpartum psychosis: the role of life events and inflammation. Psychoneuroendocrinology. 2020;113:104558. https://doi.org/10.1016/j.psyneuen.2019.104558.
28. Hazelgrove K, Biaggi A, Waites F, Fuste M, Osborne S, Conroy S, Howard LM, Mehta MA, Miele M, Nikkheslat N, Seneviratne G, Zunszain PA, Pawlby S, Pariante CM, Dazzan P. Risk factors for postpartum relapse in women at risk of postpartum psychosis: the role of psychosocial stress and the biological stress system. Psychoneuroendocrinology. 2021;128:105218. https://doi.org/10.1016/j.psyneuen.2021.105218.
29. Dazzan P, Fusté M, Davies W. Do defective immune system-mediated myelination processes increase postpartum psychosis risk? Trends Mol Med. 2018;24:942–9. https://doi.org/10.1016/j.molmed.2018.09.002.
30. Dazzan P. The biology of postpartum psychosis. A hypothetical model. In: Pariante CM, Conroy S, Dazzan P, Howard LM, Pawlby S, Seneviratne G, editors. The legacy of Channi Kumar. Oxford: Oxford University Press; 2014.
31. Kumar C, McIvor RJ, Davies T, Brown N, Papadopoulos A, Wieck A, Checkley SA, Campbell IC, Marks MN. Estrogen administration does not reduce the rate of recurrence of affective psychosis after childbirth. J Clin Psychiatry. 2003;64(2):112–8. https://doi.org/10.4088/JCP.v64n0202.
32. Wisner KL, Stowe ZN. Psychobiology of postpartum mood disorders. Semin Reprod Endocrinol. 1997;15(1):77–89. https://doi.org/10.1055/s-2008-1067970.
33. Jones I. Postpartum psychosis-important clues to the aetiology of mood disorders. In: Pariante CM, Conroy S, Dazzan P, Howard LM, Pawlby S, Seneviratne G, editors. The legacy of Channi Kumar. Oxford: Oxford University Press; 2014.
34. Bergink V, Burgerhout KM, Weigelt K, Pop VJ, De Wit H, Drexhage RC, Kushner SA, Drexhage HA. Immune system dysregulation in first-onset postpartum psychosis. Biol Psychiatry. 2013;73:1000–7. https://doi.org/10.1016/j.biopsych.2012.11.006.
35. Fusté M, Pauls A, Worker A, Reinders AATS, Simmons A, Williams SCR, Haro JM, Hazelgrove K, Pawlby S, Conroy S, Vecchio C, Seneviratne G, Pariante CM, Mehta MA, Dazzan P. Brain structure in women at risk of postpartum psychosis: an MRI study. Transl Psychiatry. 2017;7:1286. https://doi.org/10.1038/s41398-017-0003-8.
36. Sambataro F, Cattarinussi G, Lawrence A, Biaggi A, Fusté M, Hazelgrove K, Mehta MA, Pawlby S, Conroy S, Seneviratne G, Craig MC, Pariante CM, Miele M, Dazzan P. Altered dynamics of the prefrontal networks are associated with the risk for postpartum psychosis: a functional magnetic resonance imaging study. Transl Psychiatry. 2021;11(1):238. https://doi.org/10.1038/s41398-021-01351-5.
37. Oates MR. Perinatal psychiatric syndromes: clinical features. Psychiatry. 2009;8:1–6. https://doi.org/10.1016/j.mppsy.2008.10.014.
38. Doucet S, Dennis CL, Letourneau N, Blackmore ER. Differentiation and clinical implications of postpartum depression and postpartum psychosis. J Obstet Gynecol Neonatal Nurs. 2009;38(3):269–79. https://doi.org/10.1111/j.1552-6909.2009.01019.x.
39. O'Hara MW, Wisner KL. Perinatal mental illness: definition, description and aetiology. Best Pract Res Clin Obstet Gynaecol. 2014;28(1):3–12. https://doi.org/10.1016/j.bpobgyn.2013.09.002.
40. Bergink V, Rasgon N, Wisner KL. Postpartum psychosis: madness, mania, and melancholia in motherhood. Am J Psychiatry. 2016;173(12):1179–88.

41. Biaggi A, Hazelgrove K, Waites F, Fuste M, Conroy S, Howard LM, Mehta MA, Miele M, Seneviratne G, Pawlby S, Pariante CM, Dazzan P. Maternal perceived bonding towards the infant and parenting stress in women at risk of postpartum psychosis with and without a postpartum relapse. J Affect Disord. 2021;294:210–9. https://doi.org/10.1016/j.jad.2021.05.076.
42. Bergink V, Bouvy PF, Vervoort JSP, Koorengevel KM, Steegers EAP, Kushner SA. Prevention of postpartum psychosis and mania in women at high risk. Am J Psychiatry. 2012;169:609–15. https://doi.org/10.1176/appi.ajp.2012.11071047.
43. Austin MP. Puerperal affective psychosis: is there a case for lithium prophylaxis? Br J Psychiatry. 1992;161:692–4.
44. Stewart DE, Klompenhouwer JL, Kendell RE, van Hulst AM. 1991. Prophylactic lithium in puerperal psychosis. The experience of three centres. Br J Psychiatry. 1991;158:393–7.
45. Hogan CS, Freeman MP. Adverse effects in the pharmacologic Management of Bipolar Disorder during Pregnancy. Psychiatr Clin North Am. 2014;39(3):465–75.
46. Viguera AC, Nonacs R, Cohen LS, Tondo L, Murray A, Baldessarini RJ. Risk of recurrence of bipolar disorder in pregnant and nonpregnant women after discontinuing lithium maintenance. Am J Psychiatry. 2000;157(2):179–84. https://doi.org/10.1176/appi.ajp.157.2.179.
47. Goodwin GM, Consensus Group of the British Association for Psychopharmacology. Evidence-based guidelines for treating bipolar disorder: revised second edition—recommendations from the British Association for Psychopharmacology. J Psychopharmacol. 2009;23(4):346–88.
48. Cohen LS, Viguera AC, McInerney KA, Freeman MP, Sosinsky AZ, Moustafa D, et al. Reproductive safety of second-generation antipsychotics: current data from the Massachusetts General Hospital National Pregnancy Registry for atypical antipsychotics. Am J Psychiatry. 2016;173(3):263–70.
49. Dazzan P. Schizophrenia during pregnancy. Curr Opin Psychiatry. 2021;34(3):238–44. https://doi.org/10.1097/YCO.0000000000000706.
50. Habermann F, Fritzsche J, Fuhlbruck F, Wacker E, Allignol A, Weber-Schoendorfer C, et al. Atypical antipsychotic drugs and pregnancy outcome: a prospective, cohort study. J Clin Psychopharmacol. 2013;33(4):453–62.
51. Tinkelman A, Hill EA, Deligiannidis KM. Management of new onset psychosis in the postpartum period. J Clin Psychiatry. 2017;78(9):1423–4. https://doi.org/10.4088/JCP.17ac11880.
52. Meltzer-Brody S, Colquhoun H, Riesenberg R, Epperson CN, Deligiannidis KM, Rubinow DR, Li H, Sankoh AJ, Clemson C, Schacterle A, Jonas J, Kanes S. Brexanolone injection in post-partum depression: two multicentre, double-blind, randomised, placebo-controlled, phase 3 trials. Lancet. 2018;392(10152):1058–70. https://doi.org/10.1016/S0140-6736(18)31551-4.
53. Babu GN, Thippeswamy H, Chandra PS. Use of electroconvulsive therapy (ECT) in postpartum psychosis—a naturalistic prospective study. Arch Womens Ment Health. 2013;16(3):247–51.
54. Lawson A, Dalfen A. Examination of a four-step treatment algorithm for postpartum psychosis. Evid Based Ment Health. 2016;19(1):25. https://doi.org/10.1136/eb-2015-102107.
55. Heron J, McGuinness M, Blackmore ER, Craddock N, Jones I. Early postpartum symptoms in puerperal psychosis. BJOG. 2008;115:348–53. https://doi.org/10.1111/j.1471-0528.2007.01563.x.
56. Nager A, Szulkin R, Johansson SE, Johansson LM, Sundquist K. High lifelong relapse rate of psychiatric disorders among women with postpartum psychosis. Nord J Psychiatry. 2013;67(1):53–8.
57. O'Hara MW. Post-partum "blues," depression, and psychosis: A review. J Psychosom Obstet Gynecol. 1987;7(3):205–27. https://doi.org/10.3109/01674828709040280.

Childhood Trauma and Mental Health: Never Too Early to Intervene

5

Antonella Trotta

The Child is father of the Man [...]
　　—William Wordsworth, My heart leaps up, 1802

5.1　The Burden of Childhood Trauma

Approximately one billion children have experienced physical, sexual or emotional violence or neglect in the past year [1]. The average lifetime incidence cost of childhood trauma from social care, short-term health and long-term labour market outcomes has been estimated at £89,390 [2].

For the purposes of this chapter, a broad concept of the term childhood trauma will be used, which includes child maltreatment by adults (all forms of physical and/or emotional ill-treatment, sexual abuse, neglect or negligent treatment or commercial or other exploitation), peer victimisation (e.g. bullying), experiences of parental loss and separation, war-related trauma, natural disasters and witnessing domestic or non-domestic violence [3] and adverse childhood experiences [4]. The National Society for the Prevention of Cruelty to Children [5] describes childhood trauma as resulting in 'actual or potential harm to the child's health, survival, development or dignity in the context of a relationship of responsibility, trust or power'.

It is striking to think that, so far, there are no systematic methods of classifying trauma; different criteria are employed for the severity, frequency, persistence and age of exposure to such experiences making comparisons of findings between

A. Trotta (✉)
School of Health and Social Care, University of Essex, Colchester, UK

Lambeth Directorate, South London & Maudsley NHS Foundation Trust, London, UK

Social, Genetic & Developmental Psychiatry Centre, Institute of Psychiatry, Psychology & Neuroscience, King's College London, London, UK
e-mail: atrott@essex.ac.uk

© The Author(s), under exclusive license to Springer Nature Switzerland AG 2022
M. Colizzi, M. Ruggeri (eds.), *Prevention in Mental Health*,
https://doi.org/10.1007/978-3-030-97906-5_5

different studies or research groups very difficult [6, 7]. For example, findings from nationally representative samples of young adults aged 18–24, asked retrospectively about childhood adverse experiences, displayed decreases over 10 years in reports of physical abuse (from 13.1% in 1998–1999 to 9.8% in 2009), sexual abuse (6.8–5%) and verbal abuse (14.5–6%) [8]. In contrast, Gilbert and colleagues found no changes in trends in childhood trauma, suggesting that these figures could alternatively indicate a decline in overall prevalence accompanied by an increase in recognition and recording [9].

Over the past 40 years, there has been increased responsiveness to childhood adversity in many Western countries. Expansion of definitions of trauma include emotional abuse and the witnessing of intimate partner violence, and the change of thresholds for moving from recognition to recording and action, which consequently might increase the number of reported cases throughout the system [9]. Existing research of how childhood adversity is changing in developing countries is conflicting. Studies that rely on officially recorded or substantiated adversity measure only a small part of the bigger picture. Most childhood adversity is still hidden and not recognised by professionals dealing with children; it might also be that professionals consistently report to child protection agencies only a proportion of children whom they recognise as being maltreated [3, 10]. Self-reported or parent-reported incidents of trauma probably come closest to a true measurement of the incidence of trauma, although these studies might still underestimate the severity of the problem [11, 12].

Another ongoing debate is whether it is the frequency or the specific nature of traumatic experiences that impact the most on children's development. For example, the Adverse Childhood Experiences (ACE) study, a retrospective study of 13,494 adults, has suggested that it is the number of adverse life events that most influence development, not the nature of these events [4]. In contrast, other studies have shown that threatening events, such as physical abuse, impact the child's mind and body differently than experiences of absence of caregiving (e.g. neglect [13]). Furthermore, the type of threat (e.g. physical abuse vs. verbal abuse) or the type of deprivation (e.g. lack of caregiving vs. lack of visual or auditory input) likely impacts development differently [14].

In the following sections, the impact of trauma on children's mental and physical health will be discussed in some detail, also considering the nature and the timing of the traumatic experience. An overview of current evidence-based early interventions that proceed according to children's developmental needs will then be provided.

5.2 The Link Between Childhood Trauma and Health Outcomes

5.2.1 Mental Health

Approximately 241 million young people around the world are affected by a mental disorder. The worldwide-pooled prevalence has been estimated of 13.4% for any mental disorder [15], with the prevalence of any mental disorder in very young children between 14.0 and 26.4% [16]. Only in the last few decades has substantial research evidence accumulated sufficiently to show that a variety of traumatic experiences in childhood are associated with psychiatric disorders later in life. A national survey in Britain, conducted among 2869 young adults aged 18–24, reported that severe childhood maltreatment had been experienced by 16% of the sample [10]; this was associated with poorer emotional wellbeing, self-harm, suicidal ideation and delinquent behaviour [17]. Childhood trauma has been claimed to predict over 32% of all psychiatric disorders [18], including depression, anxiety disorders, post-traumatic stress disorder (PTSD), eating disorders, substance misuse, sexual dysfunction and personality and dissociative disorders at all life-course stages [19–22].

Many years before evidence has become available, Sigmund Freud [23], recalling the expression 'The Child Is the Father of the Man', underlined the impact of early experiences on adulthood and how the subject's vulnerability to psychopathology is always the result of the inevitable interplay between objective and subjective, external and internal reality [24]. Shengold [25] used the evocative expression 'soul murder' to describe traumatic experiences of child abuse and deprivation, those instances of repetitive and chronic overstimulation alternating with emotional deprivation that are deliberately brought about by another individual. Soul murder is a crime characterised by man's inhumanity to man: one man uses his power over another to crush his individuality, his dignity and his capacity to feel deeply (joy, love, hate) and to impair the victim's capacity to think rationally and to test reality. Moreover, the earlier the trauma, the more devastating is the effect on the developing mental apparatus and sense of identity and tends to interfere with full, free emotional and intellectual development [25]. Referring to the etymology of the word trauma (from the Greek verb *diatitreno*), Garland defines as traumatic an event which 'breaks through or overrides the discriminatory, filtering process, and overrides any temporary denial or patch-up of the damage' ([26], p. 10). The child's mind is flooded with stimulation that is far more than it can make sense of or manage. Trauma causes in the child a breaking of the psychic and bodily envelope and causes a massive disruption in functioning, a breakdown of established beliefs and defensive organisation; it stirs up primitive fears and paranoid beliefs, impulses and anxieties; the world becomes an unpredictable place, as well as there being no trust in any good object [26].

Consequently, children exposed to trauma show signs of psychopathology earlier in life and have a higher number of associated comorbidities, as well as a poorer response to both pharmacological and psychological treatment [27–32].

The issue of causality between trauma and mental health problems has been addressed in longitudinal twin studies, which are methodologically more robust as they allow to prospectively measure the impact of trauma and take into account all of the unmeasured shared environmental or genetic factors that might impact both the exposure and the outcome of interest. Prospective cohort studies have in fact shown evidence of causality between trauma and psychiatric diagnosis from childhood to adulthood [33] and that the effects of childhood trauma seem to be nonspecific, predicting a wide range of internalising and externalising psychopathology by age 18 [34].

However, studies that have measured trauma retrospectively have interestingly shown that psychopathology is more strongly associated with the retrospective recall of childhood trauma than the actual exposure to the traumatic event [35], highlighting the key role of subjective experience in interpreting and working through the traumatic event *après coup*.[1]

Furthermore, the more 'complex' is the trauma, the higher is the risk of negative consequences for mental health. The modern definition of complex trauma includes severe multiple experience of interpersonal assaults or threats, such as physical or sexual abuse, occurring in childhood or adolescence [37]. On average, one in four trauma-exposed children develop PTSD by age 18, with a lifetime prevalence of 4.7–7.8% in the general population [38, 39]. Children exposed to complex traumas have poorer cognitive function and are at higher risk of harming themselves and of harming others because of aggression and risk taking, and the odds of suicide attempt are ten times higher compared to peers who have not been exposed to complex traumas [40–45].

Increasing interest has also been shown in the relationship between early trauma and the risk of experiencing psychotic symptoms in adolescence as well as full-blown psychotic disorders in adulthood [46–53]. There are a large number of studies of psychiatric inpatients, and of outpatients in which a majority have a psychotic disorder, that suggest the prevalence of childhood trauma in these populations is high [54–56]. Large-scale general population studies hint at a potentially causal relationship, as the effect becomes stronger with cumulative exposure [57, 58]. Moreover, studies focusing on the possible influence of the type of trauma experienced reported stronger associations between abuse and psychosis, compared with neglect [59, 60]. However, there is now emerging evidence that childhood adversities are related to specific symptoms of psychosis, particularly hallucinations and paranoid delusions [54, 61–63], and, differently from psychosis diagnosis, the association remains significant regardless of the type of trauma (i.e. sexual abuse and growing up in foster care; [64]). These findings have also been summarised in a quantitative review and meta-analysis of the available empirical literature which reported a strong significant association between childhood adversity and increased risk for psychosis (odds ratio = 2.78), regardless of the specific type of exposure and study design [65].

5.2.2 Physical Health

The ACE study was the first to highlight a dose-response relationship between the number of adverse experiences occurring in childhood and negative physical outcomes later in life [4]. Individuals who experience multiple childhood adversities were at higher risk of both health-harming behaviours (e.g. alcohol and drug abuse,

---

[1] Term frequently used by Freud to describe how memories of traumatic experiences may be revised at a later stage of development and assimilated into a new meaning according to present circumstances (Laplanche and Pontalis [36]).

risky sexual behaviours) and chronic life-threatening diseases, such as stroke, cardiovascular disease and cancer compared to those who experienced lower frequencies of adversities or no trauma in childhood [4, 66, 67].

A recent meta-analysis confirmed the ACE study findings by showing significant effect of cumulative childhood adversity on adult cardiometabolic disease [68]. Children exposed to early life stressors not only have greater risk of common diseases of childhood, including otitis media, viral infections, asthma, dermatitis, urticaria, intestinal infectious diseases and urinary tract infections [69], but also show higher risk of poor selfreported health and elevated rates of diabetes, autoimmune disorders and premature mortality in adulthood [14, 70, 71]. Early exposure to adversities is associated with linear growth failure, high cortisol levels, reduced brain volume and altered functional connectivity [72–74].

Prospective cohort studies also support the evidence of an effect between severe victimisation early in life and higher inflammation levels [75, 76]. Our research group has shown that a history of childhood trauma may have a significant role in explaining the co-occurrence of depression [77], psychotic phenomena [78] and elevated inflammation in adolescence and young adulthood [79, 80].

Poorer physical health is, in turn, linked to increased health-care use [81, 82]. A recently published Danish population-based cohort study, using data from nationwide registers covering more than half a million children (aged 0–15), showed that those who were exposed to adversities of deprivation, family loss and negative family dynamics had a markedly higher rate of hospitalisations across all ages, compared to those children in the low adversity group [83]. The trajectory of poor health for those with a high level of early life adversity was significantly higher in those aged 16–24, suggesting a pathway from birth to adult life [83].

These findings highlight the importance of considering the individual's psychological and biological maturation, which influences sensitivity to the proximal environment over the child and adolescent years. Therefore, as well as the nature of early adversities, recent reports have begun to consider the importance of the timing of early experiences and their putative effect on the mind and the body [84].

5.3 The Timing of Exposure and Developmental Sequelae of Trauma

The question of whether a sensitive period of risk exists during which exposure to trauma is particularly likely to be associated with worse clinical and health outcomes remains understudied. Animal models have provided the first evidence that childhood maltreatment occurring earlier in life and continuing for a longer duration is associated with the worst outcomes. This phenomenon has been described as 'allostatic load', a process through which an individual's failure to adapt to conditions of repeated or chronic stress leads to wear and tear on the body and mind [85–88]. For examples, rodents separated from the mother during the early postnatal days, but not later, showed behaviours associated with anxiety and depression in adulthood [89]. A similar pattern seems to delineate in human beings, where exposure to early maltreatment during preschool (i.e. between 3 and 5 years of age) has been found to be most strongly associated with depression and suicidal ideation [90, 91].

When trauma occurs in the first few years of life, children are more sensitive to developing traumatic stress reactions including hypervigilance, re-experiencing through nightmares, flashbacks, traumatic play, emotional arousal and avoidance [92]. The psychological effects of exposure to trauma in the preschool years also include feelings of helplessness, worthlessness and hopelessness, low self-esteem, feeling responsible for bad things that happen, behavioural problems and poor social skills [93–95]. If untreated, in the long term, they translate into learning difficulties and academic challenges [96], as well as anxiety, depression, substance abuse and offending behaviours [97–99].

A sensitive period occurring around 2 years of age has been identified for the development of a secure attachment relationship: the majority of institutionalised children placed into stable family care after 2 years fail to develop secure attachments [100]. Insecure attachment relationships also affect the child's neurobiological development, including hyperreactivity of the autonomic nervous system and hypothalamic-pituitary-adrenal (HPA) axis to the environment [101]. The first years of life also represent a sensitive period for language and personality development. A recent study including data for over 2000 children in cities across the United States found that those children who experienced emotional, cognitive and/or social deprivation and those exposed to threatening events (such as physical or emotional abuse and domestic or community violence) by 3 years of age were more likely to display internalising and externalising symptoms during childhood and adolescence [102].

Nevertheless, the impact of trauma could be traced back to the antenatal period of life. Parents' unresolved childhood traumas, as well as in prior generations, may trigger intergenerational transmission of trauma in offspring, particularly in the absence of protective relationships during development [103, 104]. Parents exposed to traumas in childhood have higher risk of PTSD symptoms during adulthood, pregnancy and early parenthood [105, 106]. Maternal depression, especially when it occurs antenatally, has a stronger effect on the infant's cognitive development and cortisol levels [107–109].

In line with the allostatic load model or cumulative effect hypothesis, research has shown that early childhood and adolescent victimisation each contribute independently to the prediction of young adult mental health general liability to psychopathology, also known as 'p factor', including internalising, externalising and thought disorders [31]. Similarly, using data from the Avon Longitudinal Study of Parents and Children (ALSPAC), a large population-based birth cohort, researchers found that exposure to traumatic experiences during childhood and adolescence was associated with the development of psychotic experiences by early adulthood [110]. These findings could be explained perhaps by developmental differences in adolescence (e.g. development of neural circuitry known to play a role in the generation of psychiatric symptoms [33]). With a peak in the onset of mental disorder, adolescence may therefore function as a critical period for the negative mental health consequences of traumatic events.

Taken together, increasing evidence has shown that trauma has the most robust effects on long-term health during phases of rapid psychoneurobiological development (e.g. early childhood and adolescence [108]), and suggests that interventions at these crucial phases might be the most effective method of remediating these associations.

5.4 Prevention and Early Interventions for Trauma

Most children exposed to a traumatic experience typically present transient distress and subsequently return to their previous level of functioning with support from sensitive and consistent caregivers [111, 112]. However, for a significant minority of these children, the distress becomes persistent and can have ongoing impact on child development and well-being [113]. Particularly if the primary caregiver is emotionally and/or physically unavailable, or if they are involved in the traumatic experience (e.g. a parent who abused or neglected the child), there is higher risk of overwhelming a young child's internal resources for coping [114].

The aim of early intervention is to prevent or reduce the onset, persistence and severity of traumatic stress responses and to promote children's resilience and full emotional recovery after exposure to a potentially traumatic event [115]. Although a growing body of research describes how interventions in early childhood generate higher returns than interventions offered later in life [116–118], many children exposed to trauma who develop psychopathology go undetected and do not access treatment in time. In the past year, only 20% of trauma-exposed children sought help from general practitioners or mental health practitioners, and only 10% accessed mental health services [119, 120].

Identifying children at risk is therefore the first step in prevention and early interventions; however, there are several barriers to health-care use that still need to be overcome [121]. On one side, early screening to identify precursors of severe mental health issues is a feasible and generally acceptable practice [122], but on the other side, the current screening instruments present significant limitations. Firstly, the diagnostic specificity and sensitivity of screening tools have not yet been established [123, 124], which limits their predictive validity for trauma-related psychopathology [38]. Secondly, objective and subjective measures of childhood adversity identify different subgroups of individuals [125] and, thus, may be associated with health outcomes via different pathways. Listening to the subjectivity of the experience, through conversations with patients and their families, is therefore particularly important in capturing the complex individual needs associated with childhood trauma, which are often underdiagnosed or misdiagnosed [126].

Furthermore, screening is useful only if it informs and is part of evidence-based interventions, and also if it takes into account the role of protective factors [127]. Vice versa, early interventions, especially immediately after trauma, can be ineffective in preventing psychological sequelae if not thoughtfully developed and evaluated [128, 129].

Evidence from a recent meta-analysis supports the benefits of two-generational approaches that actively involve both children and parents in the intervention [130, 131]. For example, children who received a four-session intervention focused on psychoeducation about trauma and supporting the communication in the family, delivered within 30 days of exposure to a potentially traumatic event, were 65% less likely to meet criteria for PTSD at the 3-month follow-up than children who received the comparison condition [132]. Parents also showed increased responsiveness to their children and enhanced self-understanding when providers explained the links between parents' childhood experiences, parenting practices and satisfaction with parenting [133, 134].

However, there is still a big gap in the knowledge of which interventions are effective for whom and when. Most of the existing studies on early interventions for children exposed to trauma have focused on school-age children and adolescents, and the heterogeneity of studies makes it difficult to draw clear conclusions about effective elements [131]. Recent reviews of interventions for children exposed to disaster [135] or armed conflict [136], and of school-based interventions for PTSD symptoms [137], reveal almost no rigorous studies of interventions delivered in the early post-trauma period to prevent the development of negative psychological outcomes. A recent study suggested that assessment in early adolescence may capture adversity-exposed youth on a trajectory for the greatest health risks in adulthood [138].

Interventions for trauma can be offered at three levels and at different developmental stages [139]. Figure 5.1 summarises the early interventions with more robust evidence bases for preventing childhood trauma and/or reducing the effect of traumatic experiences. The first level is represented by *universal screening and interventions* and includes those activities provided to the general population and that do not require screening or referrals. Examples of universal screenings are *perinatal mental health screening* with instruments with proven validity, like the Edinburgh Postnatal Depression Scale [140], and *perinatal intimate partner violence (IPV) screening and advice* to increase mothers' awareness of abusive intimate partner behaviours and reduce their risk of further victimisation. Universal strategies also include *social-emotional learning interventions* at school to promote children's emotional resilience and reduce risks of health-harming behaviours and peer victimisation [141], interventions promoting parental bonding during pregnancy and *co-parenting support* for couples to offer support at crucial phases of their children's development.

A second level of early interventions is represented by *targeted selective interventions* for children and families identified as at risk of adversity, like the Family Nurse Partnership programme for teenage mothers that has shown evidence of preventing child maltreatment and domestic abuse. Early intervention also includes secondary prevention introduced when there are early distressing symptoms that indicate risk of subsequent psychiatric disorders. At a third level of interventions, there are *targeted indicated interventions* to reduce trauma-related psychopathology in children and family with a history of adversity which include interventions for parents at risk of maltreating their child (Incredible Years and Triple P series), psychotherapeutic support for parents and parents and children who are at risk of child

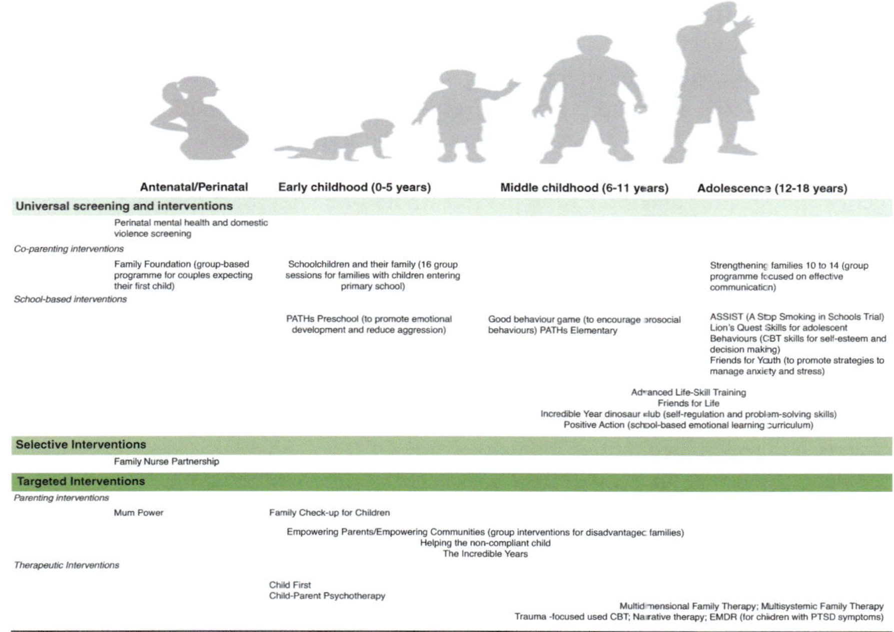

Fig. 5.1 Evidence-based early intervention for childhood trauma (adapted from [139]). *CBT* cognitive behavioural therapy, *EMDR* eye movement desensitization and reprocessing, *PTSD* post-traumatic stress disorder

maltreatment (Child-Parent Psychotherapy and the Child First programme), interventions focused on attachment relationships to promote sensitivity and healthy attachment and foster family resilience in the context of traumas.

Child-Parent Psychotherapy (CPP [133]) is an evidence-based intervention for traumatised children up to 5 years of age and their caregivers that utilises techniques such as the reframing of children's negative beliefs and attributions and somatic processing of traumatic experiences, developmental guidance and co-regulation of distress. CPP also offers help to parents to process and recover from their trauma, with the aim of fostering secure parent-child attachment [142]. Mom Power [143, 144] is a group based on CPP techniques addressing the parent-child attachment relationship with the rationale that parents with histories of trauma and untreated mental health problems are at risk for impaired caregiving.

Targeted therapeutic interventions for young people who are at risk of going into care and their families are the Multisystemic Therapy (MST), Functional Family Therapy (FFT), Multidimensional Family Therapy and Multisystemic Therapy for Child Abuse and Neglect (MST-CAN). Individualised therapeutic intervention with causal evidence of reducing symptoms related to trauma and increasing children's resilience are Trauma-Focused Cognitive Behavioural Therapy (CBT [145]), narrative therapy and Eye Movement Desensitization and Reprocessing (EMDR [146, 147]).

5.5 Conclusions

Early interventions are key to improving well-being throughout the child's life, and need to be offered at the appropriate level in the community, health and education systems. Trauma-informed care has started to be implemented widely in schools, GP practices and mental health services, with the aim of bridging the gap between theory and practice and increasing the sensitivity of health practitioners to the consequences of trauma on children's mental and physical health [148].

A wide range of initiatives falls under the umbrella of trauma-informed care, such as training practitioners about the impact of early trauma on the individual's development, screening practices to assess trauma symptoms and service redefinition to facilitate a sense of safety and empowerment [149]. Trauma-informed care should also inform governments on implementing evidence-informed policies to address the underlying social drivers of childhood adversities, including childhood poverty and social inequalities in health [150].

Clinical settings, like hospitals, could serve as an entry point for the identification of social problems and the identification of vulnerable children who would benefit from additional support [151]. Socio-economic interventions such as income supplementation and housing interventions, legal assistance, food vouchers and alcohol or drug treatment programmes have shown effectiveness in reducing the effects of traumatic events among children and adolescents living in adverse circumstances and promoting resilience and change [152]. Supporting parents, caregivers and families in providing nurturing care and protection for children [153] will help to foster their developmental potential.

References

1. Hillis S, Mercy J, Amobi A, Kress H. Global prevalence of past-year violence against children: a systematic review and minimum estimates. Pediatrics. 2016;137(3):e20154079. https://doi.org/10.1542/peds.2015-4079.
2. Conti G, Pizzo E, Morris S, Melnychuk M. The economic costs of child maltreatment in UK. Health Econ. 2021;30(12):3087–105. https://doi.org/10.1002/hec.4409.
3. World Health Organization (WHO). Preventing child maltreatment: a guide to taking action and generating evidence/World Health Organization and International Society for Prevention of Child Abuse and Neglect. World Health Organization; 2006. Available from: https://apps.who.int/iris/handle/10665/43499
4. Felitti VJ, Anda RF, Nordenberg D, Williamson DF, Spitz AM, Edwards V, et al. Relationship of childhood abuse and household dysfunction to many of the leading causes of death in adults: The Adverse Childhood Experiences (ACE) Study. Am J Prev Med. 1998;14(4):245–58.
5. National Society for the Prevention of Cruelty to Children (NSPCC). In: Meadows P, Tunstill J, George A, Dhudwar A, Kurtz Z, editors. The costs and consequences of child maltreatment: literature review for the NSPCC. London: NSPCC; 2011.
6. Cicchetti D. Editorial: advances and challenges in the study of the sequelae of child maltreatment. Dev Psychopathol. 1994;6:1–3.
7. Manly JT, Cicchetti D, Barnett D. The impact of subtype, frequency, chronicity, and severity of child maltreatment on social competence and behaviour problems. Dev Psychopathol. 1994;6:121–43.

8. Radford L, Corral S, Bradley C, Fisher H. Trends in child maltreatment. Lancet. 2012;379(9831):2048.
9. Gilbert R, Widom CS, Browne K, Fergusson D, Webb E, Janson S. Burden and consequences of child maltreatment in high-income countries. Lancet. 2009;373:68–81.
10. May-Chahal C, Cawson P. Measuring child maltreatment in the United Kingdom: a study of the prevalence of child abuse and neglect. Child Abuse Negl. 2005;29(9):969–84. https://doi.org/10.1016/j.chiabu.2004.05.009.
11. Leeb RT, Paulozzi L, Melanson C, Simon T, Arias I. Child maltreatment surveillance: uniform definitions for public health and recommended data elements, version 1.0. Atlanta: Centers for Disease Control and Prevention, National Center for Injury Prevention and Control; 2008.
12. Nelson EC, Heath AC, Madden PA, Cooper ML, Dinwiddie SH, Bucholz KK, et al. Association between self-reported childhood sexual abuse and adverse psychosocial outcomes: results from a twin study. Arch Gen Psychiatry. 2002;59(2):139–45. https://doi.org/10.1001/archpsyc.59.2.139.
13. McLaughlin KA, Sheridan MA, Lambert HK. Childhood adversity and neural development: deprivation and threat as distinct dimensions of early experience. Neurosci Biobehav Rev. 2014;47:578–91.
14. Nelson CA, Scott RD, Bhutta ZA, Harris NB, Danese A, Samara M. Adversity in childhood is linked to mental and physical health throughout life. BMJ. 2020;371:m3048. https://doi.org/10.1136/bmj.m3048.
15. Polanczyk GV, Salum GA, Sugaya LS, Caye A, Rohde LA. Annual research review: a meta-analysis of the worldwide prevalence of mental disorders in children and adolescents. J Child Psychol Psychiatry. 2015;56:345–65.
16. Vasileva M, Graf RK, Reinelt T, Petermann U, Petermann F. Research review: a meta-analysis of the international prevalence and comorbidity of mental disorders in children between 1 and 7 years. J Child Psychol Psychiatry. 2021;62(4):372–81.
17. Radford L, Corral S, Bradley C, Fisher H, Bassett C, Howat N, Collishaw S. Child abuse and neglect in the UK today. London: NSPCC; 2011.
18. Green JG, Berglund P, Gruber MJ, McLaughlin KA, Sampson NA, Zaslavsky AM, et al. Childhood adversities and adult psychopathology in the National Comorbidity Survey Replication (NCS-R). I: associations with first onset of DSM–IV disorders. Arch Gen Psychiatry. 2010;67:113–23.
19. Kilpatrick DG, Ruggiero KJ, Acierno R, Saunders BE, Resnick HS, Best CL. Violence and risk of PTSD, major depression, substance abuse/dependence, and comorbidity: results from the national survey for adolescents. J Consult Clin Psychol. 2003.71:692–700.
20. Lobbestael J, Arntz A, Bernstein DP. Disentangling the relationship between different types of childhood maltreatment and personality disorders. J Pers Disord. 2010;24(3):285–95.
21. Ruchkin V, Henrich CC, Jones SM, Vermeiren R, Schwab-Stone M. Violence exposure and psychopathology in urban youth: the mediating role of posttraumatic stress. J Abnorm Child Psychol. 2007;35(4):578–93.
22. Wasserman GA, McReynolds LS. Contributors to traumatic exposure and posttraumatic stress disorder in juvenile justice youths. J Trauma Stress. 2011;24(4):422–9.
23. Freud S. The aetiology of hysteria. Standard Edition, vol. 3. Gesammelte Werke; 1896. p. 191–221.
24. Ferenczi S, Confusion of tongues between adults and the child. In: Ferenczi S. editor. Final contributions to the problems and methods of psychoanalysis. London: Hogarth Press; 1933. p. 1955.
25. Shengold LL. Child abuse and deprivation: soul murder. J Am Psychoanal Assoc. 1979;27(3):533–59. https://doi.org/10.1177/000306517902700302.
26. Garland C. Understanding trauma: a psychoanalytical approach. 1st ed. London: Routledge; 1998. https://doi.org/10.4324/9780429484575.
27. Agnew-Blais J, Danese A. Childhood maltreatment and unfavourable clinical outcomes in bipolar disorder: a systematic review and meta-analysis. Lancet Psychiatry. 2016;3(4):342–9. https://doi.org/10.1016/S2215-0366(15)00544-1.

28. Nanni V, Uher R, Danese A. Childhood maltreatment predicts unfavorable course of illness and treatment outcome in depression: a meta-analysis. Am J Psychiatry. 2012;169(2):141–51.
29. Nemeroff CB. Paradise lost: the neurobiological and clinical consequences of child abuse and neglect. Neuron. 2016;89(5):892–909. https://doi.org/10.1016/j.neuron.2016.01.019.
30. Putnam KT, Harris WW, Putnam FW. Synergistic childhood adversities and complex adult psychopathology. J Trauma Stress. 2013;26(4):435–42.
31. Schaefer JD, Moffitt TE, Arseneault L, Danese A, Fisher HL, Houts R, et al. Adolescent victimization and early-adult psychopathology: approaching causal inference using a longitudinal twin study to rule out noncausal explanations. Clin Psychol Sci. 2018;6(3):352–71. https://doi.org/10.1177/2167702617741381.
32. Widom CS, DuMont K, Czaja SJ. A prospective investigation of major depressive disorder and comorbidity in abused and neglected children grown up. Arch Gen Psychiatry. 2007;64(1):49–56. https://doi.org/10.1001/archpsyc.64.1.49.
33. Kim-Cohen J, Caspi A, Moffitt TE, Harrington H, Milne BJ, Poulton R. Prior juvenile diagnoses in adults with mental disorder: developmental follow-back of a prospective-longitudinal cohort. Arch Gen Psychiatry. 2003;60(7):709–17.
34. Meehan AJ, Latham RM, Arseneault L, Stahl D, Fisher HL, Danese A. Developing an individualized risk calculator for psychopathology among young people victimized during childhood: a population-representative cohort study. J Affect Disord. 2020;262:90–8. https://doi.org/10.1016/j.jad.2019.10.034.
35. Danese A, Widom CS. Objective and subjective experiences of child maltreatment and their relationships with psychopathology. Nat Hum Behav. 2020;4:811–8. https://doi.org/10.1038/s41562-020-0880-3.
36. Laplanche J, Pontalis JB. The language of psycho-analysis. New York: W.W. Norton; 1973.
37. UK Trauma Council. Complex trauma. London: UKTC; 2021. Available from: https://uktraumacouncil.org/trauma/complex-trauma. Accessed 30 Oct 2021.
38. Lewis SJ, Arseneault L, Caspi A, Fisher HL, Matthews T, Moffitt TE, et al. The epidemiology of trauma and post-traumatic stress disorder in a representative cohort of young people in England and Wales. Lancet Psychiatry. 2019;6(3):247–56. https://doi.org/10.1016/S2215-0366(19)30031-8.
39. McLaughlin KA, Koenen KC, Hill ED, Petukhova M, Sampson NA, Zaslavsky AM, et al. Trauma exposure and posttraumatic stress disorder in a national sample of adolescents. J Am Acad Child Adolesc Psychiatry. 2013;52(8):815–30. https://doi.org/10.1016/j.jaac.2013.05.011.
40. Cloitre M, Garvert DW, Brewin CR, Bryant RA, Maercker A. Evidence for proposed ICD-11 PTSD and complex PTSD: a latent profile analysis. Eur J Psychotraumatol. 2013;4:20706.
41. Danese A. Annual research review: rethinking childhood trauma-new research directions for measurement, study design and analytical strategies. J Child Psychol Psychiatry. 2020;61(3):236–50. https://doi.org/10.1111/jcpp.13160.
42. Lewis S, Koenen K, Ambler A, Arseneault L, Caspi A, Fisher H, et al. Unravelling the contribution of complex trauma to psychopathology and cognitive deficits: a cohort study. Br J Psychiatry. 2021;219(2):448–55.
43. Op den Kelder R, Ensink JBM, Overbeek G, Maric M, Lindauer RJL. Executive function as a mediator in the link between single or complex trauma and posttraumatic stress in children and adolescents. Qual Life Res. 2017;26(7):1687–96. https://doi.org/10.1007/s11136-017-1535-3.
44. van der Kolk BA, Roth S, Pelcovitz D, Sunday S, Spinazzola J. Disorders of extreme stress: the empirical foundation of a complex adaptation to trauma. J Trauma Stress. 2005;18:389–99.
45. Wamser-Nanney R, Vandenberg BR. Empirical support for the definition of a complex trauma event in children and adolescents. J Trauma Stress. 2013;26:671–8.
46. Arseneault L, Cannon M, Fisher HL, Polanczyk G, Moffitt TE, Caspi A. Childhood trauma and children's emerging psychotic symptoms: a genetically sensitive longitudinal cohort study. Am J Psychiatry. 2011;168:65–72.
47. Fisher HL, Jones PB, Fearon P, Craig TK, Dazzan P, Morgan K, et al. The varying impact of type, timing and frequency of exposure to childhood adversity on its association with adult psychotic disorder. Psychol Med. 2010;40(12):1967–78.

48. Kelleher I, Keeley H, Corcoran P, Ramsay H, Wasserman C, Carli V, et al. Childhood trauma and psychosis in a prospective cohort study: cause, effect and directionality. Am J Psychiatry. 2013;170(7):734–41.
49. Morgan C, Kirkbride J, Leff J, Craig T, Hutchinson G, McKenzie K, et al. Parental separation, loss and psychosis in different ethnic groups: a case- control study. Psychol Med. 2007;37(4):495–503.
50. Trotta A, Di Forti M, Iyegbe C, Green P, Dazzan P, Mondelli V, et al. Familial risk and childhood adversity interplay in the onset of psychosis. BJPsych Open. 2015;1(1):6–13. https://doi.org/10.1192/bjpo.bp.115.000158.
51. Trotta A, Di Forti M, Mondelli V, Dazzan P, Pariante C, David A, et al. Prevalence of bullying victimisation amongst first-episode psychosis patients and unaffected controls. Schizophr Res. 2013;150:169–75.
52. Trotta A, Murray RM, David AS, Kolliakou A, O'Connor J, Di Forti M, et al. Impact of different childhood adversities on one-year outcomes of psychotic disorder in the GAP study. Schizophr Bull. 2016;42(2):464–75. https://doi.org/10.1093/schbul/sbv131.
53. Trotta A, Murray RM, Fisher HL. The impact of childhood adversity on the persistence of psychotic symptoms: a systematic review and meta- analysis. Psychol Med. 2015;45(12):2481–98.
54. Bebbington PE, Bhugra D, Brugha T, Singleton N, Farrell M, Jenkins R, et al. Psychosis, victimisation and childhood disadvantage: evidence from the second British National Survey of Psychiatric Morbidity. Br J Psychiatry. 2004;185:220–6.
55. Morgan C, Fisher H. Environment and schizophrenia: environmental factors in schizophrenia: childhood trauma—a critical review. Schizophr Bull. 2007;33:3–10.
56. Schäfer I, Fisher HL. Childhood trauma and psychosis—what is the evidence? Dialogues Clin Neurosci. 2011;13:360–5.
57. Read J, van Os J, Morrison AP, Ross CA. Childhood trauma, psychosis and schizophrenia: a literature review with theoretical and clinical implications. Acta Psychiatr Scand. 2005;112:330–50.
58. van Winkel R, Stefanis NC, Myin-Germeys I. Psychosocial stress and psychosis. A review of the neurobiological mechanisms and the evidence for gene-stress interaction. Schizophr Bull. 2008;34(6):1095–105.
59. Heins M, Simons C, Lataster T, Pfeifer S, Versmissen D, Lardinois M, et al. Childhood trauma and psychosis: a case-control and case-sibling comparison across different levels of genetic liability, psychopathology, and type of trauma. Am J Psychiatry. 2011;168:1286–94.
60. Shevlin M, Dorahy MJ, Adamson G. Trauma and psychosis: an analysis of the National Comorbidity Survey. Am J Psychiatry. 2007;164(1):166–9.
61. Bentall RP, de Sousa P, Varese F, Wickham S, Sitko K, Haarmans M, et al. From adversity to psychosis: pathways and mechanisms from specific adversities to specific symptoms. Soc Psychiatry Psychiatr Epidemiol. 2014;49(7):1011–22.
62. Matheson SL, Shepherd AM, Pinchbeck RM, Laurens KR, Carr VJ. Childhood adversity in schizophrenia: a systematic meta-analysis. Psychol Med. 2013;43(2):225–38.
63. Read J, Agar K, Argyle N, Aderhold V. Sexual and physical assault during childhood and adulthood as predictors of hallucinations, delusions and thought disorder. Psychol Psychother. 2003;76:1–22.
64. Van Nierop M, Lataster T, Smeets F, Gunther N, van Zelst C, de Graaf R, et al. Psychopathological mechanisms linking childhood traumatic experiences to risk of psychotic symptoms: analysis of a large, representative population-based sample. Schizophr Bull. 2014;40(2):S123–30.
65. Varese F, Smeets F, Drukker M, Lieverse R, Lataster T, Viechtbauer W, et al. Childhood adversities increase the risk of psychosis: a meta-analysis of patient-control, prospective- and cross-sectional cohort studies. Schizophr Bull. 2012;38(4):661–71.
66. Appleton AA, Holdsworth E, Ryan M, Tracy M. Measuring childhood adversity in life course cardiovascular research: a systematic review. Psychosom Med. 2017;79(4):434–40.

67. Hughes K, Bellis MA, Hardcastle KA, Sethi D, Butchart A, Mikton C, et al. The effect of multiple adverse childhood experiences on health: a systematic review and meta-analysis. Lancet Public Health. 2017;2(8):e356–66. https://doi.org/10.1016/S2468-2667(17)30118-4.
68. Jakubowski KP, Cundiff JM, Matthews KA. Cumulative childhood adversity and adult cardiometabolic disease: a meta-analysis. Health Psychol. 2018;37(8):701–15.
69. Miller BJ, Buckley P, Seabolt W, Mellor A, Kirkpatrick B. Meta-analysis of cytokine alterations in schizophrenia: clinical status and antipsychotic effects. Biol Psychiatry. 2011;70(7):663–71.
70. Flaherty EG, Thompson R, Dubowitz H, Harvey EM, English DJ, Proctor LJ, et al. Adverse childhood experiences and child health in early adolescence. JAMA Pediatr. 2013;167(7):622–9. https://doi.org/10.1001/jamapediatrics.2013.22.
71. Flaherty EG, Thompson R, Litrownik AJ, Zolotor AJ, Dubowitz H, Runyan DK, et al. Adverse childhood exposures and reported child health at age 12. Acad Pediatr. 2009;9(3):150–6. https://doi.org/10.1016/j.acap.2008.11.003.
72. Karlén J, Ludvigsson J, Hedmark M, Faresjö Å, Theodorsson E, Faresjö T. Early psychosocial exposures, hair cortisol levels, and disease risk. Pediatrics. 2015;135:e1450–7. https://doi.org/10.1542/peds.2014-2561.
73. Turesky TK, Jensen SKG, Yu X, Kumar S, Wang Y, Sliva DD, et al. The relationship between biological and psychosocial risk factors and resting-state functional connectivity in 2-month-old Bangladeshi infants: a feasibility and pilot study. Dev Sci. 2019;22:e12841. https://doi.org/10.1111/desc.12841.
74. Xie W, Jensen SKG, Wade M, Kumar S, Westerlund A, Kakon SH, et al. Growth faltering is associated with altered brain functional connectivity and cognitive outcomes in urban Bangladeshi children exposed to early adversity. BMC Med. 2019;17:199. https://doi.org/10.1186/s12916-019-1431-5.
75. Baldwin JR, Arseneault L, Caspi A, Fisher HL, Moffitt TE, Odgers CL, et al. Childhood victimization and inflammation in young adulthood: a genetically sensitive cohort study. Brain Behav Immun. 2018;67:211–7. https://doi.org/10.1016/j.bbi.2017.08.025.
76. Rasmussen LJH, Moffitt TE, Arseneault L, Danese A, Eugen-Olsen J, Fisher HL, et al. Association of Adverse Experiences and Exposure to Violence in Childhood and Adolescence With Inflammatory Burden in Young People. JAMA Pediatr. 2020;174(1):38–47. https://doi.org/10.1001/jamapediatrics.2019.3875.
77. Danese A, Caspi A, Williams B, Ambler A, Sugden K, Mika J, et al. Biological embedding of stress through inflammation processes in childhood. Mol Psychiatry. 2011;16(3):244–6. https://doi.org/10.1038/mp.2010.5.
78. Trotta A, Arseneault L, Danese A, Mondelli V, Rasmussen LJH, Fisher HL. Associations between childhood victimization, inflammatory biomarkers and psychotic phenomena in adolescence: a longitudinal cohort study. Brain Behav Immun. 2021;98:74–85. https://doi.org/10.1016/j.bbi.2021.08.209.
79. Danese A, Baldwin JR. Hidden wounds? Inflammatory links between childhood trauma and psychopathology. Annu Rev Psychol. 2017;68:517–44. https://doi.org/10.1146/annurev-psych-010416-044208.
80. Danese A, Moffitt TE, Harrington H, Milne BJ, Polanczyk G, Pariante CM, et al. Adverse childhood experiences and adult risk factors for age-related disease: depression, inflammation, and clustering of metabolic risk markers. Arch Pediatr Adolesc Med. 2009;163(12):1135–43.
81. Chartier MJ, Walker JR, Naimark B. Separate and cumulative effects of adverse childhood experiences in predicting adult health and health care utilization. Child Abuse Negl. 2010;34:454–64.
82. Sonu S, Post S, Feinglass J. Adverse childhood experiences and the onset of chronic disease in young adulthood. Prev Med. 2019;123:163–70.
83. Rod NH, Bengtsson J, Elsenburg LK, Taylor-Robinson D, Rieckmann A. Hospitalisation patterns among children exposed to childhood adversity: a population-based cohort study of half a million children. Lancet Public Health. 2021;S2468-2667(21):00158-4. https://doi.org/10.1016/S2468-2667(21)00158-4.

84. Narayan AJ, Englund MM, Egeland B. Developmental timing and continuity of exposure to interparental violence and externalizing behavior as prospective predictors of dating violence. Dev Psychopathol. 2013;25(4):973–90. https://doi.org/10.1017/S095457941300031X.
85. Danese A, McEwen BS. Adverse childhood experiences, allostasis, allostatic load, and age-related disease. Physiol Behav. 2012;106:29–39. https://doi.org/10.1016/j.physbeh.2011.08.019.
86. De Kloet ER, Joëls M, Holsboer F. Stress and the brain: from adaptation to disease. Nat Rev Neurosci. 2005;6:463–75. https://doi.org/10.1038/nrn1683.
87. McEwen BS. Stress, adaptation, and disease. Allostasis and allostatic load. Ann N Y Acad Sci. 1998;840:33–44. https://doi.org/10.1111/j.1749-6632.1998.tb09546.x.
88. Chen Y, Baram TZ. Toward understanding how early-life stress reprograms cognitive and emotional brain networks. Neuropsychopharmacology: official publication of the American College of Neuropsychopharmacology, 2016;41(1):197–206. https://doi.org/10.1038/npp.2015.181.
89. Eachus H, Choi MK, Ryu S. The effects of early life stress on the brain and behaviour: insights from zebrafish models. Front Cell Dev Biol. 2021;9:657591. https://doi.org/10.3389/fcell.2021.657591.
90. Dunn EC, Mclaughlin KA, Slopen N, Rosand J, Smoller JW. Developmental timing of child maltreatment and symptoms of depression and suicidal ideation in young adulthood: results from the National Longitudinal Study of Adolescent Health. Depress Anxiety. 2013;30:955–64.
91. Tracy M, Salo M, Slopen N, Udo T, Appleton AA. Trajectories of childhood adversity and the risk of depression in young adulthood: results from the Avon Longitudinal Study of Parents and Children. Depress Anxiety. 2019;36(7):596–606. https://doi.org/10.1002/da.22887.
92. Bartlett JD, Smith S. The role of early care and education in addressing early childhood trauma. Am J Community Psychol. 2019;64(3–4):359–72. https://doi.org/10.1002/ajcp.12380.
93. Howse RB, Calkins SD, Anastopoulos AD, Keane SP, Shelton TL. Regulatory contributors to children's kindergarten achievement. Early Educ Dev. 2003;14:101–19.
94. Huaging QC, Kaiser AP. Behavior problems of pre-school children from low-income families: review of literature. Top Early Child Spec Educ. 2003;23:188–216.
95. Reiland S, Lauterbach D. Effects of trauma and religiosity on self-esteem. Psychol Rep. 2008;102:779–90.
96. Dyregrov A. Educational consequences of loss and trauma. Educ Child Psychol. 2004;21:77–84.
97. Chu AT, Lieberman AF. Clinical implications of traumatic stress from birth to age five. Annu Rev Clin Psychol. 2010;6:469–94. https://doi.org/10.1146/annurev.clinpsy.121208.131204.
98. Dunn EC, Nishimi K, Powers A, Bradley B. Is developmental timing of trauma exposure associated with depressive and post-traumatic stress disorder symptoms in adulthood? J Psychiatr Res. 2017;84:119–27. https://doi.org/10.1016/j.jpsychires.2016.09.004.
99. Kaplow JB, Widom CS. Age of onset of child maltreatment predicts long-term mental health outcomes. J Abnorm Psychol. 2007;116:176–87.
100. Smyke AT, Zeanah CH, Fox NA, Nelson CA, Guthrie D. Placement in foster care enhances quality of attachment among young institutionalized children. Child Dev. 2010;81:212–23. https://doi.org/10.1111/cdev.2010.81.issue-1.
101. McLaughlin KA. Future directions in childhood adversity and youth psychopathology. J Clin Child Adolesc Psychol. 2016;45(3):361–82. https://doi.org/10.1080/15374416.2015.1110823.
102. Miller AB, Machlin L, McLaughlin KA, Sheridan MA. Deprivation and psychopathology in the fragile families study: a 15-year longitudinal investigation. J Child Psychol Psychiatry. 2021;62(4):382–91.
103. Fonagy P, Steele M, Moran G, Steele H, Higgitt A. Measuring the ghost in the nursery: an empirical study of the relation between parents' mental representations of childhood experi-

ences and their infants' security of attachment. J Am Psychoanal Assoc. 1993;41(4):957–89. https://doi.org/10.1177/000306519304100403.

104. Narayan AJ, Lieberman AF, Masten AS. Intergenerational transmission and prevention of adverse childhood experiences (ACEs). Clin Psychol Rev. 2021;85:101997. https://doi.org/10.1016/j.cpr.2021.101997.

105. Atzl VM, Narayan AJ, Rivera LM, Lieberman AF. Adverse childhood experiences and prenatal mental health: type of ACEs and age of maltreatment onset. J Fam Psychol. 2019;33:304–14. https://doi.org/10.1037/fam0000510.

106. Davis EP, Narayan AJ. Pregnancy as a period of risk, adaptation, and resilience for mothers and infants. Dev Psychopathol. 2020 Dec;32(5):1625–39. https://doi.org/10.1017/S0954579420001121.

107. Evans J, Melotti R, Heron J, Ramchandani P, Wiles N, Murray L, Stein A. The timing of maternal depressive symptoms and child cognitive development: a longitudinal study. J Child Psychol Psychiatry. 2012;53(6):632–40. https://doi.org/10.1111/j.1469-7610.2011.02513.x.

108. Kuhlman KR, Boyle CC, Irwin MR, Ganz PA, Crespi CM, Asher A, et al. Childhood maltreatment, psychological resources, and depressive symptoms in women with breast cancer. Child Abuse Negl. 2017;72:360–9. https://doi.org/10.1016/j.chiabu.2017.08.025.

109. Slopen N, Kubzansky LD, McLaughlin KA, Koenen KC. Childhood adversity and inflammatory processes in youth: a prospective study. Psychoneuroendocrinology. 2013;38:188–200. https://doi.org/10.1016/j.psyneuen.2012.05.013.

110. Croft J, Heron J, Teufel C, Cannon M, Wolke D, Thompson A, et al. Association of Trauma Type, age of exposure, and frequency in childhood and adolescence with psychotic experiences in early adulthood. JAMA Psychiat. 2019;76(1):79–86. https://doi.org/10.1001/jamapsychiatry.2018.3155.

111. Foa EB, Meadows EA. Psychosocial treatments for posttraumatic stress disorder: a critical review. Annu Rev Psychol. 1997;48:449–80. https://doi.org/10.1146/annurev.psych.48.1.449.

112. Rothbaum BO, Davis M. Applying learning principles to the treatment of post-trauma reactions. Ann N Y Acad Sci. 2003;1008:112–21. https://doi.org/10.1196/annals.1301.012.

113. Copeland WE, Keeler G, Angold A, Costello EJ. Traumatic events and posttraumatic stress in childhood. Arch Gen Psychiatry. 2007;64(5):577–84. https://doi.org/10.1001/archpsyc.64.5.577.

114. Lieberman A, Chu A, Van Horn P, Harris W. Trauma in early childhood: empirical evidence and clinical implications. Dev Psychopathol. 2011;23(2):397–410. https://doi.org/10.1017/S0954579411000137.

115. Kassam-Adams N. Design, delivery, and evaluation of early interventions for children exposed to acute trauma. Eur J Psychotraumatol. 2014;5 https://doi.org/10.3402/ejpt.v5.22757.

116. Almond D, Currie J, Duque V. Childhood circumstances and adult outcomes: act II. J Econ Lit. 2018;56:1360–446.

117. Huttenlocher PR. Neural plasticity: the effects of environment on the development of the cerebral cortex. Cambridge: Harvard University Press; 2002.

118. Shonkoff JP, Phillips DA. From neurons to neighborhoods: the science of early childhood development. Washington, DC: National Academies Press; 2000.

119. Jichlinski A. Defang ACEs: end toxic stress by developing resilience through physician-community partnerships. Pediatrics. 2017;140(6):e20172869.

120. Kerker BD, Storfer-Isser A, Szilagyi M, Stein RE, Garner AS, O'Connor KG, Hoagwood KE, Horwitz SM. Do pediatricians ask about adverse childhood experiences in pediatric primary care? Acad Pediatr. 2016;16(2):154–60. https://doi.org/10.1016/j.acap.2015.08.002.

121. Gulliver A, Griffiths KM, Christensen H. Perceived barriers and facilitators to mental health help-seeking in young people: a systematic review. BMC Psychiatry. 2010;10:113. https://doi.org/10.1186/1471-244X-10-113.

122. Conn AM, Szilagyi MA, Jee SH, Manly JT, Briggs R, Szilagyi PG. Parental perspectives of screening for adverse childhood experiences in pediatric primary care. Fam Syst Health. 2018;36(1):62–72. https://doi.org/10.1037/fsh0000311.

123. Barnes AJ, Anthony BJ, Karatekin C, Lingras KA, Mercado R, Thompson LA. Identifying adverse childhood experiences in pediatrics to prevent chronic health conditions. Pediatr Res. 2020;87(2):362–70. https://doi.org/10.1038/s41390-019-0613-3.

124. Murphy D, Bartlett J. Childhood adversity screenings are just one part of an effective policy response to childhood trauma. 2019. Available from: https://www.childtrends.org/publications/childhood-adversity-screenings-are-just-one-part-of-an-effective-policy-response-to-childhood-trauma-2. Accessed 30 Oct 2021.
125. Baldwin JR, Reuben A, Newbury J, Danese A. Agreement between prospective and retrospective measures of childhood victimization: a systematic review and meta-analysis. JAMA Psychiat. 2019;76(6):584–93.
126. Abram KM, Teplin LA, Charles DR, Longworth SL, McClelland GM, Dulcan MK. Posttraumatic stress disorder and trauma in youth in juvenile detention. Arch Gen Psychiatry. 2004;61:403–10. https://doi.org/10.1001/archpsyc.61.4.403.
127. Narayan AJ, Ippen CG, Harris WW, Lieberman AF. Protective factors that buffer against the intergenerational transmission of trauma from mothers to young children: a replication study of angels in the nursery. Dev Psychopathol. 2019;31(1):173–87. https://doi.org/10.1017/S0954579418001530.
128. Roberts NP, Kitchiner NJ, Kenardy J, Bisson JI. Systematic review and meta-analysis of multiple-session early interventions following traumatic events. Am J Psychiatry. 2009;166(3):293–301. https://doi.org/10.1176/appi.ajp.2008.08040590.
129. Rose S, Bisson J, Churchill R, Wessely S. Psychological debriefing for preventing post traumatic stress disorder (PTSD). Cochrane Database Syst Rev. 2001.3:CD000560. https://doi.org/10.1002/14651858.CD000560. Update in: Cochrane Database Syst Rev. 2002;2:CD000560.
130. Berkowitz SJ, Stover CS, Marans SR. The Child and Family Traumatic Stress Intervention: secondary prevention for youth at risk of developing PTSD. J Child Psychol Psychiatry. 2011;52(6):676–85. https://doi.org/10.1111/j.1469-7610.2010.02321.x.
131. Kramer DN, Landolt MA. Characteristics and efficacy of early psychological interventions in children and adolescents after single trauma: a meta-analysis. Eur J Psychotraumatol. 2011;2 https://doi.org/10.3402/ejpt.v2i0.7858.
132. Bartlett JD, Smith S., Bringewat E. Helping young children who have experienced trauma: policies and strategies for early care and education. 2017. Available from: https://www.childtrends.org/wp-content/uploads/2017/04/2017-19ECETrauma.pdf. Accessed 30 Oct 2021.
133. Lieberman AF, Ghosh Ippen C, Van Horn P. Don't hit my mommy: a manual for child-parent psychotherapy with young children exposed to violence and other trauma. 2nd ed. Washington, DC: Zero to Three; 2015.
134. Sperlich M, Seng J. Survivor moms: women's stories of birthing, mothering, and healing after sexual abuse. Eugene: Motherbaby Press; 2008.
135. La Greca AM, Silverman WK, Lochman JE. Moving beyond efficacy and effectiveness in child and adolescent intervention research. J Consult Clin Psychol. 2009;77(3):373–82. https://doi.org/10.1037/a0015954.
136. Peltonen K, Punamäki RL. Preventive interventions among children exposed to trauma of armed conflict: a literature review. Aggress Behav. 2010;36(2):95–116.
137. Rolfsnes ES, Idsoe T. School-based intervention programs for PTSD symptoms: a review and meta-analysis. J Trauma Stress. 2011;24(2):155–65.
138. Kuhlman KR, Robles TF, Bower JE, Carroll JE. Screening for childhood adversity: the what and when of identifying individuals at risk for lifespan health disparities. J Behav Med. 2018;41(4):516–27.
139. Asmussen K, Fischer F, Drayton E., T. McBride. Adverse childhood experiences: what we know, what we don't know, and what should happen next. 2020. Available from: https://www.eif.org.uk/report/adverse-childhood-experiences-what-we-know-what-we-dont-know-and-what-should-happen-next. Accessed 31 Oct 2021.
140. Cox JL, Holden JM, Sagovsky R. Detection of postnatal depression. Development of the 10-item Edinburgh Postnatal Depression Scale. Br J Psychiatry. 1987;150:782–6. https://doi.org/10.1192/bjp.150.6.782.
141. Durlak JA, Weissberg RP, Dymnicki AB, Taylor RD, Schellinger KB. The impact of enhancing students' social and emotional learning: a meta-analysis of school-based universal interventions. Child Dev. 2011;82(1):405–32.

142. Lieberman AF, Ghosh Ippen C, Horn PVAN. Child-parent psychotherapy: 6-month follow-up of a randomized controlled trial. J Am Acad Child Adolesc Psychiatry. 2006;45(8):913–8. https://doi.org/10.1097/01.chi.0000222784.03735.92.
143. Rosenblum K, Lawler J, Alfafara E, Miller N, Schuster M, Muzik M. Improving maternal representations in high-risk mothers: a randomized, controlled trial of the Mom Power parenting intervention. Child Psychiatry Hum Dev. 2018;49(3):372–84.
144. Rosenblum KL, Muzik M, Morelen DM, Alfafara EA, Miller NM, et al. A community-based randomized controlled trial of Mom Power parenting intervention for mothers with interpersonal trauma histories and their young children. Arch Womens Ment Health. 2017;20(5):673–86.
145. Deblinger E, Mannarino AP, Cohen JA, Steer RA. A follow-up study of a multisite, randomized, controlled trial for children with sexual abuse-related PTSD symptoms. J Am Acad Child Adolesc Psychiatry. 2006;45(12):1474–84.
146. National Institute for Health and Care Excellence. Post-traumatic stress disorder (NICE guideline NG116). 2018. Available from: https://www.nice.org.uk/guidance/ng116. Accessed 31 Oct 2021.
147. Smith P, Dalgleish T, Meiser-Stedman R. Practitioner review: posttraumatic stress disorder and its treatment in children and adolescents. J Child Psychol Psychiatry. 2019;60:500–15. https://doi.org/10.1111/jcpp.12983.
148. Sweeney A, Taggart D. (Mis)understanding trauma-informed approaches in mental health. J Ment Health. 2018;27(5):383–7. https://doi.org/10.1080/09638237.2018.1520973.
149. Elliott DE, Bjelajac P, Fallot RD, Markoff LS, Reed BG. Trauma-informed or trauma-denied: principles and implementation of trauma-informed services for women. J Community Psychol. 2005;33(4):461–77.
150. World Health Organization (WHO) Nurturing care for early childhood development. 2018. Available from: https://apps.who.int/iris/bitstream/handle/10665/272603/9789241514064-eng.pdf. Accessed 31 Oct 2021.
151. Garg A, Byhoff E, Wexler MG. Implementation considerations for social determinants of health screening and referral interventions. JAMA Netw Open. 2020;3:e200693.
152. Ochoa ER Jr, Nash C. Community engagement and its impact on child health disparities: building blocks, examples, and resources. Pediatrics. 2009;124(suppl 3):S237–45.
153. Britto PR, Lye SJ, Proulx K, Yousafzai AK, Matthews SG, Vaivada T, et al. Nurturing care: promoting early childhood development. Lancet. 2017;389(10064):91–102. https://doi.org/10.1016/S0140-6736(16)31390-3.

Promoting Positive Parenting to Prevent Mental Health Problems

6

Rosalinda Cassibba and Gabrielle Coppola

6.1 Introduction

Based on evidence from multiple disciplines, frequently collected in large retrospective studies [1 for a review] or longitudinal ones following developmental trajectories across decades [2], it has become increasingly clear that the origins of many mental health problems lie in childhood. Mental well-being in childhood is considered a prerequisite for a healthy psychological development, which allows the individual to build well-functioning social relationships, to learn and achieve adequate levels of personal autonomy, to enjoy good physical health and to be productive for the society [3].

An increasing number of studies indicate that the first signals of psychological problems can appear as early as infancy and toddlerhood. Some difficulties tend to show up in specific ages, as a signal that there might be a failure in succeeding with the main developmental task of that period. For example, during the first years of life, attachment disorders characterized by difficulties in parent–child bond, poor emotion regulation and difficulties in social development might occur in infants and young children. Most children with attachment disorders have had severe problems in their early relationships. They may have been physically or emotionally abused or neglected by their parents; some have experienced inadequate care in out-of-home placement or have had multiple traumatic losses or changes in their primary caregiver.

In early childhood, when the achievement of self-regulation is the main developmental challenge, behaviour problems appear to be the most common mental health

R. Cassibba (✉) · G. Coppola
Department of Educational Sciences, Psychology, Communication,
University of Bari Aldo Moro, Bari, Italy
e-mail: rosalinda.cassibba@uniba.it; gabrielle.coppola@uniba.it

M. Colizzi, M. Ruggeri (eds.), *Prevention in Mental Health*,
https://doi.org/10.1007/978-3-030-97906-5_6

problem affecting 5–10% of children aged 4–6. While these difficulties may be transient for some children, for others they persist and increase the likelihood of a wide range of negative outcomes including school failure, antisocial behaviour, relationship difficulties and physical and mental issues. In late childhood, between 12 and 18 years of age, mental and behavioural problems caused by the use of psychoactive substances can arise. In many cases, addictions can take root early and compromise life.

Many factors can impact child's and adolescent's mental health: these so-called risk factors interfere with the quality of the individuals' adaptation and functioning and might increase the likelihood to develop psychopathology. Instead, protective factors buffer the negative effects of the exposure to risky conditions and enhance coping strategies and resilience in the face of adversities. Risk and protective factors should not be conceived as causal ones, but as conditions that might increase or decrease the probability to develop a clinical condition: the transactional model proposed by developmental psychopathology [4, 5] is a useful theoretical framework to understand their action—risky developmental pathways can be explained as a complex and dynamic interplay of risk and protective factors related both to the child and to caregiving environment, and at any point, new risk conditions may worsen previous ones in a so-called cascade effect, and, at the same time, intervening protective conditions may compensate pre-existent conditions of disadvantage. As such, psychopathology is the result of a complex and dynamic interplay of multiple factors acting in a developing organism [6].

Risk and protective factors can belong to the child's biology (i.e. temperament, sex, family aggregation for mental disorders); other factors might be related to his/her psychological functioning (i.e. age-related, emotional or social) or to the environmental context, both the proximal one, as that related to the parents and family functioning, and the distal one (i.e. community context, socio-economic status, availability of services, lifestyles). The co-occurrence of more risk or protective factors can increase or decrease the likelihood of resilience or risk of maladaptive outcomes [7].

Research aimed at identifying early precursors of psychopathological issues and the risk factors associated with their stability highlights that a central role is played by factors related to the affective relationship with the primary caregivers such as family disruption, poor couple functioning, parenting distress, maternal psychopathology and lack of social support. As such, parenting can be conceptualized as a crucial protective or risk factor in the development of psychopathology [i.e. 1, 7–9].

Crucially, parenting is not stable but indeed susceptible to change: this means that in the presence of dysfunctional parenting which might put at risk the infant's developmental outcomes, attempts to enhance parenting can be effective, especially when intervening at a very early stage, when the infants' bio-behavioural systems are developing. Early interventions to prevent or support dysfunctional parenting are therefore privileged means to prevent maladaptive developmental outcomes and prevent mental health issues in childhood and at later ages. It becomes clear why early interventions to support parenting have such tremendous clinical and economic implications, as they allow to reduce the burden placed on public health services, social and education systems related to the treatment of mental issues among children and youth. The priority of investing in primary prevention programmes is now reflected across a number of policy guidelines and best practices, given the impact that this kind of preventive action can have [10].

In light of the many reasons supporting the interest to implement preventive programmes, the present chapter will review the main evidenced-based programmes to promote positive parenting. After a brief introduction to the concept of parenting, we will present the main intervention programmes to support parents' skills in infancy up to preschool age, for which sufficient evidence meeting the standards of evidence is thus far available [11].

6.2   The Dimensions of Parenting

Parenting is not easy to define as it refers to a very wide construct. Independently of the theoretical framework and the areas of application, this label is used to refer to the caregivers' fundamental function of supporting the child's physical, emotional, social and cognitive development. This role implies a complete dependency of the infant on the caregiver who provides primary care and support for his/her development; therefore parenting is typically characterized by the asymmetry of roles between the caregiver and the child, due to disparities in responsibility, accessibility to resources and knowledge, competences and duties [12].

Bornstein (1995) distinguishes different aspects of parenting: the *nurturant* and the *material caregiving*, which have to do with the parents' ability to meet the biological, physical and health needs of children, as well as to provide an adequate organization *and arrangement of the* child's physical world (i.e. toys, books, tools). The *didactic and social caregiving* satisfy the child's psychological needs: the first refers to the strategies parents use to stimulate children to engage, understand the environment and learn from their experiences and social interactions, while *social caregiving* refers to meeting the child's socio-emotional needs, through engaging emotionally in interpersonal exchanges and supporting the child to organize and regulate affect and emotions, in order to enjoy socio-emotional relationships and engage appropriately in them [13]. Following by we will attempt to focus on two main dimensions of parenting, both crucial for child development and therefore targeted by diverse intervention protocols.

6.2.1   The Affective Dimension of Parenting

Attachment theory and research developed from John Bowlby's speculations (1969) has focused mainly on the affective dimension of parenting, and has provided the main evidence of the significance of the affective relationship with caregiver for the child's healthy socio-emotional development and its devastating and disorganizing effect when it has a dysfunctional quality [14]. According to attachment theory, significant adults are perceived as wiser and stronger by the infant, and they act as "secure bases" from which the infant can departure to explore the physical and social world. This attachment figure is a safe haven to return in order to receive support, comfort in times of needs and to share experiences and feelings. This balance between the attachment and exploration systems is biologically based, but because this balance can work properly and lead to a healthy development, the adult is expected to be sensitive and responsive, that is, to perceive the infant's signals and needs, interpret them appropriately and respond to them in an adequate and contingent manner [15, 16]. When this happens, the infant will develop eagerness and pleasure to explore and learn from the physical and social world, thanks to the confidence of the availability of the caregiver in times of need, which over time will become self-confidence and self-efficacy. Over time, this virtuous circle promotes increasing levels of autonomy and enhances the opportunity for the child to develop skills and acquire knowledge: these are the essential features of attachment security and explain why security is associated with adaptive developmental outcomes in many domains, such as socio-emotional, socio-cognitive and communicative-linguistic [17, for a review].

Indeed, in the presence of parental insensitivity, such as the cases of dysfunctional and vulnerable parenting, the infant can develop an imbalance between exploration and attachment which leads to an insecure attachment pattern, or even to a collapse of the attachment system, as in the case of disorganized attachment: consistent evidence has shown that insecure attachment is a risk factor and disorganized attachment an early precursor of later psychopathological outcomes [8, 9].

During the lifespan, this relational process accommodates constantly, as a function of the caregivers' protection, on one side, and the offspring's increasing need of autonomy and exploration, on the other. The infant's Self develops within this process, in which the caregiver supports the infant's development by being emotionally and physically available [18], and, at the same time, structuring the environment through "sensitive discipline" strategies [19]. Indeed, besides the affective function of parenting, the regulatory one is equally important: this dimension and its developmental implications will be analysed in the next section.

6.2.2 The Regulatory Dimension of Parenting

Self-regulation is defined as the ability to act in accordance with social norms and rules and to regulate accordingly one's behaviour and emotional reactions [20]. This appears to be the main developmental task during the first years of life, as children transition from external regulation (or co-regulation) to the internalization of caregivers' norms, starting from the third year on, to be capable of complying with external "Dos" and "Don'ts" type of requests and to be able to delay on request, also in the absence of adult's monitoring.

There is no doubt that this developmental pathway is the result of a complex interplay between the child's neurobiology and caregiving environment: on one side, through early co-regulation, it supports the organization of the infants' neurobiological systems related to attachment, affiliation, arousal, stress and emotions.

On the other side, neurobiology defines the threshold of infants' sensitivity to parental influences, making them differentially susceptible to these influences [21].

With this complex picture in mind and without minimizing the importance of child's neurobiology and temperamental contribution to this developmental outcome (i.e. fearfulness, surgency, effortful control, callous-unemotional trait, sensitivity just to quote some of the temperamental traits mostly related to the development of self-regulation), in the present section, we will briefly focus on parental caregiving behaviours and practices that may promote self-regulation.

Sensitive and responsive parenting has been shown to predict effective self-regulation and prevent dysregulation issues [22–24]. Depending on their children's age, effective parental strategies vary from physical contact to provide comfort at earlier ages to more distal ways of interaction, though which the parent scaffolds the emerging child's regulatory skill: through verbal dialogues, the caregiver labels and validates the child's experience, shares meaning of what is going on and at the same time provides appropriate support should the child's own regulatory or problem-solving resources prove inadequate to the task [2, 25].

To promote adequate self-regulation, parental behaviour includes also the ability to set limits for appropriate child behaviour and/or misbehaviour [18]. These qualities may be observed in the parent's establishing rules and requesting or demanding compliance with them: this typically occurs in the *Do* contexts which require the child to engage in an unpleasant and/or tedious activity, and in the *Don't* contexts, which involve suppressing a behaviour which will lead to a pleasant result [20]. Limit-letting also involves proactive interventions to protect the child from dangers in a firm and not dysregulated matter, as parents are essential guides for children to learn about potential dangers in their environments [18, 26].

When such parental functions fail, there is an increased risk for the child to develop dysregulation problems, especially externalizing ones, such as conduct disorder (CD), oppositional defiant disorder (ODD) and attention-deficit hyperactivity disorder (ADHD) [27]. Aetiological mechanisms for these disorders are best explained by multifactorial processes in which biological, neurodevelopmental, temperamental, parental and other proximal and distal ecological factors might concur. Restricting the focus to the parental domain, which is the focus of the present sections, specific traits have been shown to increase the risk for child's externalizing dysregulated behaviour although bidirectional and reciprocal influences have also been supported [28, 29]. Among the parental dysfunctional behaviours increasing the risk for dysregulated externalizing problems, there is the combination of high levels of restrictive control, high levels of negativity and low levels of warmth, well identified as an authoritative parenting style [29], harsh behaviour [30] and reactive hostility expressed verbally and physically, which might lead into physical punishment [31]. Also lack of supervision and manipulative, coercive, hyper-protective and anxious parenting behaviours have been shown to be predictive of externalizing problems [21, for a review].

In conclusion, the conjunction of the affective and regulatory functions of parenting as the condition promoting the most effective developmental outcomes finds indirect empirical support in research testing whether attachment security is related to self-regulation. In fact, attachment security and self-regulation are the main developmental outcomes of each of the parental functions described above. Meta-analytic findings show that attachment security is related to positive and adaptive emotion regulation strategies [32], while a massive longitudinal study over a period of 10 years has shown that early attachment predicted emotion regulation in pre-school age, which was related to broader measures of behavioural and socio-emotional regulation in preadolescence [20].

It becomes clear, therefore, why identifying early parental vulnerabilities and risk conditions in order to target them through effective intervention programmes is equivalent to promoting a positive adaptation and development for the child and the future adult.

6.3 Types of Intervention

There is a wide range of intervention to support parenting skills, which vary according to the parental dimension on which they intervene, the duration, the theoretical framework and the evidence available thus supporting their efficacy. Stewart-Brown and Schrader-McMillan (2011) examined 52 systematic reviews of interventions to promote parenting, and organized the results according to their type and efficacy as follows: (a) antenatal parent programmes (focused on the transition to parenthood, relationship issues and preparation for new roles) and perinatal maternal mental health programmes (skin-to-skin contact, kangaroo care, advice on infant capabilities and prevention, infant massage, prevention identification and treatment of maternal depression, etc.); (b) parenting support programmes in infancy and early years focused on enhancing caregiver sensitivity and infant attachment security (they covered a wide range of attachment-based interventions including one-to-one and group-based programmes, parent training, home visiting, parent-infant psycho-therapy, etc.); (c) parenting programmes focused on children's behaviour aimed at improving the capacity of parents to support their children's behavioural and emotional development (these programmes are supported by a range of theoretical approaches, often combined (social learning, cognitive behavioural training and relationship-based education are the most common)); and (d) parenting support for highest risk groups in which parents suffer from mental illness or alcohol or drug abuse and parents that have already abused their children. In these cases, interventions are aimed to reduce some of the most hurtful effects on the psychological health of children and abuse escalation or recurrence [33].

In the following sections, we will focus particularly on some examples of intervention programmes belonging respectively to the (b) group, which aim at supporting especially the affective function of parenting, and from the (c) group, which target the regulatory function of parenting in order to prevent externalizing disorders among the offspring.

The standards of *evidence-based* interventions guided our selection: according to these standards, intervention programmes are required to be efficacious, which refers to the benefits the programme is able to produce in controlled and optimal conditions; the next step (effectiveness) requires the test in the real world, taking into account the multiple variations that can occur and that might moderate the benefits, in face of a manualized and standardized procedure to release the intervention. As to the third step, scale-up and dissemination must be possible, in order to make an impact on the entire population, in terms of enhancing health, education and well-being on a large scale, through community interventions [11]. Although the process from translational research to population impact has been now conceptualized as a recursive and circular process, with reciprocal influences between the three steps [34], we believe that the programmes described below have made significant advances through these three steps, and are worthy to be illustrated.

6.3.1 Video-Feedback Interventions and Their Efficacy

Interventions that use video-feedback methods as a mean to promote positive parenting are getting widespread over time. These interventions typically involve the video recording of parent-child interactions in different situations (e.g. playing together, cuddles, mealtimes, bath time) which are then reviewed with an intervenor to highlight episodes of positive interaction. Video-feedback intervention can take different several forms; the two most often used are known as Video Interaction Guidance (VIG) [35–37] and Video-feedback Intervention to promote Positive Parenting (VIPP). Although both are very intriguing, we will focus mainly on the second, as there are more empirical evidence supporting its efficacy.

Most video-feedback research is based on trials of the Leiden *VIPP* (Video-feedback Intervention to promote Positive Parenting), an evidence-based intervention for enhancing parental sensitivity and security [19]. Therefore, the intervention is focused on enhancing the parents' ability to orient and perceive the infant's non-verbal and emotional signals. This kind of work allows to interpret the signals in a more accurate way and avoid distortions due to one's own personal emotions: parents are guided to empathize with the child's needs and desires, in order to be able to easily select the appropriate reaction.

The VIPP protocol is a brief, home-based intervention involving six visits aimed at promoting positive parent-child relationships. There are specific themes for each session, and guidelines for each session are described in a detailed protocol. At each visit, the intervenor preliminary identifies and selects video fragments functional to address the theme of each session, accompanied with specific feedback to prompt the caregiver to observe and reflect on the proposed theme (i.e. differentiate and identify attachment and exploration signals, emotional labelling, emotional attunement, etc.). While watching the video clips with the mother, the intervenor provides positive feedback for effective parental behaviours and prompts the parent to find an alternative in the face of unsuccessful behaviours or for managing difficult behaviour. The rationale is that each parent is the best expert of his/her child, and therefore the identification of appropriate behaviours should result from the parent's insight, instead of being suggested by the intervenor, who has the role to guide the caregivers' reflective thinking. The ultimate goal is to support the parent in perceiving and interpreting their child's behaviour, emotions and signals, and to respond to them in a sensitive way. Feedbacks are also combined with brochures on sensitive responding in daily situations.

Attachment theory has further highlighted that the behaviours parents display in interaction with the infant are guided and filtered by internal working models [25]: these representations are built upon repeated experiences of interaction with the attachment figures and reflect the degree of security and confidence within intimate relationships. These representations accomplish a very important adaptive function by providing a personal framework to regulate behaviour, emotions and expectations both in present relationships and as new ones are constructed [38].

These internal working models based on one's personal affective history drive the intergenerational transmission of attachment and parenting styles [39]. It has been shown, in fact, that it is very likely that parents will re-experience with the infant the interactive and communicative patterns that they have experienced with their own caregivers in the past [38, 39]. Given the importance of the internal working models in regulating parental behaviours, intervention efforts have also been directed at the representational level. With this respect, the *VIPP-R* represents a valid alternative intervention modality which associates with the video-feedback strategy in targeting the behavioural dimension of parenting, offering additional discussions on parental attachment representations, in order to promote a reorganization of mental representations towards security with subsequent behavioural changes. In this intervention modality, the video feedback and brochures used in the VIPP are followed by discussions about the parent's relationship experiences in her own childhood. Each intervention session starts with video feedback and continues with the discussion part, stimulated by specific prompt material and addressing a specific attachment relevant topic (i.e. anxiety for separation from attachment figures, autonomy from one's own parents, continuity and discontinuity with the past). This intervention modality is particularly relevant for parents with insecure representations of attachment; in these cases, in fact, discussions about past and present attachments may allow mothers to reconsider their childhood experiences and look into the links between those past experiences and the current relationship with their child.

As a further intervention modality, the VIPP has been combined with an additional focus on sensitive discipline (*VIPP-SD*); this alternative programme has been developed to support parents who have to deal with challenging child problem behaviours. This intervention programme is particularly suitable for parents dealing with toddlers' behavioural issues, mainly with an externalizing quality (i.e. tantrums, aggressive, disruptive, oppositional behaviours). Indeed, these children are particularly at risk to develop an insecure attachment relationship in the presence of insensitive parents [40]. The VIPP-SD is based on the integration of attachment theory [14] and coercion theory [41], an extension of social learning theory [42], which focuses on the cycle whereby parents unintentionally reinforce their child's difficult behaviours, which generates a negative reaction in the parent and so on, either the child or parent gives in. For coercion theory, harsh discipline strategies give rise to exchanges that reinforce and increase aggressive and disruptive behaviour. VIPP-SD intervention seeks to improve caregivers' ability to deal with their children's behaviour by praising/rewarding positive behaviour, setting appropriate limits and applying consistent consequences for undesirable or unwanted behaviour. In this intervention modality, the sessions follow the standard VIPP procedure of filming, reviewing, commenting and discussing video fragments with the mother; however, additional guidelines and intervention themes are added for the discipline part of the intervention. Four themes are specific of VIPP-SD: (a) inductive discipline and distraction as non-coercive responses to difficult child behaviour, (b) praising the child for positive behaviour and ignoring negative attention seeking, (c) the use of sensitive time-out to de-escalate temper tantrums and (d) empathy with the child in consistent discipline and clear limit setting [19].

VIPP protocols have been gone through more than two decades of validation studies, involving over time samples with diverse cultural backgrounds and risk conditions related to both the child, such as prematurity, atopic dermatitis, autism, intellectual disability, international adoption and externalizing problems, and the parents, as insecure attachment representations, harsh discipline, low SES status, eating disorders, social isolation, maltreatment and ethnic minority [43]. Short- and long-term effects have been widely reported, related to increasing parental sensitivity, infant's attachment security and a variety of other positive indicators of child functioning [i.e. 43–45 for a complete review]. Restricting the focus to the VIPP-SD protocol, which is currently released by training courses and thus widely disseminated, recent meta-analytic evidence supports the efficacy of the protocol in enhancing parental sensitivity and positive child outcomes [43]. Overall, we feel confident in stating that based on the state of art of the literature, the VIPP protocol is on a good way to become a community-based tool: currently, in fact, dissemination is promoted through training courses organized in different countries, and this protocol has been included in the list of the Home Visiting Evidence of Effectiveness (HomVEE) of the US Department of Health and Human Services (HHS).

6.3.2 Parent Training Programmes and Their Efficacy

By parent training (PT) or parent management training (PMT), we refer to a wide group of protocols mainly inspired to the cognitive behavioural theoretical perspective. Starting from the seventies, based on behavioural and social learning principles, it became clear that not only trained therapists could promote children's behaviour change, but parents too could be agents of change, leading to a growing understanding of how parents contribute to their children's adaptive or maladaptive behaviours [46]. As such, behavioural problems started to be no longer conceived as individual but relational issues, originated from dysfunctional learning processes within the caregiving environment, such as modelling or reinforcement.

Since then, PT programmes are delivered in different forms (e.g. clinic-based therapy, community-based group sessions, individual home visits). Moreover, PT is now widely used to support parenting in the presence of many different at-risk conditions, besides externalizing problems, such as ADHD, autistic spectrum disorders, mood disorders and many different psychosocial risk conditions [47, 48].

Besides the variety of the programmes [e.g. 49, for a review], the main ingredients of these programmes are parents' active involvement and learning; manualized and standardized protocols; highly focused and limited in time interventions, according to the lesson that "less is more"; and the use of cognitive behavioural techniques such modelling, shaping, role playing, video feedback and homework assignments to train parents to use alternative techniques to regulate child's behaviours. Group discussions prompted by ad hoc materials with a psycho-educational approach are also very frequent, in order to teach parents important concepts of developmental psychology as well as effective problem-solving skills and alternative discipline strategies that may reduce the use of harsh discipline practices.

Following Lambruschi and colleagues [47], we will illustrate the main steps of PT intervention which are commonly shared by the different programmes. Firstly, a particular attention should be devoted to the group composition: usually, it should include parents going through the same kind of management issues with children more or less of the same age—this will increase the likelihood that parents will comply and experience alliance in the group. Both parents are encouraged to participate in order to promote between the two a shared view of the child and alliance in the use of alternative caregiving and discipline strategies; usually, groups should not exceed five or six couples of parents.

As to the first phase of the work, the intervenor aims at favouring a full understanding of the child's functioning; this includes also a description of the disorder, such as the deficits in executive functions, impulsiveness and difficulties in waiting and delaying gratification. At the same time, parents are encouraged to recoup and value the positive aspect of their children, so to promote an integrated and differentiated mental representation of the child, in which the disorder is no longer excessively emphasized, with the remaining parts of the child put on the ground. This kind of work implies "mentalizing in third person" [30 , p. 119], that is, assuming the child's mental perspective and reflecting on his/her mental states [50]: this reflective function has been shown to be such an important protective factor for mental health and parenting [51].

The next step is the contextual and operational redefinition of the child's problematic behaviours: parents are guided to understand that problematic behaviours are usually stabilized within a specific context because of their successfulness for the child in reaching advantages (i.e. avoiding unpleasant tasks and requests, obtaining benefits, receiving others' attention). By teaching parents the principles of functional analyses, parents learn to identify the antecedents of problematic behaviours (the so-called *A*s), describe frequency and intensity of the problematic behaviour (the so-called *B*s) and focus on the consequences that somewhat maintain the dysfunctional behaviour (the so-called *C*s). The assignment of A-B-C homework helps parents to enhance their observational and reflective skills in the home context and highlight mechanisms regulating dysfunctional behaviours; also, by learning to contextualize bad behaviour, parents are supported to reduce their generalizations ("My child *always* misbehaves!"), which inevitably pave the way to dysfunctional self-perceptions, such as low-self efficacy and learned helpless.

By learning to contextualize and operationalize problematic behaviours, parents discover the ways to act on these dysfunctional mechanisms. Positive parental practices are then promoted by teaching parents to prevent and reorganize the antecedents (i.e. preventing arousing situations, distracting the child) and master the consequences (i.e. by ignoring undesired behaviours, token economy, differential reinforcement, etc.). The definition of a caregiving context based on new rules might also be made explicit through a behavioural contract between parents and child, which helps both parts to feel in charge of the desired change.

As a last possible step, parents are supported to reflect on their own mental states, beliefs and emotions and eventually find their origin in past childhood experiences with their own significant others: this is what the authors label as "mentalizing in first person" [47 , p. 128]. This kind of reflective work helps parents to regulate more effectively their emotional reactions during challenging interaction with the child, reorganize their beliefs and expectations so to meet more realistically the child functioning, enjoy positive interaction with the child and develop self-efficacy in managing difficult caregiving situations.

There is no doubt that parent training can be defined as an evidence-based intervention, as decades of empirical findings support efficacy in randomized controlled trials, effectiveness, as it has been tested across a variety of different samples for clinical conditions and cultural background and dissemination, as it appears thus far to be world-widely used. Restricting the focus to the prevention and treatment of externalizing disorders, consistent meta-analytic findings support the efficacy of these programmes in reducing the child's externalizing problems, especially disruptive behaviours, compared to waitlist control conditions, although the efficacy is moderated by the study design [52–54]. Review and meta-analytic evidence also supports the positive impact on parental dimensions, as it decreases parental stress, improves perceptions and mental health indicators and enhances positive parent-child relationship [55, 56].

Meta-analytic evidence shows that PT programmes need to be highly focused on both the affective and regulatory dimensions of parenting, instead of other dimensions, in order to be highly effective: Kaminski and colleagues (2008), in fact, report that targeting positive parent-child interactions and emotional communication skills, teaching parents to use time out and consistent discipline and requiring them to practice new skills with their children appear to be the most effective. Conversely, shifting the focus to other goals, such as teaching parents to promote children's cognitive, academic or social skills, might lead to reduced efficacy [46].

Besides strategies and focuses, other factors moderating the effectiveness of parent training programmes are child's genetic and temperamental predisposition, such as differential susceptibility and emotional reactivity [57, 58], together with low parental education, occupation and family income, more severe pretreatment child behaviour symptoms and maternal psychopathology [59], as a confirmation that self-regulation depends on a complex interplay between individual and environmental factors.

It is worthy to cite briefly that there is recent interest to promote dissemination through innovative parent training programmes in order to increase PT accessibility and use and make them community-based tools. One example is self-directed (SD) parenting interventions, which provide parents with the materials necessary to teach behavioural strategies to themselves, at home and at the most convenient time to them, through a variety of formats (e.g. manual, Internet, videotape, DVD). Tarver and colleagues' [60] meta-analysis supports the effectiveness of SD PT programmes, as they seem to reduce child's externalizing problems, and improve parental behaviour, mood and self-efficacy. As to a second example of dissemination, meta-analytic findings also support online parent programmes, with significant effects on children's behavioural and emotional problems and parental mental health problems [61].

In conclusion, despite scholars auspicate for the future a convergence of methodological choices in order to facilitate meta-analytic syntheses, such as blinded measures, randomized control trials and standardized protocols, there is no doubt about the state of art of the literature supporting thus far the usefulness of these programmes to enhance vulnerable parenting.

6.4 Conclusions

The present chapter meant to highlight the importance of positive parenting for the child's healthy functioning and development. The commons rationale of these interventions is seeking not only to reduce the impact of risk factors but also to empower the protective factors, by reinforcing the parenting role. Indeed, for many years, scholars have been investigating how the family ecology and the quality of parenting shape the child's well-being; nowadays, research has become more translational, as it has shifted to the identification of the resources and capabilities that parents should bring into the parenting task and their multiple needs for support [62].

Researchers have given a great contribution to test the efficacy and effectiveness of these intervention programmes, as well as professionals and policy makers to deliver the best evidence-based programmes aimed at supporting parents [63–65]. Both groups of interventions to which we devoted attention in the chapter are good examples of how the standards of evidence can be met, thanks to the implementation of manualized and standardized protocols, and appropriate research designs to test their efficacy, based on randomized control trials with control group and follow-up assessments [11, 34].

Following by are a few recommendations that can support the translational research of preventive intervention programmes to support parenting and child's positive development. Firstly, it is important to guarantee the coherence between theory and application, with respect to targets and outcomes: both programmes presented in the chapter underwent multiple empirical tests across multiple risk conditions, which allowed to highlight their differential effects as a function of both child and parents' conditions.

As to a second recommendation, one key component is the quality of the relationship between the intervenor and the parent, as the first act as an attachment figure and a secure base for the second, from whom the parent can depart to explore one personal distressing themes [66]. Indeed, interventions to support parenting aim at empowering fragile parents' social network, so that they can rely also on relational resources to cope with difficulties. In such cases, the intervenors might encounter some difficulties when relating with difficult parents and try to build alliance with them, and therefore adequate training and supervision of the intervenors is of fundamental importance to guarantee successful outcomes. Supervision might also include the exploration of one's own emotional reactions prompted by those difficult parents, in order to help intervenors to become aware of their own relational patterns.

In conclusion, we hope to raise awareness of how important are the early phase of life for healthy human development and the investment in this early stage of life in order to prevent and treat early risk conditions. Early prevention will have not only immediate psychological benefits for parents and children but also long-term ones, in terms of reducing the economic, social and educational burden of treating maladaptive youth and adults.

References

1. Asmundson JG, Afifi TO. Adverse childhood experiences using evidence to advance research, practice, policy, and prevention. Elsevier Science, London: Academic Press; 2020.
2. Sroufe LA, Egelend B, Carlson EA, Collins WA. The development of the person. The Minnesota study of risk and adaptation from birth to adulthood. New York: Guilford Press; 2006.
3. Dawes A, et al. Child and adolescent mental health. In: Foster D, Freeman M, Pillay Y, editors. Mental health policy issues for South Africa. Cape Town: Multimedia Publications; 1997.
4. Cicchetti DE, Cohen DJ. Developmental psychopathology. Theory and methods, vol. 1. New York: Wiley; 1995.
5. Sameroff AJ, Fiese BH. Models of development and developmental risk. In: Zeanah C, editor. Handbook of infant mental health. 2nd ed. New York: Guilford Press; 2000. p. 3–19.
6. Drabick DA, Kendall PC. Developmental psychopathology and the diagnosis of mental health problems among youth. Clin Psychol Sci Pract. 2010;17(4):272–80.
7. Zeanah C. Handbook of infant mental health. 4th ed. New York: Guilford Press; 2019.
8. DeKlyen M, Greenberg MT. Attachment and psychopathology in childhood. In: Cassidy J, Shaver PH, editors. Handbook of attachment. Theory, research and clinical applications. New York: Guilford Press; 2017. p. 637–65.
9. Lyons-Ruth K, Jacobwitz D. Attachment disorganization: genetic factors, parenting contexts, and developmental transformation from infancy to adulthood. In: Cassidy J, Shaver PH, editors. Handbook of attachment. Theory, research and clinical applications. New York: Guilford Press; 2017. p. 666–97.
10. Heckman JJ, Masterov DV. The productivity agreement for investing in young children. Appl Econ Perspect Policy. 2007;29:446–93.
11. Flay BR, Biglan A, Boruch RF, Castro FG, Gottfredson D, Kellam S, Mościcki EM, Schinke S, Valentine JC, Ji P. Standards of evidence: criteria for efficacy, effectiveness and dissemination. Prev Sci. 2005;6(3):151–75.
12. Lambruschi F, Lionetti F. La genitorialità. Strumenti di valutazione e interventi di sostegno. Roma: Carocci Editore; 2015.
13. Bornstein MH, editor. Handbook of parenting. Mahwah: Lawrence Erlbaum Associates; 1995.
14. Bowlby J. Attachment and loss, Attachment, vol. 1. New York: Penguin Books; 1969.
15. Ainsworth MD, S., Blehar M. C., Waters E., Wall S. Patterns of attachment. A psychological study of the strange situation. Hillsdale, NJ: Laureance Erlbaum; 1978.

16. Powell B, Cooper G, Hoffman K, Marvin B. The circle of security intervention. Enhancing attachment in early parent-child relationship. New York: Guilford Press; 2014.
17. Thompson R. Early attachment and later development: familiar questions, new answers. In: Cassidy J, Shaver PH, editors. Handbook of attachment. Theory, research and clinical applications. New York: Guilford Press; 2008. p. 348–65.
18. Zeynep B, Derscheid D, Vliegen N, Closson L, Easterbrooks MA. Emotional availability (EA): theoretical background, empirical research using the EA Scales, and clinical applications. Dev Rev. 2014;34(2):114–67.
19. Juffer F, Bakermans-Kranenburg MJ, van IJzendoorn M. H., editors. Promoting positive parenting. An attachment-based intervention. New York, NY: Lawrence Erlbaum Associates; 2008.
20. Boldt LJ, Goffin KC, Kochanska G. The significance of early parent-child attachment for emerging regulation: a longitudinal investigation of processes and mechanisms from toddler age to preadolescence. Dev Psychol. 2020;56(3):431–43.
21. Miller JG, Hastings PD. Parenting, neurobiology, and prosocial development. In: Laible DJ, Carlo G, Padilla-Walker LM, editors. The Oxford handbook of parenting and moral development. Cape Town: Multimedia Publications; 2019.
22. Thompson RA, Meyer S. Socialization of emotion regulation in the family. In: Gross JJ, editor. Handbook of emotion regulation. New York: Guilford Press; 2007. p. 249–68.
23. Chronis AM, Lahey BB, Pelham WE Jr, Williams SH, Baumann BL, Kipp H, Jones HA, Rathouz PJ. Maternal depression and early positive parenting predict future conduct problems in young children with attention-deficit/hyperactivity disorder. Dev Psychol. 2007;43(1):70–82. https://doi.org/10.1037/0012-1649.43.1.70.
24. Calkins SD, Hill A. Caregiver influences on emerging emotion regulation: biological and environmental transactions in early development. In: Gross JJ, editor. Handbook of emotion regulation. New York: Guilford Press; 2007. p. 229–48.
25. Kopp CB. Regulation of distress and negative emotions: a developmental view. Dev Psychol. 1989;25:343–54. https://doi.org/10.1037/0012-1649.25.3.343.
26. Snyder J. Coercive family processes in the development of externalizing behavior: incorporating neurobiology into intervention research. In: Beauchaine TP, Hinshaw SP, editors. The Oxford handbook of externalizing spectrum disorders. Oxford: Oxford University Press; 2016. p. 286–302. https://doi.org/10.1093/oxfordhb/9780199324675.013.009.
27. Lambruschi F, Muratori P. Psicopatologia e psicoterapia dei disturbi della condotta. Rome: Carocci; 2013.
28. Deater-Deckard K. The social environment and the development of psychopathology. In: Zelazo PD, editor. The Oxford handbook of developmental psychology, Self and other, vol. 2. Oxford: Oxford University Press; 2013. https://doi.org/10.1093/oxfordhb/9780199958474.013.0021.
29. Rothenberg WA, Lansford JE, Alampay LP, Al-Hassan SM, Bacchini D, Bornstein MH, Chang L, Deater-Deckard K, Di Giunta L, Dodge KA, Malone PS, Oburu P, Pastorelli C, Skinner AT, Sorbring E, Steinberg L, Tapanya S, Tirado LMU, Yotanyamaneewong S. Examining effects of mother and father warmth and control on child externalizing and internalizing problems from age 8 to 13 in nine countries. Dev Psychopathol. 2020;32(3):1113–37.
30. Di Giunta L, Rothenberg WA, Lunetti C, Lansford JE, Pastorelli C, Eisenberg N, Thartori E, Basili E, Favini A, Yotanyamaneewong S, Peña Alampay L, Al-Hassan SM, Bacchini D, Bornstein MH, Chang L, Deater-Deckard K, Dodge KA, Oburu P, Skinner AT, et al. Longitudinal associations between mothers' and fathers' anger/irritability expressiveness, harsh parenting, and adolescents' socioemotional functioning in nine countries. Dev Psychol. 2020;56(3):458–74.
31. Lansford JE, Chang L, Dodge KA, Malone PS, Oburu P, Palmérus K, Bacchini D, Pastorelli C, Bombi AS, Zelli A, Tapanya S, Chaudhary N, Deater-Deckard K, Manke B, Quinn N. Physical discipline and children's adjustment: cultural normativeness as a moderator. Child Dev. 2005;76(6):1234–46.
32. Zimmer-Gembeck MJ, Webb HJ, Pepping CA, Swan K, Merlo O, Skinner EA, Avdagic E, Dunba M. Review: is parent–child attachment a correlate of children's emotion regulation and coping? Int J Behav Dev. 2017;41(1):74–93.

33. Stewart-Brown SL, Schrader-McMillan A. Parenting for mental health: what does the evidence say we need to do? Report of Workpackage 2 of the DataPrev project. Health Promot Int. 2011;26(1):110–28.
34. Gottfredson DC, Cook TD, Gardner FEM, Gorman-Smith D, Howe GW, Sandler IN, Zafft KM. Standards of evidence for efficacy, effectiveness, and scale-up research in prevention science: next generation. Prev Sci. 2015;16(7):893–926.
35. Doria MV, Kennedy H, Strathie C, et al. Explanations for the success of video interaction guidance (VIG). Fam J. 2013;22(1):78–87.
36. Rackett PMB. "Fun with Mum": using video interaction guidance to enhance early relationships and diminish maternal postnatal depression. Educ Child Psychol. 2014;31(4):82–9.
37. Ryan R, O'Farrelly C, Ramchandani P. Parenting and child mental health. London J Prim Care. 2017;9:86–94.
38. Main M, Kaplan N, Cassidy J. Security in infancy, childhood and adulthood: a move to the level of representation. Monogr Soc Res Child Dev. 1985;50:66–104.
39. Van IJzendoorn MH, Juffer F, Duyvesteyn MGC. Breaking the intergenerational cycle of insecure attachment: a review of the effects of attachment-based interventions on maternal sensitivity and infant security. J Child Psychol Psychiatry. 1995;36:225–48.
40. Erickson MF, Sroufe LA, Egeland B. Attachments past and present: implications for therapeutic intervention with mother-infant dyads. Special issue: developmental approaches to prevention and intervention. Dev Psychopathol. 1985;64:22–31.
41. Patterson GR. Coercive family process. Eugene, OR: Castilia; 1982.
42. Bandura A, Walters RH. Social learning theory. New York: General Learning Press; 1971.
43. Juffer F, Bakermans-Kranenburg M, Van Ijzendoorn MH. Video-feedback intervention to promote positive parenting and sensitive discipline (VIPP-SD). In: Steele H, Steele M, editors. Handbook of attachment-based intervention. New York, NY: The Guidford Press; 2018. p. 1–26.
44. Cassibba R, Castoro G, Costantino E, Sette G, Van Ijzendoorn MH. Enhancing maternal sensitivity and infant attachment security with video feedback: an exploratory study in Italy. Infant Ment Health J. 2015;36(1):53–61.
45. Cassibba R., Van Ijzendoorn M.H., Coppola G., Bruno S., Costantini A., Gatto S., Elia L., & Tota A. (2008). Supporting families with preterm children and children suffering from dermatitis. In F. Juffer, M. J. Bakermans-Kranenburg, & M. H. van IJzendoorn (Eds.), Promoting positive parenting: an attachment-based intervention. (pp. 91–110). Taylor & Francis Group/ Lawrence Erlbaum AssociatesOxfordshire
46. Kaminski JW, Valle LA, Filene JH, Boyle CL. A meta-analytic review of components associated with parent training program effectiveness. J Abnorm Child Psychol. 2008;36(4):567–89.
47. Lambruschi F, Muratori P, Polidori L. Il parent training nell'ottica cognitivo-comportamentale. In: Lambruschi F, Lionetti F, editors. La genitorialità. Strumenti di valutazione e interventi di sostegno. Roma: Carocci Editore; 2015.
48. Benedetto L. Il parent training. Nuova Edizione. Roma: Carocci Editore; 2017.
49. Kendall PC, Peterman JS, Villabø MA, Mychailyszyn M, O'Neil KA. Treating children and adolescents. In: Maguth Nezu C, Nezu AM, editors. The Oxford handbook of cognitive and behavioral therapies. Oxford: Oxford University Press; 2015. https://doi.org/10.1093/oxfordhb/9780199733255.013.18.
50. Meins E. Security of attachment and the social development of cognition. Hove: Psychology Press; 1997.
51. Fonagy P, Gergely G, Jurist EL, Target M. Affect regulation, mentalization and the development of the self. New York: Other Press; 2002.
52. Buchanan-Pascall S, Gray KM, Gordon M, Melvin GA. Systematic review and meta-analysis of parent group interventions for primary school children aged 4–12 years with externalizing and/or internalizing problems. Child Psychiatry Hum Dev. 2018;49(2):244–67.
53. Maughan DR, Christiansen E, Jenson WR, Olympia D, Clark E. Behavioral parent training as a treatment for externalizing behaviors and disruptive behavior disorders: a meta-analysis. Sch Psychol Rev. 2005;34(3):267–86.

54. Michelson D, Davenport C, Dretzke J, Barlow J, Day C. Do evidence-based interventions work when tested in the "real world?" A systematic review and meta-analysis of parent management training for the treatment of child disruptive behavior. Clin Child Fam Psychol Rev. 2013;16(1):18–34.

55. Colalillo S, Johnston C. Parenting cognition and affective outcomes following parent management training: a systematic review. Clin Child Fam Psychol Rev. 2016;19(3):216–35. https://doi.org/10.1007/s10567-016-0208-z.

56. Weber L, Kamp-Becker I, Christiansen H, Mingebach T. Treatment of child externalizing behavior problems: a comprehensive review and meta–meta-analysis on effects of parent-based interventions on parental characteristics. Eur Child Adolesc Psychiatry. 2019;28(8):1025–36.

57. Shaw DS, Galán CA, Lemery-Chalfant K, Dishion TJ, Elam KK, Wilson MN, Gardner F. Trajectories and predictors of children's early-starting conduct problems: child, family, genetic, and intervention effects. Dev Psychopathol. 2019;31(5):1911–21.

58. Weeland J, Chhangur RR, Jaffee SR, van der Giessen D, Matthys W, Orobio De Castro B, Overbeek G. Does the incredible years reduce child externalizing problems through improved parenting? The role of child negative affectivity and serotonin transporter linked polymorphic region (5-HTTLPR) genotype. Dev Psychopathol. 2018;30(1):93–112.

59. Reyno SM, McGrath PJ. Predictors of parent training efficacy for child externalizing behavior problems—a meta-analytic review. J Child Psychol Psychiatry. 2006;47(1):99–111.

60. Tarver J, Daley D, Lockwood J, Sayal K. Are self-directed parenting interventions sufficient for externalising behaviour problems in childhood? A systematic review and meta-analysis. Eur Child Adolesc Psychiatry. 2014;23(12):1123–37.

61. Thongseiratch T, Leijten P, Melendez-Torres GJ. Online parent programs for children's behavioral problems: a meta-analytic review. Eur Child Adolesc Psychiatry. 2020;29(11):1555–68.

62. Rodrigo MJ, Almeida A, Spiel C, Koops W. Introduction: evidence-based parent education programmes to promote positive parenting. Eur J Dev Psychol. 2012;9(1):2–10.

63. Bakermans-Kranenburg MJ, van IJzendoorn MH, Juffer F. Less is more: meta-analyses of sensitivity and attachment interventions in early childhood. Psychol Bull. 2003;129(2):195–215.

64. Reicle B, Backes S, Dette-Hagenmeyer DE. Positive parenting the preventive way: transforming research into practice with an intervention for new parents. Eur J Dev Psychol. 2012;9(1):33–46.

65. Steele H, Steele M. Handbook of attachment-based intervention. New York, NY: The Guidford Press; 2018.

66. Bowlby J. A secure base: parent-child attachment and healthy human development. New York: Basic Books; 1988.

Neurodevelopmental Disorders and Psychosocial Issues Later in Life

Leonardo Zoccante, Giulia Antolini, Laura Passarella, Elena Puttini, Valentina Rizzo, and Marco Colizzi

7.1 Introduction

Neurodevelopmental disorders are a group of conditions broadly defined as being characterised by abnormalities in the development of the central nervous system. The term refers to a wide array of neurologic and psychiatric disorders, ranging from cerebral palsy to dyslexia. They are brought together by some defining features, such as childhood onset, a steady course—rather than being characterised by remitting and relapsing episodes which instead are typical of many adulthood psychiatric conditions—and the tendency to more commonly affect male individuals [1]. Even though they are heterogeneous in terms of clinical, aetiological and therapeutical aspects and outcome, the vast overlapping between these disorders can make it difficult to define them as separate clinical entities (Fig. 7.1).

The section dedicated to neurodevelopmental disorders in the DSM-5 includes intellectual disability (ID), communication disorders, autism spectrum disorder (ASD), attention deficit hyperactivity disorder (ADHD), specific learning disorders and motor disorders encompassing developmental coordination disorder, stereotypic movement disorder and tic disorders such as Gilles de la Tourette syndrome (TS) [2]. The prevalence of these disorders has been estimated to be up to 15% in industrialised countries [3]. Changing diagnostic criteria, methodological limitations of earlier epidemiological surveys and cultural factors make it challenging to estimate the exact prevalence of such disorders [4]. ADHD appears to be the most prevalent neurodevelopmental condition, and recent studies show that its worldwide

L. Zoccante (✉) · G. Antolini · L. Passarella · E. Puttini · V. Rizzo · M. Colizzi
Maternal-Child Integrated Care Department, Integrated University Hospital of Verona, Verona, Italy
e-mail: leonardo.zoccante@aovr.veneto.it; elena.puttini@aovr.veneto.it; marco.colizzi@uniud.it

M. Colizzi, M. Ruggeri (eds.), *Prevention in Mental Health*,
https://doi.org/10.1007/978-3-030-97906-5_7

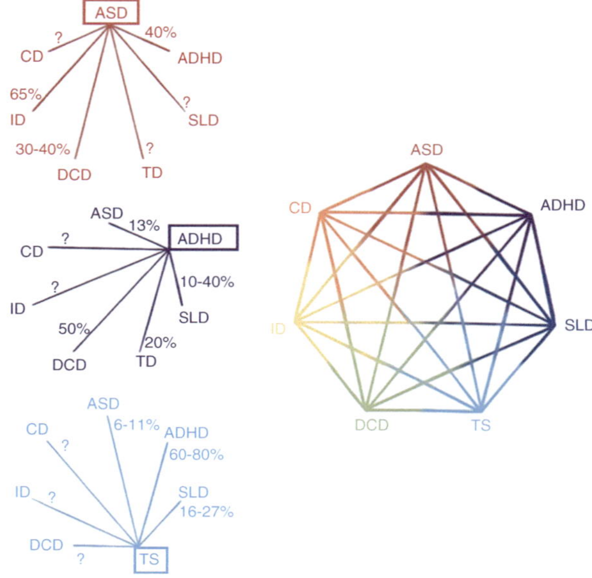

Fig. 7.1 This picture constitutes an attempt at showing the complexity and overlapping of neurodevelopmental phenotypes [10–12]. *ASD* autism spectrum disorder, *ADHD* attention deficit hyperactivity disorder, *SLD* specific learning disabilities, *TS* Tourette syndrome, *DCD* developmental coordination disorder, *ID* intellectual disability, *CD* conduct disorder

prevalence is around 5% [5, 6]. ASD was once regarded as a "rare disease" (2–5/10,000) [7], whereas more recent data show an increasing trend with prevalence rates as high as 1 in 68 in the United States [8]. TS prevalence is estimated to be around 1% [9].

Neurodevelopmental disorders have been shown to be highly heritable, with ASD, ADHD and TS displaying 91% [13], 70–80% [14] and 77% [15] heritability, respectively. More than 900 genes have so far been implicated in the genesis of neurodevelopmental disorders [16, 17]. Many environmental factors have also been discovered to influence neurodevelopment, such as maternal alcohol consumption and smoking, advanced maternal age, infections during pregnancy (especially rubella and cytomegalovirus), maternal psychosocial stress and obesity as well as gestational diabetes and hypertension, use of medication during pregnancy such as valproic acid, preterm birth, perinatal asphyxia, postnatal infections, childhood traumatic brain injury, exposure to toxic substances and gut dysbiosis [18–28]. To further complicate matters, even when a specific genetic variant is found, in most cases, pleiotropy and variable expressivity give rise to multiple phenotypes.

Studies support the involvement of the dopaminergic system in the aetiology of ADHD, emphasising the association of the disorder with the gene for dopamine beta-hydroxylase and the gene for dopamine receptor type 2 (DRD2) [29]. Structural neuroimaging studies have shown that people with ADHD have an approximately 5% reduction in total brain volume and a 10–12% reduction in the size of brain regions implicated in behavioural control functions [30]. These studies reveal anatomical differences at the level of the prefrontal cortex, cingulate cortex, basal ganglia, cerebellum and corpus callosum, while other work points to the involvement of the thalamus, amygdala, hippocampus and hypothalamus [31–33].

According to available literature, neurophysiological features of ASD include reduced long-distance connectivity and increased short-distance connectivity in different brain areas, an imbalance between excitatory and inhibitory neuronal activity due to altered GABA-ergic neuron function, dysfunction in the "social areas" of the brain such as amygdala and fusiform gyrus, anomalous fronto-striatal activity (typically involved in behavioural stereotypies), reduced hemispherical lateralisation (involved in expressive language function) and mirror neuron dysfunction [34–36].

Neuroimaging studies in patients with TS have shown alterations in the cortico-striatal-thalamic-cortical circuits, as well as a reduction in the volume of basal ganglia, corpus callosum and sensory motor cortex [37–41].

While many of the problems associated with neurodevelopmental disorders tend to improve with age, such that in many cases they may no longer be diagnosable in adulthood, follow-up studies highlight the persistence of significant impairment throughout adulthood and the onset of novel issues [1]. Therefore, when evaluating psychiatric manifestations in adults, the likelihood of a pre-existing neurodevelopmental condition should always be considered.

7.2 Developmental Trajectories

An increasing body of evidence seems to show that early life events contribute to the development of mental illness during adulthood. Many of the same risk factors associated with neurodevelopmental disorders have also been implicated in psychiatric issues later in life. For instance, prematurity has been known to correlate with psychosis since the 1930s [42]. Even though the association between neurodevelopmental disorders and many adult psychiatric conditions has already been established (Table 7.1), not enough research has been carried out so far to quantify how much of a pathophysiological continuum there could be throughout the lifespan, and whether neurodevelopmental factors might modulate psychopathology later in life (Fig. 7.2).

Most psychiatric conditions have their peak of onset during adolescence; however, the initial risk events may have occurred as early as in the prenatal stage of life. According to different studies, adolescence is characterised by many psychological and behavioural changes which reflect the completion of central nervous system maturation [43]. During this critical period, relevant changes occur in the dopaminergic projections from the midbrain, resulting in increased dopamine levels [44], as well as a substantial elimination of synapses [45], and a change in the response to GABA-ergic neurons [46]. These modifications make the adolescent brain more susceptible to stress and other environmental factors, as confirmed by preclinical evidence of the effects of stress on brain maturation [47]. It is thus plausible that a neurodevelopmental alteration of these circuits may increase subsequent susceptibility to environmental stressors (Fig. 7.3).

Table 7.1 Prevalence estimates on adult psychiatric comorbidities in neurodevelopmental disorders

	Intellectual disability	Autism spectrum disorder	Attention deficit hyperactivity disorder		Tourette syndrome
Psychotic disorders	8.4% [48]	6.4% [49]	–		No correlation [12]
Bipolar disorder	0.8% [48]	6–20% [50]	9.5% [51]		No correlation [12]
Depressive disorders	2.8% [52]	23% [53]	35–50% [51]		13–76% [12]
Anxiety disorders	5–6% [52, 54]	27% [53]	40–60% [51]		16–37% [12]
Obsessive-compulsive disorder	2.2% [52]	24% [53]	~2% [55]		40–60% [12]
Eating disorders	1–35% [56]	↑ [57]	3–9% [51]		–
Sleep-wake disorders	9.2% [58]	↑ [59]	↑ [51]		25–30% [12]
Gender dysphoria	–	↑ [60]	–		–
Addiction disorders	–	–	50% [51]		↑ [12]
Personality disorders:	2.8% [54]	[61]	[61]	[61]	64% [12]
– Paranoid		25.5%	25.9%	22.2%	
– Schizotypal		23.4%	11.1%	4.9%	
– Schizoid		31.9%	22.2%	12.3%	
– Histrionic					
– Narcissistic		6.4%	3.7%	3.7%	
– Borderline		10.6%	14.8%	37%	
– Antisocial			18.5%	30.9%	
– Avoidant		34%	11.1%	22.2%	
– Dependent		8.5%	22.2%	25.9%	
– Obsessive-compulsive		42.6%	29.6%	13.6%	
– Depressive		19.1%	18.5%	25.9%	
– Passive-aggressive		8.5%	14.8%	8.6%	

Where no clear estimate was available, the general trend reported in available literature is shown by arrows

7.2.1 Attention Deficit Hyperactivity Disorder (ADHD)

ADHD age of onset is placed within the 12th year of life, although the disorder may be detected as early as 3–4 years, as symptoms of behavioural self-regulation deficits can be identified during the preschool period. A meta-analysis conducted among preschool ADHD children indicates that parental behavioural interventions carry significant benefits, and such treatment represents an excellent alternative upon

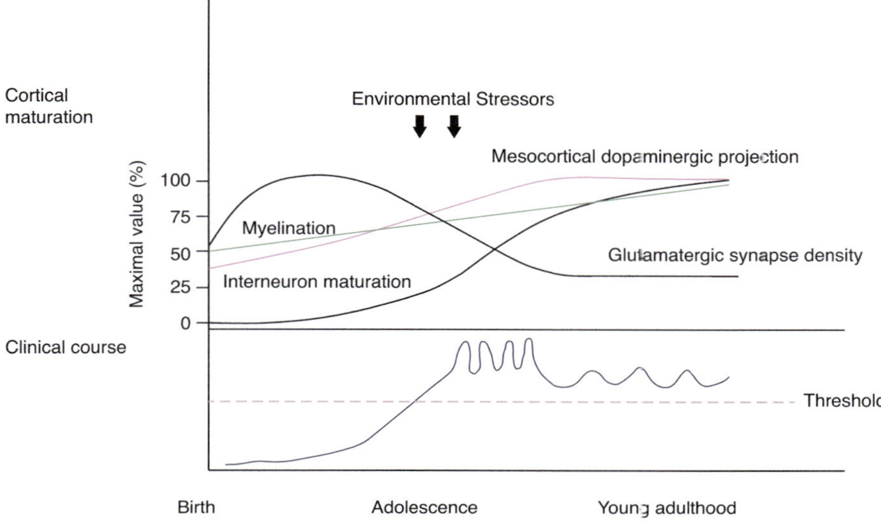

Fig. 7.2 Changes that the brain goes through during childhood and adolescence, making it more susceptible to environmental stressors

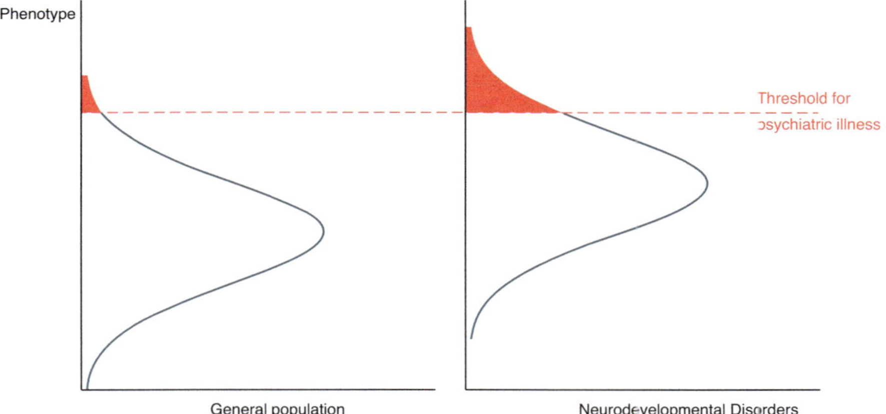

Fig. 7.3 Individuals with neurodevelopmental disorders might be more susceptible to environmental factors associated with adult psychiatric issues in the general population

refusal to start psychostimulant medications [62]. Although ADHD was originally described as a disorder limited to childhood, prospective clinical studies conducted through follow-ups of children with ADHD indicate that approximately 15% of children with ADHD will continue to meet all diagnostic criteria, while 50% will continue to experience ADHD symptoms in varying forms in adolescence and early adulthood [63, 64], even though of reduced severity [65–67].

ADHD developmental course can be divided into five stages, each characterised by a specific pattern of symptoms: (i) the prenatal stage during which risk for the disorder onset can be estimated; (ii) the 3–6-year-old, preschool phase; (iii) the school-age phase; (iv) the late childhood and preadolescent phase; and (v) the adolescent and early adulthood phase [68].

In the first years of life, elements that can be perceived as precursors of a structuring disorder should be considered as developmental and modifiable. In such preschool phase, reactivity to contextual factors is particularly high, which may bias diagnosis when based on limited observation of the individual's overall behaviour. Early identification of the disorder is not straightforward, since even primary symptomatic characteristics of ADHD may turn out to be transitory, especially for those children exposed to a less structured environment. Consequently, it should be emphasised that any early diagnostic procedure has a high risk of resulting into false positives [69].

Attention should be posed to when children move to primary school, as they have to learn new skills and competences that require attention, prolonged cognitive effort, organisation and planning skills and behaviours appropriate to a more structured school setting. The more complex demands of the school-age phase expose ADHD subjects to potential difficulties in both the scholastic and relational domains. Such difficulties may be evident also in other social contexts, with ADHD children struggling to behave appropriately with peers. As a consequence, a feeling of frustration and inadequacy may arise, increasing the risk of developing depressive reactions.

During childhood and preadolescence, school, family and social conflicts become more relevant. Motor hyperactivity generally subsides in this phase, but symptoms of inattention and impulsivity may remain. Also, psychiatric comorbidities may frequently occur at this stage, resulting in a worse outcome compared to those that will continue to present the core symptoms of ADHD only [68]. In fact, self-esteem and mood problems may arise, not necessarily related to the school context, affecting social relations more widely. Furthermore, about 25% of ADHD adolescents will develop clinically significant depression associated with decreased hope for academic and professional success [68].

During adolescence, persisting core symptoms of ADHD increase the risk of developing addictive behaviours such as gambling addiction (GA), pathological video gaming (PVG) and Internet addiction disorder (IAD), although studies are not yet completely concordant. Longitudinal studies support the role of impulsivity in the onset of GA [70–72], with ADHD adolescents being more likely to develop problem gambling than non-ADHD adolescents, while the role of inattention symptoms is less clear [73].

Regarding PVG, both hyperactivity/impulsivity and inattention have been associated with pathological use of video games [74]. Finally, also IAD has been associated with both inattention and hyperactivity/impulsivity [75, 76]. While evidence indicates a role of hyperactivity/impulsivity and attentional difficulties in the development of addictive behaviours during adolescents, further studies will have to clarify the contribution of comorbid difficulties, such as learning problems, aggression and conflicting family relationships.

With regard to the evolution of the disorder into adulthood, longitudinal evidence indicates that a significant proportion of subjects diagnosed with ADHD during childhood/adolescence will continue to show significant difficulties in executive functions, social relations, self-esteem, risky behaviours as well as psychopathological vulnerability [67]. Follow-up studies indicate that those ADHD adolescents with persisting hyperactive features are particularly vulnerable to such broader problems [77].

Historically, it has been believed that ADHD would disappear with time; however, current evidence supports different developmental trajectories into adulthood: (i) in about 40% of cases, the disorder would remit; (ii) in another 40%, the condition would affect social competences, emotional regulation and occupational integration; and (iii) in a remaining 20%, the persistence of nuclear symptoms will impact on social, academic and occupational performance, with a higher risk of presenting with substance use and other psychiatric problems [78].

In conclusion, the specific pattern of ADHD comorbidities and symptomatology changes substantially over time [79]. While in children with ADHD oppositional defiant disorder (ODD) and conduct disorder (CD) are the most common comorbid conditions, in adolescence and early adulthood, substance use disorder and other addictions, anxiety disorders, mood disorders, obsessive-compulsive and related disorders, sleep disorders and personality disorders [80] as well as somatic disorders [81] are frequently reported. The ADHD developmental trajectory, risk factors and comorbidities occurring across the lifespan are currently only partially known and require future longitudinal studies to strengthen the evidence.

7.2.2 Autism Spectrum Disorder (ASD)

Even though the prevalence of ASD in the general population is estimated to be around 1%, knowledge of its manifestations during adulthood is still limited compared to other psychiatric conditions. It is one of the latest additions to the DSM and thus many adults, especially those with a higher cognitive level, have so far gone undiagnosed. There are many issues with diagnosing ASD in adulthood, such as difficulties in obtaining anamnestic details, the possibility that adaptation may have allowed individuals to camouflage some typical features of the disorder (for instance, overcoming eye contact avoidance) and overlapping of symptoms with other psychiatric conditions [82]. Even though symptoms tend to get better with age, ASD is a lifelong condition with variable developmental trajectories and outcomes in terms of employment, independent living, general health and ageing and even early death [82]. Previous studies have identified some predictors of outcome, such as receptive language, motor skills, verbal and motor imitation, higher IQ, gender, early diagnosis and therapeutic interventions [83].

Only about one-third of people with ASD with and without ID in a 2004 UK study find some type of employment, out of which almost 20% in sheltered employment [84]. Survey data from larger, more recent studies showed that only about half of higher functioning ASD individuals are employed with IT, education, retail, healthcare, food services and government being the most frequently listed fields. Out of the lower functioning subjects, only about 20% hold paid employment, in most cases with support [85, 86]. Other studies found that many people with ASD on average work reduced hours and occupy fewer permanent positions compared to the general population, and have a lower rate of employment than individuals with other developmental disabilities [87, 88]. Predictors of more competitive employment include older age, male gender, intellectual and communication skills, higher levels of education and fewer psychiatric and general comorbidities [89]. The gender effect may be exacerbated by a selection bias caused by underdiagnosing in females.

Fewer individuals with ASD live independently compared even to subjects with other developmental disorders, including ID, showing that intellectual functioning is not the main factor in determining outcome in ASD [90]. Longitudinal studies show that over 50% of adults with ASD are in residential placement, including about nearly a quarter of individuals without ID [91]. Many other individuals live with their families, as well [90]. A frequent concern in clinical settings is the difficulty in coping with changes in living situations caused by ageing or loss of family caregivers and subsequential transition into residential homes [82].

Frequent childhood co-occurrences of ASD include seizure disorders, gastrointestinal problems and immunological conditions [82]. Large-scale studies have found nearly all major chronic medical conditions to be more common in adult individuals with ASD, particularly those already found in children and metabolic issues such as hypertension, obesity, dyslipidemia, vitamin deficiencies, diabetes and, consequently, cardiovascular events. Parkinson's disease and sensory impairments are also more commonly found in ASD [92]. The higher susceptibility to metabolic issues may be explained by reduced access to healthcare and lower levels of physical activity due to social and communication impairment as well as diet selectivity stemming from sensory issues and adverse effects of neuroleptic medications often prescribed to ASD patients [93, 94].

A high prevalence of psychiatric comorbidities is consistently reported in adults with ASD, with a high rate of variability which could be explained by lack of standard assessment protocols, non-representative study samples and the aforementioned difficulty in discriminating overlapping manifestations of ASD and other psychiatric conditions. In adults with ASD without ID, lifetime rates between 69 and 89% have been reported [95–97]. Lower rates are generally seen in adults with ASD and ID [96, 98, 99]. Furthermore, ASD adults without ID are commonly (in 40–60% of cases) prescribed psychiatric medication [96, 97], although it may be challenging to ascertain whether this is due to additional symptoms or those of ASD itself. Individuals with ASD and ID are prescribed medications mainly for behavioural problems and as often as in 44% of cases [100]. ASD individuals with ID appear to have an increased psychiatric risk compared to the general population, although much lower than those with higher functioning profile. A Swedish register study found that those diagnosed with what was formerly called Asperger's syndrome had an odds ratio for needing psychiatric care almost seven times higher than that of people diagnosed with "childhood autism" [101].

Mood disorders are listed as the most prevalent co-occurring psychiatric diagnoses in adults with ASD, with rates as high as 50–70%, the most common conditions being major depression, dysthymia and premenstrual dysphoric disorder [86, 92, 96, 97, 102]. A recent systematic review and meta-analysis of studies of anxiety and depression in adults with ASD reported a lifetime prevalence of depression of 37%, and current depression diagnosis or moderate to severe depressive symptoms of 23% [53]. Moreover, a clinical cohort study of more than 350 individuals with an adult first-time diagnosis of Asperger syndrome found that one-third had a self-reported history of depression, two-thirds had experienced suicidal ideation and one-third had planned or attempted suicide. Age and gender didn't seem to influence these findings [103]. Alexithymia, or other specific processes sustaining suicidal ideation in ASD individuals, may be responsible for the higher rates of suicidal ideation compared to the general population, in the context of a history of depression [82].

Anxiety seems to be present with a frequency comparable to that of mood disorders, with a high likelihood of having both [86, 92, 96, 97, 102, 104]. A recent meta-analysis (though with a high inter-study heterogeneity) revealed a current anxiety disorder prevalence of 27%. Lifetime prevalence of any anxiety disorder was 42%, of which 26% for GAD, 20% for social anxiety disorder and 18% for panic disorder/agoraphobia. The presence of ID did not appear to have a significant impact on prevalence of anxiety [53]. The reported rates for psychotic disorders range between 10 and 17% [105, 106].

Substance use disorders are generally less frequent in ASD compared to the general population, occurring almost exclusively in "high-functioning" adults [93, 104].

Executive function, information processing and working memory, already implicated in physiological ageing [107], have also been shown to be significantly impaired in children and adolescents with ASD [108]. These impairments seem to persist into adulthood, but no significant correlation has so far been found between ASD and predisposition to age-related cognitive decline [109–111]. Neuroimaging studies of ASD individuals throughout ageing have been performed, but they yielded inconsistent findings and were limitedly informative in terms of clinical correlates.

Since the late 1990s, ASD has been associated with an increased risk of premature mortality, two up to ten times higher, or 36 years earlier than the general population [112–114]. A large population-based Swedish registry study found increased odds of mortality, independent of gender and psychosocial functioning, for all the analysed causes of death except for infectious diseases. Mean age of death for the ASD group was 53.87 years (39.5 for low-functioning, 58.39 high-functioning) compared to 70.2 years for those in the general population. The most frequent cause of death was a nervous system disease (odds ratio = 7.49), specifically epilepsy in the low-functioning group and suicide (odds ratio = 7.55) in the high-functioning group [115].

Many factors could contribute to the difficulty in identifying therapeutic strategies with a significant effect on long-term outcomes in ASD, such as clinical, genetic and environmental heterogeneity, small study sample sizes, relatively short follow-up and lack of standardised outcome measures. Although some specific randomised controlled clinical trials have been performed [116], only two antipsychotics (risperidone and aripiprazole) have been approved by the FDA as pharmacological treatments for ASD, although their longer-term effects are unclear [117]. Intensive early behavioural interventions are often the first-line treatment in autistic children, and are supported by most available evidence in terms of ameliorating social, emotional and behavioural problems [118, 119], but their long-term effects have not yet been adequately investigated.

7.2.3 Tourette Syndrome (TS) and Other Tic Disorders

Tic disorders are arguably the least studied neurodevelopmental disorders, even though they significantly affect quality of life in terms of self-esteem, social relationships and academic and work performance even in the absence of comorbidities [120] (a rare occurrence, given that up to 90% of individuals with TS have concomitant psychopathologies [121]). Tic severity in TS typically follows a waxing and waning course, with a peak around 10–12 years followed by a steady decline during and after adolescence [37]. Smaller caudate volumes have been correlated to a poorer prognosis in terms of persistence of tic manifestation into adulthood [41]. Poor fine motor skills in childhood have also been associated with an increased risk of tic persistence [122]. For individuals with mild to moderate tics not impacting social life and functioning in school/work environments, psycho-educational interventions usually suffice in providing coping strategies. Behavioural interventions constitute the first-line treatment in most cases warranting some type of therapy [123]. European and American guidelines suggest that pharmacological treatments should be reserved to cases in which tics cause pain or injury, social and emotional issues or functional impairments in daily life. No strong recommendations are made with regard to comparative efficacy of different medications because of limitations in existing literature; however, most available evidence supports the use of molecules with an action on dopaminergic metabolism (particularly those blocking post-synaptic D2 receptors) [124–126].

The element with the largest impact on longitudinal outcomes is the presence of obsessive-compulsive manifestations in up to 60–90% of TS subjects, justifying a concurrent obsessive-compulsive disorder (OCD) diagnosis in about 40% of cases [12]. As for the general population, OCD appears to correlate with higher IQ in TS patients. Compulsive symptoms have been shown to significantly decline with age, while obsessive symptoms may persist into adulthood [9]. OCD patients with comorbid tics tend to have greater rates of symmetry and numerical obsessions [127]. Obsessive-compulsive symptoms have been reported to be at their worst about 2 years after tic manifestation has reached its peak [128]. As for tic severity, smaller caudate nucleus volumes, as indexed at structural imaging, have been associated with increased obsessive-compulsive symptomatology in early adulthood [41]. Tic-related OCD has been shown to have a less satisfactory response to SSRIs and a more favourable response to antipsychotics, when compared to OCD without comorbid tics, while no differences have been found in terms of cognitive behavioural therapy [129, 130].

A longitudinal study of the predictors of clinical course in TS showed that the most severe tics and OCD in childhood are such symptoms in early adulthood. Family history and psychosocial stress have also been implicated in modulating TS outcome. Evidence does not suggest childhood tic severity to be a strong predictor of later comorbidities, while female gender and severe childhood comorbid ADHD have been associated with future emotional disorders [131]. Other frequently reported comorbidities of TS include mood and anxiety disorders, conduct disorders, personality disorders, migraines and elimination disorders [12, 132]. Further studies are necessary to better understand whether any clinical or psychosocial characteristics would predict the onset of such disorders later in life.

7.3 Conclusions

As already mentioned, neurodevelopmental disorders encompass a spectrum of overlapping and diverging phenotypes, which often outlie present diagnostic criteria. So far, research has struggled to incorporate this heterogeneity into study designs, raising uncertainty regarding clinical outcomes and therapeutic perspectives for these conditions. To date, only a few studies [83] have included subjects older than 40 years, and information is particularly poor for female adults, resulting in limited data regarding the overall outcome during adulthood.

Furthermore, little evidence is available on the long-term effect of approved pharmacological treatments. In terms of non-pharmacological interventions, some evidence suggests that small-group activities and augmentative and alternative communication (AAC) may be effective in improving interpersonal skills during adolescence, and preventing behavioural issues in adulthood, in ASD [133, 134]. Also, while interventions have been evaluated in terms of child outcome, their impact on parents and families' well-being is rarely considered. Having a child with ASD has been associated with high rates of divorce and lower family well-being [135], suggesting that family issues may have a role in the long-term effects of therapeutic options. Finally, transition to adult psychiatric services should also be carefully planned, ensuring access to the most appropriate services for the individual's age and needs, as inadequacies or failure in transition preparation may result in non-adherence to treatment, loss to follow-up and poor outcome.

A close look at available literature points towards the presence of a pathophysiological continuum between atypical neurodevelopment and psychiatric issues emerging later in life. Presently, this continuum is not translated into clinical practice, where much more rigid categorisations prevail. This gap could possibly be causing a significant loss of health and quality of life for patients, due to failure to account for additional subthreshold symptoms and developmental trajectories into adulthood. Future studies will need to focus more on the environmental, clinical and pathophysiological aspects involved in the persistence of neurodevelopmental disorders into adulthood and their outcome. Therapeutical options should follow suit. As we gain more understanding of the psychobiological mechanisms underlying brain development and related behaviour, clinical practice should be constantly updated in order to support patients throughout their lifespan.

References

1. Thapar A, Cooper M, Rutter M. Neurodevelopmental disorders. Lancet Psychiatry. 2017;4:339–46.
2. APA. Diagnostic and Statistical Manual of Mental Disorders, 5th ed. Arlington, TX, USA: American Psychiatric Publishing; 2013.
3. WHO. https://www.who.int/ceh/capacity/neurodevelopmental.pdf
4. Masi A, DeMayo MM, Glozier N, Guastella AJ. An overview of autism spectrum disorder, heterogeneity and treatment options. Neurosci Bull. 2017;33:183–93.
5. Polanczyk GV, Willcutt EG, Salum GA, Kieling C, Rohde LA. ADHD prevalence estimates across three decades: an updated systematic review and meta-regression analysis. Int J Epidemiol. 2014;43:434–42.
6. Sayal K, Prasad V, Daley D, Ford T, Coghill D. ADHD in children and young people: prevalence, care pathways, and service provision. Lancet Psychiatry. 2018;5:175–86.
7. Rutter M. Incidence of autism spectrum disorders: changes over time and their meaning. Acta Paediatr Int J Paediatr. 2005;94:2–15.
8. CDC. https://www.cdc.gov/mmwr/volumes/69/ss/ss6904a1.htm
9. Groth C. Tourette syndrome in a longitudinal perspective. Clinical course of tics and comorbidities, coexisting psychopathologies, phenotypes and predictors. Dan Med J. 2018;65(4):B5465.
10. Persico A. Manuale di Neuropsichiatria Infantile e dell'Adolescenza. 2018th ed. Seu, editor. Roma; 2018. 1420 p.
11. Antshel KM, Russo N. Autism spectrum disorders and ADHD: overlapping phenomenology, diagnostic issues, and treatment considerations. Curr Psychiatry Rep. 2019;21(5):34.
12. Robertson MM. A personal 35 year perspective on Gilles de la Tourette syndrome: prevalence, phenomenology, comorbidities, and coexistent psychopathologies. Lancet Psychiatry. 2015;2:68–87.
13. Tick B, Bolton P, Happé F, Rutter M, Rijsdijk F. Heritability of autism spectrum disorders: a meta-analysis of twin studies. J Child Psychol Psychiatry Allied Discip. 2016;57:585–95.
14. Williams B, Jalilianhasanpour R, Matin N, Fricchione GL, Sepulcre J, Keshavan MS, Perez DL. Individual differences in corticolimbic structural profiles linked to insecure attachment and coping styles in motor functional ne, 230–237. Discovery of the first genome-wide significant risk loci for attention deficit/hyperactivity disorder. Physiol Behav. 2019;176:139–48.
15. Mataix-Cols D, et al. Familial risks of tourette syndrome and chronic tic disorders a population-based cohort study. JAMA Psychiat. 2015;72:787–93.
16. Chiurazzi P, Pirozzi F. Advances in understanding—genetic basis of intellectual disability. F1000 Res. 2016;5:1–16.
17. Wright CF, et al. Genetic diagnosis of developmental disorders in the DDD study: a scalable analysis of genome-wide research data. Lancet. 2015;385:1305–14.
18. Leckman JF. Tourette's syndrome. 2002;360:1577–86.
19. Roessner V, Hoekstra PJ. European multicenter tics in children studies (EMTICS): exploring the onset and course of tic disorders. Eur Child Adolesc Psychiatry. 2013;22:451–2.
20. Kalkbrenner AE, et al. Maternal smoking during pregnancy and the prevalence of autism spectrum disorders, using data from the autism and developmental disabilities monitoring network. Environ Health Perspect. 2012;120:1042–8.
21. Veroniki AA, et al. Comparative safety of antiepileptic drugs for neurological development in children exposed during pregnancy and breast feeding: a systematic review and network meta-analysis. BMJ Open. 2017;7:1–11.
22. Atladóttir HÓ, et al. Maternal infection requiring hospitalization during pregnancy and autism spectrum disorders. J Autism Dev Disord. 2010;40:1423–30.
23. Maher GM, et al. Association of hypertensive disorders of pregnancy with risk of neurodevelopmental disorders in offspring a systematic review and meta-analysis. JAMA Psychiat. 2018;75:809–19.

24. Ornoy A, Becker M, Weinstein-Fudim L, Ergaz Z. Diabetes during pregnancy: a maternal disease complicating the course of pregnancy with long-term deleterious effects on the offspring. A clinical review. Int J Mol Sci. 2021;22:1–38.
25. Carlsson T, Molander F, Taylor MJ, Jonsson U, Bölte S. Early environmental risk factors for neurodevelopmental disorders—a systematic review of twin and sibling studies. Dev Psychopathol. 2020;33:1–48. https://doi.org/10.1017/S0954579420000620.
26. Burchi E, Pallanti S. Diagnostic issues in early-onset obsessive-compulsive disorder and their treatment implications. Curr Neuropharmacol. 2019;17(8):672–80.
27. Andreo-Martínez P, Rubio-Aparicio M, Sánchez-Meca J, Veas A, Martínez-González AE. A meta-analysis of gut microbiota in children with autism. J Autism Dev Disord. 2022;52(3):1374–87. https://doi.org/10.1007/s10803-021-05002-y.
28. Al-Dewik N, et al. Overview and introduction to autism spectrum disorder (ASD). Adv Neurobiol. 2020;24:3–42.
29. Nyman ES, et al. ADHD candidate gene study in a population-based birth cohort: association with DBH and DRD2. J Am Acad Child Adolesc Psychiatry. 2007;46:1614–21.
30. Gallo EF, Posner J. Moving towards causality in attention-deficit hyperactivity disorder: overview of neural and genetic mechanisms. Lancet Psychiatry. 2016;3:555–67.
31. Vogt BA. Cingulate impairments in ADHD: comorbidities, connections, and treatment. Handb Clin Neurol. 2019;166:297–314.
32. Vieira de Melo BB, Trigueiro MJ, Rodrigues PP. Systematic overview of neuroanatomical differences in ADHD: definitive evidence. Dev Neuropsychol. 2018;43:52–68.
33. He N, et al. Neuroanatomical deficits correlate with executive dysfunction in boys with attention deficit hyperactivity disorder. Neurosci Lett. 2015;600:45–9.
34. Chen R, Jiao Y, Herskovits EH. Structural MRI in autism spectrum disorder. Bone. 2014;23:1–7.
35. Foster NEV, et al. Structural gray matter differences during childhood development in autism Spectrum disorder: a multimetric approach. Pediatr Neurol. 2015;53:350–9.
36. Supekar K, et al. Deficits in mesolimbic reward pathway underlie social interaction impairments in children with autism. Brain. 2018;141:2795–805.
37. Logan PGB and GD. 基因的改变NIH Public Access. Bone. 2014;23;1–7.
38. Rizzo R, Gulisano M, Calì PV, Curatolo P. Long term clinical course of Tourette syndrome. Brain Dev. 2012;34:667–73.
39. Paschou P, Fernandez TV, Sharp F, Heiman GA, Hoekstra PJ. Genetic susceptibility and neurotransmitters in Tourette syndrome. Int Rev Neurobiol. 2013;112:155–77.
40. Muellner J, et al. Altered structure of cortical sulci in gilles de la Tourette syndrome: further support for abnormal brain development. Mov Disord. 2015;30:655–61.
41. Bloch MH, Leckman JF, Zhu H, Peterson BS. Caudate volumes in childhood predict symptom severity in adults with Tourette syndrome. Neurology. 2005;65:1253–8.
42. Rosanoff AJ, Handy LM, Plesset IR, Brush S. The etiology of so-called schizophrenic psychoses, with special reference to their occurrence in twins. AJP. 1934;91:247–86.
43. Lockhart S, Sawa A, Niwa M. Developmental trajectories of brain maturation and behavior: relevance to major mental illnesses. J Pharmacol Sci. 2018;137:1–4.
44. Lambe EK, Krimer LS, Goldman-Rakic PS. Differential postnatal development of catecholamine and serotonin inputs to identified neurons prefrontal cortex of rhesus monkey. J Neurosci. 2000;20:8780–7.
45. McGlashan TH, Hoffman RE. Schizophrenia as a disorder of developmentally reduced synaptic connectivity. Arch Gen Psychiatry. 2000;57:637–48.
46. Tseng KY, O'Donnell P. Dopamine modulation of prefrontal cortical interneurons changes during adolescence. Cereb Cortex. 2007;17:1235–40.
47. Niwa M, et al. Adolescent stress–induced epigenetic control of dopaminergic neurons via glucocorticoids. Science. 2013;339(6117):335–9.
48. Morgan VA, Leonard H, Bourke J, Jablensky A. Intellectual disability co-occurring with schizophrenia and other psychiatric illness: population-based study. Br J Psychiatry. 2008;193:364–72.

49. Lugo Marín J, et al. Prevalence of schizophrenia spectrum disorders in average-IQ adults with autism spectrum disorders: a meta-analysis. J Autism Dev Disord. 2018;48:239–50.
50. Vannucchi G, et al. Bipolar disorder in adults with Asperger's syndrome: a systematic review. J Affect Disord. 2014;168:151–60.
51. Sobanski E. Psychiatric comorbidity in adults with attention-deficit/hyperactivity disorder (ADHD). Eur Arch Psychiatry Clin Neurosci. 2006;256:i26–31.
52. Maïano C, et al. Prevalence of anxiety and depressive disorders among youth with intellectual disabilities: a systematic review and meta-analysis. J Affect Disord. 2018;236:230–42.
53. Hollocks MJ, Lerh JW, Magiati I, Meiser-Stedman R, Brugha TS. Anxiety and depression in adults with autism spectrum disorder: a systematic review and meta-analysis. Psychol Med. 2019;49:559–72.
54. Mazza MG, Rossetti A, Crespi G, Clerici M. Prevalence of co-occurring psychiatric disorders in adults and adolescents with intellectual disability: a systematic review and meta-analysis. J Appl Res Intellect Disabil. 2020;33:126–38.
55. Abramovitch A, Dar R, Mittelman A, Wilhelm S. Comorbidity between attention deficit/hyperactivity disorder and obsessive-compulsive disorder across the lifespan: a systematic and critical review. Harv Rev Psychiatry. 2015;23:245–62.
56. S., G. Eating disorders in adults with intellectual disability. J Intellect Disabil Res. 2000;44:625–37.
57. Westwood H, Tchanturia K. Autism spectrum disorder in anorexia nervosa: an updated literature review. Curr Psychiatry Rep. 2017;19:41.
58. Van de Wouw E, Evenhuis HM, Echteld MA. Prevalence, associated factors and treatment of sleep problems in adults with intellectual disability: a systematic review. Res Dev Disabil. 2012;33:1310–32.
59. Morgan B, Nageye F, Masi G, Cortese S. Sleep in adults with autism spectrum disorder: a systematic review and meta-analysis of subjective and objective studies. Sleep Med. 2020;65:113–20.
60. Glidden D, Bouman WP, Jones BA, Arcelus J. Gender dysphoria and autism spectrum disorder: a systematic review of the literature. Sex Med Rev. 2016;4:3–14.
61. Anckarsäter H, et al. The impact of ADHD and autism spectrum disorders on temperament, character, and personality development. Am J Psychiatry. 2006;163:1239–44.
62. Mulqueen JM, Bartley CA, Bloch MH. Meta-analysis: parental interventions for preschool ADHD. J Atten Disord. 2015;19:118–24.
63. Shaw P, Sudre G. Adolescent attention-deficit/hyperactivity disorder: understanding teenage symptom trajectories. Biol Psychiatry. 2021;89:152–61.
64. Philipsen A, Döpfner M. ADHD in the transition to adulthood: prevalence, symptoms, risks, and care. Bundesgesundheitsblatt Gesundheitsforsch Gesundheitsschutz. 2020;63:910–5.
65. Laufer MW, Denhoff E. Hyperkinetic behavior syndrome in children. J Pediatr. 1957;50:463–74.
66. Biederman J, Mick E, Faraone SV. Age-dependent decline of symptoms of attention deficit hyperactivity disorder: impact of remission definition and symptom type. Am J Psychiatry. 2000;157:816–8.
67. Faraone SV, Biederman J, Mick E. The age-dependent decline of attention deficit hyperactivity disorder: a meta-analysis of follow-up studies. Psychol Med. 2006;36:159–65.
68. Marzocchi GM, Sclafani M, Rinaldi R, Giangiacomo A. ADHD in pediatria: guida operativa. Erickson, editor. 2012. 155 p.
69. Fedeli D. Il disturbo da deficit di attenzione e iperattività. Carocci, editor. 2013. 207 p.
70. Dussault F, Brendgen M, Vitaro F, Wanner B, Tremblay RE. Longitudinal links between impulsivity, gambling problems and depressive symptoms: a transactional model from adolescence to early adulthood. J Child Psychol Psychiatry Allied Discip. 2011;52:130–8.
71. Pagani LS, Derevensky JL, Japel C. Predicting gambling behavior in sixth grade from kindergarten impulsivity: a tale of developmental continuity. Arch Pediatr Adolesc Med. 2009;163:238–43.

72. Faregh N, Derevensky J. Gambling behavior among adolescents with attention deficit/hyperactivity disorder. J Gambl Stud. 2011;27:243–56.
73. Canu WH, Schatz NK. A weak association between traits of attention-deficit/hyperactivity disorder and gambling in college students. J Coll Stud Psychother. 2011;25:334–43.
74. Gentile DA, Swing EL, Lim CG, Khoo A. Video game playing, attention problems, and impulsiveness: evidence of bidirectional causality. Psychol Pop Media Cult. 2012;1:62–70.
75. Hee JY, et al. Attention deficit hyperactivity symptoms and Internet addiction. Psychiatry Clin Neurosci. 2004;58:487–94.
76. Dalbudak E, Evren C. The relationship of Internet addiction severity with Attention Deficit Hyperactivity Disorder symptoms in Turkish University students; impact of personality traits, depression and anxiety. Compr Psychiatry. 2014;55:497–503.
77. Kooij JJS, et al. Distinguishing comorbidity and successful management of adult ADHD. J Atten Disord. 2012;16:3S–19S.
78. Ianes D, Marzocchi GN, Sanna G. Facciamo il punto su... L'iperattività. Aspetti clinici e interventi psicoeducativi. Erickson, editor. 2009. 104 p.
79. Costello EJ, Mustillo S, Erkanli A, Keeler G, Angold A. Prevalence and development of psychiatric disorders in childhood and adolescence. Arch Gen Psychiatry. 2003;60:837–44.
80. Jacob CP, et al. Co-morbidity of adult attention-deficit/hyperactivity disorder with focus on personality traits and related disorders in a tertiary referral center. Eur Arch Psychiatry Clin Neurosci. 2007;257:309–17.
81. Instanes JT, Haavik J, Halmøy A. Personality traits and comorbidity in adults with ADHD. J Atten Disord. 2016;20:845–54.
82. Wise EA. Aging in autism spectrum disorder. Am J Geriatr Psychiatry. 2020;28:339–49.
83. Posar A, Visconti P. Long-term outcome of autism spectrum disorder. Turk Pediatr Ars. 2019;54:207–12.
84. Howlin P, Goode S, Hutton J, Rutter M. Adult outcome for children with autism. J Child Psychol Psychiatry Allied Discip. 2004;45:212–29.
85. Ohl A, et al. Predictors of employment status among adults with autism spectrum disorder. Work. 2017;56:345–55.
86. Gotham K, et al. Characterizing the daily life, needs, and priorities of adults with autism spectrum disorder from Interactive Autism Network data. Autism 2015;19:794–804.
87. Baldwin S, Costley D, Warren A. Employment activities and experiences of adults with high-functioning autism and Asperger's disorder. J Autism Dev Disord. 2014;44:2440–9.
88. Zwicker J, Zaresani A, Emery JCH. Describing heterogeneity of unmet needs among adults with a developmental disability: an examination of the 2012 Canadian Survey on Disability. Res Dev Disabil. 2017;65:1–11.
89. Lawer L, Brusilovskiy E, Salzer MS, Mandell DS. Use of vocational rehabilitative services among adults with autism. J Autism Dev Disord. 2009;39:487–94.
90. Hewitt AS, et al. Characteristics of adults with autism spectrum disorder who use residential services and supports through adult developmental disability services in the United States. Res Autism Spectr Disord. 2017;34:1–9.
91. Ballaban-Gil K, Rapin I, Tuchman R, Shinnar S. Longitudinal examination of the behavioral, language, and social changes in a population of adolescents and young adults with autistic disorder. Pediatr Neurol. 1996;15:217–23.
92. U.S. Census Bureau Website. https://www.census.gov. Accessed July 3, 2021.
93. Croen LA, et al. The health status of adults on the autism spectrum. Autism. 2015;19:814–23.
94. Kral TVE, Eriksen WT, Souders MC, Pinto-Martin JA. Eating behaviors, diet quality, and gastrointestinal symptoms in children with autism spectrum disorders: a brief review. J Pediatr Nurs. 2013;28:548–56.
95. Howlin P, Magiati I. Autism spectrum disorder: outcomes in adulthood. Curr Opin Psychiatry. 2017;30:69–76.
96. Buck TR, et al. Psychiatric comorbidity and medication use in adults with autism spectrum disorder. J Autism Dev Disord. 2014;44:3063–71.

97. Lever AG, Geurts HM. Psychiatric co-occurring symptoms and disorders in young, middle-aged, and older adults with autism spectrum disorder. J Autism Dev Disord. 2016;46:1916–30.
98. Howlin P, Moss P. Adults with autism spectrum disorders. Can J Psychiatr. 2012;57:275–83.
99. Cervantes PE, Matson JL. Comorbid symptomology in adults with autism spectrum disorder and intellectual disability. J Autism Dev Disord. 2015;45:3961–70.
100. Kats D, Payne L, Parlier M, Piven J. Prevalence of selected clinical problems in older adults with autism and intellectual disability. J Neurodev Disord. 2013;5:27.
101. Nylander L, Axmon A, Björne P, Ahlström G, Gillberg C. Older adults with autism spectrum disorders in Sweden: a register study of diagnoses, psychiatric care utilization and psychotropic medication of 601 individuals. J Autism Dev Disord. 2018;48:3076–85.
102. Howlin P. Outcome in adult life for more able individuals with autism or Asperger syndrome. Autism. 2000;4:63–83.
103. Cassidy S, et al. Suicidal ideation and suicide plans or attempts in adults with Asperger's syndrome attending a specialist diagnostic clinic: a clinical cohort study. Lancet Psychiatry. 2014;1:142–7.
104. Hofvander B, et al. Psychiatric and psychosocial problems in adults with normal-intelligence autism spectrum disorders. BMC Psychiatry. 2009;9:1–9.
105. Joshi G, et al. Psychiatric comorbidity and functioning in a clinically referred population of adults with autism spectrum disorders: a comparative study. J Autism Dev Disord. 2013;43:1314–25.
106. Stahlberg O, Soderstrom H, Rastam M, Gillberg C. Bipolar disorder, schizophrenia, and other psychotic disorders in adults with childhood onset AD/HD and/or autism spectrum disorders. J Neural Transm. 2004;111:891–902.
107. Deary IJ, et al. Age-associated cognitive decline. Br Med Bull. 2009;92:135–52.
108. Lord C, Elsabbagh M, Baird G, Veenstra-Vanderweele J. Autism spectrum disorder. Clin Child Neurol. 2018;392(10146):508–20.
109. Lever AG, Geurts HM. Age-related differences in cognition across the adult lifespan in autism spectrum disorder. Autism Res. 2016;9:666–76.
110. Davids RCD, Groen Y, Berg IJ, Tucha OM, van Balkom IDC. Executive functions in older adults with autism spectrum disorder: objective performance and subjective complaints. J Autism Dev Disord. 2016;46:2859–73.
111. Wise EA, Smith MD, Rabins PV. Correlates of daily functioning in older adults with autism spectrum disorder. Aging Ment Health. 2020;24:1754–62.
112. Isager T, Mouridsen SE, Rich B. Mortality and causes of death in pervasive developmental disorders. Autism. 1999;3:7–16.
113. Mouridsen SE, Brønnum-Hansen H, Rich B, Isager T. Mortality and causes of death in autism spectrum disorders: an update. Autism. 2008;12:403–14.
114. Guan J, Li G. Injury mortality in individuals with autism. Am J Public Health. 2017;107:791–3.
115. Hirvikoski T, et al. Premature mortality in autism spectrum disorder. Br J Psychiatry. 2016;208:232–8.
116. Yatawara CJ, Einfeld SL, Hickie IB, Davenport TA, Guastella AJ. The effect of oxytocin nasal spray on social interaction deficits observed in young children with autism: a randomized clinical crossover trial. Mol Psychiatry. 2016;21:1225–31.
117. Food and Drug Administration Website. http://www.fda.gov/cder/approval/index.htm. Accessed July 4, 2021.
118. Eldevik S, et al. Meta-analysis of early intensive behavioral intervention for children with autism. J Clin Child Adolesc Psychol. 2009;38:439–50.
119. Wang X, et al. Cognitive behavioral therapy for autism spectrum disorders: a systematic review. Pediatrics. 2021;147:e2020049880.
120. Leckman JF, Bloch MH, King RA, Scahill L. Phenomenology of tics and natural history of tic disorders. Adv Neurol. 2006;99:1–16.
121. Robertson MM. Gilles de la tourette syndrome: the complexities of phenotype and treatment. Br J Hosp Med. 2011;72:100–7.

122. Bloch MH, Sukhodolsky DG, Leckman JF, Schultz RT. Fine-motor skill deficits in childhood predict adulthood tic severity and global psychosocial functioning in Tourette's syndrome. J Child Psychol Psychiatry Allied Discip. 2006;47:551–9.
123. Robertson MM, et al. Gilles de la Tourette syndrome. Nat Rev Dis Prim. 2017;3:16097.
124. Verdellen C, et al. European clinical guidelines for Tourette syndrome and other tic disorders. Part III: Behavioural and psychosocial interventions. Eur Child Adolesc Psychiatry. 2011;20:197–207.
125. Roessner V, et al. European clinical guidelines for Tourette syndrome and other tic disorders. Part II: pharmacological treatment. Eur Child Adolesc Psychiatry. 2011;20:173–96.
126. Tamara P, et al. Practice guideline: the treatment of tics in people with Tourette syndrome and chronic tic disorders. Neurology. 2019;92(19):896–906.
127. Leckman JF, et al. TIC-related obsessive compulsive disorder. Anxiety. 1994;215:208–15.
128. Bloch MH, et al. Adulthood outcome of tic and obsessive-compulsive symptom severity in children with Tourette syndrome. Arch Pediatr Adolesc Med. 2006;160:65–9.
129. March JS, et al. Tics moderate treatment outcome with sertraline but not cognitive-behavior therapy in pediatric obsessive-compulsive disorder. Biol Psychiatry. 2007;61:344–7.
130. Bloch MH, et al. A systematic review: antipsychotic augmentation with treatment refractory obsessive-compulsive disorder. Mol Psychiatry. 2006;11:622–32.
131. Groth C, Skov L, Lange T, Debes NM. Predictors of the clinical course of Tourette syndrome: a longitudinal study. J Child Neurol. 2019;34:913–21.
132. Hirschtritt ME, et al. Lifetime prevalence, age of risk, and etiology of comorbid psychiatric disorders in Tourette syndrome. JAMA Psychiat. 2015;72:325–33.
133. Rose V, Paynter J, Vivanti G, Keen D, Trembath D. Predictors of expressive language change for children with autism spectrum disorder receiving AAC-infused comprehensive intervention. J Autism Dev Disord. 2020;50:278–91.
134. Iacono T, Trembath D, Erickson S. The role of augmentative and alternative communication for children with autism: current status and future trends. Neuropsychiatr Dis Treat. 2016;12:2349–61.
135. Karst JS, van Hecke AV. Parent and family impact of autism spectrum disorders: a review and proposed model for intervention evaluation. Clin Child Fam Psychol Rev. 2012;15:247–77.

Migration and Mental Health: From Vulnerability to Resilience

Michela Galatolo, Ruben Biagini, Giuseppe D'Andrea, and Ilaria Tarricone

8

8.1 The Migration Phenomenon Worldwide

8.1.1 Migration: Trends and Definitions

According to the latest estimates, the absolute number of international migrants has increased over the last five decades, from 84 million back in 1970 to 272 million in 2019 [1]. The number of migrants has already surpassed the predicted estimates for 2050, which were for 230 million [1]. However, despite the increase in absolute numbers, one should note that the change in the proportion of international migrants

M. Galatolo · G. D'Andrea
Psychiatry Unit, Department of Biomedical and Neuro-motor Sciences (DIBINEM), University of Bologna, Bologna, Italy

Bologna Transcultural Psychosomatic Team, Department of Medical and Surgical Sciences, University of Bologna, Bologna, Italy
e-mail: michela.galatolo@studio.unibo.it; giuseppe.dandrea6@studio.unibo.it

R. Biagini
Department of Medical and Surgical Sciences (DIMEC), University of Bologna, Bologna, Italy
e-mail: ruben.biagini@studio.unibo.it

I. Tarricone (✉)
Bologna Transcultural Psychosomatic Team, Department of Medical and Surgical Sciences, University of Bologna, Bologna, Italy

Department of Medical and Surgical Sciences (DIMEC), University of Bologna, Bologna, Italy

Department of Mental Health and Pathological Addiction, Local Health Authority, Bologna, Italy
e-mail: ilaria.tarricone@unibo.it

M. Colizzi, M. Ruggeri (eds.), *Prevention in Mental Health*, https://doi.org/10.1007/978-3-030-97906-5_8

among the global population has only risen by 1.2% in the aforementioned time span (from 2.3% in 1970 to 3.5% in 2019). It is also worth mentioning that a great majority of people who migrate are internal migrants: in 2009 the estimate was of 740 million people [2].

At an international level, there is no universally accepted definition for "migration". According to the World Health Organization, migration can be defined as "the movement of a person or a group of persons, either across an international border or within a State. It is a population movement, encompassing any kind of movement of people, whatever its length, composition and causes; it includes migration of refugees, displaced persons, economic migrants, and persons moving for other purposes, including family reunification" [3]. Thus, "migration" and "migrants" are umbrella terms, which encompass a broad and heterogeneous population, making it difficult to provide a clear and coherent categorization of the phenomenon. However, within such a definition it is useful to bear in mind some pivotal distinctions such as international vs internal migrants, labour migrants, and forcibly displaced migrants (refugees and asylum seekers) [4].

The drivers of migration can be identified at various levels and include the main features of the country of origin (the macro-level: political, social, environmental, economic, and demographic factors), which interact with the availability of migratory facilitators (local policies, cost of travel), as well as with individual characteristics (the micro-level) to determine the individual's decision to migrate [5].

The whole migratory process can be divided into three phases: pre-migration, migration, and post-migration. The pre-migration comprises the decision to move and preparation to do so. The migration phase corresponds to the physical relocation of individuals from one place to another. Finally, the post-migration represents the "absorption of the immigrant within the social and cultural framework of the new society" [6].

8.2 Mental and General Health Outcomes of Migration

8.2.1 Migration and Health

The theme of migrants' mental and physical health and the capacity of the health services to adapt and respond to the needs of this "new" population represent a current and topical issue. Many studies have observed the so-called healthy migrant effect [7–9], based on the observation of lower mortality rates among migrants compared to native counterparts in the country of resettlement. This observation led to the hypothesis of a positive selection mechanism, that is, only the healthiest individuals migrated and kept their healthier conditions once resettled. Nevertheless, a recent meta-analysis [10], while confirming the lower mortality rates in migrants, questions the generalizability of this finding, limiting its applicability to those who migrated to high-income countries, since most of the qualitatively valuable data come from studies conducted in these countries. This finding, therefore, while it might offer a reliable picture of the health of labour migrants and international students, is not valid for other more disadvantaged categories such as refugees, asylum seekers, or undocumented migrants and does not consider the complexity and multifactoriality of the migratory process. In fact, factors like age and type of migration, social class, and public health policies in the resettlement country have proved to be significant determinants of the outcome of migration in terms of general health [11]. Furthermore, there is evidence that the reported "advantage" in terms of lower mortality rates tends to reduce over time [12, 13].

Whether migrants experience improvement or worsening of their health status largely depends on the interaction between the various factors determining their health before, during, and after migration. Such factors, known as "social determinants of health", include possibility of a safe transit (airplane travel rather than walking across deserts or hiding in trucks), adequate accommodation, and access to health care, considering that before or during the journey migrants may be exposed to many potentially harmful situations and different pathogens (malaria, tuberculosis, dehydration, violence, etc.) [4]. The field of migratory health should thus encompass all the health problems arising from human mobility and should address all aspects of well-being in the context of migration, including migrants' families and the public health of the communities with which migrants interact during the phases of the migratory journey [14].

Health vulnerability and resilience factors are dynamic. Migrants are not intrinsically vulnerable to health issues, but the conditions within the different migration stages significantly shape their health and well-being [15].

8.2.2 Barriers to Health Care

Health is a human right. Guided by the principles of non-discrimination and equal treatment of all, countries should ensure that health facilities are available, accessible, and of good quality. Despite this, many migrants still encounter obstacles in accessing health care, including language barriers, discrimination, cost differentials, and bureaucratic issues [16]. There is established evidence that migrants tend to underutilize health services, experiencing serious delays in diagnosis and treatment [17]. This might be due to poor awareness of the organization of local health care and the welfare system, especially when migrants come from countries with severely disrupted health systems [18]. Available evidence thus points to the need for intervention aimed to improve migrants' knowledge of health-care facilities and health literacy [19, 20]. This holds true not only for refugees and asylum seekers but also for labour migrants. For instance, the International Organization for Migration (IOM) states that "migrant workers are among the most vulnerable workers in the world, often subject to exploitation, discrimination and abuse, lacking access to mechanisms for remedy and redress and in constant fear of deportation" [21]. A systematic literature review on the challenges faced in providing appropriate health care for migrants and refugees in high-income countries has identified three major issues: communication, confidence, and continuity of care (the "3C model") [22].

In relation to communication, migrants may have difficulty explaining their reasons for seeking medical help and understanding information about symptoms, diagnostic tests required, and treatment, due to limited proficiency in the host country's primary language [22]. For this reason, health care needs to be integrated with a cultural mediation service. By facilitating communication and helping health professionals to understand and be aware of migrants' cultural practices, a cultural mediator may contribute to a more reliable diagnostic workout [23]. For instance, one of the commonest conditions encountered among migrants receiving primary care, somatization, is recognized as tying up with one's cultural models [24, 25]. There is evidence to suggest that somatization among migrants may lie behind an under-recognized post-traumatic condition [26]; somatic syndrome has proved to be the main psychopathological dimension among migrants diagnosed with psychotic disorders [27].

With respect to confidence and continuity of care in mental health settings, it seems that a bad starting interaction with services may adversely affect proper engagement, by people coming from culturally diverse backgrounds, resulting in potentially harmful delay in help-seeking [28]. It is therefore important to make services culturally accessible; training mental health professionals to improve their cultural competency will significantly improve the quality of assistance provided. A set of useful and precious recommendations for policymakers, service providers, and clinicians is available [29].

8.2.3 Mental Disorders in Migrants

Some psychiatric disorders have a higher incidence in migrant populations such as depression [30], post-traumatic stress disorder (PTSD) [31], and psychosis [32]. We will make a brief examination about the first two disorders, to focus later on psychosis that results the mental disorder in which the migrant population is most at risk.

Depression is a mood disorder rating in natives from 3% (severe depression) to 32.5% (minor depression) and in migrant from 0 to 74% [33]. Despite the higher incidence in the migrant population, depression may be underdiagnosed within the migrant population [34] for many factors, including the absence of words to describe depression in many cultures and the fact that in some countries depression is not considered an illness but a natural mood swing [35]. Cultural shock and cultural bereavement are listed among the most important factors accountable for the onset of distress and depression in migrants [36]. Oberg [37] defined cultural shock as the sense of loss and rejection by members of the new culture. Cultural bereavement is defined as a "grief reaction" to the loss of one's social structure and culture [38]. All these factors contribute to the development of an identity crisis that may be only transitory if the migrant has enough self-confidence and good social support [39]. The interplay between cultural identity and cultural congruity is believed to be crucial in this adaptation phase [36].

Post-traumatic stress disorder (PTSD) has an overall prevalence of 47% in migrant populations [31], while its prevalence in the general population varies between 1.9 and 8.8% [40]. It is therefore clear that migrant populations are more susceptible to develop it. This can be due to the quantitative effect mentioned in various studies, i.e. the greater the number of traumas suffered, the higher the relative risk of developing PTSD.

Research on PTSD among migrants has focused mainly on asylum seekers and refugees. They are indeed often exposed to traumatic events and psychosocial stress factors during the pre-migratory, migratory [41], and post-migratory phases [42]. Particularly, it seems that post-migratory traumatic events play a role of fundamental importance in the development of PTSD [43–45] and include social precariousness, poverty, discrimination, and the persisting fear of being repatriated [41].

In these populations traumas are often perpetrated over time and may lead to the development of so-called complex PTSD [46]. This disorder includes the classic signs of PTSD (intrusive symptoms, signs of avoidance and negative alterations of thoughts and emotions associated with the event), but affective, relational, and somatic domains are also affected. The diagnosis is difficult to formulate, since the available diagnostic tools are calibrated on Western populations [47] and have limited validity when applied to culturally different people.

8.3 Migration and Psychosis: From Vulnerability to Resilience

8.3.1 Relative Risk of Psychosis among Migrants

Over the years, mounting evidence has shown that migrants have a higher risk of psychotic disorders than do natives or fellow countrymen without a history of migration. A recent meta-analysis [32] found that in European countries, the relative risk (RR) of non-affective psychosis among first- and second-generation migrants of non-European origin is three times higher than among native counterparts (RR = 2.94, 95% CI 2.63–3.29). Migrants of European provenance had a lower, but still significantly increased, risk (RR = 1.88, 95% CI 1.62–2.18). The RR was the highest among blacks (RR = 4.19, 95% CI 3.42–5.14). In Israel and Canada, however, migrants did not have a RR of psychosis greater than natives. This finding reflects the results from another recent work by the EUropean Network of National Schizophrenia Networks Studying Gene-Environment Interactions (EU-GEI) group [48]: this multinational study [49] found that the incidence risk ratio (IRR) of psychotic disorders among migrants or ethnic minorities varied by study catchment site and was the lowest in Valencia (IRR = 0.70, 95% CI 0.32–1.53) and the highest in Paris (IRR = 2.47, 95% CI 1.66–3.69). The IRR of psychosis among migrants and ethnic minorities, from site to site, was higher where the IRR of psychosis among the reference population (natives) was higher and vice versa. Overall, the IRR of psychosis was higher for migrants from non-Western countries (pooled IRR = 2.12, 95% CI 1.88–2.40) than migrants from Western countries (pooled IRR = 1.09, 95% CI 0.91–1.32). Those with the highest IRR were from sub-Saharan Africa (IRR = 3.23, 95% CI 2.66–3.93). In a study conducted by Tarricone et al. [50], rates of psychosis were found to be considerably elevated in internal migrants as well (IRR = 1.93, 95% CI 1.19–3.13).

8.3.2　Possible Explanations of the Phenomenon

Despite many years of dedicated research, the causes of such increased rates of psychotic disorders among migrants and ethnic minorities remain largely ununderstood.

One of the first hypotheses to explain this phenomenon was that of a higher incidence of psychosis in the countries of origin. Nevertheless, studies conducted in Jamaica [51], Trinidad [52], Barbados [53], Surinam [54], India, and China [55] failed to demonstrate this hypothesis. This implies that the excess of psychosis among migrants cannot be explained only in terms of biological predisposition or genetic vulnerability.

Odegaard [56] proposed the hypothesis of "selective migration", meaning that the individuals carrying the highest risk of psychosis were more likely to migrate. This hypothesis was refuted by subsequent studies [57, 58]. Notwithstanding the aforementioned limitations, however, some evidence seems to support a mechanism of positive selection (the so-called healthy migrant effect). Also, host countries with strict immigration policies may tend to reinforce such a mechanism.

Some authors have suggested that the increased rates of psychosis in migrants could be due to misdiagnosis [59, 60]. Again, the hypothesis failed to be supported by later evidence: for instance, a study comparing diagnoses formulated by British and Jamaican psychiatrists on the same group of patients did not find differences in the rates of psychotic disorder diagnosis [61]. Nevertheless, in the light of the potential negative effect of a wrong diagnosis, it is of fundamental importance not to introduce such biases in epidemiological studies.

Another possible explanation is substance-induced psychosis. It is a fact that abuse of psychotropic substances is considerably more frequent among men than women. However, evidence as to the possible greater risk of psychosis among migrants of male than female gender proves to be heterogeneous and inconclusive: for example, in the meta-analysis conducted by Selten et al. [32], there were no significant sex differences in the RR of psychosis, while another meta-analysis found that, among migrants from the Maghreb resettled in Europe, the risk of psychosis was greater for men [62]. Due to the lack of conclusive evidence, Selten et al. [32] conclude that abuse of psychotropic substances does not play a major role in explaining the excess of psychosis in migrants. In a multicentric study conducted in Italy, none of the migrants recruited was diagnosed with substance-related psychosis [63].

Finally, some authors have highlighted the possible role of exposure to biological risk factors before, during, and after migration. These include infections, obstetric complications, and vitamin D deficiency. Again, the evidence supporting the role of these factors in populations of migrants is weak or limited [54, 64–66].

Taken together, the data available suggest that the factors that mainly condition the mental health of migrants are social in the first place.

Among the main aetiopathogenic models taking into account the social determinants of psychosis, it is worth citing the "neuro-sociodevelopmental model" proposed by Morgan et al. [67, 68]. According to this model, exposure to social stressors (social adversities and childhood abuse), before or during migration, may interact with genetic susceptibility or other factors which can impair the neurodevelopment (perinatal infections, obstetric complications, etc.) generating a liability to psychosis. The cumulative effect of further stressors or environmental adversities, including substance abuse, may then lead to full-blown psychosis.

Another hypothesis is that of "social defeat", which is defined as "the long-term experience of a subordinate position or outsider status" [69, 70]. The prolongated experience of "social defeat" is believed to lead to sensitization of the mesolimbic dopaminergic system, which is linked to psychosis. Neurobiological evidence derived from animal models [71] and from a Canadian study conducted on migrants (healthy volunteers, subjects at clinical high risk of psychosis, and patients with schizophrenia) [72] would seem to support this hypothesis.

8.3.3 Vulnerability Factors in Migrants

A history of migration across the three stages (pre-migration, migration, and post-migration) may itself significantly contribute to the excess of psychosis in migrants, given the exposure to adversity and social disadvantages which, cumulatively, may lead to a 14-fold increase in the odds of psychosis [73]. In their study, conducted over a sample of first-generation migrants recruited from six different countries, Tarricone et al. [73] tried to disentangle the timing of the social disadvantages across the three phases of migration, finding an increase of about 1.5 in the odds of first-episode psychosis for each additional disadvantage (on a scale from 1 to 3) in the pre-migratory phase (OR = 1.61, 95% CI 1.06–2.44) and about two-fold for each additional disadvantage (range from 1 to 3) in the post-migratory phase (OR = 1.89, 95% CI 1.02–3.51). This study adds further evidence that the most significant risk factors for the onset of psychosis in migrants lie in the post-migration phase. Previous studies had already identified a pre-eminent role for the post-migration social disadvantages, such as difficulties of integration in the host society [74, 75], higher levels of perceived discrimination [76–78], reduced "social capital" [79, 80], mismatch between expectations prior to migration and achievements once resettled in a new country [81], and a worse quality of general health [63, 82]. In their study, Tarricone and colleagues claim that effective social and public health strategies should be adopted to address the social drivers of high rates of psychosis among migrants [73].

8.3.4 Resilience Factors in Migrants

However, despite the possibly high potential exposure to several risk factors, not all migrants go on to develop a psychotic disorder. Thus, we also must consider resilience factors that may counterbalance the negative effects of migration-related stressors and protect the individuals from the development of psychosis. Among the factors that may exert a protective effect, the literature available to date lists age of migration [83], family network (with gender specificities) [84], premorbid levels of psychosocial functioning [63], proficiency in the host country main language [85], and living in high-ethnic density neighborhoods [86].

Concerning age of migration, a meta-analysis has shown that those who migrate after the age of 18 have a significantly lower risk of psychosis compared to those who migrate during childhood or adolescence [83]. This suggests that the effects of international migration stressors may have a greater impact on a brain that is still under development. Thus, minor migrants deserve special attention and require specific intervention to promote their resilience and prevent psychosis onset.

A recent study found a significant association between family networks during migration and post-migration psychosis, and the association was influenced by gender [84]: for females it was protective to migrate with the family or to rejoin it, while for males this represented a risk factor. This is probably due to the difference in terms of perceived role and expectations about the migration. Males might feel the burden of having to care and support their families and perceive this as a strong post-migration stress (risk was higher when they also had dependent children). On the other hand, it is known that women encounter more difficulties to enter the labour market, risking obtaining exploitative jobs, and to integrate into the new society [87–89]; for this reason, they may have more benefit from a supportive family network.

There is evidence to support that migrants diagnosed with psychotic disorders may have higher levels of premorbid functioning and better occupational outcomes than native counterparts [63, 90]. In a multicentric Italian study [63], many migrants with first-episode psychosis presented with a "high functioning portrait": that is to say, they were highly educated, employed, and in a past or current stable affective relationship. This is in contrasts with common findings among natives with psychosis from the same country [91, 92]. Adjunctively, another study from Tarricone et al. [90] found that 12 months after the onset of first-episode psychosis, migrants were more likely than natives to have resumed studies or work activity. The personal resources are an important factor of resilience, and migrants diagnosed with psychosis should receive support and rehabilitative treatments to maintain adequate psychosocial functioning.

Recent findings from a EU-GEI study [85] highlighted the role of the linguistic distance (expressed as a combination of one's language proficiency and distance on a language tree between one's first language and the majority language in the country of arrival). Migrant with greater linguistic distance had significantly increased odds of psychosis. Language proficiency is pivotal for the integration in the new country and seems essential to promote resilience with respect to migrants' mental health.

Finally, there is established evidence that migrants living in neighbourhoods with high ethnic density have lower psychosis risk [86], possibly due to reduced social stress, better social support, and increased social capital.

8.4   Conclusions

Migrants have a higher prevalence of severe mental disorders, including psychosis. The excess of such disorders among migrants has been widely recognized and defined as a "public tragedy" for its human and social costs. But migrants still face health inequalities when it comes to seeking and receiving timely and appropriate treatment. It is of crucial importance that we make further progress in understanding where exactly the vulnerabilities of migrants lie, from the early phases of migration to the definitive resettlement stage. Years of research have already identified several factors, and most of them are environmental and social in nature. Policymakers and service providers should be aware of these findings and implement effective strategies in terms of both prevention and treatment of mental disorders in migrants.

> **Key Points**
> - Migration is an ever-painful process with the potential to expose individuals to several life stressors and disadvantages which may be responsible for the excess of mental disorders in migrants.
> - Notwithstanding the well-documented higher risk of psychosis and other serious mental disorders, migrants still encounter several barriers and inequalities in receiving prompt and adequate mental health care.
> - Future research should focus not only on the factors that make migrants more vulnerable but also on the factors that may promote their resilience in order to implement effective and evidence-based psychosocial prevention strategies.

References

1. International Organization for Migration (IOM). World Migration Report. Published online 2020.
2. United Nations Development Programme (UNDP). Human development report 2009|Human development reports: overcoming barriers: human mobility and development; 2009. http://hdr.undp.org/en/content/human-development-report-2009
3. World Health Organization (WHO). WHO|Definitions. Published online 2017. http://www.who.int/migrants/about/definitions/en/
4. Abubakar I, Aldridge RW, Devakumar D, et al. The UCL–Lancet Commission on migration and health: the health of a world on the move. Lancet. 2018;392(10164):2606–54. https://doi.org/10.1016/S0140-6736(18)32114-7.
5. Castelli F. Drivers of migration: why do people move? J Travel Med. 2018;25(1):1–7. https://doi.org/10.1093/jtm/tay040.
6. Bhugra D, Gupta S, Bhui K, et al. WPA guidance on mental health and mental health care in migrants. World Psychiatry. 2011;10(1):2–10. https://doi.org/10.1002/j.2051-5545.2011.tb00002.x.

7. Juárez SP, Revuelta-Eugercios BA. Exploring the 'healthy migrant paradox' in Sweden. A cross sectional study focused on perinatal outcomes. J Immigr Minor Health. 2016;18(1):42–50. https://doi.org/10.1007/s10903-015-0157-5.

8. Blair AH, Schneeberg A. Changes in the "healthy migrant effect" in Canada: are recent immigrants healthier than they were a decade ago? J Immigr Minor Health. 2014;16(1):136–42. https://doi.org/10.1007/s10903-013-9813-9.

9. Speciale AM, Regidor E. Understanding the universality of the immigrant health paradox: the Spanish perspective. J Immigr Minor Health. 2011;13(3):518–25. https://doi.org/10.1007/s10903-010-9365-1.

10. Aldridge RW, Nellums LB, Bartlett S, et al. Global patterns of mortality in international migrants: a systematic review and meta-analysis. Lancet. 2018;392(10164):2553–66. https://doi.org/10.1016/S0140-6736(18)32781-8.

11. Moullan Y, Jusot F. Why is the "healthy immigrant effect" different between European countries? Eur J Pub Health. 2014;24(Suppl 1):80–6. https://doi.org/10.1093/eurpub/cku112.

12. Abraído-Lanza AF, Chao MT, Flórez KR. Do healthy behaviors decline with greater acculturation? Implications for the Latino mortality paradox. Soc Sci Med. 2005;61(6):1243–55. https://doi.org/10.1016/j.socscimed.2005.01.016.

13. Fuller-Thomson E, Noack AM, Usha G. Health decline among recent immigrants to Canada: findings from a nationally-representative longitudinal survey. Can J Public Health. 2011;102(4):273–80. https://doi.org/10.1007/bf03404048.

14. Lougarre C. Using the right to health to promote universal health coverage: a better tool for protecting non-nationals' access to affordable health care? Health Hum Rights. 2016;18(2):35–47.

15. Agbata EN, Padilla PF, Agbata IN, et al. Migrant healthcare guidelines: a systematic quality assessment. J Immigr Minor Health. 2019;21(2):401–13. https://doi.org/10.1007/s10903-018-0759-9.

16. Hiam L, Gionakis N, Holmes SM, McKee M. Overcoming the barriers migrants face in accessing health care. Public Health. 2019;172:89–92. https://doi.org/10.1016/j.puhe.2018.11.015.

17. Suphanchaimat R, Kantamaturapoj K, Putthasri W, Prakongsai P. Challenges in the provision of healthcare services for migrants: a systematic review through providers' lens. BMC Health Serv Res. 2015;15(1):390. https://doi.org/10.1186/s12913-015-1065-z.

18. Setia MS, Quesnel-Vallee A, Abrahamowicz M, Tousignant P, Lynch J. Access to health-care in Canadian immigrants: a longitudinal study of the National Population Health Survey. Health Soc Care Community. 2011;19(1):70–9. https://doi.org/10.1111/j.1365-2524.2010.00950.x.

19. Baumeister A, Aldin A, Chakraverty D, et al. Interventions for improving health literacy in migrants. Cochrane Database Syst Rev. 2019;2019(4):CD013303. https://doi.org/10.1002/14651858.cd013303.

20. Pottie K, Batista R, Mayhew M, Mota L, Grant K. Improving delivery of primary care for vulnerable migrants: Delphi consensus to prioritize innovative practice strategies. Can Fam Physician. 2014;60(1):e32. www.ccirhken.ca

21. International Organization for Migration (IOM). International Migration, Health and Human Rights; 2013. www.iom.int

22. Brandenberger J, Tylleskär T, Sontag K, Peterhans B, Ritz N. A systematic literature review of reported challenges in health care delivery to migrants and refugees in high-income countries-the 3C model. BMC Public Health. 2019;19(1):755. https://doi.org/10.1186/s12889-019-7049-x.

23. Martín MC, Phelan M. Interpreters and cultural mediators-different but complementary roles. Translocat Migr Soc Chang. 2010;6(1):1–19.

24. Ferrari S, Burian R, Hahn E, et al. Somatization among ethnic minorities and immigrants: why does it matter to consultation liaison psychiatry? J Psychosom Res. 2015;79(1):85–6. https://doi.org/10.1016/j.jpsychores.2015.02.011.

25. Kirmayer LJ, Sartorius N. Cultural models and somatic syndromes. Psychosom Med. 2007;69:832–40. https://doi.org/10.1097/PSY.0b013e31815b002c.

26. Aragona M, Catino E, Pucci D, et al. The relationship between somatization and post-traumatic symptoms among immigrants receiving primary care services. J Trauma Stress. 2010;23(5):615–22. https://doi.org/10.1002/jts.20571.

27. Braca M, Berardi D, Mencacci E, et al. Understanding psychopathology in migrants: a mixed categorical-dimensional approach. Int J Soc Psychiatry. 2014;60(3):243–53. https://doi.org/10.1177/0020764013484237.

28. Morgan C, Mallett R, Hutchinson G, Leff J. Negative pathways to psychiatric care and ethnicity: the bridge between social science and psychiatry. In: Social science and medicine, vol. 58. Elsevier Ltd; 2004. p. 739–52. https://doi.org/10.1016/S0277-9536(03)00233-8.

29. Schouler-Ocak M, Graef-Calliess IT, Tarricone I, Qureshi A, Kastrup MC, Bhugra D. EPA guidance on cultural competence training. Eur Psychiatry. 2015;30(3):431–40. https://doi.org/10.1016/j.eurpsy.2015.01.012.

30. Juhasz G, Eszlari N, Pap D, Gonda X. Cultural differences in the development and characteristics of depression. Neuropsychopharmacol Hung. 2012;14(4):259–65.

31. Lindert J, von Ehrenstein OS, Priebe S, Mielck A, Brähler E. Depression and anxiety in labor migrants and refugees—a systematic review and meta-analysis. Soc Sci Med. 2009;69(2):246–57. https://doi.org/10.1016/j.socscimed.2009.04.032.

32. Selten JP, Van Der Ven E, Termorshuizen F. Migration and psychosis: a meta-analysis of incidence studies. Psychol Med. 2019;50(2):303–13. https://doi.org/10.1017/S0033291719000035.

33. Ilaria T. Ethnic variation in the prevalence of depression and anxiety in primary care: a systematic review and meta-analysis. Psychiatry Res. 2012;195(3):91–105.

34. Antoniades J, Mazza D, Brijnath B. Efficacy of depression treatments for immigrant patients: results from a systematic review. BMC Psychiatry. 2014;14:176. https://doi.org/10.1186/1471-244X-14-176.

35. Bhugra D, Gupta S, Schouler-Ocak M, et al. EPA guidance mental health care of migrants. Eur Psychiatry. 2014;29(2):107–15. https://doi.org/10.1016/j.eurpsy.2014.01.003.

36. Bhugra D, Becker MA. Migration, cultural bereavement and cultural identity. World Psychiatry. 2005;4(1):18–24. https://doi.org/10.1016/j.critrevonc.2017.12.007.

37. Oberg K. Cultural shock: adjustment to new cultural environments. Pract Anthropol. 1960;os-7(4):177–82. https://doi.org/10.1177/009182966000700405.

38. Eisenbruch M. From post-traumatic stress disorder to cultural bereavement: diagnosis of Southeast Asian refugees. Soc Sci Med. 1991;33(6):673–80. http://www.ncbi.nlm.nih.gov/pubmed/1957187

39. Bhugra D. Migration and mental health. Acta Psychiatr Scand. 2004;109(4):243–58. https://doi.org/10.1046/j.0001-690X.2003.00246.x.

40. Bisson JI, Cosgrove S, Lewis C, Roberts NP. Post-traumatic stress disorder. BMJ. 2015;351:h6161. https://doi.org/10.1136/bmj.h6161.

41. Priebe D, El-Nagib R, Giacco S. Public health aspects of mental health among migrants and refugees: a review of the evidence on mental health care for refugees, Asylum seekers and irregular migrants in the WHO European Region. World Health Organization. Regional Office for Europe; 2016. https://apps.who.int/iris/handle/10665/326308

42. Nosè M, Turrini G, Imoli M, et al. Prevalence and correlates of psychological distress and psychiatric disorders in asylum seekers and refugees resettled in an Italian catchment area. J Immigr Minor Health. 2018;20(2):263–70. https://doi.org/10.1007/s10903-017-0629-x.

43. Fazel M, Wheeler J, Danesh J. Prevalence of serious mental disorder in 7000 refugees resettled in western countries: a systematic review. Lancet. 2005;365(9467):1309–14. https://doi.org/10.1016/S0140-6736(05)61027-6.

44. Abbott A. The mental-health crisis among migrants. Nature. 2016;538(7624):158–60. https://doi.org/10.1038/538158a.

45. Aragona M, Castaldo M, Cristina Tumiati M, et al. Influence of post-migration living difficulties on post-traumatic symptoms in Chinese asylum seekers resettled in Italy. Int J Soc Psychiatry. 2020;66(2):129–35. https://doi.org/10.1177/0020764019888960.

46. Herman JL. Complex PTSD: a syndrome in survivors of prolonged and repeated trauma. J Trauma Stress. 1992;5(3):377–91. https://doi.org/10.1002/jts.2490050305.

47. Kleinman A. Anthropology and psychiatry: the role of culture in cross-cultural research on illness. Br J Psychiatry. 1987;151(4):447–54. https://doi.org/10.1192/bjp.151.4.447.

48. European Network of National Networks studying Gene-Environment Interactions in Schizophrenia (EU-GEI), van Os J, Rutten BP, et al. Identifying gene-environment interac-

tions in schizophrenia: contemporary challenges for integrated, large-scale investigations. Schizophr Bull. 2014;40(4):729–36. https://doi.org/10.1093/schbul/sbu069.

49. Termorshuizen F, Van Der Ven E, Tarricone I, et al. The incidence of psychotic disorders among migrants and minority ethnic groups in Europe: Findings from the multinational EU-GEI study. Psychol Med. 2020:1–10. https://doi.org/10.1017/S0033291720003219.

50. Tarricone I, Boydell J, Kokona A, et al. Risk of psychosis and internal migration: results from the Bologna First Episode Psychosis study. Schizophr Res. 2016;173(1–2):90–3. https://doi.org/10.1016/j.schres.2016.02.032.

51. Hickling FW, Rodgers-Johnson P. The incidence of first contact schizophrenia in Jamaica. Br J Psychiatry. 1995;167(2):193–6. https://doi.org/10.1192/bjp.167.2.193.

52. Bhugra D, Hilwig M, Hossein B, et al. First-contact incidence rates of schizophrenia in Trinidad and one-year follow-up. Br J Psychiatry. 1996;169(5):587–92. https://doi.org/10.1192/bjp.169.5.587.

53. Mahy GE, Mallett R, Leff J, Bhugra D. First-contact incidence rate of schizophrenia on Barbados. Br J Psychiatry. 1999;175(1):28–33. https://doi.org/10.1192/bjp.175.1.28.

54. Selten JP, Slaets J, Kahn R. Prenatal exposure to influenza and schizophrenia in Surinamese and Dutch Antillean immigrants to the Netherlands. Schizophr Res. 1998;30(1):101–3. https://doi.org/10.1016/S0920-9964(97)00105-9.

55. Baxter AJ, Charlson FJ, Cheng HG, Shidhaye R, Ferrari AJ, Whiteford HA. Prevalence of mental, neurological, and substance use disorders in China and India: a systematic analysis. Lancet Psychiatry. 2016;3(9):832–41. https://doi.org/10.1016/S2215-0366(16)30139-0.

56. Odegaard O. Emigration and insanity. Acta Psychiatr Neurol Scand Suppl. 1932;4:1–206.

57. Van Der Ven E, Dalman C, Wicks S, et al. Testing Ødegaard's selective migration hypothesis: a longitudinal cohort study of risk factors for non-affective psychotic disorders among prospective emigrants. Psychol Med. 2015;45(4):727–34. https://doi.org/10.1017/S0033291714001780.

58. Cantor-Graae E, Selten J-P. Schizophrenia and migration: a meta-analysis and review. Am J Psychiatry. 2005;162(I):12–24. https://doi.org/10.1021/jf1031026.

59. Fernando S. Mental health, race and culture. London: Macmillan Education UK; 1991. https://doi.org/10.1007/978-1-349-21644-4

60. Littlewood R, Lipsedge M. Aliens and alienists: ethnic minorities and psychiatry. 3rd ed. London: Routledge; 1997.

61. Hickling FW, McKenzie K, Mullen R, Murray R. A Jamaican psychiatrist evaluates diagnoses at a London psychiatric hospital. Br J Psychiatry. 1999;175(September):283–5. https://doi.org/10.1192/bjp.175.3.283.

62. van der Ven E, Veling W, Tortelli A, et al. Evidence of an excessive gender gap in the risk of psychotic disorder among North African immigrants in Europe: a systematic review and meta-analysis. Soc Psychiatry Psychiatr Epidemiol. 2016;51(12):1603–13. https://doi.org/10.1007/s00127-016-1261-0.

63. Tarricone I, D'Andrea G, Storbini V, et al. First-episode psychosis and migration in Italy: results from a study in the Italian Mental Health Services (Pep-Ita Study). J Immigr Minor Health. 2021;23(3):519–27. https://doi.org/10.1007/s10903-021-01168-w.

64. Selten JP, Van Vliet K, Pleyte W, Herzog S, Hoek HW, Van Loon AM. Borna disease virus and schizophrenia in Surinamese immigrants to the Netherlands. Med Microbiol Immunol. 2000;189(2):55–7. https://doi.org/10.1007/PL00008256.

65. O'Neill SM, Curran EA, Dalman C, et al. Birth by caesarean section and the risk of adult psychosis: a population-based cohort study. Schizophr Bull. 2016;42(3):633–41. https://doi.org/10.1093/schbul/sbv152.

66. Huibers MHW, Visser DH, Deckers MML, Van Schoor NM, Van Furth AM, Wolf BHM. Vitamin D deficiency among native Dutch and first- and second-generation non-Western immigrants. Eur J Pediatr. 2014;173(5):583–8. https://doi.org/10.1007/s00431-013-2198-x.

67. Morgan C, Charalambides M, Hutchinson G, Murray RM. Migration, ethnicity, and psychosis: toward a sociodevelopmental model. Schizophr Bull. 2010;36(4):655–64. https://doi.org/10.1093/schbul/sbq051.

68. Morgan C, Knowles G, Hutchinson G. Migration, ethnicity and psychoses: evidence, models and future directions. World Psychiatry. 2019;18(3):247–58. https://doi.org/10.1002/wps.20655.
69. Selten JP, Van Der Ven E, Rutten BPF, Cantor-Graae E. The social defeat hypothesis of schizophrenia: an update. Schizophr Bull. 2013;39(6):1180–6. https://doi.org/10.1093/schbul/sbt134.
70. Selten J, Cantor-Graae E. Social defeat: risk factor for schizophrenia? Br J Psychiatry. 2005;187(2):101–2. https://doi.org/10.1192/bjp.187.2.101.
71. Hammels C, Pishva E, De Vry J, et al. Defeat stress in rodents: from behavior to molecules. Neurosci Biobehav Rev. 2015;59:111–40. https://doi.org/10.1016/j.neubiorev.2015.10.006.
72. Egerton A, Howes OD, Houle S, et al. Elevated striatal dopamine function in immigrants and their children: a risk mechanism for psychosis. Schizophr Bull. 2017;43(2):293–301. https://doi.org/10.1093/schbul/sbw181.
73. Tarricone I, D'Andrea G, Jongsma HE, et al. Migration history and risk of psychosis: results from the multinational EU-GEI study. Psychol Med. 2021:1–13. https://doi.org/10.1017/s003329172000495x.
74. Kirkbride JB, Morgan C, Fearon P, Dazzan P, Murray RM, Jones PB. Neighbourhood-level effects on psychoses: re-examining the role of context. Psychol Med. 2007;37(10):1413–25. https://doi.org/10.1017/S0033291707000499.
75. Van Os J, Hanssen M, Bijl RV, Vollebergh W. Prevalence of psychotic disorder and community level of psychotic symptoms: an urban-rural comparison. Arch Gen Psychiatry. 2001;58(7):663–8. https://doi.org/10.1001/archpsyc.58.7.663.
76. Berg AO, Melle I, Rossberg JI, et al. Perceived discrimination is associated with severity of positive and depression/anxiety symptoms in immigrants with psychosis: a cross-sectional study. BMC Psychiatry. 2011;11:77. https://doi.org/10.1186/1471-244X-11-77.
77. Cooper C, Morgan C, Byrne M, et al. Perceptions of disadvantage, ethnicity and psychosis. Br J Psychiatry. 2008;192(3):185–90. https://doi.org/10.1192/bjp.bp.107.042291.
78. Misra S, Gelaye B, Williams DR, et al. Perceived major experiences of discrimination, ethnic group, and risk of psychosis in a six-country case–control study. Psychol Med. 2021:1–9. https://doi.org/10.1017/S0033291721000453.
79. Allardyce J, Gilmour H, Atkinson J, Rapson T, Bishop J, McCreadie RG. Social fragmentation, deprivation and urbanicity: relation to first-admission rates for psychoses. Br J Psychiatry. 2005;187:401–6. https://doi.org/10.1192/bjp.187.5.401.
80. Kirkbride JB, Jones PB. The prevention of schizophrenia—what can we learn from eco-epidemiology? Schizophr Bull. 2011;37(2):262–71. https://doi.org/10.1093/schbul/sbq120.
81. Reininghaus UA, Morgan C, Simpson J, et al. Unemployment, social isolation, achievement–expectation mismatch and psychosis: findings from the ÆSOP Study. Soc Psychiatry Psychiatr Epidemiol. 2008;43(9):743–51. https://doi.org/10.1007/s00127-008-0359-4.
82. Tarricone I, Atti AR, Salvatori F, et al. Psychotic symptoms and general health in a socially disadvantaged migrant community in Bologna. Int J Soc Psychiatry. 2009;55(3):203–13. https://doi.org/10.1177/0020764008093445.
83. Anderson KK, Edwards J. Age at migration and the risk of psychotic disorders: a systematic review and meta-analysis. Acta Psychiatr Scand. 2020;141(5):410–20. https://doi.org/10.1111/acps.13147.
84. Dykxhoorn J, Hollander AC, Lewis G, Dalman C, Kirkbride JB. Family networks during migration and risk of non-affective psychosis: a population-based cohort study. Schizophr Res. 2019;208:268–75. https://doi.org/10.1016/j.schres.2019.01.044.
85. Jongsma HE, Gayer-Anderson C, Tarricone I, et al. Social disadvantage, linguistic distance, ethnic minority status and first-episode psychosis: results from the EU-GEI case-control study. Psychol Med. 2021;51(9):1536–48. https://doi.org/10.1017/S003329172000029X.
86. Schofield P, Thygesen M, Das-Munshi J, et al. Ethnic density, urbanicity and psychosis risk for migrant groups—a population cohort study. Schizophr Res. 2017;190:82–7. https://doi.org/10.1016/j.schres.2017.03.032.

87. Llácer A, Victoria Zunzunegui M, del Amo J, Mazarrasa L, Bolůmar F. The contribution of a gender perspective to the understanding of migrants' health. J Epidemiol Community Health. 2007;61:4–10. https://doi.org/10.1136/jech.2007.061770.
88. Milewski N, Struffolino E, Bernardi L. Migrant status and lone motherhood—risk factors of female labour force participation in Switzerland. Cham: Springer; 2018. p. 141–63. https://doi.org/10.1007/978-3-319-63295-7_7.
89. Riaño Y, Baghdadi N. Understanding the labour market participation of skilled immigrant women in Switzerland: the interplay of class, ethnicity, and gender. J Int Migr Integr. 2007;8(2):163–83. https://doi.org/10.1007/s12134-007-0012-1.
90. Tarricone I, Morgan C, Boydell J, et al. Occupation and first episode psychosis in Northern Italy: better outcomes for migrants. Early Interv Psychiatry. 2017;11(6):522–5. https://doi.org/10.1111/eip.12325.
91. Tarricone I, Mimmi S, Paparelli A, et al. First-episode psychosis at the West Bologna Community Mental Health Centre: results of an 8-year prospective study. Psychol Med. 2012;42(11):2255–64. https://doi.org/10.1017/S0033291712000335.
92. Lasalvia A, Bonetto C, Tosato S, et al. First-contact incidence of psychosis in North-Eastern Italy: influence of age, gender, immigration and socioeconomic deprivation. Br J Psychiatry. 2014;205(2):127–34. https://doi.org/10.1192/bjp.bp.113.134445.

Tackling Urbanicity and Pollution in Mental Health Prevention Strategies

9

Antonio Ventriglio, João Mauricio Castaldelli-Maia, Julio Torales, Domenico De Berardis, and Dinesh Bhugra

9.1 Setting the Scene

The modern era has been characterized by a rapid globalization leading to cultural and economic exchanges between countries with an increase of urbanization, mega-cities, and metropolitan areas characterized by a higher level of industrialization [1]. It has been largely argued that these changes have led to new challenges for mental health globally: living in urban or metropolitan areas as well as being exposed to higher levels of pollution may impact on citizens' psychological balance and lead to distress [2].

A. Ventriglio (✉)
Department of Clinical and Experimental Medicine, University of Foggia, Foggia, Italy
e-mail: a.ventriglio@libero.it

J. M. Castaldelli-Maia
Department of Neuroscience, Medical School, Fundação do ABC, Santo André, SP, Brazil

Department of Psychiatry, Medical School, University of São Paulo, São Paulo, SP, Brazil

J. Torales
Department of Psychiatry, School of Medical Sciences, National University of Asunción, Asunción, Paraguay

D. De Berardis
Department of Mental Health, Teramo, Italy

University of Chieti, Chieti, Italy
e-mail: domenico.deberardis@aslteramo.it

D. Bhugra
Institute of Psychiatry, King's College, London, UK
e-mail: dinesh.bhugra@kcl.ac.uk

M. Colizzi, M. Ruggeri (eds.), *Prevention in Mental Health*,
https://doi.org/10.1007/978-3-030-97906-5_9

9.2   Introduction

9.2.1   Urbanization

Urbanization is a global process characterized by the shift of population from rural areas to cities or towns as a direct consequence of globalization. It includes some other processes as industrialization and social migration as well as cultural and economic exchanges [3]. It has been argued that urbanization leads to changes in the environment and society with an impact on social determinants of health and mental health [2]: in fact, many conditions such as economic resources, job opportunities, and access to the health-care system as well as pollution, lack of contact with nature (green and blue spaces), and social interactions (neighborhood structure) may be affected by the process of urbanization. Marmot pointed out that social stratification, political power and the economic factors directly affect the individual development, health status, as well as social determinants of health may be recognized as mediators between the macro-context and the individual balance [4].

It has been estimated that the percentage of world population living in the urban areas will increase rapidly in the following decades reaching 67% in 2050 [5].

In the 1990s, Faris and Dunham [6] proposed an association between the structure of neighborhood and the relative risk of developing schizophrenia in the city of Chicago, USA. More recently, March et al. [7] in their article entitled "Psychosis and Place" confirmed a set of associations between factors related to the neighborhood, such as living conditions, economic status and level of poverty, distributions of green areas or access to the rivers or sea, and mental health of inhabitants. Also, it has been observed that moving from rural to urban areas during childhood may be a risk factor for schizophrenia in vulnerable subjects with lower intelligence quotient (IQ) at baseline [8]. Nonetheless, behavioral and mental disorders among children may be prevalent in rural areas because of the lack of psychological and medical assistance as well as poor social and financial support [9].

In fact, social support is considered to be a protective factor in the prevention of mental illness [3]. In urban areas the rhythm of city life, long distances, the need to travel, and daily commitments do not promote social integration and interactions. New technology and social networks replace the direct interactions among people (in *flesh and bone*) with poorer social and emotional support: this may also be due to a major perceived insecurity in the cities and increase the level of it in a vicious circle [3, 10]. In fact, perceived insecurity and the risk of violence are higher in urban areas and may affect negatively social interactions and psychological well-being of the general population and mentally ill patients [11]. Also, the level of social integration may largely vary across urban and rural areas. For instance, mega-cities are inclusive and based on a globalized culture, with an "open-minded" approach to different cultures, ethnical variations, or minorities (including mentally ill patients). Thus, levels of stigma should be reduced in the urban setting, but there may be a lack of interpersonal support and high levels of lowliness especially for those people who are not able to work or not living with their own family [3]. Conversely, stigma in rural areas may be higher due to cultural closeness and discrimination of those people considered as minorities for any reason (migrants, sexual variants, etc.). Nonetheless, social distance and levels of interpersonal support may be higher [3].

Finally, a set of environmental factors impact on mental health in rural as well as urban settings such as the availability of green spaces (gardens, parks, etc.), access to the sea and rivers (blue spaces), access to services, vehicular traffic, air pollution, and noise [12]. It has been argued that the lack of green and blue spaces impacts negatively on mental health as well as the high level of pollution [12].

9.2.2 Pollution

Pollution has been increasing over the centuries in parallel with the process of industrialization worldwide. Even if the effect of pollution on human health in general is well described, there is poor evidence on the consequences of pollutant agents in terms of psychological distress and psychopathological issues. The term *pollution* refers to the action of noxious elements on the ecosystem mostly derived from the work of man and human industrialization [13]. It has been argued that pollution may affect the central nervous system as an *exogenous* agent and lead to mental illness through the interaction with the gene expression and neural system (*gene x environment interaction model*) or, alternatively, as a *psychogenic* agent as source of psychological long-term stress leading to mental disorders [14]. In fact, some authors have reported that the consequences of pollution on human health, physical as well as mental, are better described in the long term since all mechanisms of genetic mutation but also stress-related processes occur over the months or years [15]. Thus, two pathogenic mechanisms are proposed in the framework of mental disorders related to pollution: (a) *direct effect* due to biochemical mechanisms of interaction between pollutant agents and tissues or cells and (b) *indirect effect* due to the production of a stressful prolonged condition impacting on the hypothalamic-pituitary-adrenal axis and psychological balance [15].

9.3 Urban Mental Health

In the last decade, there has been a growing interest in the literature on the epidemiology of mental disorders across urban and rural settings. In 2010 a large study describing the results of 20 adult-population surveys conducted from 1985, authors reported higher rates of mental disorders in urban areas than rural ones, in particular anxiety and depressive disorders, ranging from 21% to 38% of prevalence [16].

A large study from India, conducted by the National Mental Health Survey of India, confirmed that the prevalence of mood disorders and stress-related conditions were two to three times higher in urban areas than in rural and semi-rural ones with a general rate of 37–50% for the urban setting [17].

According to the explanatory model based on the socio-environmental hypothesis of mental illness, it has been argued that a number of factors related to urbanicity

Table 9.1 Socio-environmental factors related to mental illness in urban areas

Environmental	Socioeconomic	Sociocultural	Urban design
Vehicular traffic	Welfare	Social support	Crowding and neighborhood structure
Factories	Employment	Social capital	Green spaces
Air pollution	Housing	Segregation and marginalization	Blue spaces
Noise pollution	Migration	Stigma and discrimination	Long distances
Light pollution	Health facilities (including mental health services)	Violence and crimes	Public transportation

may trigger the observed increased incidence and prevalence of mental disorders in the urban areas. All factors are acting as pathogenic agents leading to psychological as well as biological stress. We report in Table 9.1 some putative triggering factors as recognized by the literature [18–25].

Physical environmental factors such as air and noise pollution, mostly related to the industrialization index and the vehicular traffic volumes, are responsible for both biological and psychological stress since they may act as noxious and psychogenic agents on the central nervous system, as discussed in the following section of this chapter.

The socioeconomic pressure on the individual health balance is also relevant. Urban areas may be based on a welfare state, which promotes the economic and social well-being of any citizen with equal opportunity, distribution of wealth, and minimal provisions for a good life. In this case, job opportunities as well a housing and access to health-care systems are facilitated at any level of society with positive consequences on mental health; conversely, if social welfare programs are not appropriate, people who are less advantaged in terms of socioeconomic position will have worse opportunities (job, house, health care, etc.) and poorer health [3].

As already discussed, also the cultural milieu in the cities and social beliefs may impact on an individual's mental health: urban societies generally are emancipated and show an "open-minded" approach to minorities (migrants, poverty, homeless people) or variants (sexual variants, political variants, religious variants) with lower levels of stigma and discrimination [3]. Nonetheless, cities do not promote social interactions, and, as discussed, social support and social capital may be lower than in rural settings in some cases. This may lead to a marginalization of people who are economically disadvantaged or minorities with possible conducts of segregation (poor people, ethnical groups, or sexual variants may be marginalized in specific areas of the cities) [3].

Urbanicity and psychosis: In the 1990s, Faris and Duham presented a very interesting report on the risk of psychosis in the city of Chicago related to the neighborhood structure, confirming a higher incidence of mental health problems in the urban setting [20]. Many other following studies based on a large population from different countries have been conducted (UK, Germany, USA, North Europe; [26–34]).

The higher prevalence of schizophrenia and psychosis in the cities has been discussed and explained through some hypotheses such as "the social drift," the "gene x environmental" interaction as discussed, and the detection bias in the rural setting [3]. The drift hypothesis points out that schizophrenia patients show a chronic and progressive clinical outcome with impaired social functioning leading to a shift towards lower social classes and poorer life condition: they also may move to more deprived urban areas or live as homeless [20]. Several studies describing the polygenic risk score in schizophrenia have pointed out that socio-environmental factors (as recognized for other common disorders) may impact on the rate of psychosis onset, in particular poverty, perinatal risk (e.g., obstetric complications), social stress, and pollution, all related to urbanicity [3, 35, 36]. Also, substance abuse impacts significantly on the onset of psychosis [37]. It has been reported that the rate of substance abuse, above all novel psychoactive substances such as methamphetamine, salvia divinorum, and desomorphine, is higher in the urban settings, as well as the access to bars, discos, drug-dealing hotspots, and information about substances (peer to peer or Internet) [37]. Also, 48% of people aged 16–24 years old in the cities report alcohol consumption [37]. Substances abuse in the rural areas may be mostly due to isolation, unemployment, and difficulty in accessing therapeutic programs [37].

In addition, the detection of psychosis, above all the early stages of illness as well as at-risk mental states, may be lower in rural areas than in urban ones, and this may affect the different prevalence among the two settings. In particular, early-intervention units for the diagnosis and treatment of psychosis are missing in the rural zones, and psychoses may be underestimated or under-detected for a lack of surveillance [38].

Urbanicity and suicide: Life in urban areas has been associated with higher rates of suicidality even if the prevalence may vary widely over the reports. Some studies described a higher rate of suicide in the cities in the last decades in some countries (Europe, USA, New Zealand, China, and Canada), whereas the trend was reverse in Australia with higher rates in rural settings [39, 40]. Reasons for suicidality in these areas may be due to social isolation, socioeconomic difficulties, lack of mental health services, and climate challenges [41]. Conversely, reasons for suicide in urban setting may be unemployment, marginalization, socioeconomic pressure, and stressful lifestyle [3]. Interestingly, methods of suicide may be different in the two settings, with a prevalent employment of pesticides or jumping into a river or lake in rural setting *versus* jumping from a height or throwing oneself in front of a train in cities: urban designers should improve place security protecting buildings, bridges, railways, and subways, and social integration and public welfare should be promoted [42].

Homelessness and marginalization in the cities: The rapid urbanization in the last decades has led to the development of megacities around the globe with a variable range of socioeconomic inequalities as well as poverty and marginalization in the lower social classes [3]. In fact, the sociocultural and economic development does not necessarily follow the flux of urbanization, and preexisting disparities in the society may increase [3]. Megacities are characterized by some major challenges: social and occupational unmet needs, competition for job opportunities and resources, housing issues and homelessness, ethnical/cultural/religious/political minorities and their marginalization, and immigration [3]. A set of factors have been associated with homelessness in the cities as history of trauma in adolescence, migration, job loss, etc. [43]. According to evidence from Stergioupulos et al. [44], 72% of homeless people living in six larger urban areas in Canada report cognitive impairment related to mental disorders (mostly mood and psychotic disorders), substance abuse, or poor quality of life: mental disorders and substance abuse are also associated with a higher risk of infections, trauma, and a higher mortality among these vulnerable subjects. Health problems and homelessness are in a bidirectional relationship since substance abuse and childhood traumas may be leading causes for homelessness. In addition, homeless people have no health insurance and poor access to the care system, education, and resources in general [45]. Priebe and colleagues [46] proposed a set of actions for reaching vulnerable and marginalized people in the European countries: outreach programs for engaging marginalized people into the care system, facilitating access to services, integration between primary and secondary care, and informative campaigns about mental illness among marginalized people. It has also been proposed that community-based treatments are effective for this population such as contingency management, cognitive behavioral intervention, and motivational interviewing; an assertive community treatment (ACT) may improve the access to services, the case management, crisis interventions [47]. Sociopolitical polices are needed for supporting housing and employment and relocating resources for those people who report marginalization, and social discrimination should be contrasted in order to reduce *social stress* against the minorities and improve social resilience [48]. Discrimination and social marginalization may affect also the LGBTQI (lesbian, gay, bisexual, transgender, queer, and intersex) population reporting a significant *minority stress* leading to a higher risk of psychological distress and mental illness [48]. Specific services should be promoted in order to approach specific health problems related to their condition in the cities. In fact, sexual variants tend to migrate from rural zones to larger cities since the *social* and *minority* pressure should be less impacting, even if they may experience marginalization as well with following depression, anxiety, substance abuse, and risk of suicide: in 2013, a large study from the USA reported no differences in mental illness rates and related quality of life among sexual minorities living in the urban and rural settings [49].

Urbanicity and neuroscience: In the *environment x gene* framework, it has been proposed that rural and urban environmental factors may impact on mental illness differently. The ecological hypothesis of psychosis, in fact, reports a direct impact of external environmental stimuli to brain neural mechanisms [50]. Neural regions identified as involved in the reaction to the external stimuli are the premotor cortex and perigenual anterior caudal cortex (pACC); also, the right dorsolateral prefrontal cortex (rDLPFC) is involved in ecological perception [51]. In fact, the pACC seems to be connected to the limbic emotional reactions to the social stimuli, whereas the rDLPFC may be related to the spatial representation in the working memory of urban/rural setting with a higher visual complexity for the urban one. Consequently, an increased activity of the amygdale may be due to a higher self-involvement in the city context: a putative mechanism might involve the pACC; in social interactions, the amygdale, modulating the salience of external stimuli, and the rDLPFC are possibly involved in processing complex spatial elements and affordances. Even if evidence is not conclusive, it is emerging that environmental factors may impact directly on brain functioning and plasticity and may play a triggering action on mental disorders [3].

Urban design and mental health: As mentioned above, the ecological hypothesis of mental illness suggests that environmental factors may impact on subjective well-being and brain functioning. According to this evidence, urban design may be responsible for some determinants of health and mental health. The availability of places for recreational and physical activity, relaxation, and social interaction in the urban setting may be relevant for the physical and mental health [3]. Also, urban design may influence, secondarily, the access to the health-care system [3].

The Centre for Urban Design and Mental Health proposed the GAPS framework for improving health and mental health in the urban settings: Green, Active, Pro-social, and Safe places [52]. Green and blue spaces (parks, woods, public gardens, and lakes and access to rivers and seas in the city) are all suggested as factors impacting positively on mental health [52]. In 2019, Labib and colleagues systematically reviewed the impact of green-blue spaces on human health and well-being confirming the positive influence on mental health outcomes and quality of life with a reduction of stress and improvement of subjective well-being [53]. Three models have been proposed for explaining the benefits of green spaces: the *biophilia* theory arguing that green spaces bring out the biological attitude to be in touch with the nature; the stress reduction theory, according to which green reduces urban stress with a *dose-response* effect; and the attention restoration theory based on the evidence that green reduces attention and concentration which are much higher in the urban setting because of a multitude of external stressful stimuli [54–56]. According to the second point of the framework, *Active*, green spaces promote physical activity and exercise with improvements in physical and psychological balance. Parks and gardens need to be publicly accessible and walkable, and bicycle paths should be introduced [3]. *Pro-social and safe places* should be promoted introducing public spaces for meetings and improving the structure of neighborhoods with squares and gardens; also, video-surveillance system and a higher control of the territory with regular rounds of police should be guaranteed for increasing public security [3].

9.4   Pollution and Its Impact on Mental Health

9.4.1   Air Pollution

Air pollution is due to the chemical emissions derived from various urban and industrial activities and vehicular traffic with suggested consequences on human neurodevelopmental processes and on the central nervous system (CNS) [57]. Also, air pollutants may have a synergistic impact on the neuroendocrine system, the pro-inflammatory immune pathways, and the human redox balance [58]. In fact, experimental evidence reported the association between air pollutants and chronic inflammation of neural tissues with alterations of the microglia and white matter [59]. Outdoor pollution may activate an immunological process with systemic inflammation, neuroinflammation, oxidative stress, and immune-dysregulation. In particular, children seem to be at a higher risk of health consequences if exposed to pollutants because of the immaturity of metabolic enzyme systems and susceptibility of the brain [60]. Such evidence has suggested a possible role of pollution in the neurodevelopment of autism or pathogenesis of psychoses [60].

Annavarapu et al. [57] explored the possible association between exposure to vehicular pollution from 2005 to 2015 among children and the prevalence of neuro-degeneration, neurodysfunction, ADHD (attention-deficit/hyperactivity disorder), and autism. Similarly, Sunyer et al. [61] reported an association between exposure to air pollutants and inflammatory reaction in the prefrontal cortex and striatum, possibly responsible for cognitive deficits among children.

Recently, de Prado Bert and colleagues [62] systematically reported on evidence regarding the effect of traffic-related air pollution integrating epidemiological and neuroimaging findings. They found an association between long-term exposure to air pollutants and alterations in the brain white matter and brain functioning as indexed by MRI (magnetic resonance imaging) techniques [62].

Carbon monoxide (CO): It is a product of incomplete combustion of hydrocarbons, included in vehicle-related pollution, gas stove pollution, and tobacco smoke. It has been associated with alterations of neurodevelopment in case of exposure during the perinatal period with cognitive deficits later in childhood [63]. It has been supposed a possible action through the programmed cell-death pathways of the brain tissues as confirmed in mice models exposed to CO in the perinatal period [64].

PM$_{2.5}$ (fine particulate matter, PM): Particles with a diameter of $\leq$2.5 μm (PM2.5) are considered an important risk factor for neurodegenerative disorders and neurological development disorders including autism: it has been described that PM2.5 particles involve the redox balance with a decrease in GSH/GSSG (glutathione/oxidized glutathione) level and abnormal DNA methylation possibly associated with cognitive deficits or behavioral disorders [65]. Jones and Thomsen [66] have described an association between air pollution and the increase of pro-inflammatory markers and depression-like behaviors in animals. Some other studies have suggested an association between air pollution and depression with and increased risk of suicide even if findings are not conclusive [67, 68].

Environmental ultrafine particles (UFP): It has been hypothesized on the base of mice models that UFP may impact on neurogenesis in the first trimester of pregnancy with an increased risk for schizophrenia, attention deficit disorder, and periventricular leukomalacia [69]. Also, a short-term exposure to ultrafine particles has been associated with exacerbations of psychiatric conditions in children as observed at Cincinnati Children's Hospital Medical Center emergency department for psychiatric issues [59].

Heavy metals: Heavy metals may impact on early neurodevelopment even if their long-term effects are not properly described. They are mostly derived from electronic waste: silver, copper, platinum, and palladium but also iron, aluminum, and small amounts of heavy metals like mercury, lead, and cadmium. Grant et al. [70] described side effects in the thyroid function, worsening in the neonatal health, increases in spontaneous abortions, premature births, and reduction of the lung functionality after exposure. Data regarding mental health are not conclusive. An early exposure to lead (Pb) impacts on gene expression for dopaminergic and glutamatergic neurotransmission (Pb is a noncompetitive antagonist of the N-methyl-D-aspartate receptor and disrupts neuronal processes depending on NMDAR activation), influencing the risk of psychosis [71]. Mercury as other heavy metals can employ the sulfur-dependent detoxification system and glutathione reserves in particular. It has been described that brain pathophysiology in autism shows similarities with those abnormalities found in mercury intoxication [72]. Cadmium impacts on the brain and increases reactive oxygen species damaging antioxidant defense systems with resulting neurotoxicity [73].

Ionizing radiation (IRs): IRs have a direct impact on biological processes of the CNS with specific damages to DNA, proteins, and lipids, leading to the production of highly reactive free radicals. However, the awareness of being exposed to radiations with the consequent perception of risk is also an important source of psychological distress for healthy subjects. In Western countries, radiodiagnostics and nuclear medicine are the main sources of exposure to IRs, and most of the evidence concerning the exposure to IRs may be collected from patients exposed to radiotherapy [74].

It has been proposed that persons exposed to IRs may develop schizophrenia spectrum disorders as observed among subjects involved in the Chernobyl accident, atomic bombing, nuclear weapons tests, environmental contamination by radioactive waste, and radiotherapy [75]. Supposed pathogenesis includes induced limbic dysfunctions and damages at molecular level as well as alterations of neurodevelopment if exposure occurs during the first trimester of pregnancy [75]. IRs may have a role in inducing mood disorders as well. Depression, in particular, has been described among the long-term effects of nuclear accidents with an increased prevalence of depression among Chernobyl survivors of 18% and cases of suicide [76]. In these cases, a biological mechanism of damage alongside personal vulnerability for depression and reaction to the traumatic experience has been proposed.

IRs are responsible for neurological issues as well. In particular, a significant increase of cerebrovascular diseases had been described among nuclear workers, and an association between cerebrovascular characteristics and neurodegenerative patterns of Alzheimer's disease has been found such as cerebral beta-amyloidosis and cerebral amyloidal angiopathy with amyloid-β plaque production [77].

There is also increasing evidence on the effect of IRs on cognitive deficits in patients treated with radiotherapy for brain tumors. Radiations seem to affect executive functions, verbal and nonverbal memory, sustained attention, and information processing speed, and the brain structures most affected by radiation damages are the prefrontal cortex and hippocampus [78].

Organophosphate (OP) pesticides: These are commonly used as insecticides and are particularly toxic to humans in rural and urban areas. Acute intoxications are mostly due to inhalation with inhibition of acetylcholinesterase enzyme with neurological syndromes or ingestion with affection of the gastrointestinal tract [79]. Chronic exposure leads to debilitating neuropsychiatric conditions such as anxiety, depression, and suicide [79].

9.4.2 Light Pollution

Light is an important vital *zeitgeber* for humans, animals, and plants, allowing the synchronization of day/night rhythms and activities, of behavioral and biological processes. The introduction of electric light has led to a global exposure to an unnatural light. These changes obviously have biological impacts. Artificial light, in particular, may have a role in influencing circadian rhythm and mood. In fact, any unnatural timing of light exposure can cause a desynchronization between internal biological processes and the external environment, leading to mood alterations. The different exposure to light may lead to depression in the seasonal switches in nearly 10% of the population: in these cases, morning bright light therapy, particularly blue wavelengths, may have a therapeutic role [80]. Also, in shift workers population, the higher prevalence of mood disorders is due to sleep deprivation with a consequence on the monoaminergic system but also to the exposure to unnatural light at night which may alter neurotrophin and neurotransmitter systems [81]. Also, according to the World Health Organization (WHO), recently shift work has been proposed as a probable carcinogen factor [82].

Noise pollution: Acoustic pollution is caused by work environment and household appliances, planes, and city traffic and acts through direct biological mechanisms that involve CNS tissues (ears, brain) as well as by generating stress impacting on psychological well-being and mental health. People, in particular children, living in noisy areas may report cognitive deficits as reduction of problem-solving skills, impaired hearing, poor reading, and frustration: noise may affect neurotransmitters in different parts of the brain resulting in consequences on cognition and memory, increased stress and corticosteroids, and neuronal damages [83]. Additionally, it has been demonstrated that noise may have negative effects on working memory and verbal domains in schizophrenia patients: this may add more distress and lead to poorer outcomes in patients with preexisting compromised cognition due to psychosis [84].

Environmental catastrophes: Loss of pipelines, damages to oil extraction platforms, and contamination of forests and ecosystems may produce enormous psychological distress even if evidence on these disastrous events are few.

Some studies have demonstrated higher levels of depression, anxiety, and stress in individuals and communities either exposed to oil or financially impacted by the spill in Louisiana (USA) in 2010 when the mobile offshore drilling unit Deepwater Horizon exploded [85, 86]. Long-term effects were associated with distress as well as sense of injustice and desperation.

Rung et al. [87] analyzed mental distress and depression among Louisiana women exposed to the Deepwater Horizon Oil Spill. A part of them reported symptoms of depression, others severe mental distress, others an increase in the number of fights with their partners, and a small part an increase in the intensity of fights with partner. Depressive symptoms were associated with both economic and physical exposures, whereas only physical exposure was associated with mental distress. Additionally, social capital and support both appeared beneficial for depression post-oil spill: authors concluded that social capital and support are helpful coping resources for contrasting post-disaster depression.

9.5   New Strategies and Challenges

Urbanicity may affect mental health according to evidence shown in this chapter. Associated factors may include social stress, substance abuse, social isolation, marginalization and loneliness, noise and pollution, crime and insecurity, crowding and reduced privacy, economic stress, poor physical activity, transport conditions, and inadequate access to health-care system and nature (green and blue spaces).

According to Litman, in his *Urban Sanity* [88], possible strategies may be employed in order to reduce the impact of urbanicity on mental health, as an *urban remediation* program. *Targeted social services* should be promoted in order to reduce social stress due to some factors like poverty, housing (homelessness), minorities and immigrants' isolation etc.; *affordability* of housing and transportation should be improved; *pro-social places* need to be considered by urban designers such as parks and public buildings, in order to promote community interactions and facilitate contact with nature and physical activity. Also, policy makers and urban designers together need to adopt strategies in order to reduce air, light, and noise pollution and promote walking, cycling, and accessible public transportation and health-care services as well as social contractedness in reasonably sized and well-organized neighborhoods and common spaces. Finally, research studies in this field should be encouraged in order to define globally accepted guidelines, for both policy makers and urban designers, for improving mental health and mental health-care facilities in the cities and rural settings.

Conflict of Interests None.

References

1. Bhugra D, Castaldelli-Maia JM, Torales J, et al. Megacities, migration, and mental health. Lancet Psychiat. 2019;6(11):884–5.
2. Ventriglio A, Torales J, Castaldelli-Maia JM, De Berardis D, Bhugra D. Urbanization and emerging mental health issues. CNS Spectr. 2021;26(1):43–50. https://doi.org/10.1017/S1092852920001236. Epub 2020 Apr 6
3. Bhugra D, Ventriglio A, Castaldelli-Maia JM, et al. Urban mental health. Oxford University Press; 2019. ISBN-13: 9780198804949
4. Marmot M. The health gap: The challenge of an unequal world. London: Bloomsbury; 2016.
5. United Nations. World Urbanization Prospects. The 2014 Revision. Available at: https://esa.un.org/unpd/wup/Publications/Files/WUP2014-Highlights.pdf (accessed 17 November 2019).
6. Faris REL, Dunham HW. Mental disorders in urban areas: An ecological study of Schizophrenia and other psychoses. Chicago, IL: University of Chicago Press; 1939.
7. March D, Hatch SL, Morgan C, et al. Psychosis and place. Epidemiol Rev. 2008;30:84–100.

8. Toulopoulou T, Picchioni M, Mortensen PB, et al. IQ, the urban environment, and their impact on future schizophrenia risk in men. Schizophr Bull. 2017;43:1056–63.

9. Robinson LR, Holbrook JR, Bitsko RH, et al. Differences in health care, family, and community factors associated with mental, behavioral, and developmental disorders among children aged 2–8 years in rural and urban areas—United States, 2011–2012. MMWR Surveill Summ. 2017;66(8):1–11.

10. Schomerus G, Heider D, Angermeyer MC, et al. European Schizophrenia Cohort. Residential area and social contacts in schizophrenia. Results from the European Schizophrenia Cohort (EuroSC). Soc Psychiatry Psychiatr Epidemiol. 2007;42:617–22.

11. Luciano M, De Rosa C, Del Vecchio V, et al. Perceived insecurity, mental health and urbanization: Results from a multicentric study. Int J Soc Psychiatry. 2016;62(3):252–61.

12. Litman T. Urban sanity: Understanding urban mental health impacts and how to create saner, happier cities. Victoria, Canada: Victoria Transport Policy Institute; 2016.

13. Crutzen P. (2005). Benvenuti nell'Antropocene. L'uomo ha cambiato il clima, la Terra entra in una nuova era. Mondadori. ISBN 88-04-53730-2.

14. Khan A, Plana-Ripoll O, Antonsen S, et al. Environmental pollution is associated with increased risk of psychiatric disorders in the US and Denmark. PLoS Biol. 2019; https://doi.org/10.1371/journal.pbio.3000353.

15. Anakwenze U, Zuberi D. Mental health and poverty in the inner City. Health Social Work. 2014;38(3):147–57.

16. Peen J, Schoevers RA, Beekman AT, et al. The current status of urban–rural differences in psychiatric disorders. Acta Psychiatr Scand. 2010;121:84–93.

17. Desai NG, Tiwari SC, Nambi S, et al. Urban mental health services in India: how complete or incomplete? Ind J Psychiatr. 2004;46:195–212.

18. Abbott A. Stress and the city: urban decay. Nature. 2012;490:162–4.

19. Park RE, Burgess EW. The city. Chicago, IL: Chicago University Press; 1925.

20. Faris R, Dunham H. Mental disorders in urban areas. Chicago, IL: University of Chicago Press; 1939.

21. American Psychological Association. Task force on urban psychology toward an urban psychology: research, action, and policy. Washington, DC: American Psychological Association; 2005.

22. Adli M. Urban stress and mental health. London: London School of Economics; 2011. Available at: https://lsecities.net/media/objects/articles/urban-stress-and-mental-health/en-gb/ (accessed 17 October 2019)

23. Houtman I, Jettinghoff K, Cedillo L. Raising awareness of stress at work in developing countries: a modern hazard in a traditional working environment: advice to employers and worker representatives. Protecting workers' health, series no 6. World Health Organization; 2007.

24. World Health Organization (WHO). Why urban health matters. Geneva: WHO; 2010.

25. Kessler RCP, Chiu WTA, Demler OM, et al. Prevalence, severity, and comorbidity of 12-month DSMIV disorders in the National Comorbidity Survey Replication. Arch Gen Psychiatr. 2005;62:617–27.

26. Hare EH. Mental illness and social condition in Bristol. J Ment Sci. 1956;102:349–57.

27. Giggs JA, Cooper JE. Ecological structure and the distribution of schizophrenia and affective psychoses in Nottingham. Br J Psychiatry. 1987;151:627–33.

28. Giggs JA. Distribution of schizophrenics in Nottingham. Trans Inst Br Geogr. 1973;59:5–76.

29. Giggs JA. Mental disorders and ecological structure in Nottingham. Soc Sci Med. 1986;23:945–61.

30. Maylaih E, Weyerer S, Hafner H. Spatial concentration of the incidence of treated psychiatric disorders in Mannheim. Acta Psychiatr Scand. 1980;80:650–6.

31. Hafner H, Reimann H. Spatial distribution of mental disorders in Mannheim, 1965. In: Hare EH, Wing JK, editors. Psychiatric epidemiology. London: Oxford University Press; 1970. p. 341–54.

32. Loffler W, Hafner H. Ecological patterns of first admitted schizophrenics to two German cities over 25 years. Soc Sci Med. 1999;49:93–108.

33. Mintz NL, Schwartz DT. Urban ecology and psychosis: community factors in the incidence of schizophrenia and manic-depression among Italians in Greater Boston. Int J Soc Psychiatr. 1964;10:101–18.

34. Oh H, Susser E, Koyanagi A, et al. Urban birth and psychotic experiences in the United States. Acta Psychiatr Scand. 2019; https://doi.org/10.1111/acps.13106. [Epub ahead of print]

35. van Os J, Hannssen M, Bak M, et al. Do urbanicity and familial liability coparticipate in causing psychosis? Am J Psychiatr. 2003;160:477–82.

36. van Os J, Hanssen M, Bijl RV, Vollebergh W. Prevalence of psychotic disorder and community level of psychotic symptoms: an urban-rural comparison. Arch Gen Psychiatr. 2011;58:663–8.

37. Martinotti G, Lupi M, Carlucci L, et al. Novel psychoactive substances: use and knowledge among adolescents and young adults in urban and rural areas. Hum Psychopharmacol. 2015;30(4):295–301. https://doi.org/10.1002/hup.2486.

38. Schelin EM, Munk-Jorgensen P, Olesen AV, et al. Regional differences in schizophrenia incidence in Denmark. Acta Psychiatr Scand. 2000;101:293–9.

39. Taylor R, Page A, Morrell S, et al. Social and psychiatric influences on urban–rural differentials in Australian suicide. Suicide Life Threat Behav. 2005;35:277–90.

40. Cheung YTD, Spittal MJ, Pirkis J, et al. Spatial analysis of suicide mortality in Australia: investigation of metropolitan-rural-remote differentials of suicide risk across states/territories. Soc Sci Med. 2012;75:1460–8.

41. Knipe DW, Padmanathan P, Muthuwatta L, et al. Regional variation in suicide rates in Sri Lanka between 1955 and 2011: a spatial and temporal analysis. BMC Pub Health. 2017;17:193.

42. Barker E, Kolves K, De Leo D. Rail-suicide prevention: systematic literature review of evidence-based activities. Asia Pac Psychiatry. 2017;9:e12246.

43. Ventriglio A, Mari M, Bellomo A, et al. Homelessness and mental health: a challenge. Int J Soc Psychiatry. 2015;61(7):621–2.

44. Stergiopoulos V, Cusi A, Bekele T, et al. Neurocognitive impairment in a large sample of homeless adults with mental illness. Acta Psychiatr Scand. 2015;131(4):256–68.

45. Krausz M, Strehlau V, Choi F, et al. Urbanization and marginalization. In: Bhugra D, Ventriglio A, Castaldelli-Maia JM, et al., editors. Urban mental health. Oxford University Press; 2019. ISBN-13:9780198804949.

46. Priebe S, Matanov A, Schor R, et al. Good practice in mental health care for socially marginalised groups in Europe: a qualitative study of expert views in 14 countries. BMC Pub Health. 2012;12:248.

47. Nelson G, Aubry T, Lafrance A. A review of the literature on the effectiveness of housing and support, assertive community treatment, and intensive case management interventions for persons with mental illness who have been homeless. Am J Orthopsychiatr. 2007;77:350–61.

48. Ventriglio A, Bhugra D. Social justice for the mentally ill. Int J Soc Psychiatry. 2015;61(3):213–4.

49. Wienke C, Hill G. Does place of residence matter? Rural–urban differences and the wellbeing of gay men and lesbians. J Homosex. 2013;60:1256–79.

50. Krabbendam L, van Os J. Schizophrenia and urbanicity: a major environmental influence—conditional on genetic risk. Schizophr Bull. 2005;31:795.

51. Rizzolatti G, Craighero L. The mirror neuron system. Ann Rev Neurosci. 2004;27:169–92.

52. The Centre for Urban Design and Mental Health. At: https://www.urbandesignmentalhealth.com/# (accessed 17 November 2019).

53. Labib SM, Lindley S, Huck JJ. Spatial dimensions of the influence of urban green-blue spaces on human health: A systematic review. Environ Res. 2019;2:108869. https://doi.org/10.1016/j.envres.2019.108869. [Epub ahead of print]

54. Wilson EO. Biophilia—the human bond with other species. Cambridge, MA: Harvard University Press; 1984.

55. Ulrich RS. Aesthetic and affective responses to natural environment. In: Altman I, Wohlwill J, editors. Behaviour and the natural environment. New York: Plenum Press; 1983. p. 85–125.

56. Kaplan R, Kaplan S. The experience of nature. A psychological perspective. Cambridge: Cambridge University Press; 1983.

57. Annavarapu RN, Kathi S. Cognitive disorders in children associated with urban vehicular emissions. Environ Pollut. 2016;208:74–8.
58. Wright RJ. Moving towards making social toxins mainstream in children's environmental health. Curr Opin Pediatr. 2009;21(2):222.
59. Brokamp C, Strawn JR, Beck AF, Ryan P. Pediatric psychiatric emergency department utilization and fine particulate matter: a case-crossover study. Environ Health Perspect. 2019;127(9):097006. https://doi.org/10.1289/ehp4815.
60. Perera F, Ashrafi A, Kinney P, Mills D. Towards a fuller assessment of benefits to children's health of reducing air pollution and mitigating climate change due to fossil fuel combustion. Environ Res. 2018; https://doi.org/10.1016/j.envres.2018.12.016.
61. Sunyer J, Esnaola M, Alvarez-Pedrerol M, et al. Association between traffic-related air pollution in schools and cognitive development in primary school children: a prospective cohort study. PLoS Med. 2015;12(3):e1001792.
62. de Prado BP, Mercader EMH, Pujol J, et al. The effects of air pollution on the brain: a review of studies interfacing environmental epidemiology and neuroimaging. Curr Environ Health Reports. 2018;5:351–64.
63. Levy RJ. Carbon monoxide pollution and neurodevelopment: a public health concern. Neurotoxicol Teratol. 2015;49:31–40.
64. Cheng Y, Thomas A, Mardini F, et al. Neurodevelopmental consequences of sub-clinical carbon monoxide exposure in newborn mice. PLoS One. 2012;7:e32029.
65. Wei H, Liang F, Meng G, et al. Redox/methylation mediated abnormal DNA methylation as regulators of ambient fine particulate matter-induced neurodevelopment related impairment in human neuronal cells. Sci Rep. 2016;14(6):33402.
66. Jones KA, Thomsen C. The role of the innate immune system in psychiatric disorders. Mol Cell Neurosci. 2013;53:52–62.
67. Thompson AM, Zanobetti A, Silverman F, et al. Baseline repeated measures from controlled human exposure studies: associations between ambient air pollution exposure and the systemic inflammatory biomarkers IL-6 and fibrinogen. Environ Health Perspect. 2010;118(1):120–4.
68. Kim C, Jung SH, Kang DR, et al. Ambient particulate matter as a risk factor for suicide. Am J Psychiatry. 2010;167(9):1100–7.
69. Allen JL, Oberdorster G, Morris-Schaffer K, et al. Developmental neurotoxicity of inhaled ambient ultrafine particle air pollution: parallels with neuropathological and behavioral features of autism and other neurodevelopmental disorders. Neurotoxicology. 2017;59:140–54.
70. Grant K, Goldizen FC, Sly PD, et al. Health consequences of exposure to e-waste: a systematic review. Lancet Glob Health. 2013;1(6):e350–61. https://doi.org/10.1016/S2214-109X(13)70101-3.
71. Guilarte TR, Miceli RC. Age-dependent effects of lead on [3H]-MK-801 binding to the NMDA receptor-gated ionophore: in vitro and in vivo studies. Neurosci Lett. 1992;148:27–30.
72. Kern JK, Geier DA, Audhya T, P.G., et al. Evidence of parallels between mercury intoxication and the brain pathology in autism. Acta Neurobiol Exp (Warsz). 2012;72:113–53.
73. Vaziri ND. Mechanisms of lead-induced hypertension and cardiovascular disease. Am J Physiol Heart Circ Physiol. 2008;295:H454–65.
74. Marazziti D, Baroni S, Lombardi A, et al. Psychiatric effects of ionizing radiation. Clin Neuropsychiatry. 2014;11(2):61–7.
75. Loganovsky KN, Volovik SV, Manton KG, et al. Whether ionizing radiation is a risk factor for schizophrenia spectrum disorders? World J Biol Psychiatry. 2005;6:212–30.
76. Bolt MA, Helming LM, Tintle NL. The associations between self-reported exposure to the Chernobyl nuclear disaster zone and mental health disorders in Ukraine. Front Psych. 2018;15(9):32. https://doi.org/10.3389/fpsyt.2018.00032. eCollection 2018
77. Zlokovic BV. The blood–brain barrier in health and chronic neurodegenerative disorders. Neuron. 2008;57:178–201.
78. Agbahiwe H, Rashid A, Horska A, et al. A prospective study of cerebral, frontal lobe, and temporal lobe volumes and neuro psychologic al performance in children with primary brain tumors treated with cranial radiation. Cancer. 2017;123(1):161–8.

79. Stephens R, Sreenivasan B. Neuropsychological effects of long-term low-level organophosphate exposure in orchard sprayers in England. Arch Environ Health. 2004;59:556–74.
80. Glickman G, Byrne B, Pineda C, et al. Light therapy for seasonal affective disorder with blue narrow-band light-emitting diodes (LEDs). Biol Psychiatry. 2006;59:502–7.
81. Scott AJ, Monk TH, Brink LL. Shiftwork as a risk factor for depression: a pilot study. Int J Occup Environ Health. 1997;3:S2–9.
82. Stevens RG, Hansen J, Costa G, et al. Considerations of circadian impact for defining 'shift work' in cancer studies: IARC Working Group Report. Occup Environ Med. 2011;68:154–62.
83. Cohen S. After effects of stress on human performance and social behavior: a review of research and theory. Psychol Bull. 1980;88:82–108.
84. Wright B, Peters E, Ettinger U, et al. Effects of environmental noise on cognitive (dys) functions in schizophrenia: a pilot within-subjects experimental study. Schizophr Res. 2016;173(1–2):101–8. https://doi.org/10.1016/j.schres.2016.03.017.
85. Chung S, Kim E. Physical and mental health of disaster victims: a comparative study on typhoon and oil spill disasters. J Prev Med Public Health. 2010;43(5):387–95.
86. Sabucedo JM, Arce C, Senra C, et al. Symptomatic profile and health-related quality of life of persons affected by the Prestige catastrophe. Disasters. 2010;34(3):809–20.
87. Rung AL, Gaston S, Robinson WT, et al. Untangling the disaster-depression knot: the role of social ties after deepwater horizon. Soc Sci Med. 2017;177:19–26.
88. Litman T. Urban sanity: understanding urban mental health impacts and how to create saner, happier cities. Victoria Transport Policy Institute; 2017. (www.vtpi.org); at www.vtpi.org/urban-sanity.pdf

Is There Room for Anti-stigma Interventions in Mental Health Preventive Programmes?

10

Antonio Lasalvia

10.1 Introduction

One of the most promising ways to reduce the high personal, familial, societal, clinical and economic costs of mental disorders is prevention [1]. The traditional public health classification differentiates between primary, secondary and tertiary prevention. The three forms of prevention are placed along a continuum in terms of when intervention is offered in relation to problem development: Primary prevention seeks to prevent the onset (incidence) of mental disorders by addressing risk factors; secondary prevention seeks to lower the rate of established cases of mental disorders in the population (prevalence) through early detection and treatment; tertiary prevention includes interventions that reduce disability, enhance rehabilitation and prevent relapses and recurrences. Because tertiary prevention is often confused with treatment, the Institute of Medicine (IoM) [2] has recommended that only interventions occurring before the onset of disorders (i.e. primary and secondary prevention) can be considered as prevention. Therefore, the IoM has proposed a classification of prevention in relation to the specific target group: *Universal prevention* is defined as those interventions that are targeted at the general public; *selective prevention* targets individuals or subgroups of the population whose risk of developing a mental disorder is significantly higher than average; *indicated prevention* targets high-risk people who are identified as having minimal but detectable signs or symptoms foreshadowing mental disorder or biological markers indicating predisposition for mental disorder, but who do not meet diagnostic criteria for any mental disorder.

A. Lasalvia (✉)

Section of Psychiatry, Department of Neuroscience, Biomedicine and Movement Sciences, University of Verona, Verona, Italy

e-mail: antonio.lasalvia@univr.it

© The Author(s), under exclusive license to Springer Nature Switzerland AG 2022

M. Colizzi, M. Ruggeri (eds.), *Prevention in Mental Health*, https://doi.org/10.1007/978-3-030-97906-5_10

Literature has provided evidence of effectiveness for a wide range of preventive interventions for mental disorders. These have been found to reduce risk factors, strengthen protective factors and decrease psychiatric symptoms and disability and the onset of some mental disorders [3]. However, these interventions are still insufficiently implemented in routine public health or mental health service programmes [4]. Lack of awareness of the significant economic savings from preventive interventions for mental disorders; the need for an initial investment in training and investment of time by professionals, often with no short-term return; and the stigma of mental disorders explain the lack of interest in mental health prevention as compared with other areas of medicine [5]. Indeed, among possible factors, stigma and discrimination associated with mental disorders do act as barriers for both prevention and treatment of mental disorders [6]. Stigma keeps individuals from seeking out services that can improve their health or, in some cases, save their lives. Stigma and fear of stigma discourage people from disclosing their mental health status, seeking care and adhering to treatment. Family members and friends of people with mental disorders, together with mental health providers, also experience stigma and discrimination (i.e. 'associative stigma'). On the other hand, literature shows that stigma reduction is crucial to the success of prevention, care and treatment efforts for mental disorders [7]. This chapter aims to discuss how stigma and discrimination hinder preventive interventions in mental health and how the efficacy of preventive actions may be enhanced by addressing stigma and discrimination.

10.2   The Problem of Mental Health Stigma

There are virtually no societies or cultures all over the world in which people with mental disorders are as equally valued as people who do not suffer from these conditions [8]. People with mental disorders generally experience in their everyday life the negative effect of stigma, which arises from society stereotypes and misconceptions on mental disorders (e.g. dangerousness, unpredictability, incompetence) and the consequent prejudicial reactions. Subjective accounts of people with mental disorders testify that effects of stigma are often perceived as more burdensome and distressing than the primary condition itself (stigma is often referred to as 'second disorders').

The term stigma refers to a social devaluation of a person due to an 'attribute that is deeply discrediting' [9]. The WHO define stigma as a 'mark of shame, disgrace or disapproval which results in an individual being rejected, discriminated against, and excluded from participating in a number of different areas of society' [10].

In a sociological perspective, the so-called modified labelling theory [11] emphasises two aspects. First, as a precondition of stigma, differences between persons have to be noticed, to be regarded as relevant and to be labelled accordingly. Labelling implies a separation of 'us' from 'them'. This separation easily leads to the belief that 'they' are fundamentally different from 'us' and that 'they' even are the thing they are labelled. 'They' become fundamentally different from those who do not share a negative label, so that 'they' appear to be a completely different sort of people. The second condition is that the stigmatising group has to be in a more powerful position than the stigmatised group. These processes can operate in a number of settings and are evident through various direct and indirect social interactions.

In a public health perspective, stigma can be conceptualised as an overarching term consisting of three main problems:

(a) Problems of knowledge (ignorance or misinformation). Most people do not know very much about mental disorders, and much of what they do know – or think they know – is inaccurate.
(b) Problems of attitudes (prejudice). People fear and avoid other people with mental disorders; people with mental disorders anticipate fear and avoidance from other people.
(c) Problems of behaviour (discrimination). The general public acts towards people with mental disorders in ways that are unjust and unfair [12].

The behavioural component of stigma – discrimination – has the most detrimental effect in the life of people with mental disorders and leads to disadvantages under many respects. At an individual level, it leads to social distance [13], exclusion from employment opportunities [14] and reduction of intimate relationships and parenting [15]. At a structural and societal level, negative views and attitudes are related to discrimination, e.g. in equal civil rights, medical insurance coverage, parenting or serving jury duty, access to housing or employment or reliance on jails, prisons and homeless shelters as the focus of care for the most severely ill [16].

As a further complication, most people with mental disorders accept the stereotypes and prejudices about mental health issues held by the general population and turn them against themselves. This process is referred to as 'self-stigma' or internalised sigma [17]. As a result of the internalised stigma, some people with mental disorders may come to accept the discrediting prejudices held against them and so lose self-esteem, leading to feelings of shame, a sense of alienation and social withdrawal [18]. Therefore, people with mental disorders often expect to be treated in a discriminatory way ('anticipated discrimination') and try to hide their disorders or stop themselves from taking up life opportunities [19].

In summary, stigma can express itself in three main ways: (a) *public stigma*, when members of the general public endorse prejudice and discrimination against people with mental disorders; (b) *self-stigma*, when people with mental disorders agree with and internalise prejudice and negative stereotypes, leading to low self-esteem, shame, demoralisation and giving up life goals; and (c) *structural stigma*, which refers to rules and regulations in society that intentionally or unintentionally disadvantage people with mental disorders.

The following paragraphs will discuss how these three forms of stigma may impair the three different types of preventive interventions – universal, selective and indicated – as outlined by the IoM [2]. Table 10.1 summaries how the three types of stigma can hinder the different types of prevention. Consistent with Rüsch and Thornicroft [6], selective and indicated preventions have been collapsed into one category, referring to as prevention for individuals at elevated risk to develop mental disorders, as compared with the general population.

Table 10.1 Examples of how the three main different type of stigma may hinder the different types of prevention and related possible intervention strategies

	Public stigma		Self-stigma		Structural stigma	
	Examples	Intervention	Examples	Intervention	Examples	Intervention
Universal prevention	– Unwillingness to participate in or implement prevention due to prejudice against people with mental illness – Pessimism about success of prevention in mental health	'Mental health literacy' interventions targeting general population to improve knowledge on mental health issues (by e.g. community campaigns, interventions in educational settings, information websites, social media)	–	–	– Allocation of fewer resources to prevention in mental health – Negative media portrayals of people with mental illness that discourage prevention	*– Awareness raising and* communication *campaigns;* *human rights advocacy* *– Anti-stigma interventions* *on media professionals;* *media-monitoring* projects; development of reporting guidelines

Selective/ indicated prevention	– Avoidance of early recognition/ intervention due to fear of public stigma -Pessimism about success of early intervention – Labelling as unintended consequence of prevention, leading to stigma-related stress – Avoidance of service use due to fear of public stigma	– Use of new, hope-oriented labels aimed at distancing "at risk" state from psychosis; – Accurate information about the "at risk" state to reduce negative reactions and misconceptions; – Educational campaigns to general public to give evidence of effectiveness of early intervention; – Implement youth-friendly, stigma-free specialized services for young people separate from institutions for patients with *established* disorders	– Avoidance of early recognition/ intervention because of self-stigma/ shame – Self-labelling as unintended consequence of prevention, leading to shame and demoralisation – Avoidance of service use because of self-stigma/ shame – Demoralisation, 'why try', and social isolation as consequences of self-stigma	– *Strategies* for individuals with *mental disorders* to self-*disclose their mental health problems*, to promote personal empowerment, to enhance self-esteem – Interventions for individuals with *mental disorders* aimed at reducing social isolation; – Self-help groups; peer support programmes	– Low financial resources for early intervention services may lead to poor implementation of such services, low quantity of available services and poor quality of interventions provided (e.g., untrained and unskilled staff)	– Campaigns by mental health advocacy groups/user associations targeting policy makers, legislators, health administrators; – Monitoring groups of legislative activity

10.3   Stigma as a Barrier for Universal Prevention in Mental Health

Universal prevention targets generic risk and protective factors for the onset of mental disorders that are in the general population. Such interventions are aimed to reducing the overall probability of developing psychiatric disorders. A holistic approach to health, integrating social, psychological and physical aspects of well-being, may be especially valuable in this regard [5]. Universal prevention in mental health should be therefore integrated within a public policy approach that encompasses horizontal action through different public sectors, such as the environment, housing, social welfare, employment, education, criminal justice and human rights. Actions and policies that improve the protection of basic human rights represent a powerful preventive strategy for mental disorders [3].

Mental disorders are inextricably linked to human rights issues. The stigma, discrimination and human rights violations that individuals and families affected by mental disorders suffer are intense and pervasive [20]. At least in part, these phenomena are consequences of a general perception that no effective preventive or treatment modalities exist against these disorders. Effective prevention can do a lot to alter these perceptions and hence change the way mental disorders are looked upon by society. Human rights issues go beyond the specific violations that people with mental disorders are exposed to, however. In fact, limitations on the basic human rights of vulnerable individuals and communities may act as powerful determinants of mental disorders. Hence, it is not surprising that many of the effective preventive measures are harmonious with principles of social equity, equal opportunity and care of the most vulnerable groups in society, that people with mental disorders undoubtedly are [3].

10.3.1 The Effect of Public Stigma on Universal Prevention

Stigmatisation of mental disorders and poor or inaccurate knowledge on mental health-related issues usually lead to an underestimation of the need for prevention from the general population. With specific reference to universal prevention, the general public usually has a poor knowledge about risk and protective factors for mental disorders. Moreover, pessimism about the success of prevention that is related to poor knowledge of mental disorders, together with unwillingness to participate in or implement prevention due to prejudice against people with mental disorders, may hinder universal prevention efforts.

The term 'mental health literacy' was coined to define the 'knowledge and beliefs about mental disorders that aid their recognition, management or prevention' [21]. Therefore, according to this notion, mental health literacy is more than the absence of erroneous stereotypes and includes the recognition of a developing disorder as well as knowledge about prevention and effective interventions. Mental health literacy has the potential to influence help-seeking behaviour and holds serious implications for adherence to treatment [21, 22]. A number of studies have been conducted addressing mental health literacy [23, 24]. There is evidence from surveys in several countries for deficiencies in (a) the public's knowledge of how to prevent mental disorders, (b) recognition of when a disorder is developing, (c) knowledge of help-seeking options and treatments available, (d) knowledge of effective self-help strategies for milder problems and (e) first aid skills to support others affected by mental health problems [25].

Universal prevention will likely be more difficult to implement among members of the general population who have poor knowledge about mental health, who distance themselves from people with mental disorders, who hold pessimistic views about the benefits of prevention and treatment of mental disorders and who are opposed to channelling resources towards mental health [6, 26].

Nevertheless, there is also evidence that a range of interventions can improve mental health literacy among the general population, including whole-of-community campaigns, interventions in educational settings and information websites [25]. It should be noted that the majority of anti-stigma interventions implemented worldwide so far are education-based, half of which are stand-alone interventions specifically aimed at promoting mental health literacy [27].

10.3.2 The Effect of Structural Stigma on Universal Prevention

Structural (or institutional) stigma refers to policies of private and/or governmental institutions that either intentionally restrict the opportunities of stigmatised individuals or unintentionally yield consequences for them [28]. A prominent example of intentional structural stigma from the private sector is the predominantly negative representations of people with mental disorders in the news media. A large body of literature reveals a major contribution by mass media in reinforcing common stereotypes of people with mental disorders by providing a negative image of such people, who are often labelled as dangerous, violent or unpredictable [29, 30]. Mass communication sources, including the news media, provide fundamental frameworks through which most people come to perceive and understand the contemporary world. Unfortunately, when the news media frames a group in a negative light, it propagates prejudice and discrimination. Hence, whether it is intentional or not, mass media become social structures for perpetuating stigma [31]. Within this context, when a newspaper or a television publishes negative and/or prejudicial portraits of people with mental disorders, it becomes a strong source of structural stigma. Media representations of mental disorders can have a detrimental impact on people with mental disorders by reducing their level of self-esteem, discouraging help-seeking behaviours and increasing their lived experience of discrimination and their possibility to recover [32]. Moreover, media depiction of mental disorders contributes to the level of fear, hostility and intolerance in the general population [33, 34]. In addition, negative media portrayals of people with mental disorders may discourage universal prevention efforts [6].

On the other hand, mass media may be also viewed as a formidable ally in helping to challenge public prejudices, initiate public debate and project positive, human interest stories about people who live with mental health problems [35, 36]. Media professionals may be eager and responsive targets for anti-stigma interventions and proactive lobbying particularly if this improves communication between reporters, mental health providers and service users and facilitates access to better information [37]. National anti-stigma campaigns targeting negative portrayal of mental disorders in the media, in which media professionals are included as a target group, have shown to effectively reduce stigma and disseminate positive mental health messages [38, 39, 40].

10.4　Stigma as a Barrier for Selected and Indicated Prevention in Mental Health

Selective interventions aim at preventing the manifestation of psychiatric symptoms in individuals or subpopulation whose risk of developing a mental disorder is significantly higher than the rest of the population while still being asymptomatic [3]. Overall these interventions aim to strengthen abilities in these individuals to prevent future development of psychiatric conditions. The identification of these risk groups may be based on biological, psychological or social risk factors. Children of parents with mental disorders or substance use disorders represent one of the populations at highest risk for psychiatric problems [41]. Group programmes for children of parents with mental disorders have shown to be especially helpful [42].

Conceptually related to selective intervention is indicated prevention. It is again targeted to individuals at high risk for the development of a mental disorder, but in this case such individuals also show early minimal but detectable clinical manifestations. Indicated interventions aim to treat subclinical manifestations in these people and to strengthen their coping abilities to prevent transition to full-blown psychiatric disorders. Also for this kind of intervention, the identification of at-risk individuals is based on biological, psychological or social risk factors.

The prototype of indicated prevention in mental health is intervention targeting young people at clinical high risk for psychosis (i.e. those showing attenuated psychotic symptoms and a recent decline in functioning). Literature has found that indicated interventions on people at risk for psychosis may have positive effects not only in reducing the presenting symptoms but also in improving other areas of psychosocial adjustment [43]. Research also suggests that the development of services for indicated prevention has met the objectives of strengthening treatment engagement, reducing the duration of untreated disorders and liaising with secondary prevention interventions in this specific population [3]. However, the 'at risk' state for psychosis may be associated with stigma [44]. This is relevant, also in light of stigma potentially affecting all individuals referring to early intervention services for psychosis independent of whether they ever progress to full-blown psychosis [45]. Within 2–2.5 years from identification, only 30–35% of people at risk for psychosis eventually develop the disorder [46]; and the transition rates seem to have further declined over the years, possibly because of earlier referral and intervention [47]. Thus, the large majority of people at risk for psychosis may be exposed to stigma for a condition they will never develop.

An increasing number of studies have weighted harms *and benefits* associated with early intervention services for people at risk of developing psychosis in terms of stigma and related consequences for patients and their families [48]. An early review specifically addressing pathways to mental healthcare among people in the psychosis-risk state found that stigma does have a detrimental effect on help-seeking process [49]. In addition, a more recent review confirms that the psychosis risk condition may trigger stigmatising processes and that young people at risk of psychosis experiencing stigma are more likely to show poor mental health outcomes and suicidal behaviour, develop full-blown psychosis, disengage from services and have family members distressed by associative stigma [50].

10.4.1 The Effect of Public Stigma on Indicated Prevention

Overall, most people at risk for psychosis report being aware of psychosis' negative image in the public opinion and the media as well as of stereotypes associated to this condition, preferring not to disclose their 'at risk' status due to expected negative reactions by others [51]. Public stigma towards people 'at risk' for psychosis is higher among the general public compared to mental health professionals as well as in people with an intermediate level of education (e.g. diploma), who have never worked or volunteered in mental health and who have frequently encountered in the public someone who appeared to be mentally ill [52].

Conceptually related to public stigma are the effects of the labelling process. A psychiatric label sets into action cultural stereotypes and negative images about mental disorders that are applied to the person by others and by the person to himself or herself [18]. Similarly to full-blown mental disorders [53], the labelling process may produce differing effects also in people at risk for psychosis. Early studies report that the 'at risk' label may elicit feelings of validation and relief in people experiencing this condition [54], thus increasing mental health service use [55]. Studies of comparison with other labels suggest that the 'at risk' label elicits only slightly more [56] or no different stigma [57] than other labels (e.g. 'breakup') among young healthy population and has a lower impact than non-psychotic labels (e.g. depression or anxiety) on at-risk individuals [58]. Moreover, symptom-related stigma seems to have a greater impact than labelling-related stigma on at-risk individuals, suggesting that labelling-related stigma, if present, does not fully permeate self-concept at this early stage [59]. In contrast, other studies found that being labelled as 'at risk' is associated with a higher stigma and with a number of potential adverse health effects [60, 61]. In particular, in studies conducted among college students [62], patients with full-blown mental disorders [63], as well as members of the general public and mental health professionals [52, 63], indicate that the 'at risk' label may elicit similar [63] or greater [52, 62] status loss, discrimination and stigma than non-psychotic disorders such as major depression and generalised anxiety disorder. The misconception that the 'at risk' state might be a long-lasting or irreversible condition contributes to a high level of stigma [52], which in some cases does not differ from that endorsed for schizophrenia [62]. Also, at-risk individuals who have transitioned to psychosis or with a family history of psychosis find the identification of the 'at risk' state of little help, reporting more stigma associated to it [64].

10.4.2 The Effect of Self-Stigma on Indicated Prevention

When stigma towards the 'at risk' condition arises among the general public [52, 65], 'at risk' persons become aware of it, tend to agree with it and thus may experience self-stigma and related negative emotions. Research indicates that 'at risk' individuals do experience negative thoughts and emotions about themselves more frequently than 'healthy' subjects [66] and do report a higher stereotype awareness related to their condition compared to patients with non-psychotic disorders [59]. Also, the higher the stereotype awareness, the higher is the agreement with them, which in turn is associated with the experience of negative emotions [59]. At-risk individuals reporting internalised stigma, negative appraisals of their unusual experiences, reduced social acceptance of such experiences and shame are more likely to experience high levels of distress related to their condition [67] and to misattribute fear to non-fearful stimuli [68]. Also, internalised stigma is reported to become a stressful condition when stigma-related harm is perceived as exceeding the person's coping resources ('stigma stress') [55]. In turn, high levels of stigma stress among at-risk individuals are associated with higher shame [60], and the persistence of increased stigma stress over time is also associated with a higher likelihood of self-labelling as mentally ill [61]. When such negative emotions, such as shame, fear and self-labelling as mentally ill, exceed the person's coping resources, a stressful state arises that in turn amplifies these negative reactions and negatively influences *the help-seeking behaviour* [55].

Professionals involved in indicated prevention, such as those working in services for young people at risk for psychosis, must be cognisant of the problem of stigma, reconciling the interests and feelings of the young individuals with those of their parents as well as facilitating any attempt to break down public stigma in the community. In order to avoid emotional risks of stigma associated with the 'at risk' label, diagnostic or prognostic information should be tailored to each individual's characteristics, including age, social context, identity formation, cognitive capacity and comorbidities [50]. Moreover, addressing the stigma of the 'at risk' label at the public health level, even by simply providing accurate information about the 'at risk' state, may significantly reduce negative reactions and misconceptions about the condition [62]. Finally, hope-oriented labels distancing the 'at risk' state from a prodromal phase inevitably leading to psychosis should be preferred [48, 52].

10.4.3 The Effect of Structural Stigma on Indicated Prevention

One of the main implementation barriers for both selective [69] and indicated preventive interventions [70, 71] is the lack of resources, both in terms of experienced and trained professionals and of financial resources. The issue of insufficient allocation of funding and financial resources for mental health is a critical one and may be an aspect of structural stigma. In fact, structural stigma may be represented by the fact that mental healthcare is not covered by insurance companies to the same extent as other medical care (i.e. parity) and that governments may not prioritise mental health funding. The allocation of healthcare resources and services may not be intended to discriminate against those with mental disorders by prioritising funding for physical diseases, but that prioritisation can lead to lower amounts of funding, and fewer healthcare facilities and staff, which ultimately disadvantages those with mental disorders [72]. In most Western countries, the steady increase in costs for healthcare has resulted in an urgent need for cost containment, raising the question as to whether in times of scarce financial resources psychiatric patients are at greater risk of having financial resources withheld than patients with other medical conditions [26]. Many low- and middle-income countries currently allocate less than 2% − or even 1% − of the health budget to the treatment and prevention of mental disorders. This is not remotely proportionate to the burden they cause and appears to place a very low value on the psychological or emotional well-being of populations. Most of the funds that are made available by governments are specifically directed to the operational costs of outdated mental hospitals that are commonly associated with isolation, human rights violations and poor outcomes [73].

With regard to specialised services/programmes for young people at risk for psychosis, they have been neglected for a long time in most parts of the world. Traditionally, public mental health services worldwide are poorly designed, grossly under-resourced and typically unfriendly to young people. Only the last 20 years have seen significant gains in developing and implementing early intervention services tailored to the specific needs of young people [74]. Unfortunately, these services have not been successfully implemented in all parts of the world, and in many countries their implementation still remains a challenging issue. A nationwide survey conducted in Italy aiming at collecting evidence about the process of implementation and development of early intervention services/programmes across the country found a wide variability, with southern regions showing poor availability of such services [75]. The lack of funding and of trained staff was among the main reasons for the heterogeneous diffusion of these services across the Italian territory. At the time of the Italian survey, a delay in the implementation of the early intervention model had been also observed in many other countries. Even in Australia − where the revolution of early intervention started − a slow and variable implementation of services for at-risk people was reported, due again to insufficient allocation of funds [76]. However, recent economic analyses found that investment in early intervention services not only help reduce some of the long-term costs and consequences of mental disorders to the healthcare system but also produce broader economic benefits that strengthen the potential cost savings to society [77]. In addition, interventions in early life to protect the mental health and well-being of children, as well as their parents, can generate substantive positive returns on investment not just for health but for other sectors such as education, criminal justice and social welfare [78]. Mental health professionals should therefore bring this evidence on the desk of policymakers and health administrators and to the attention of the general public in order to correct biased assumptions and misconceptions on funding allocation for mental disorders and tackle this form of structural stigma.

10.5 Conclusions

Taken together, literature discussed here provides good evidence that the reducing of *stigma* associated with *mental disorders* represents a critical step for the successful implementation of prevention programmes both in public health and clinical settings. Stigma reduction initiatives should be therefore urgently undertaken at multiple levels and sustained over time [79].

Approaches to changing stigma have been divided into protest, education and contact strategies [80]. Protest relies on an appeal to a moral authority, leading to a call for suppressing these thoughts. Education seeks to decrease stigmatising myths of mental disorders by contrasting them with facts. Contact tries to erase the prejudice and discrimination of mental disorders through interactions between the 'public' and people experiencing mental disorders in recovery. However, education has little impact on the prejudice and discrimination limiting people's rightful opportunities, while contact yields significantly greater change in attitudes [81]. Finally, programmes meant to erase stigma should be underpinned by an explicit equalities- and human rights-based approach. Erasing stigma, in fact, is not enough; people need to replace prejudice with affirming attitudes and behaviours. Affirming attitudes promote recovery and pursuit of individual goals based on ideas of hope, empowerment and self-determination. Affirming behaviours are community actions that firm up recovery and self-determination. People with lived experience of mental health problems need to drive this effort and set policies and actions that may improve their lives.

References

1. Fusar-Poli P, Bauer M, Borgwardt S, Bechdolf A, Correll CU, Do KQ, Domschke K, et al. European College of Neuropsychopharmacology network on the prevention of mental disorders and mental health promotion (ECNP PMD-MHP). Eur Neuropsychopharmacol. 2019;29:1301–11.
2. Mrazek PJ, Haggerty RJ, editors. Reducing risks for mental disorders: Frontiers for preventive intervention research. Washington: National Academy Press; 1994.
3. World Health Organization. Prevention of mental disorders. Effective interventions and policy options. Geneva: Department of Mental Health and Substance Abuse; 2004.
4. Colizzi M, Lasalvia A, Ruggeri M. Prevention and early intervention in youth mental health: is it time for a multidisciplinary and trans-diagnostic model for care? Int J Ment Health Syst. 2020;14:23.
5. Arango C, Díaz-Caneja CM, McGorry PD, Rapoport J, Sommer IE, Vorstman JA, et al. Preventive strategies for mental health. Lancet Psychiatry. 2018;5:591–604.
6. Rüsch N, Thornicroft G. Does stigma impair prevention of mental disorders? Br J Psychiatry. 2014;204:249–51.
7. Rüsch N, Angermeyer MC, Corrigan PW. Mental disorders stigma: concepts, consequences, and initiatives to reduce stigma. Eur Psychiatry. 2005;20:529–39.
8. Thornicroft G. Shunned discrimination against people with mental disorders. New York: Oxford University Press; 2006.
9. Goffmann E. Stigma: notes on the management of spoiled Identity. Englewood Cliffs, NJ: Prentice-Hall; 1963.

10. World Health Organization. The world health report 2001—mental health: new understanding, new hope. Geneva: WHO; 2001.
11. Link B, Struening E, Cullen F, Shrout P, Dohrenwend B. A modified labeling theory approach to mental disorders – an empirical assessment. Am Sociol Rev. 1989;54:400–23.
12. Thornicroft G, Rose D, Kassam A, Sartorius N. Stigma: ignorance, prejudice or discrimination? Br J Psychiatry. 2007;190:192–3.
13. Müller B, Nordt C, Lauber C, Rössler W. Changes in social network diversity and perceived social support after psychiatric hospitalisation: results from a longitudinal study. Int J Soc Psychiatry. 2007;53:564–75.
14. Stuart H. Mental disorders and employment discrimination. Curr Opin Psychiatry. 2006;19:522–6.
15. Hinshaw SP. The stigmatization of mental disorders in children and parents: developmental issues, family concerns, and research needs. J Child Psychol Psychiatry. 2005;46:714–34.
16. Lauber C, Nordt C, Falcato L, Rössler W. Community psychiatry: results of a public opinion survey. Int J Soc Psychiatry. 2006;52:234–42.
17. Corrigan PW, Watson AC. The paradox of self-stigma and mental illness. Clin Psychol Sci Pract. 2002;9:35–53.
18. Link BG, Struening EL, Neese-Todd S, Asmussen S, Phelan JC. Stigma as a barrier to recovery: The consequences of stigma for the self-esteem of people with mental disorders. Psychiatr Serv. 2001;52:1621–6.
19. Ritsher JB, Otilingam PG, Grajales M. Internalized stigma of mental disorders: psychometric properties of a new measure. Psychiatry Res. 2003;121:31–49.
20. Lasalvia A, Ventriglio A, Colizzi M, Bellomo A. Stigma as the main obstacle in health care and human rights among people with mental disorders. A rights-based ethics approach. Rivista Sperimentale di Freniatria. 2019;3:133–53.
21. Jorm A, Korten AE, Jacomb PA, Christensen H, Rodgers B, Pollitt P. "Mental health literacy": a survey of the public's ability to recognise mental disorders and their beliefs about the effectiveness of treatment. Med J Aust. 1997;166:182–6.
22. Wright A, Jorm A, Harris M, McGorry P. What's in a name? Is accurate recognition and labeling of mental disorders by young people associated with better help-seeking and treatment preferences? Soc Psychiatry Psychiatr Epidemiol. 2007;42:244–50.
23. Angermeyer MC, Dietrich S. Public beliefs about and attitudes toward people with mental disorders: a review of population studies. Acta Psychiatr Scand. 2006;113:163–79.
24. Hugo CJ, Boshoff DL, Traut A, Zungu-Dirwayi N, Stein DJ. Community attitudes toward and knowledge of mental disorders in South Africa. Soc Psychiatry Psychiatr Epidemiol. 2003;38:715–9.
25. Jorm AF. Mental health literacy: empowering the community to take action for better mental health. Am Psychol. 2012;67:231–43.
26. Schomerus G, Matschinger H, Angermeyer MC. Preferences of the public regarding cutbacks in expenditure for patient care: are there indications of discrimination against those with mental disorders? Soc Psychiatry Psychiatr Epidemiol. 2006;41:369–77.
27. Walsh DAB, Foster JLH. A call to action. A critical review of mental health related anti-stigma Campaigns. Front Public Health. 2021;8(8):569539.
28. Corrigan PW, Markowitz FE, Watson AC. Structural levels of mental disorders stigma and discrimination. Schizophr Bull. 2004;30:481–91.
29. Angermeyer MC, van der Auwera S, Carta MG, Schomerus G. Public attitudes towards psychiatry and psychiatric treatment at the beginning of the 21st century: a systematic review and meta-analysis of population surveys. World Psychiatry. 2017;16:50–61.
30. Schomerus G, Stolzenburg S, Angermeyer MC. Impact of the Germanwings plane crash on mental disorders stigma: results from two population surveys in Germany before and after the incident. World Psychiatry. 2015;14:362–3.
31. Corrigan PW, Watson AC, Gracia G, et al. Newspaper stories as measures of structural stigma. Psychiatr Serv. 2005;56:551–6.

32. Lyons AC. Examining media representations: benefits for health psychology. J Health Psychol. 2000;5:349–58.
33. Hallam A. Media influences on mental health policy: long-term effects of the Clunis and Silcock cases. Int Rev Psychiatry. 2002;14:26–33.
34. Wahl OF. Mental health consumers' experiences of stigma. Schizophr Bull. 1999;25:467–78.
35. Benbow A. Mental disorders, stigma, and the media. J Clin Psychiatry. 2007;68(Suppl. 2):31–5.
36. Klin A, Lemish D. Mental disorders stigma in the media: review of studies on production, content, and influences. J Health Commun. 2008;13:434–49.
37. Cutcliffe JR, Hannigan B. Mass media, 'monsters' and mental health clients: the need for increased lobbying. J Psychiatr Ment Health Nurs. 2001;8:315–21.
38. Vaughan G, Hansen C. 'Like Minds, Like Mine': a New Zealand project to counter the stigma and discrimination associated with mental disorders. Australas Psychiatry. 2004;12:113–7.
39. Stuart H. Media portrayal of mental disorders and its treatments: what effect does it have on people with mental disorders? CNS Drugs. 2006;20:99–106.
40. Clement S, Lassman F, Barley E, et al. Mass media interventions for reducing mental health-related stigma. Cochrane Database Syst Rev. 2013;7:CD009453.
41. Rasic D, Hajek T, Alda M, Uher R. Risk of mental disorders in offspring of parents with schizophrenia, bipolar disorder, and major depressive disorder: a meta-analysis of family high-risk studies. Schizophr Bull. 2014;40:28–38.
42. Sommer IE, Bearden CE, van Dellen E, et al. Early interventions in risk groups for schizophrenia: what are we waiting for? NPJ Schizophr. 2016;2:16003.
43. Conley CS, Shapiro JB, Kirsch AC, Durlak JA. A meta-analysis of indicated mental health prevention programs for at-risk higher education students. J Couns Psychol. 2017;64:121–40.
44. Corcoran C, Malaspina D, Hercher L. Prodromal interventions for schizophrenia vulnerability: the risks of being "at risk". Schizophr Res. 2005;73:173–84.
45. Yang L, Wonpat-Borja A, Opler M, Corcoran C. Potential stigma associated with inclusion of the psychosis risk syndrome in the DSM-V: an empirical question. Schizoph Res. 2010;120:42–8.
46. Fusar-Poli P, Bonoldi I, Yung AR, Borgwardt S, Kempton MJ, Valmaggia L, et al. Predicting psychosis: meta-analysis of transition outcomes in individuals at high clinical risk. Arch Gen Psychiatry. 2012;69:220–9.
47. Riecher-Rössler A, Studerus E. Prediction of conversion to psychosis in individuals with an at-risk mental state: a brief update on recent developments. Curr Opin Psychiatry. 2017;30:209–19.
48. Moritz S, Gawęda Ł, Heinz A, Gallinat J. Four reasons why early detection centers for psychosis should be renamed and their treatment targets reconsidered: we should not catastrophize a future we can neither reliably predict nor change. Psychol Med. 2019;49:2134–40.
49. Gronholm PC, Thornicroft G, Laurens KR, Evans-Lacko S. Mental health-related stigma and pathways to care for people at risk of psychotic disorders or experiencing first-episode psychosis: a systematic review. Psychol Med. 2017;47:1867–79.
50. Colizzi M, Ruggeri M, Lasalvia A. Should we be concerned about stigma and discrimination in people at risk for psychosis? A systematic review. Psychol Med. 2020;50:705–26.
51. Uttinger M, Koranyi S, Papmeyer M, Fend F, Ittig S, Studerus E, et al. Early detection of psychosis: helpful or stigmatizing experience? A qualitative study. Early Interv Psychiatry. 2018;12:66–73.
52. Lee EH, Hui CL, Ching EY, Lin J, Chang WC, Chan SK, Chen EY. Public stigma in China associated with Schizophrenia, depression, attenuated psychosis syndrome, and psychosis-like experiences. Psychiatr Serv. 2016;67:766–70.
53. Link BG, Phelan JC. Labeling and stigma. In: Scheid TL, Brown TN, editors. A handbook for the study of mental health: social contexts, theories and systems. New York: Cambridge University Press; 2010. p. 571–87.
54. Welsh P, Tiffin PA. Observations of a small sample of adolescents experiencing an at-risk mental state (ARMS) for psychosis. Schizophr Bull. 2012;38:215–8.

55. Rush N, Heekeren K, Theodoridou A, Dvorsky D, Muller M, Paust T, et al. Attitudes towards help-seeking and stigma among young people at risk for psychosis. Psychiatry Res. 2013;210:1313–5.
56. Trask CL, Kameoka VA, Schiffman J, Cicero DC. Perceptions of attenuated psychosis in a diverse sample of undergraduates. Early Interv Psychiatry. 2019;13:922–7.
57. Parrish EM, Kim NS, Woodberry KA, Friedman-Yakoobian M. Clinical high risk for psychosis: the effects of labelling on public stigma in a undergraduate population. Early Interv Psychiatry. 2019;13:874–81.
58. Yang LH, Woodberry KA, Link BG, Corcoran CM, Bryant C, Shapiro DI, et al. Impact of "psychosis risk" identification: examining predictors of how youth view themselves. Schizophr Res. 2019;208:300–7.
59. Yang LH, Link BG, Ben-David S, Gill KE, Girgis RR, Brucato G, et al. Stigma related to labels and symptoms in individuals at clinical high-risk for psychosis. Schizophr Res. 2015;168:9–15.
60. Rüsch N, Corrigan PW, Heekeren K, Theodoridou A, Dvorsky D, Metzler S, et al. Well-being among persons at risk of psychosis: the role of self-labeling, shame, and stigma stress. Psychiatr Serv. 2014;65:483–9.
61. Rüsch N, Müller M, Heekeren K, Theodoridou A, Metzler S, Dvorsky D, et al. Longitudinal course of self-labeling, stigma stress and well-being among young people at risk of psychosis. Schizophr Res. 2014;158:82–4.
62. Yang LH, Anglin DM, Wonpat-Borja AJ, Opler MG, Greenspoor M, Corcoran CM. Public stigma associated with psychosis risk syndrome in a college population: implications for peer intervention. Psychiatr Serv. 2013;64:284–8.
63. Baba Y, Nemoto T, Tsujino N, Yamaguchi T, Katagiri N, Mizuno M. Stigma toward psychosis and its formulation process: prejudice and discrimination against early stages of schizophrenia. Compr Psychiatry. 2017;73:181–6.
64. Kim SW, Polari A, Melville F, Moller B, Kim JM, Amminger P, et al. Are current labeling terms suitable for people who are at risk of psychosis? Schizophr Res. 2017;188:172–7.
65. He E, Eldeeb SY, Cardemil EV, Yang LH. Psychosis risk stigma and help-seeking: attitudes of Chinese and Taiwanese residing in the United States. Early Interv Psychiatry. 2020;14:97–105.
66. Saleem MM, Stowkowy J, Cadenhead KS, Cannon TD, Cornblatt BA, McGlashan TH, et al. Perceived discrimination in those at clinical high risk for psychosis. Early Interv Psychiatry. 2014;8:77–81.
67. Baer LH, Shah JL, Lepage M. Anxiety in youth at clinical high risk for psychosis: a case study and conceptual model. Schizophr Res. 2019;208:441–6.
68. Larsen EM, Herrera S, Bilgrami ZR, Shaik RB, Crump F, Sarac C, et al. Self-stigma related feelings of shame and facial fear recognition in individuals at clinical high risk for psychosis: a brief report. Schizophr Res. 2019;208:483–5.
69. Kumpfer KL, Fowler MA. Parenting skills and family support programs for drug-abusing mothers. Semin Fetal Neonatal Med. 2007;12:134–42.
70. Selick A, Durbin J, Vu N, O'Connor K, Volpe T, Lin E. Barriers and facilitators to implementing family support and education in Early Psychosis Intervention programmes: a systematic review. Early Interv Psychiatry. 2017;11:365–74.
71. Ince P, Haddock G, Tai S. A systematic review of the implementation of recommended psychological interventions for schizophrenia: rates, barriers, and improvement strategies. Psychol Psychother. 2016;89:324–50.
72. Schomerus G, Matschinger H, Angermeyer MC. Familiarity with mental disorders and approval of structural discrimination against psychiatric patients in Germany. J Nerv Ment Dis. 2007;195:89–92.
73. World Health Organization. Investing in mental health: evidence for action. Geneva: WHO; 2013.
74. McGorry PD, Mei C. Ultra-high-risk paradigm: lessons learnt and new directions. Evid Based Ment Health. 2018;21:131–3.

75. Cocchi A, Cavicchini A, Collavo M, Ghio L, Macchi S, Meneghelli A, Preti A. Implementation and development of early intervention in psychosis services in Italy: a national survey promoted by the Associazione Italiana Interventi Precoci nelle Psicosi. Early Interv Psychiatry. 2018;12:37–44.
76. McGorry P. Evidence, early intervention and the tipping point. Early Interv Psychiatry. 2010;4:1–3.
77. Park AL, McCrone P, Knapp M. Early intervention for first-episode psychosis: broadening the scope of economic estimates. Early Interv Psychiatry. 2016;10:144–51.
78. Skokauskas N, Lavelle TA, Munir K, Sampaio F, Nystrand C, McCrone P, et al. The cost of child and adolescent mental health services. Lancet Psychiatry. 2018;5:299–300.
79. Thornicroft G, Metha N, Clement S, et al. Evidence for effective interventions to reduce mental health-related stigma and discrimination. Lancet. 2016;387:1123–32.
80. Corrigan PW, Penn DL. Lessons from social psychology on discrediting psychiatric stigma. Am Psychol. 1999;54:765–76.
81. Corrigan PW, Morris SB, Michaels PJ, Rafacz JD, Rüsch N. Challenging the public stigma of mental illness: a meta-analysis of outcome studies. Psychiatr Serv. 2012;63:963–73.

Combined Prevention for Substance Use and Mental Health Problems in Youth: A Glance at Two Conditions at High Risk for Addiction

Fabio Lugoboni and Biagio Tinghino

11.1 Prologue

There is a child, less frequently a girl, with attention deficit. This will unfortunately increase exposure to adversity and trauma, starting with school failures which represent a formidable glue to group "losers" together. Among such children, cigarettes will appear, much earlier than among their peers, and then problematic alcohol use and illicit drugs. Alcohol and drugs will also be used by many of the "good" students, but while the latter will stop soon because they will become involved in other interests (study, sport, relationships, hobbies), our unfortunate boy/girl will go further and further down [1]. At that point, we can only wish for him/her to meet the right therapists, which is not so obvious [2].

11.2 The Gateway Theory: Is It Just a Theory?

The idea that the consumption of a drug (even once) can lead to subsequent use of other and stronger substances has long been suggested. Such belief has been raised in the popular imagination by events without a solid scientific basis, even if—paradoxically—research has recently proved that some substances can indeed sensitize brain areas involved in addiction, thus exposing to further addictive behaviors.

The first attempt to legitimize the so-called drug gateway theory dates back to the late 1930s, when Harry Anslinger—a US official—was trying to ban the use of

F. Lugoboni (✉)
Department Medicine, University Hospital of Verona, Verona, Italy
e-mail: fabio.lugoboni@aovr.veneto.it

B. Tinghino
Department of Psychiatry, Addiction Clinic of Vimercate, Monza-Brianza, Italy

M. Colizzi, M. Ruggeri (eds.), *Prevention in Mental Health*,
https://doi.org/10.1007/978-3-030-97906-5_11

cannabis through well-designed propaganda operations, which highlighted the damage that it could have on health. Posters in public areas associated the use of marijuana with death and serious illness and warned citizens against the danger of the drug being put, without their knowledge, in tea, drinks, and tobacco for cigarettes. The first in-depth study to verify Anslinger's alarmist claims was promoted in 1938 by the mayor of New York, Fiorello La Guardia, who appointed a commission of experts, who in 1944 produced the La Guardia Committee Report. The report said that the use of cannabis did not favor heroin or cocaine addiction and that it could not be considered to facilitate the commission of crimes. In a nutshell, the report denied the theory that there are "gateway" drugs, capable of subsequently facilitating the consumption of "heavy" substances. It was even concluded that marijuana could be useful for treating alcohol and heroin addiction.

The conflict between the two positions, however, did not stop, and Anslinger asked the American Medical Association to produce a report that reversed the La Guardia Committee Report. This happened promptly, in the direction requested by the client, also through the use of racial considerations (it was disputed that the sample was composed mainly of "blacks" and so on). The confusion obviously increased, and the argument remained debated. These events have possibly affected our ability to draw valid scientific conclusions until today. We still suffer the consequences of what happened one hundred years ago, as the debate continues to be addressed at the level of political factions and not—as it should—left to the conclusions of scientists.

11.3 The Return of the Theory

In the early 1960s, also due to the spread of drugs such as heroin, the problem became topical again. After several unsuccessful attempts, Denise Kandel managed to complete a longitudinal study on 1325 high school students, in order to understand if there were a connection between the use of some substances and others. Subsequent studies [3, 4] led Kandel to believe that some substances might indeed lead to the use of other drugs, even if data have never been explained in deterministic (cause-effect) terms, but in probabilistic and correlation terms.

These studies showed a well-defined sequence in the use of drugs, which started with licit substances (alcohol and tobacco) and continued with illicit substances (cocaine, marijuana, MDMA, heroin). On the other hand, human studies that had tried to deny the gateway effect have frequently given negative results [5]. Investigations have also focused on identifying the age at which first use occurs and its correlation with use/addiction in adulthood [6, 7]. Some have found a positive correlation with alcohol use at age 15, but not with tobacco or marijuana [7], while others—conducted among a sample of twins—have indicated a correlation with cannabis use [8].

Further studies among populations found correlations between the daily consumption of tobacco and the use of cannabis as well as illicit drugs [9]. Degenhardt and others performed a very large study in 2010, conducted in 17 countries, which found that young age and previous drug use are the main determinants of subsequent addiction to psychotropic substances. As a whole, data seem to confirm that drugs taken in adolescence somehow facilitate subsequent experiences and possibly the onset of addiction [10].

11.4   Not Just Substances

A further level of complexity in this field of research is given by the multiplicity of factors that can intervene in facilitating the early use and progression in the use of substances. It is in fact known how important are familial, demographic, social, and psychological factors, as well as genetic vulnerability and—finally—the concomitant presence of frailty/psychiatric disorders. Another limitation of the available studies is their duration and the difficulty of following participants from adolescence to adulthood, in order to demonstrate a correlation between the described phenomena.

Many considerations prevent us from thinking of a deterministic pattern in the progression towards addiction. Not all individuals who use a drug become addicted. Only 30% of those who take cocaine will become long-term addicts. Individuals also differ in their susceptibility to the same substance and doses [11, 12].

Genetic factors are important in modulating the susceptibility and vulnerability to addiction [11–14]. Other factors recognized as having an effect on patterns of drug use are sex hormones (gender differences), duration of drug exposure, periodicity (regularity and intermittence), route of intake (e.g., venous or inhalation), and level of cognitive dissonance.

On the other hand, the presence of life skills (but also of family skills) is now universally accepted as one of the most powerful protective factors against the use and dependence on substances or addictive behaviors. Once the use of a substance or behavior is memorized as having a high positive effect, and reinforcement is established, the transition from an experimental/social use phase to a phase of addiction becomes easier. When the addictive behavior is structured, psychological factors (all-or-nothing) take over the control function on behavior.

11.5   Neurochemical Aspects

Predisposing factors and early consumption of one substance or another result in a modification of brain structures. It is therefore important to deepen the knowledge on how these changes occur, how relevant they are and how they can affect subsequent behaviors. In recent years, basic research has reserved many surprises and has made it possible to re-evaluate the drug gateway theory, providing unexpected data [15, 16].

Substance use induces alterations of different areas of the central nervous system (CNS) at the synaptic level, also altering the structural plasticity. Morphological alterations of the neurons are measurable and depend on the modulation of intracellular signals responsible for the growth and survival of the neurons themselves. These plastic modifications represent a form of adaptation that reinforces the mechanisms underlying the development and maintenance of addiction. A first concept connected to the drug gateway theory is that the repeated use of stimulants does not attenuate the gratifying effect, but amplifies it. We are talking about the so-called sensitization or reverse tolerance. This phenomenon goes in the opposite direction to what occurs during tolerance, that is, when the body "gets used" to the use of a substance, which is reflected in a less intense effect with repeated consumption. Sensitization seems to occur for all addictive substances and tends to persist even after the cessation of use, being one of the main causes of relapse, showing also cross-sensitivity among similar substances, and is modulated by psychic phenomena such as stress or intense emotional situations, even if positive. The table below shows the characteristics and mechanisms of "wanting," intended as a pathological progression of the more physiological "liking" [17–19].

The "wanting" mechanism

- It is the most represented and is mediated mostly by dopamine
- Dopamine probably does not mediate pleasure, but desire, which is little connected to cognitive goals and more closely related to reward stimuli
- Dopamine makes these signals attractive and salient
- Addiction causes an amplified state of incentive salience, so any emotional situation (e.g., positive or negative stressful events) can promote relapse
- It is mediated by mesocorticolimbic areas that involve dopamine projections to the nucleus accumbens or other parts of the striatum
- The stronger the stimuli of the external cues, the stronger is the craving, even though the trigger can also be produced by subliminal ("unconscious") stimuli
- The dopamine system is susceptible to sensitization by many drugs (amphetamines, nicotine, cocaine, etc.)
- Sensitization acts against tolerance, i.e., it induces an increase in the effect of subsequent doses/drugs
- Sensitization occurs especially if drugs are taken repeatedly, in high doses and intermittently
- Once induced, it lasts for a long time and perhaps forever
- Sensitization also occurs in addictions without the use of substances (e.g., gambling)

The mechanisms of liking are more delicate and probably quite different than those of wanting. This means that in some subjects, the pleasurable sensations of the consumption of psychotropic substances can be disentangled from necessity or at least can be reproduced independently of the compulsion deriving from addiction.

In theory, some subjects may decide to access the consumption of substances or initiate potentially addictive behaviors not because they are driven by need (which they do not perceive), but because the drug-use behavior is motivated by pleasure. All of this seems to happen even when the dopamine competition has been suppressed.

A common example is that of patients in whom dopamine production is artificially reduced. In these people, the need to eat is reduced but not the satisfaction or pleasure associated with food [17, 20].

The "liking" mechanism

- The liking system includes a series of interactive hedonic hotspots
- This active circuit can be shared by heterogeneous pleasures, such as human sensory, food, cultural, and social pleasures
- Hotspots are anatomically tiny, neurochemically limited, and very fragile
- The hedonic hotspot is about 10% of the nucleus accumbens, in the rat. The remaining 90% does not improve liking but wanting

---

11.6 Drug Gateway, Nicotine, and Memory Consolidation Mechanisms

The use of substances interferes with learning mechanisms, in particular by changing the salience of stimuli and experiences and their appetitive and emotional aspects. These changes are also affected by specific biological vulnerabilities, constitute measurable phenomena, and are now well described in terms of the chain of processes that lead from use to addiction. Drugs change the brain and its circuits. This occurs through a memory modification, from short-term memory (in example: the first contacts with a substance) into a more consolidated, persistent memory, therefore capable of influencing the behavior for a long time. There are experiences that are easily forgotten and others that remain firmly fixed in the brain: the consumption of psychotropic substances belongs to this second category [21]. The Nobel Prize Eric Kandel, his wife Denise, and colleagues have shown how a short experience can turn into a long-term memory. Transformation into long-term memory requires acetylation of chromatin (acetylation of histones H3 and H4), which occurs when drugs (nicotine in particular) activate a genetic transcription factor, CREB (cyclic AMP response element-binding protein), which activates a cascade of neurochemical events that promote the expression of the ΔFosB gene in the nucleus accumbens and ultimately stimulate the growth of new synapses [22]. The substance that acts most strongly in this direction is nicotine. It is capable of activating the early genes C-fos and C-jun. To reach such conclusion, the Kandels developed a model in the mouse, in collaboration with Amir Levine. This model is capable of simulating the behavioral, electrophysiological, and genetic modifications induced by some given drugs with a specific sequence. In particular, the researchers focused on two behaviors that are related to addiction in these animals: locomotor sensitization and conditioned place preference. After experimenting with different sequences in drug administration, it was found that the greatest sensitization was obtained by giving the animals first nicotine (7 days) and then cocaine and nicotine together (4 days). This resulted in a 98% enhancement of the excitatory response compared to controls. The most important aspect is that such response was obtained only if nicotine was given first compared to cocaine, and not vice versa. Awareness for other drugs is therefore not a bidirectional phenomenon between any substances. Nicotine is the drug that raises awareness for other drugs, in a cause-effect relationship. Researchers then looked at the histochemical underpinnings of such behavioral changes, by measuring the expression of the FosB gene in the nucleus accumbens, and found that the "nicotine before cocaine" sequence induced the greatest enhancement of long-term memory. In other words, it was the nicotine that induced the greatest rewarding effect for subsequent drugs of abuse [23].

To those who criticized their work because it was done only in animal models and ignored the complexity of the human sociodemographic variables, the Kandels replied that they had chosen a mice model precisely for this reason, to study the molecular aspects and mechanisms of action of drugs without other confounding factors. To this, however, they added the epidemiological consideration that, according to the National Survey on Drug Use and Health, cigarette smoking had reduced (among 18–25-year-olds) from 40.8% to 30.6% between 2002 and 2013, and in the same period, the percentage of cocaine users had also dropped from 6.7% to 4.4%. In line with the molecular data, such finding was interpreted as indicating that if the use of tobacco were reduced, we would also expect a reduction in the use of cocaine [24].

The drug gateway theory assumes greater relevance especially when applied to the period of adolescence. This phase of life represents a unique period of vulnerability to the action of nicotine with respect to the possibility of reprogramming brain synapses and the development of rewarding neuronal circuits. The addictive effects of nicotine last for a very long time. Adermark et al. [25] demonstrated (and photographed) that nicotine administration increases the density of dendritic spines in the striated spine (DMS) after only 3 weeks. Italian authors [26] have also seen that the administration of nicotine induces an increase in the length of the dendrites. How much nicotine sensitization affects liking is yet to be fully understood. Certainly, this substance has a robust dopaminergic action. This means that when you start smoking, the need to smoke (craving for nicotine) rises very quickly compared to that of simple hedonic pleasure, which can be controlled and relegated to a voluptuous habit. People think that they smoke because they "like it" (and this is partly true), but they continue mainly because they need it. We are therefore witnessing a set of data that lead us to confirm the drug gateway theory, except for the fact that the direction of the studies leads us to different conclusions than those that had been initially hypothesized. Clinicians, but also policy makers, should begin to take these findings into account when suggesting or deciding on the promotion of nicotine products other than traditional cigarettes, such as smokeless tobacco or electronic cigarettes. It is no coincidence that the 2014 article in which Eric and Denise Kandel reported their extraordinary discoveries ends with these above recommendations.

11.7 ADHD and SUDs

Attention-deficit hyperactivity disorder (ADHD) is a neurodevelopmental disorder in children and adolescents, persisting into adulthood in a majority of them. ADHD and SUDs commonly co-occur in the clinical adult population. The higher-than-normal prevalence rates of SUDs in people with ADHD indicate increased risk for developing SUD.

The prevalence of ADHD in children and adolescents is estimated to be between 2 and 7%, whereby some studies found prevalence rates up to 16% in certain age groups [27]. The prevalence rates vary depending on the underlying classification system, and males are diagnosed about two to three times more often than females [8, 28]. ADHD is a multifactorial, clinically heterogeneous neurodevelopmental condition caused by an interplay between genetic and environmental factors [27]. It is assumed to result from suboptimal dopamine levels in the synaptic cleft due to overexpression of the presynaptic dopamine transporter (DAT) [29]. Environmental risk factors include, but are not limited to, prenatal exposure to alcohol and tobacco, premature birth, critical birth circumstances, and difficulties in the parent-child interaction [30]. People with ADHD show deficits in attention intensity and selectivity, in executive inhibitory control (e.g., controlling motor action or overbearing responses) and therefore in self-regulation, as well as in memory functions, especially in short-term/working memory. They therefore struggle with continuous vigilance and attention, are easily distracted by internal and/or external stimuli, experience themselves as "forgetful," and express difficulty in self-organizing and performing their daily routines. Other neurocognitive performances are usually not affected [27].

Co-occurring ADHD and SUDs are routinely encountered in clinical settings. Studies have shown that the prevalence rates of SUDs are two to four times higher in people with ADHD than in the general population [31, 32]. In clinical samples, one-fifth of all alcohol-dependent and up to one-third of all cocaine-dependent patients meet the criteria for adult ADHD [27]. Drug-dependent individuals suffering also from ADHD have significantly higher problem severity scores, lower quality-of-life scores, more comorbid SUDs, and psychiatric disorders [33]. More complex and chronic drug dependence has been found in treatment-seeking SUD patients who screen positive for ADHD [34].

11.8 ADHD and Nicotine Smoking

Having established that the substance that acts as a "Trojan horse" towards cocaine and, probably, also towards other substances is nicotine, it is necessary to clarify how these recent acquisitions may have a more or less important role in ADHD. The presence of ADHD during neurodevelopment has been shown to significantly increase the prevalence of substance use, anticipate the age of onset of use, and increase the likelihood of developing a greater degree of dependence and is associated with a more complex therapeutic path and a greater likelihood of relapse [32, 35, 36]. The scientific literature has long reported a strong correlation between ADHD and smoking, although these reports have very little influenced the attention and clinical practice of neuropsychiatry services. In particular, it has long been proven that individuals with ADHD have a higher probability of smoking in adolescence and adulthood [37–39], but this has only recently led to further studies on the patterns of smoking in this population, i.e., quantity, degree of dependence, and difficulty in quitting, although it is undoubtedly clear that smoking is the first avoidable cause of death in the world. One of these studies found that adults with ADHD, compared to smokers without such condition, present with a higher consumption of cigarettes, a greater degree of dependence, more attempts to quit, and more severe withdrawal symptoms, all factors that result in greater difficulty to quit. The group of smokers with ADHD reported an earlier contact with cigarettes than the control group and a more rapid progression to compulsive cigarette use [40]. A prospective, multicenter study confirmed these data, underlining the fact that smoking in childhood correlates with more severe symptoms of ADHD in adulthood [41–43]. It was also reported that pregnant women diagnosed with ADHD smoke more than controls and quit in a significantly lower percentage of cases [44]. These studies also stressed out that the scientific literature, with few exceptions, continues to overlook the implications of smoking in individuals with ADHD [45]. If we analyze the specific behavioral changes of people with ADHD, it is easy to understand how this disorder can affect early exposure to smoke, which, per se, occurs very frequently in youth. This experience can provoke a "reinforcement," that is, a particularly positive experience, in a more intense way in those with ADHD, and, due to a greater degree of impulsivity, a high level of tolerance (and therefore dependence) may quickly arise resulting in greater difficulties in controlling smoking and a higher rate of relapse in cases of cessation. It should be taken into account that the two elements that characterize any addiction are the "positive reinforcement" (predominant at the beginning) and the avoidance of negative effects, the so-called withdrawal symptoms.

11.9 ADHD-Related Symptoms and Their Role in Nicotine Use

Inattention is a pivotal symptom of ADHD that persists in 60% of cases even in adulthood and is expressed as difficulty in maintaining attention, organizing activities, giving oneself priority tasks, and maintaining a valid working memory activity. Nicotine, due to its cholinergic activity, improves attentional skills and therefore may reduce, at least initially, such ADHD-related difficulties [40]. Impulsiveness, which often correlates with hasty choices and risky behaviors due to failure to evaluate the possible consequences, is one of the driving forces that leads very young smokers with ADHD to develop early tolerance for nicotine, becoming heavy smokers rapidly [43]. Hyperactivity, which usually leads to diagnosis in childhood and tends to lessen in adulthood, can also find an initial benefit from tobacco use and therefore be a reason for positive reinforcement following smoking [40]. Executive dysfunctions, including impairments in working memory (forgetting things, important appointments), task-shifting (inability to complete a task, maintaining attention for an adequate time), self-monitoring (inability to prioritize assigned tasks), initiation (difficulty applying to a task, procrastinating), and self-inhibition (difficulty in controlling oneself), can be positively influenced, at least initially, by nicotine [46–48]. It should be noted that they are all reported, to varying degrees, as possible disturbances in nicotine withdrawal [49].

Emotional dysregulation, including mood instability, irritability, outbursts of anger, and low tolerance to frustrations, is a hallmark of ADHD. Even in this case, it is easy to understand how nicotine can bring relief from these symptoms which are instead found in smoking abstinence [49]. Although literature on ADHD and SUDs, including smoking, begins to accumulate, it still remains scarce, from both the theoretical and therapeutic points of view, also in light of the role of nicotine in the gateway drug theory discussed above.

Our vision, as a natural consequence of several decades of experience in the study and treatment of smoking and SUDs, which in recent years has increasingly involved the evaluation of the impact of adult ADHD on all behaviors of abuse [32, 50, 51], leads us to summarize the problem of the relationship between ADHD, smoking, and SUDs, in the following key points:

1. Early symptoms of ADHD (hyperactivity in childhood, which is often a consequence of attention deficit) lead to early frustration, especially in the school setting, if not properly diagnosed and treated.
2. Frustration leads children with ADHD to ally themselves, in a defensive way, with the "last, the worst" in the class.
3. This alliance increases the likelihood of early cigarette use.
4. The intake of nicotine (not excluding e-cigarettes and heated tobacco devices) brings a quick benefit on the pivotal symptoms of ADHD, as analyzed above.
5. Impulsiveness, however, leads to an escalation of use with consequent tolerance and dependence.
6. The use of cigarettes, as we discussed, increases the likelihood that occasional experiences with alcohol and drugs (but also other addictive behaviors such as gambling) become more and more salient and therefore lead from a behavior supported by liking to one characterized by wanting.
7. All of this worsens a harmonious development, which is already more difficult in itself.
8. The treatment of these further complications is made even more difficult by the diagnostic challenge to consider adult ADHD in psychiatric care settings and services for pathological addictions [32].

11.10 Conclusions

Tobacco gateway drug theory underlines the central role of nicotine to develop other substance addictions. Moreover, the acetylcholine mechanisms of nicotine create a strong link with ADHD symptomatology, through its effects in reducing inattention.

Nicotine addiction is often considered a minor problem by the specialist (neuropsychiatry, psychiatry, and addiction unit), but this substance can create strong links with other substances (cocaine, alcohol, cannabis, and opioids). SUDs, but we could say in a broader way any pathological addiction, generally receive less attention also from university courses, thus failing the importance they deserve. It is a "historical fault" common to most countries: you cannot teach what you don't know. What is worse, we will tend to ignore it. So we can't be surprised if neuropsychiatry services are generally unprepared to deal with early smoking in such environments, not to mention drugs. "There is nothing in medicine that combines such a strong concentration of prevalence, lethality and neglect as tobacco smoke," writes Michael Fiore in the American guidelines on smoking [52]. Over the years, partly due to a not always enlightened politics, we have seen an excessive focus on new substances, often neglecting the neurodevelopmental disorders that favor the use and then the addiction to substances. Very often, the new drugs are nothing more than derivatives of old ones, and the traditional substances are still the most pernicious, in absolute terms, for morbidity and mortality.

Highly impulsive situations compromise resilience towards substances. Also a poor resilience compromises the possibility of adequately resisting adversity, the first traumatic experiences, starting with school failures which represent a formidable glue to group losers together. Among such children, cigarettes will appear, much earlier than among their peers, and then the first hangovers and drugs. It is extremely important that neuropsychiatry services and pediatricians realize the crucial role they can play in preventing SUD, not only by diagnosing and treating neurodevelopmental disorders early, ADHD at first, but also by tackling initiation of tobacco smoking, empowering parents, and supporting them to quit if they do smoke too. That should be a good enough reason to extend your life and possibly avoid severe complications for your children.

Conflict of Interest None.

References

1. Gerra G, Benedetti E, Resce G, Potente R, Cutilli A, Molinaro S. Socioeconomic status, parental education, school connectedness and individual socio-cultural resources in vulnerability for drug use among students. Int J Environ Res Public Health. 2020;18(17):1306.
2. Shackleton N, Milne BJ, Jerrim J. Socioeconomic inequalities in adolescent substance use: evidence from twenty-four European countries. Subst Use Misuse. 2019;54:1044–9.
3. Kandel DB. Stages in adolescent involvement in drug use. Science. 1975;190:912–4.
4. Kandel DB, Logan JA. Patterns of drug use from adolescence to young adulthood: I. Periods of risk for initiation, continued use, and discontinuation. Am J Public Health. 1984;74:660–6.

5. van Gundy K, Rebellon CJ. A life-course perspective on the "gateway hypothesis". J Health Soc Behav. 2010;51:244–59.
6. Behrendt S, Wittchen HU, Höfler M, Lieb R, Beesdo K. Transitions from first substance use to substance use disorders in adolescence: is early onset associated with a rapid escalation? Drug Alcohol Depend. 2009;99:68–78.
7. Trenz RC, Scherer M, Harrell P, Zur J, Sinha A, Latimer W. Early onset of drug and poly-substance use as predictors of injection drug use among adult drug users. Addict Behav. 2012;37:367–72.
8. Chen CY, Storr CL, Anthony JC. Early-onset drug use and risk for drug dependence problems. Addict Behav. 2009;34:319–22.
9. Mayet A, Legleye S, Falissard B, Chau N. Cannabis use stages as predictors of subsequent initiation with other illicit drugs among French adolescents: use of a multi-state model. Addict Behav. 2012;37:160–6.
10. Degenhardt L, Dierker L, Chiu WT, et al. Evaluating the drug use "gateway" theory using cross-national data: consistency and associations of the order of initiation of drug use among participants in the WHO World Mental Health Surveys. Drug Alcohol Depend. 2010;108:84–97.
11. Becker JB, Perry AN, Westenbroek C. Sex differences in the neural mechanisms mediating addiction: a new synthesis and hypothesis. Biol Sex Differ. 2012;3:14.
12. Robinson TE, Berridge KC. The incentive sensitization theory of addiction: some current issues. Philos Trans R Soc Lond Ser B Biol Sci. 2008;363:3137–46.
13. Franklin TR, Wang Z, Li Y, et al. Dopamine transporter genotype modulation of neural responses to smoking cues: confirmation in a new cohort. Addict Biol. 2011;16:308–22.
14. Moeller SJ, Parvaz MA, Shumay E, et al. Goldstein Gene x abstinence effects on drug cue reactivity in addiction: multimodal evidence. J Neurosci. 2013;33:10027–36.
15. Díaz A, Pérez L. Gambling and substance use: a cross-consumption analysis of tobacco smoking, alcohol drinking and gambling. Subst Abus. 2021;2:1–6.
16. Hellberg SN, Russell TI, Robinson MJF. Cued for risk: evidence for an incentive sensitization framework to explain the interplay between stress and anxiety, substance abuse, and reward uncertainty in disordered gambling behavior. Cogn Affect Behav Neurosci. 2019;19:737–58.
17. Heinz A, Daedelow LS, Wackerhagen C, Di Chiara G. Addiction theory matters-Why there is no dependence on caffeine or antidepressant medication. Addict Biol. 2020;25:e12735.
18. Jasinska AJ, Stein EA, Kaiser J, Naumer MJ, Yalachkov Y. Factors modulating neural reactivity to drug cues in addiction: a survey of human neuroimaging studies. Neurosci Biobehav Rev. 2014;38:1–16.
19. Pisanu A, Lecca D, Valentini V, Bahi A, Dreyer JL, Cacciapaglia F, Scifo A, Piras G, Cadoni C, Di Chiara G. Impairment of acquisition of intravenous cocaine self-administration by RNA-interference of dopamine D1-receptors in the nucleus accumbens shell. Neuropharmacology. 2015;89:398–411.
20. Hardman CA, Herbert V, Brunstrom J, Munafò M, Rogers P. Dopamine and food reward: effects of acute tyrosine/phenylalanine depletion on appetite. Physiol Behav. 2012;105:1202–7.
21. Chiamulera C, Hinnenthal I, Auber A, Cibin M. Reconsolidation of maladaptive memories as a therapeutic target: pre-clinical data and clinical approaches. Front Psych. 2014;19(5):107.
22. Kandel DB, Kandel ER. A molecular basis for nicotine as a gateway drug. N Engl J Med. 2014;371:2038–9.
23. Kandel D, Kandel E. The gateway hypothesis of substance abuse: developmental, biological and societal perspectives. Acta Paediatr. 2015;104:130–7.
24. Kandel D, Johnson J, Bird HR, et al. Psychiatric comorbidity among adolescents with substance use disorders: findings from the MECA Study. J Am Acad Child Adolesc Psychiatry. 1999;38:693–9.
25. Adermark L, Morud J, Lotfi A, et al. Temporal rewiring of striatal circuits initiated by nicotine. Neuropsychopharmacology. 2016;41:3051–9.
26. Collo G, Bono F, Cavalleri L, et al. Nicotine-induced structural plasticity in mesencephalic dopaminergic neurons is mediated by dopamine D3 receptors and Akt-mTORC1 signaling. Mol Pharmacol. 2013;83:1176–89.

27. Chamakalayil S, Strasser J, Vogel M, Brand S, Walter M, Dürsteler KM. Methylphenidate for attention-deficit and hyperactivity disorder in adult patients with substance use disorders: good clinical practice. Front Psychiatry. 2021;11:540837.
28. Chen Q, Brikell I, Lichtenstein P, Serlachius E, Kuja-Halkola R, Sandin S, et al. Familial aggregation of attention-deficit/hyperactivity disorder. J Child Psychol Psychiatry. 2017;58:231–9.
29. Krause KH, Dresel SH, Krause J, Kung HF, Tatsch K. Increased striatal dopamine transporter in adult patients with attention deficit hyperactivity disorder: effects of methylphenidate as measured by single photon emission computed tomography. Neurosci Lett. 2000;285:107–10.
30. Thapar A, Cooper M, Eyre O, Langley K. What have we learnt about the causes of ADHD? J Child Psychol Psychiatry. 2013;54:3–16.
31. Cumyn L, French L, Hechtman L. Comorbidity in adults with attention-deficit hyperactivity disorder. Can J Psychiatr. 2009;54:673–83.
32. Lugoboni F, Levin FR, Monfredini M, Zamboni L, Somaini L, Gerra G. Co-occurring attention deficit hyperactivity disorder symptoms in adults affected by heroin dependence: patients characteristics and treatment needs. Psychiatry Res. 2017;250:210–6.
33. Carpentier PJ. Addiction from a developmental perspective: the role of conduct disorder and ADHD in the development of problematic substance use disorders. Tijdschr Psychiatr. 2014;56:95–105.
34. Young JT, Carruthers S, Kaye S, et al. Comorbid attention deficit hyperactivity disorder and substance use disorder complexity and chronicity in treatment-seeking adults. Drug Alcohol Rev. 2015;34:683–93.
35. Kollins SH. ADHD, substance use disorders, and psychostimulant treatment: current literature and treatment guidelines. J Atten Disord. 2008;12:115–25.
36. Paraskevopoulou M, van Rooij D, Batalla A, Chauvin R, Luijten M, Schene AH, Buitelaar JK, Schellekens AFA. Effects of substance misuse on reward-processing in patients with attention-deficit/hyperactivity disorder. Neuropsychopharmacology. 2021;46:622–31.
37. Milberger S, Biederman J, Faraone SV, Chen L, Jones J. ADHD is associated with early initiation of cigarette smoking in children and adolescents. J Am Acad Child Adolesc Psychiatry. 1997;36:37–44.
38. Molina BS, Pelham WE. Childhood predictors of adolescent substance use in a longitudinal study of children with ADHD. J Abnorm Psychol. 2003;112:497–507.
39. Sibley MH, Pelham WE, Molina BSG, et al. The role of early childhood ADHD and subsequent CD in the initiation and escalation of adolescent cigarette, alcohol, and marijuana use. J Abnorm Psychol. 2014;123:362–74.
40. Kollins SH, Sweitzer MM, McClernon FJ, Perkins KA. Increased subjective and reinforcing effects of initial nicotine exposure in young adults with attention deficit hyperactivity disorder (ADHD) compared to matched peers: results from an experimental model of first-time tobacco use. Neuropsychopharmacology. 2020;45:851–6.
41. Mitchell JT, Howard AL, Belendiuk KA, et al. Cigarette smoking progression among young adults diagnosed with ADHD in childhood: a 16-year longitudinal study of children with and without ADHD. Nicotine Tob Res. 2019;21:638–47.
42. Mitchell JT, McClernon FJ, Beckham JC, Brown RA, Lejuez CW, Kollins SH. Smoking abstinence effects on emotion dysregulation in adult cigarette smokers with and without attention-deficit/hyperactivity disorder. Drug Alcohol Depend. 2019;205:107594.
43. Sánchez-García N, González R, Ramos-Quiroga J, et al. Attention deficit hyperactivity disorder increases nicotine addiction severity in adults seeking treatment for substance use disorders: the role of personality disorders. Eur Addict Res. 2020;26:191–200.
44. Andersson A, Hegvik TA, Chen Q, et al. Attentiondeficit/hyperactivity disorder and smoking habits in pregnant women. PLoS One. 2020;15:e0234561.
45. Lee CT, McClernon FJ, Kollins SH, Fuemmeler BF. Childhood ADHD symptoms and future illicit drug use: the role of adolescent cigarette use. J Pediatr Psychol. 2018;43:162–71.
46. Becker TD, Arnold MK, Ro V, Martin L, Rice TR. Systematic review of electronic cigarette use (vaping) and mental health comorbidity among adolescents and young adults. Nicotine Tob Res. 2021;23:415–25.

47. Rhodes JD, Kennedy TM, Walther CAP, Gnagy EM, Pelham WE Jr, Molina BSG. Smoking-specific risk factors in early adulthood that mediate risk of daily smoking by age 29 for children with ADHD. J Atten Disord. 2021;26:108.
48. Zamboni L, Marchetti P, Congiu A, Giordano R, Fusina F, Carli S, Centoni F, Verlato G, Lugoboni F. ASRS questionnaire and tobacco use: not just a cigarette. A screening study in an Italian young adult sample. Int J Environ Res Public Health. 2021;18:2920.
49. Aubin HJ, Rollema H, Svensson HT, Winterer G. Smoking, quitting, and psychiatric disease: a review. Neurosci Biobehav. 2012;36:271–84.
50. Lugoboni F, Bertoldi A, Casari R, Mantovani E, Morbioli L, Tamburin S. Adult attention-deficit/hyperactivity disorder and quality of life in high-dose benzodiazepine and related Z-drug users. Eur Addict Res. 2020;22:1–9.
51. Lugoboni F, Zamboni L, Mantovani E, Cibin M, Tamburin S. Association between adult attention deficit/hyperactivity disorder and intravenous misuse of opioid and benzodiazepine in patients under opioid maintenance treatment: a cross-sectional multicentre study. Eur Addict Res. 2020;29:1–11.
52. Fiore MC, Jaen CR, Baker WC, Benowitz NL, Curry SJ, et al. Treating tobacco use and dependance: 2008 update. Clinical practice guideline. Rockville: MDUS Department of Health and Human Services; 2008.

Marcella Bellani, Niccolò Zovetti, Cinzia Perlini,
and Paolo Brambilla

12.1 Introduction

Cognitive alterations associated with mental health disorders have been studied ever since schizophrenia was known in its early conceptualizations as *dementia praecox*. According to current literature, neurocognitive impairments are now considered key features of schizophrenia, bipolar disorders and related psychotic disorders, significantly affecting patients' quality of life, functional ability, interpersonal and socio-occupational outcomes [1]. These impairments affect several key cognitive functions and processes including different aspects of attention (selective, divided, sustained and alternating), memory, reasoning, processing speed, motor coordination, theory of mind, affective processing, decision-making and language [2–6]. Specifically, more than 90% of patients suffering from psychosis perform significantly worse on

M. Bellani (✉) · N. Zovetti
Department of Neurosciences, Biomedicine and Movement Sciences, Section of Psychiatry, University of Verona, Verona, Italy
e-mail: marcella.bellani@univr.it; niccolo.zovetti@univr.it

C. Perlini
Department of Neurosciences, Biomedicine and Movement Sciences, Section of Clinical Psychology, University of Verona, Verona, Italy
e-mail: cinzia.perlini@univr.it

P. Brambilla
Department of Neurosciences and Mental Health, Fondazione IRCCS Ca' Granda Ospedale Maggiore Policlinico, Milan, Italy

Department of Pathophysiology and Transplantation, University of Milan, Milan, Italy
e-mail: paolo.brambilla1@unimi.it

M. Colizzi, M. Ruggeri (eds.), *Prevention in Mental Health*,
https://doi.org/10.1007/978-3-030-97906-5_12

203

neuropsychological tests than what would be predicted by their education level, and those who show less deficits are usually characterized by a considerably higher premorbid cognitive level [7]. Cognitive dysfunctions are thought to arise from the disruption of important neural networks encompassing cortical-cerebellar-thalamic-cortical regions [8]. As such, recent theorizations suggest that cognitive impairments can be considered a highly heritable endophenotype of psychosis characteristic of the entire spectrum [9]. Specifically, some psychiatric conditions such as schizophrenia or bipolar disorder and their auxiliary cognitive deficits are thought to be associated with genetic vulnerabilities such as catechol-O-methyltransferase or BDNF Val66Met alterations [10, 11].

More importantly, the cognitive deficits characteristic of psychotic conditions have been shown to be present even in the premorbid states by Mollon and Reichenberg [12]. In their review the authors argue that individuals who develop schizophrenia or related disorders exhibit deficit in general intelligence, several cognitive domains (i.e. attention, working memory), language, processing speed and executive functioning even in the prodromal states or before the onset of the condition. Therefore, these alterations are thought to arise from genetic vulnerabilities (e.g. COMT and its role in dopaminergic neurotransmission) and environmental factors (e.g. obstetric complications, prenatal influenza, cannabis use) that later in life contribute to the onset of schizophrenia [12].

From a global perspective, schizophrenia and related psychotic disorders account for more than 1% of the global burden of disease in European countries [13]. However, unlike conditions with a similar prevalence, psychotic disorders are associated with more disruptive effects on the patients' daily lives, independence and social integration, for example, employment rates in psychotic populations (that usually ranges between 5 and 23%), confirming that these disorders represent a great burden upon patients' social functioning and, ultimately, a great cost upon the national health system worldwide [13, 14].

Moreover, patients suffering from major mental disorders frequently face secondary problems significantly slowing their recovery and ability to reintegrate in the social structure such as social stigma, medication side effects and inadequate availability and funding of mental health services. In fact, severe mental conditions have been found to be associated with premature death, more medical organic diseases including cardiovascular diseases and generally a lower quality of life [15].

Unfortunately, the aforementioned cognitive deficits have been found to respond only moderately to pharmacotherapy; thus, research has focused on behavioural interventions aimed at improving cognitive functioning such as cognitive remediation in order to ameliorate the cognitive and social cognition impairments characteristic of major psychiatric conditions [16–18]. In the following sections, we will present the various types of interventions aimed at enhancing cognition in patients suffering from severe mental conditions, discuss their efficacy in subjects at risk and in patients in the early and chronic phases and discuss about the effectiveness of these interventions.

12.2 Intervention Paradigms

Considering the key role of the cognitive deficits in major psychiatric disorders and their predictive value of a patient's social and occupational functioning [19], the treatment of these impairments has become a relevant target in the therapy of these disorders. As previously introduced, pharmacological interventions have been shown to only partially improve the cognitive component of psychotic disorders; specifically, first-generation antipsychotics are characterized by mostly a negative impact, while new-generation antipsychotics seem to exert only a modest beneficial effect on patients' cognition [20, 21]. For this reason, research has moved towards the study of non-pharmacological clinical and rehabilitative interventions. Briefly, a first distinction can be made between cognitive-enhancing and cognitive remediation programs. The former interventions focus on the idea that the core cognitive abilities such as processing speed, working memory, perception, attention and general intelligence can be improved through repeated behavioural training [22]. Theoretically, these types of interventions could exert beneficial effects on both healthy subjects and patients suffering from cognitive dysfunctions [23]. However, in a recent review by Green and colleagues [22], the authors argue that a "gold standard" is currently missing in the domain of cognitive-enhancing programs since cognitive training is a broad term that can include many different interventions that have been previously shown to exert beneficial effects on cognition (e.g. video games, physical exercise, mindfulness). All these interventions are usually referred as "brain training", but, as Green and colleagues suggest, this can lead to a confused scenario since every cognitive-enhancing program differs in some way from all others producing different effects on cognition. In this context, it is thus difficult to discuss the exact effects and the replicability of the results of different cognitive-enhancing programs. Conversely, cognitive remediation programs were originally developed as auxiliary interventions aimed at improving cognition of patients suffering from schizophrenia [24, 25] and since their early conceptualization have been extensively studied and categorized to facilitate the replicability, reliability and generalizability of the results. Over the last few years, different strategies and specific techniques have been proposed and developed aimed at improving the cognitive performance and the clinical functioning of patients [26]. These interventions are based on the theorization that cognitive impairments are not persistent and can be, to some extent, improved through constant exercise and/or by the development of new cognitive and social skills [16, 27]. On average, these paradigms have been found to exert moderate and durable beneficial effects on cognitive performance in patients suffering from severe psychiatric conditions such as psychosis. This can be done by either restoring the cognitive functioning of key cognitive domains altered (*restorative approach*) or helping the patient develop new skills and abilities that can, somehow, replace those disrupted by the disorder (*compensatory approach*). Briefly, current literature defines cognitive remediation as a group of interventions based on behavioural training aimed at improving cognitive functions such as attention, memory, executive functioning, social cognition and metacognition with the aim of obtaining the persistence of results and their generalization in a more ecological scenario, that is, in the patients' daily lives [16]. As previously suggested, most of the current psychiatric interventions and theorizations follow a restorative approach and are based on the most recent neuroscientific findings about neuroplasticity claiming that the brain is a network capable of changing through neuronal growth, re-mapping and re-organization induced by cognitive training [28]. Specifically, neuroplasticity has been previously defined as a partial adaptation of the central nervous system to a pathological condition, in the case of schizophrenia expressed as a global alteration of limbic, prefrontal and fronto-striatal brain networks at the base of several key psychological functions including motivation, perception, cognition and emotion and behaviour regulation [29]. While most psychiatric conditions are characterized by important neurodevelopmental and polygenic risk factors, their development is also greatly influenced by experience and environmental conditions [30]. Recent evidence suggests that cognitive remediation and enhancing programs can induce notable changes in the brain of these patients at the cellular level [29] leading to white and grey matter changes localized in prefrontal, parietal and limbic areas [31, 32]. Specifically, these interventions have been shown to be associated with an increase of fractional anisotropy of several white matter structures and to exert a protective effect on the reduction of grey matter volumes characteristic of major psychiatric conditions [32]. However, the exact nature of these brain changes is still debated; for example, Vinogradov and colleagues found that schizophrenia patients undergoing cognitive remediation were characterized by a significant increase of serum brain-derived neurotrophic factor, a polypeptide responsible for the sustainment and development of brain neurons [33].

When it comes to evaluation of the clinical and neuro-social effects of these programs, it is important to make a clear distinction between the primary targets of the intervention, that is, the improvement of cognition (i.e. memory, attention), and the secondary targets such as the improvement of clinical symptoms, social functioning and social skills. While the effect of cognitive remediation on the former is established, recent studies also suggested a beneficial effect of these interventions on social functioning and several clinical measures [34, 35]. These results are important because even though the cognitive functioning of patients is a key factor disrupted by many severe psychiatric conditions, social cognition and social skills impairments significantly hinder the patients' ability to reintegrate in the social context [36]. However, other studies showed that cognitive remediation interventions exert only a limited effect on everyday functioning despite the robust effects on cognition and that, in order to obtain more generalizable and durable improvements, it is important to combine cognitive remediation programs with secondary interventions such as social skills training [37, 38]. The combination of these interventions has been shown to produce robust improvements in patients' neurocognition leading to generalization of these effects in the real-world behaviour. This is especially important as psychotic conditions are characterized by severe and persistent impairments in everyday functioning, social cognition and theory of mind.

Another important distinction within the restorative-approach class lies in the difference between "bottom-up" or "top-down" design; the former indicates a group of interventions aimed at stimulating and improving basic cognitive abilities ultimately affecting higher-order cognitive functions through generalization and abstraction. Conversely, the top-down approach directly targets more complex cognitive functions such as metacognition [25]. From both a theoretical and practical perspective, a clear and defined distinction between these variables appears excessively reductive and impractical since, for example, most models, studies and theorizations frequently employ multiple designs including compensatory, restorative, top-down and bottom-up techniques [26, 39].

Another factor that can also greatly impact on the outcomes of the intervention and that should be considered by clinicians is the patient's motivation. As a psychological construct, motivation is composed of two distinct components: intrinsic and extrinsic; intrinsic motivation refers to the desire to engage in an activity because it is intrinsically interesting, productive, desired and compelling. On the contrary, extrinsic motivation refers to the urge to learn in order to obtain a tangible extrinsic result and reward (e.g. a prize). Several evidence indicate that intrinsic motivation is associated with more durable and persistent learning, creativity and well-being when compared with its counterpart [40]. In the context of cognitive remediation, studies have found significant differences on the efficacy on the intervention when participants were divided into two groups characterized by a high or low intrinsic motivation respectively [41, 42]. Unsurprisingly, those patients in whom intrinsic motivation was high exhibited greater improvements of cognitive functioning at the end of the intervention. As such, considering the important role of intrinsic motivation in learning, it becomes crucial when designing a cognitive-enhancing program to carefully consider all those variables, actions and clinical strategies that could positively impact on a patient's intrinsic motivation. Other factors have also been shown to significantly influence the outcome of cognitive remediation interventions such as specific psychiatric conditions, treatment intensity, type of cognitive remediation program (e.g. drill and practice, strategic), therapist qualifications and baseline work habits [42]. All these factors should be considered when developing cognitive interventions.

12.3   Interventions on Chronic Patients

The first cognitive remediation interventions were originally conceptualized and developed by pioneering researchers between 1993 and 1999 (Delahunty or Wykes) and tested on schizophrenic patients. In these early studies, the authors showed that after the administration of the intervention, patients performed significantly better on neuropsychological testing evaluating executive functioning, cognitive flexibility and memory [24, 25]. Notably, the cognitive improvements induced by the interventions persisted even after 6 months. In the last 30 years, several studies and randomized trials have been conducted on patients suffering from both psychotic and other major psychiatric disorders aiming at elucidating and quantifying the exact effects induced by cognitive-enhancing programs. For example, in a recent meta-analysis by Wykes and colleagues, the authors showed that cognitive remediation exerts beneficial improvements on patients' cognitive functioning acting specifically on attention, speed of processing, verbal and working memory and executive functioning [16] (see Table 12.1).

Table 12.1 Systematic reviews and meta-analyses investigating the effects of cognitive-enhancing programs on chronic patients discussed in this chapter

Authors	Type of study	Sample size	Results
Wykes et al. [16]	Meta-analysis	2104 psychotic patients (40 studies)	The meta-analysis showed that cognitive remediation exerts a small to moderate effect on cognitive functioning of patients suffering from schizophrenia. Moreover, these effects persisted at follow-up assessments
Anaya et al. [43]	Systematic review and meta-analysis	16 studies	The meta-analysis conducted by the authors found that, on average, cognitive interventions exert a beneficial effect on the cognitive functioning of both schizophrenia and schizo-affective disorder patients (effect size: 0.32)
Motter et al. [44]	Meta-analysis	9 studies	The meta-analysis found that cognitive-enhancing interventions exert a beneficial effect on several cognitive domains in patients suffering from major depression including symptoms severity, daily functioning, attention, working memory and global functioning
Cella et al. [45]	Meta-analysis	2511 psychotic patients (41 studies)	The meta-analysis results showed that cognitive remediation programs significantly reduce patients' negative symptoms when compared with TAU or comparable interventions. Moreover, meta-analysis confirmed that cognitive remediation was superior to TAU and TAU plus active control or adjunctive treatment
Prikken et al. [46]	Meta-analysis	1262 psychotic patients (24 studies)	The meta-analysis results showed that, compared to a control condition, patients receiving computerized cognitive training improved on several cognitive functions including attention (effect size 0.31), working memory (effect size 0.38), positive symptoms (effect size 0.31) and depressive symptoms (effect size 0.37). Small but significant effect sizes were found for processing speed, verbal and visual learning and memory and verbal fluency. However, no significant effects on functional outcomes and social cognition were found
Del Fabro et al. [47]	Systematic review	189 schizophrenic patients (13 studies)	The authors concluded that olanzapine treatment is associated with a normalization of brain activity in schizophrenia during the execution of both cognitive and emotional tasks

Table 12.1 (continued)

Authors	Type of study	Sample size	Results
Ciappolino et al. [48]	Systematic review	638 psychiatric patients (8 studies)	The authors conducted this review to investigate the relationship between docosahexaenoic acid and cognitive function in relation to mental disorders. Results from few randomized controlled trials on the effects of docosahexaenoic acid (alone or in combination) in psychotic, mood and neurodevelopmental disorders are inconclusive
D'Abate et al. [49]	Systematic review	277 borderline personality disorder patients (11 studies)	The review suggests that borderline personality disorder is associated with impairments in metacognitive sub-domains of integration, differentiation and mastery. The most appropriate treatment appeared to be a long-term treatment specifically focused on metacognitive deficits
Ciappolino et al. [50]	Longitudinal	31 bipolar patients	The aim of this study was to evaluate the effects of docosahexaenoic acid supplementation on cognitive performances in euthymic bipolar disorder patients. After 12 weeks of treatment, patients undergoing treatment improved on emotion inhibition tests
Crisanti et al. [51]	Systematic review	11 studies	The review showed that ketamine induces no significant improvement on neurocognitive functions in most of the studies, with only three studies observing improvements in speed of processing, verbal learning, sustained attention and response control and verbal and working memory
Hagan et al. [52]	Meta-analysis	9 studies	The authors conducted a review to evaluate the potential impact of cognitive remediation programs on patients suffering from eating disorders. Results indicated the absence of any significant advantage of cognitive-enhancing programs compared to TAU or other therapies on any psychological outcome
Sciortino et al. [53]	Systematic review	738 bipolar disorder or schizophrenia patients (15 studies)	The review suggested that transcranic magnetic stimulation induces no significant improvements in schizophrenia patients and exerts a limited effect on bipolar disorder patients

TAU treatment as usual

Another meta-analysis was conducted on more than 1200 patients (24 studies) suffering from psychosis evaluating the effects of computerized interventions excluding thus the standard "pen and paper" approaches. Results showed that, on average, cognitive remediation exerted beneficial effects on several cognitive functions including attention, working memory, positive symptoms and depressive symptoms when compared with a control treatment [46]. Notably, the average effect size varied between 0.31 and 0.38 indicating a medium effect of these interventions on patients' cognition. Unfortunately, the meta-analysis also showed the absence of any significant effect on patients' functional outcomes and social cognition variables. These results are in line with those found in the early theorization and experimentations and suggest the importance of also including an accessory intervention aimed at improving the patients' social cognition and metacognition [54]. Notably, other meta-analyses focused on other clinical factors showing that cognitive remediation interventions also exert beneficial effects on schizo-affective and affective disorders and on patients' negative symptomatology including blunting of affect, poverty of speech and thought, apathy, anhedonia and loss of motivation [43, 45]. Interestingly, in a recent review by Biagianti et al. [55], the authors examined the predictors of the responses to cognitive remediation suggesting that the most indicative factors are younger age, shorter illness duration, lower symptoms severity, lower antipsychotic medications and the administration of synergistic interventions.

Having established the beneficial effects of cognitive-enhancing programs on schizophrenia and related psychotic disorders, other researchers aimed at evaluating the potential effects of cognitive remediation on other major psychiatric conditions. For example, Motter and colleagues conducted a meta-analysis on all the studies assessing the potential effect of cognitive remediation on patients suffering from depression, while Hagan et al. followed the same principle focusing on eating disorders [44, 52]. In the first meta-analysis, it was shown that, on average, depressed patients responded more positively when engaged in cognitive-enhancing programs when compared with standard treatment. Improvements were found in key cognitive functions such as symptoms severity, daily functioning, attention, working memory and global functioning. However, Hagan et al. did not find any significant advantage of cognitive remediation over standard treatment on patients suffering from eating disorders. D'Abate et al. and Sala and colleagues focused on patients suffering from borderline personality disorder suggesting that this condition is associated with metacognition and memory impairments [49, 56]. Other studies, meta-analyses and reviews examined the presence of neurocognitive and social cognition impairment in other major psychiatric disorders such as post-traumatic stress disorder, anxiety, bipolar disorder (with and without psychotic symptoms) and schizo-affective conditions [53, 57–61]. To some extents, all these conditions have been found associated with selective cognitive impairments, and many interventions have been proposed including transcranial magnetic stimulation [53]. Ultimately, the most preeminent deficits seem to affect working memory, attention and metacognition because all these cognitive functions are known to be regulated by frontal cortices and brain networks commonly disrupted by major psychiatric disorders [56]. Although it is unclear whether these patients could benefit from cognitive-enhancing treatments, it is reasonable to speculate that tailored interventions could help ameliorate these deficits as seen in psychotic patients. Lastly, several studies and reviews have been conducted with the aim of evaluating the potential beneficial effects of specific medications or substances on cognition [47, 48, 50, 51]. For example, ketamine has been suggested to beneficially impact on the cognition and clinical symptomatology of patients suffering from major depression although a recent review indicated that ketamine leads to a non-significant improvement of neurocognitive functioning [51]. Similarly, docosahexaenoic acid supplements have been found to exert only a marginal beneficial effect in bipolar and other major psychiatric disorders [48, 50].

12.4   Early-Phase Interventions

The improvement of neuro- and social cognition impairment of the psychotic spectrum has become a primary goal in the early intervention strategies as early application of cognitive-enhancing programs might lead to better long-term outcomes [1, 62].

When it comes to cognition-enhancing interventions in the early phases of psychotic disorders, the literature is still scarce, and only a paucity of studies has focused on the early phases of psychosis (see Table 12.2). In a review by Zaytseva et al., the authors suggested that cognitive interventions in the early phases of psychosis might exert a beneficial effect on several cognitive key functions such as learning, visual processing speed, executive functioning, working memory and attention [4]. Although this was one of the earliest reviews present in the literature, several studies confirmed the hypotheses of the authors; for example, Lee and colleagues showed that, compared to treatment as usual, even a short cognitive-enhancing intervention (10 weeks) can induce a significant improvement of learning, memory and psychosocial functioning in psychotic patients. These results have also been replicated by other studies comparing the effects of cognitive-enhancing interventions with treatment as usual or control therapies on either first-episode psychosis or early-phase psychosis patients [65, 68, 70, 72, 74] as well as by a single meta-analysis [64].

In detail, Mendella and colleagues showed that a cognitive-enhancing intervention lasting 6 months induced significant improvements in processing speed and social cognition [65]; other two studies found that cognitive remediation exerted greater improvements of processing speed, attention, vigilance, verbal learning, verbal memory and problem-solving compared with treatment as usual [70]; and, finally, two recent studies with considerably large sample size replicated these findings also showing that cognitive-enhancing programs significantly impacted on the patients' symptomatology (reduction of affective flattening, alogia, anhedonia, social isolation) and social-occupational functioning leading to a faster social and occupational reintegration [72, 74]. Notably, only a single study in the current literature did not find any difference in the cognitive improvements between a group of patients assigned to a computerized cognitive-enhancing training and a control group [71].

Table 12.2 Studies, reviews and meta-analyses investigating the effects of cognitive-enhancing programs on individuals in the first phases of psychosis discussed in this chapter

Authors	Type of study	Sample size	Results
Zaytseva et al. [9]	Review	ns	The review showed that cognitive-enhancing programs exert a beneficial effect on several cognitive functions in patients in the early phase of psychosis including attention, processing speed, executive functioning, verbal working memory, verbal learning and visual learning
Lee et al. (2013)	Longitudinal	55 early-phase patients	Patients were randomized to either TAU or a cognitive remediation program for 10 weeks. In comparison to TAU, the experimental group was associated with improvements in learning, memory and psychosocial functioning
Eack et al. [63]	Longitudinal	58 early-phase patients	Patients assigned to a cognitive remediation intervention for three months showed less reduction of grey matter volumes in the hippocampus, parahippocampal, fusiform gyrus and amygdala. These changes were associated with improved cognition
Revell et al. [64]	Systematic review and meta-analysis	11 studies (615 patients)	The meta-analysis and systematic review showed that cognitive remediation exerts a positive effect on verbal learning and memory in first-episode and early-course psychotic patients. Results also showed the presence of lesser beneficial effects on other cognitive domains including working memory, social cognition, reasoning, problem-solving and executive functioning
Mendella et al. [65]	Longitudinal	27 FEP patients	FEP patients were randomized to TAU or to a cognitive intervention (6 months duration). Results showed that, compare to TAU, patients undergoing the intervention showed improvements in processing speed and social cognition
Eack et al. [66]	Longitudinal	41 early-phase patients	Patients were assigned to a cognitive remediation intervention or to a control therapy. The former group showed greater resting functional connectivity preservation between the resting-state networks involved in emotion processing and problem-solving (i.e. fronto-temporal network) and the dorsal prefrontal cortex, the fronto-temporal network and the insula. These changes were associated with improved emotion perception and regulation
Keshavan et al. [67]	Longitudinal	41 early-phase patients	Patients randomized to a cognitive-enhancing program for 3 months showed increased resting-state activity in the dorsolateral prefrontal cortex and reduced connectivity with anterior cingulate cortex; increased activity correlated positively with neurocognitive improvements

Table 12.2 (continued)

Authors	Type of study	Sample size	Results
Breitborde et al. [68]	Longitudinal	20 FEP patients	Patients were randomized to either a computerized intervention or a computerized intervention and a metacognitive skills training. Results showed an improvement of working memory and social cognition. Patients who underwent the metacognitive skills training also showed greater improvements in processing speed, attention, vigilance, verbal learning and problem-solving
Ramsay et al. [69]	Longitudinal	86 early-phase patients	Patients were assigned to a cognitive remediation intervention or to a control therapy. The cognitive remediation intervention was associated with increases of thalamic volumes and cognitive performance
Deste et al. [70]	Longitudinal	56 patients (11 early course)	Patients were randomized to either TAU or a cognitive intervention program for 6 months. Results showed that both the early-course and the chronic groups were characterized by improvements in attention, executive functioning, verbal memory and working memory and processing speed. A significantly greater improvement was found in the early-course group
García-Fernández et al. [71]	Longitudinal	86 FEP patients	FEP patients were randomized to a computerized cognitive-enhancing program or to a control condition lasting 12 weeks. Results showed the presence of a progressive improvement in neurocognition in both groups over the course of the study, but no differences were found between the two groups
Ventura et al. [72]	Longitudinal	80 FEP patients	80 FEP patients were randomized to a cognitive intervention program or to a control intervention (healthy behaviour training) lasting 6 months. Results showed a progressive and greater improvement of cognition, social functioning and psychosis symptoms (affective flattening, alogia, anhedonia, social isolation) in the cognitive remediation group
Bellani et al. [59]	Review	4 studies (216 patients)	The authors reviewed the neurobiological correlates of cognitive-enhancing programs on early-phase and first-episode patients concluding that cognitive remediation leads to neuroplastic changes localized in the hippocampus, parahippocampus, amygdala, thalamic regions and dorsolateral and insular cortices

(continued)

Table 12.2 (continued)

Authors	Type of study	Sample size	Results
Perlini et al. [73]	Review	254 FEP or at-risk patients (9 studies)	The review suggests that mindfulness-based interventions may be considered a promising adjunctive therapy for the treatment of major psychoses in the early phases of the illness
Nuechterlein et al. [74]	Longitudinal	60 FEP patients	In a 12-month randomized study, FEP patients were either randomized to a cognitive-intervention program or to a control therapy. Results showed that cognitive remediation was superior to the control therapy in improving cognition. Moreover, cognitive remediation led to significantly greater improvement in work and/or school functioning
Haas et al. [75]	Longitudinal	35 FEP patients	The authors performed a machine learning analysis to identify neuromarkers of the response to a computerized intervention treatment

FEP first-episode psychosis, *ns* not specified, *TAU* treatment as usual

Finally, only a paucity of studies investigated the possible neuroplastic effects induced by cognitive-enhancing effects in patients in the early phases of psychosis. For example, Ramsay and colleagues conducted a structural magnetic resonance imaging study to evaluate the effects of a cognitive remediation training on grey matter volumes of patients with early schizophrenia [69]. After 40 h of training, the experimental group showed significant improvements in cognitive performance associated with volume changes in the thalamus [69]. Other three studies randomly assigned patients to a cognitive remediation training or a control therapy and treated for two years evaluating the effects on the intervention on several brain indices [63, 66, 67]. In all the three studies, patients undergoing cognitive-enhancing intervention showed greater preservation of grey matter volume in several cortical and subcortical regions, normalization of brain activity at rest and, more importantly, greater improvements of neuro and social cognition functioning that correlated with the previously mentioned brain changes. Moreover, in a recent review by our group, we suggested that cognitive-enhancing interventions lead to structural and functional brain changes localized in the medial-temporal, thalamic, dorsolateral, prefrontal and insular regions. Notably, these neuroplastic changes are usually associated with improvements in cognitive performance and emotion regulation [1]. Perlini et al. showed in a recent review that mindfulness-based interventions are effective in the treatment of negative symptoms in the early phases of non-affective psychoses and that these interventions potentially exert beneficial effects on depression and anxiety but not on manic symptoms [73]. Lastly, Haas and colleagues evaluated the effect of a computerized training on patients in the early phases of psychosis finding a beneficial effect on attention and sensory processing [75].

To conclude, cognitive interventions appear to be a promising approach in the treatment of cognitive and social deficits manifesting in the early phase of psychosis and in first-episode psychosis patients inducing improvements in memory, attention and executive functioning. However, evidence about the exact neuroplastic changes induced by cognitive-enhancing programs is still scarce, and due to the presence of several confounding factors, it is difficult to estimate the exact neurobiological correlates of these interventions. Specifically, studies present in the literature conducted in patients with early psychosis suggest that cognition-enhancing interventions are associated with structural and functional brain changes and a deceleration of brain degeneration characteristic of psychotic disorders leading in turn to a greater improvement of cognitive and social functioning. Even though the results are still scarce and only a paucity of studies have been conducted, it is reasonable to speculate that the neuroprotective and enhancing effect of cognitive interventions could be the highest the earliest the intervention is offered due to ongoing neurodevelopmental processes [76].

12.5   Interventions on High-Risk Patients

While neuropsychological and social impairments are well known to be present and stable in the first and chronic phases of psychotic disorders, it has been suggested that subtler cognitive alterations might be present also in prodromal phases of psychosis, that is, in individuals "at risk" or "ultra-high risk" [9]. The ultra-high risk status is characterized by alterations of perception, thought and language. Some individuals might occasionally experience brief psychotic episodes different from those experienced by full-blown psychosis patients. An individual generally defined as "at risk" is also characterized by attenuated positive symptomatology, genetic vulnerabilities, specific personality traits and possibly a decline in social functioning. The rate of transition from the state of risk to overt psychosis ranges approximately from 30 to 35% within a follow-up period of 1–3 years [9].

When it comes to neurocognitive and social impairments, Fusar-Poli and other authors have previously suggested that cognitive deficits are prominent in individuals at ultra-high risk for psychosis, and, more importantly, these deficits have been linked to severe functional impairments [77–79].

Having previously shown the beneficial effects of cognitive-enhancing programs on both chronic- and early-phase patients, it could be speculated that cognitive remediation might also exert an enhancing effect on individuals in the prodromal stage of psychosis due to possible ongoing neuroplastic processes [80]. As such, in this section we will review evidence about the potential beneficial effects of cognitive-enhancing intervention on individuals at risk of developing psychosis.

In one of the first studies conducted by Rauchensteiner and colleagues, a group of ultra-high-risk individuals underwent a cognitive-enhancing training for a total of ten sessions showing an improvement in long-term memory and attention [81]. Although in this specific study the control group was composed of chronic patients and the sample was relatively small (10 patients), these results were in part replicated by future studies. For example, in two studies conducted in 2014 and 2016, patients at risk of developing psychosis underwent a computerized cognitive remediation program and were found to significantly improve on visual, processing speed and verbal memory tasks compared to control groups [82, 83].

Moreover, other studies conducted with a similar approach found that cognitive-enhancing programs exerted a beneficial effect on the cognition of individuals at risk that were found to perform significantly better on executive functioning, reasoning, social cognition and processing speed neuropsychological tests after the interventions [84–86]. Notably, one study found that the rate of progression to a full-blown psychosis was significantly lower in the experimental group (3.2% vs 16.9%) of individuals at risk that were randomized to an integrated psychological intervention including cognitive remediation [87]. These results have been partially confirmed by reviews suggesting that cognitive-enhancing interventions significantly improve cognition in ultra-high-risk individuals specifically acting on verbal memory, attention, processing speed and social functioning [9, 62, 88].

Lastly, a systematic review and meta-analysis conducted by Devoe and colleagues found no beneficial effects of cognitive-enhancing programs on social functioning of youth at risk of developing psychosis [89]. However, it is important to specify that the aim of this meta-analysis was not to evaluate the effects of cognitive remediation programs on cognition as a whole but only on social functioning. The lack of any significant effect might be due to the young age of individuals included in the studies or to the fact that none of the studies included any social skills training (e.g. social skills training) in addition to the standard computer-based training. In fact, it has been previously demonstrated that a combined intervention of cognitive remediation and social skills training exerts greater beneficial effects on patients' social cognition [54].

To conclude, cognitive-enhancing interventions such as cognitive remediation or integrated psychological approaches appeared to improve cognition and functional outcome (e.g. occupational measures) of ultra-high-risk patients acting specifically on key cognitive domains such as verbal memory, executive, functioning and processing speed (see Table 12.3). However, only a paucity of studies found a positive effect on clinical symptomatology or social cognition, and, considering the negative findings of a recent meta-analysis [89], it could be theorized that cognitive-enhancing programs alone do not exert significant beneficial improvements on these two variables unless coupled with specific interventions (e.g. social skills training) as suggested by previous studies. Interestingly, if replicated, the results of the study conducted by Bechdolf indicated that cognitive remediation programs significantly reduced the rate of progression to a full-blown psychosis in patients at risk [87]. This finding is especially important as future studies integrating psychological, neuropsychological and rehabilitative programs could be used as a preventive intervention to avoid escalation from a state of risk to a full-blown major mental disorder.

Table 12.3 Studies, reviews and meta-analyses investigating the effects of cognitive-enhancing programs on individuals at risk of developing psychosis discussed in this chapter

Authors	Type of study	Sample size	Results
Rauchensteiner et al. [81]	Longitudinal	10 UHR individuals	Ten individuals at risk of developing psychosis underwent a computerized training for a total of ten sessions; results showed a significant improvement of long-term memory and attention
Bechdolf et al. [87]	Longitudinal	128 UHR individuals	UHR individuals were randomized to either TAU or an integrated psychological intervention including cognitive remediation; results showed that the rate of progression to psychosis was significantly lower in the experimental group (3.2% vs 16.9%)
Urben et al. [84]	Longitudinal	32 individuals at risk	Individuals at risk of developing psychosis were either randomized to a cognitive-enhancing program or to a control therapy for 8 weeks. When compared with the control group, individuals at risk of developing psychosis exhibited a significant improvement in executive functioning, reasoning abilities and symptomatology
Zaytseva et al. [9]	Review	ns	Despite the paucity of studies, the authors suggested that cognitive-enhancing interventions might improve the verbal memory and social skills and reduce the rate of transition to psychosis in UHR individuals
Hooker et al. [82]	Longitudinal	12	UHR individuals underwent 8 weeks of computerized cognitive-enhancing intervention and showed a significant improvement in visual and processing speed and verbal memory
Piskulic et al. [85]	Longitudinal	32 UHR individuals	UHR participants were randomized to a computerized control condition or to a computerized cognitive remediation intervention for 40 h; after the intervention, the experimental group performed significantly better in social cognition and processing speed tasks
Loewy et al. [83]	Longitudinal	83 UHR individuals	UHR participants were randomized to a computerized control condition or to a computerized cognitive remediation intervention for 40 h; after the intervention, the experimental group performed significantly better in a verbal memory task

(continued)

Table 12.3 (continued)

Authors	Type of study	Sample size	Results
Choi et al. [86]	Longitudinal	62 UHR individuals	Participants were randomized to a cognitive remediation intervention or to a control condition for 30 h; after the intervention, the experimental group performed significantly better in a processing speed task
Glenthøj et al. [88]	Review	327 UHR individuals (6 studies)	The authors conducted a systematic review and found that, despite paucity of studies, in 83% of the studies, cognitive-enhancing interventions improved cognition in UHR individuals exerting beneficial effects on verbal memory, attention, processing speed and social functioning
Devoe et al. [89]	Review and meta-analysis	1513 individuals at risk (19 studies)	The authors conducted a systematic review and meta-analysis including a total of 1513 individuals at risk of developing psychosis who underwent cognitive-enhancing interventions. The results indicated that, overall, no treatment significantly improved social functioning in youth at risk of developing psychosis

ns not specified, *TAU* treatment as usual, *UHR* ultra-high risk

12.6 Conclusions

To conclude, it appears that cognitive remediation and similar approaches exert a beneficial effect and on several cognitive functions in patients suffering from schizophrenia, related psychotic disorders or major psychiatric conditions (i.e. major depression). Average effect sizes range from 0.30 to 0.38 indicating a modest effect of these interventions on working and verbal memory, processing speed and executive functioning. These effects also manifest when examining meta-analysis including other major psychiatric conditions such as depression or schizo-affective disorders. Cognitive-enhancing programs can also be effective on high-risk or early-phase patients improving cognition and functional outcomes as seen in chronic patients. Possibly, it could be speculated that the early the intervention, the better and more durable would be the outcome as suggested by a recent study by our group [1]. However, cognitive-enhancing interventions alone do not seem to improve social cognition in most meta-analyses and systematic reviews. As such, current literature suggests the use of an integrative approach combining cognitive remediation and other interventions [54].

The beneficial effects associated with cognitive-enhancing programs are thought to arise from brain neuroplasticity as found by some studies [90]. For example, Wykes et al. evaluated the effects of cognitive remediation on the brain showing that improvements in cognition were associated with increased activations in the cortico-frontal regions, frequently associated with working memory. Recent randomized trials also confirmed these early findings showing that these interventions are associated with greater grey matter volumes and changes of the brain's activity in the prefrontal, thalamic and hippocampal regions [91, 92]. Finally, a recent review by our group suggested that cognitive remediation induces structural and functional brain changes even in the early phases of schizophrenia. These grey matter changes are localized in the hippocampus, parahippocampus, amygdala and thalamic regions [1]. As previously mentioned, recent studies suggest that cognitive interventions exert a beneficial effect on both white/grey matter structures and brain functioning leading to white and grey matter changes localized in prefrontal, parietal and limbic areas and to the normalization of several brain networks including the default and central executive networks [31, 32]. Overall, these results are not entirely surprising considering that the prefrontal network is considered a key region involved in working memory, reasoning and behaviour control and regulation that are disrupted by many psychiatric conditions ranging from psychosis to anxiety or post-traumatic stress disorder [18, 57]. The hippocampus is involved not only in memory processes but also in social cognition, and thalamic regions are frequently found disrupted in schizophrenia and psychotic disorders [93–95]. Parietal networks are involved in several cognitive and theory-of-mind processes, and limbic areas are frequently disrupted in affective psychiatric conditions [96, 97].

Having suggested the beneficial effects of cognitive remediation and enhancing programs on severe psychiatric conditions, future studies are warranted exploring the specific effects of combined interventions taking into consideration different strategies, clinical approaches and perspectives as current literature suggests that integrative approaches produce greater, more durable and generalizable improvements [54]. Furthermore, future longitudinal and controlled studies should precisely quantify and evaluate the impact of nonspecific factors (e.g. the therapist's role) which have been shown to affect and moderate the outcome of the intervention [27]. In fact, these have been poorly investigated but once understood may lead to the development of more effective interventions.

Acknowledgements This study was partially supported by grants from the Ministry of Health GR-2016-02361283 (CP).

References

1. Bellani M, Ricciardi C, Rossetti MG, Zovetti N, Perlini C, Brambilla P. Cognitive remediation in schizophrenia: the earlier the better? Epidemiol Psychiatr Sci. 2020;29:57.
2. Rossetti MG, Bonivento C, Garzitto M, Caletti E, Perlini C, Piccin S, Lazzaretti M, Marinelli V, Sala M, Abbiati V, Rossi R, Lanfredi M, Serretti A, Porcelli S, Bellani M, Brambilla P. The brief assessment of cognition in affective disorders: normative data for the Italian population. J Affect Disord. 2019;252:245–52.
3. Betz LT, Brambilla P, Ilankovic A, Premkumar P, Kim MS, Raffard S, Bayard S, Hori H, Lee KU, Lee SJ, Koutsouleris N, Kambeitz J. Deciphering reward-based decision-making in schizophrenia: a meta-analysis and behavioral modeling of the Iowa Gambling Task. Schizophr Res. 2019;204:7–15.

4. Bellani M, Bonivento C, Brambilla P. Interaction between cognition and emotion in developmental psychopathology: the role of linguistic stimuli. Epidemiol Psychiatr Sci. 2012;21(3):249–53.

5. Brambilla P, Macdonald AW, Sassi RB, Johnson MK, Mallinger AG, Carter CS, Soares JC. Context processing performance in bipolar disorder patients. Bipolar Disord. 2007;9(3):230–7.

6. Brambilla P, Perlini C, Bellani M, Tomelleri L, Ferro A, Cerruti S, Marinelli V, Rambaldelli G, Christodoulou T, Jogia J, Dima D, Tansella M, Balestrieri M, Frangou S. Increased salience of gains versus decreased associative learning differentiate bipolar disorder from schizophrenia during incentive decision making. Psychol Med. 2013;43(3):571–80.

7. Keefe RSE, Harvey PD. Cognitive impairment in schizophrenia. Novel antischizophrenia treatments. New York: Springer; 2012. p. 11–37.

8. Van Den Heuvel MP, Fornito A. Brain networks in schizophrenia. Neuropsychol Rev. 2014;24(1):32–48.

9. Zaytseva Y, Korsakova N, Agius M, Gurovich I. Neurocognitive functioning in schizophrenia and during the early phases of psychosis: targeting cognitive remediation interventions. Biomed Res Int. 2013;2013:819587.

10. Pigoni A, Lazzaretti M, Mandolini GM, Delvecchio G, Altamura AC, Soares JC, Brambilla P. The impact of COMT polymorphisms on cognition in bipolar disorder: a review: Special Section on "Translational and Neuroscience Studies in Affective Disorders" Section Editor, Maria Nobile MD, PhD. This Section of JAD focuses on the relevance of translational and neuroscience studies in providing a better understanding of the neural basis of affective disorders. The main aim is to briefly summaries relevant research findings in clinical neuroscience with particular regards to specific innovative topics in mood and anxiety disorders. J Affect Disord. 2019;243:545–51.

11. Mandolini GM, Lazzaretti M, Pigoni A, Delvecchio G, Soares JC, Brambilla P. The impact of BDNF Val66Met polymorphism on cognition in bipolar disorder: a review: Special Section on "Translational and neuroscience studies in affective disorders" Section Editor, Maria Nobile MD, PhD. This section of JAD focuses on the relevance of translational and neuroscience studies in providing a better understanding of the neural basis of affective disorders. The main aim is to briefly summaries relevant research findings in clinical neuroscience with particular regards to specific innovative topics in mood and anxiety disorders. J Affect Disord. 2019;243:552–8.

12. Mollon J, Reichenberg A. Cognitive development prior to onset of psychosis. Psychol Med. 2018;48(3):392.

13. Thornicroft G, Tansella M, Becker T, et al. The personal impact of schizophrenia in Europe. Schizophr Res. 2004;69(2-3):125–32.

14. World Health Organization. The world health report 2001: mental health: new understanding, new hope. Geneva: World Health Organization; 2001.

15. Viron MJ, Stern TA. The impact of serious mental illness on health and healthcare. Psychosomatics. 2010;51(6):458–65.

16. Wykes T, Huddy V, Cellard C, McGurk SR, Czobor P. A meta-analysis of cognitive remediation for schizophrenia: methodology and effect sizes. Am J Psychiatr. 2011;168(5):472–85.

17. Vita A, Barlati S, Bellani M, Brambilla P. Cognitive remediation in schizophrenia: background, techniques, evidence of efficacy and perspectives. Epidemiol Psychiatr Sci. 2014;23(1):21–5. https://doi.org/10.1017/S2045796013000541.

18. Bellani M, Brambilla P. Social cognition, schizophrenia and brain imaging. Epidemiol Psichiatr Soc. 2008;17(2):117–9.

19. Alptekin K, Akvardar Y, Akdede BBK, et al. Is quality of life associated with cognitive impairment in schizophrenia? Prog Neuro-Psychopharmacol Biol Psychiatry. 2005;29(2):239–44.

20. Woodward ND, Purdon SE, Meltzer HY, Zald DH. A meta-analysis of neuropsychological change to clozapine, olanzapine, quetiapine, and risperidone in schizophrenia. Int J Neuropsychopharmacol. 2005;8(3):457–72.

21. Mortimer AM, Ahmed Al-Agib AO. Quality of life in schizophrenia on conventional versus atypical antipsychotic medication: a comparative cross-sectional study. Int J Soc Psychiatry. 2007;53(2):99–107.
22. Green CS, Bavelier D, Kramer AF, et al. Improving methodological standards in behavioral interventions for cognitive enhancement. J Cogn Enhance. 2019;3(1):2–29.
23. Zhu X, Yin S, Lang M, He R, Li J. The more the better? A meta-analysis on effects of combined cognitive and physical intervention on cognition in healthy older adults. Ageing Res Rev. 2016;31:67–79.
24. Delahunty A, Morice R, Frost B. Specific cognitive flexibility rehabilitation in schizophrenia. Psychol Med. 1993;23(1):221–7.
25. Wykes T, Reeder C, Corner J, Williams C, Everitt B. The effects of neurocognitive remediation on executive processing in patients with schizophrenia. Schizophr Bull. 1999;25(2):291–307.
26. Vita A. La riabilitazione cognitiva della schizofrenia. New York: Springer; 2013.
27. Wykes T, Spaulding WD. Thinking about the future cognitive remediation therapy—what works and could we do better? Schizophr Bull. 2011;37(2):80–90.
28. Medalia A, Choi J. Cognitive remediation in schizophrenia. Neuropsychol Rev. 2009;19(3):353.
29. Cramer SC, Sur M, Dobkin BH, et al. Harnessing neuroplasticity for clinical applications. Brain. 2011;134(6):1591–609.
30. Leonardo ED, Hen R. Anxiety as a developmental disorder. Neuropsychopharmacology. 2008;33(1):134–40.
31. Penadés R, Pujol N, Catalán R, et al. Brain effects of cognitive remediation therapy in schizophrenia: a structural and functional neuroimaging study. Biol Psychiatry. 2013;73(10):1015–23.
32. Thorsen AL, Johansson K, Løberg E-M. Neurobiology of cognitive remediation therapy for schizophrenia: a systematic review. Front Psych. 2014;5:103.
33. Vinogradov S, Fisher M, Holland C, Shelly W, Wolkowitz O, Mellon SH. Is serum brain-derived neurotrophic factor a biomarker for cognitive enhancement in schizophrenia? Biol Psychiatry. 2009;66(6):549–53.
34. Sánchez P, Peña J, Bengoetxea E, et al. Improvements in negative symptoms and functional outcome after a new generation cognitive remediation program: a randomized controlled trial. Schizophr Bull. 2014;40(3):707–15.
35. Lindenmayer J-P, Khan A, McGurk SR, et al. Does social cognition training augment response to computer-assisted cognitive remediation for schizophrenia? Schizophr Res. 2018;201:180–6.
36. Penn DL, Sanna LJ, Roberts DL. Social cognition in schizophrenia: an overview. Schizophr Bull. 2008;34(3):408–11.
37. Bowie CR, McGurk SR, Mausbach B, Patterson TL, Harvey PD. Combined cognitive remediation and functional skills training for schizophrenia: effects on cognition, functional competence, and real-world behavior. Am J Psychiatr. 2012;169(7):710–8.
38. Peña J, Ibarretxe-Bilbao N, Sánchez P, et al. Combining social cognitive treatment, cognitive remediation, and functional skills training in schizophrenia: a randomized controlled trial. NPJ Schizophr. 2016;2(1):1–7.
39. Velligan DI, Kern RS, Gold JM. Cognitive rehabilitation for schizophrenia and the putative role of motivation and expectancies. Schizophr Bull. 2006;32(3):474–85.
40. Deci EL, Ryan RM. Self-determination theory: a macrotheory of human motivation, development, and health. Can Psychol. 2008;49(3):182.
41. Choi J, Medalia A. Factors associated with a positive response to cognitive remediation in a community psychiatric sample. Psychiatr Serv. 2005;56(5):602–4.
42. Medalia A, Richardson R. What predicts a good response to cognitive remediation interventions? Schizophr Bull. 2005;31(4):942–53.
43. Anaya C, Aran AM, Ayuso-Mateos JL, Wykes T, Vieta E, Scott J. A systematic review of cognitive remediation for schizo-affective and affective disorders. J Affect Disord. 2012;142(1-3):13–21.
44. Motter JN, Pimontel MA, Rindskopf D, Devanand DP, Doraiswamy PM, Sneed JR. Computerized cognitive training and functional recovery in major depressive disorder: a meta-analysis. J Affect Disord. 2016;189:184–91.

45. Cella M, Preti A, Edwards C, Dow T, Wykes T. Cognitive remediation for negative symptoms of schizophrenia: a network meta-analysis. Clin Psychol Rev. 2017;52:43–51.
46. Prikken M, Konings MJ, Lei WU, Begemann MJH, Sommer IEC. The efficacy of computerized cognitive drill and practice training for patients with a schizophrenia-spectrum disorder: a meta-analysis. Schizophr Res. 2019;204:368–74.
47. Del Fabro L, Delvecchio G, D'Agostino A, Brambilla P. Effects of olanzapine during cognitive and emotional processing in schizophrenia: a review of functional magnetic resonance imaging findings. Hum Psychopharmacol. 2019;34(3):e2693.
48. Ciappolino V, Mazzocchi A, Botturi A, Turolo S, Delvecchio G, Agostoni C, Brambilla P. The role of docosahexaenoic acid (DHA) on cognitive functions in psychiatric disorders. Nutrients. 2019;11(4):769.
49. D'Abate L, Delvecchio G, Ciappolino V, Ferro A, Brambilla P. Borderline personality disorder, metacognition and psychotherapy. J Affect Disord. 2020;276:1095–101.
50. Ciappolino V, DelVecchio G, Prunas C, Andreella A, Finos L, Caletti E, Siri F, Mazzocchi A, Botturi A, Turolo S, Agostoni C, Brambilla P. The effect of DHA supplementation on cognition in patients with bipolar disorder: an exploratory randomized control trial. Nutrients. 2020;12(3):708.
51. Crisanti C, Enrico P, Fiorentini A, Delvecchio G, Brambilla P. Neurocognitive impact of ketamine treatment in major depressive disorder: a review on human and animal studies. J Affect Disord. 2020;276:1109–18.
52. Hagan KE, Christensen KA, Forbush KT. A preliminary systematic review and meta-analysis of randomized-controlled trials of cognitive remediation therapy for anorexia nervosa. Eat Behav. 2020;2020:101391.
53. Sciortino D, Pigoni A, Delvecchio G, Maggioni E, Schiena G, Brambilla P. Role of rTMS in the treatment of cognitive impairments in bipolar disorder and schizophrenia: a review of randomized controlled trials. J Affect Disord. 2021;280(Pt A):148–55.
54. Hogarty GE, Flesher S, Ulrich R, et al. Cognitive enhancement therapy for schizophrenia: effects of a 2-year randomized trial on cognition and behavior. Arch Gen Psychiatry. 2004;61(9):866–76.
55. Biagianti B, Castellaro GA, Brambilla P. Predictors of response to cognitive remediation in patients with major psychotic disorders: a narrative review. J Affect Disord. 2021;281:264–70.
56. Sala M, Caverzasi E, Marraffini E, De Vidovich G, Lazzaretti M, d'Allio G, Isola M, Balestrieri M, D'Angelo E, Thyrion FZ, Scagnelli P, Barale F, Brambilla P. Cognitive memory control in borderline personality disorder patients. Psychol Med. 2009;39(5):845–53.
57. Dossi G, Delvecchio G, Prunas C, Soares JC, Brambilla P. Neural bases of cognitive impairments in post-traumatic stress disorders: a mini-review of functional magnetic resonance imaging findings. Front Psych. 2020;11:176.
58. Biagianti B, Conelea C, Brambilla P, Bernstein G. A systematic review of treatments targeting cognitive biases in socially anxious adolescents. J Affect Disord. 2020;264:543–51.
59. Bellani M, Biagianti B, Zovetti N, Rossetti MG, Bressi C, Perlini C, Brambilla P. The effects of cognitive remediation on cognitive abilities and real-world functioning among people with bipolar disorder: a systematic review. J Affect Disord. 2019;257:691–7.
60. Biagianti B, Merchant J, Brambilla P, Lewandowski KE. The effects of cognitive remediation in patients with affective psychosis: a systematic review. J Affect Disord. 2019;255:0165.
61. Madre M, Canales-Rodríguez EJ, Ortiz-Gil J, Murru A, Torrent C, Bramon E, Perez V, Orth M, Brambilla P, Vieta E, Amann BL. Neuropsychological and neuroimaging underpinnings of schizoaffective disorder: a systematic review. Acta Psychiatr Scand. 2016;134(1):16–30.
62. Vidarsdottir OG, Roberts DL, Twamley EW, Gudmundsdottir B, Sigurdsson E, Magnusdottir BB. Integrative cognitive remediation for early psychosis: results from a randomized controlled trial. Psychiatry Res. 2019;273:690–8.
63. Eack SM, Hogarty GE, Cho RY, et al. Neuroprotective effects of cognitive enhancement therapy against gray matter loss in early schizophrenia: results from a 2-year randomized controlled trial. Arch Gen Psychiatry. 2010;67(7):674–82.

64. Revell ER, Neill JC, Harte M, Khan Z, Drake RJ. A systematic review and meta-analysis of cognitive remediation in early schizophrenia. Schizophr Res. 2015;168(1-2):213–22.
65. Mendella PD, Burton CZ, Tasca GA, Roy P, Louis LS, Twamley EW. Compensatory cognitive training for people with first-episode schizophrenia: results from a pilot randomized controlled trial. Schizophr Res. 2015;162(1-3):108–11.
66. Eack SM, Newhill CE, Keshavan MS. Cognitive enhancement therapy improves resting-state functional connectivity in early course schizophrenia. J Soc Soc Work Res. 2016;7(2):211–30.
67. Keshavan MS, Eack SM, Prasad KM, Haller CS, Cho RY. Longitudinal functional brain imaging study in early course schizophrenia before and after cognitive enhancement therapy. NeuroImage. 2017;151:55–64.
68. Breitborde NJK, Woolverton C, Dawson SC, et al. Meta-cognitive skills training enhances computerized cognitive remediation outcomes among individuals with first-episode psychosis. Early Interv Psychiatry. 2017;11(3):244–9.
69. Ramsay IS, Fryer S, Boos A, et al. Response to targeted cognitive training correlates with change in thalamic volume in a randomized trial for early schizophrenia. Neuropsychopharmacology. 2018;43(3):590–7.
70. Deste G, Barlati S, Galluzzo A, et al. Effectiveness of cognitive remediation in early versus chronic schizophrenia: a preliminary report. Front Psych. 2019;10:236.
71. García-Fernández L, Cabot-Ivorra N, Rodríguez-García V, et al. Computerized cognitive remediation therapy, REHACOM, in first episode of schizophrenia: a randomized controlled trial. Psychiatry Res. 2019;281:112563.
72. Ventura J, Subotnik KL, Gretchen-Doorly D, et al. Cognitive remediation can improve negative symptoms and social functioning in first-episode schizophrenia: a randomized controlled trial. Schizophr Res. 2019;203:24–31.
73. Perlini C, Bellani M, Rossetti MG, Rossin G, Zovetti N, Rossi A, Bressi C, Piccolo LD, Brambilla P. Mindfulness-based interventions in the early phase of affective and non-affective psychoses. J Affect Disord. 2020;263:747–53.
74. Nuechterlein KH, Ventura J, Subotnik KL, et al. A randomized controlled trial of cognitive remediation and long-acting injectable risperidone after a first episode of schizophrenia: improving cognition and work/school functioning. Psychol Med. 2020;2020:1–10.
75. Haas SS, Antonucci LA, Wenzel J, Ruef A, Biagianti B, Paolini M, Rauchmann BS, Weiske J, Kambeitz J, Borgwardt S, Brambilla P, Meisenzahl E, Salokangas RKR, Upthegrove R, Wood SJ, Koutsouleris N, Kambeitz-Ilankovic L. A multivariate neuromonitoring approach to neuroplasticity-based computerized cognitive training in recent onset psychosis. Neuropsychopharmacology. 2021;46(4):828–35.
76. Corbera S, Wexler BE, Poltorak A, Thime WR, Kurtz MM. Cognitive remediation for adults with schizophrenia: does age matter? Psychiatry Res. 2017;247:21–7.
77. Fusar-Poli P, Deste G, Smieskova R, et al. Cognitive functioning in prodromal psychosis: a meta-analysis. Arch Gen Psychiatry. 2012;69(6):562–71.
78. Fusar-Poli P, Bonoldi I, Yung AR, et al. Predicting psychosis: meta-analysis of transition outcomes in individuals at high clinical risk. Arch Gen Psychiatry. 2012;69(3):220–9.
79. Bolt LK, Amminger GP, Farhall J, et al. Neurocognition as a predictor of transition to psychotic disorder and functional outcomes in ultra-high risk participants: findings from the NEURAPRO randomized clinical trial. Schizophr Res. 2019;206:67–74.
80. Glenthøj LB, Mariegaard LS, Fagerlund B, et al. Cognitive remediation plus standard treatment versus standard treatment alone for individuals at ultra-high risk of developing psychosis: results of the FOCUS randomised clinical trial. Schizophr Res. 2020;224:151–8.
81. Rauchensteiner S, Kawohl W, Ozgurdal S, et al. Test-performance after cognitive training in persons at risk mental state of schizophrenia and patients with schizophrenia. Psychiatry Res. 2011;185(3):334–9.
82. Hooker CI, Carol EE, Eisenstein TJ, et al. A pilot study of cognitive training in clinical high risk for psychosis: initial evidence of cognitive benefit. Schizophr Res. 2014;157:314.

83. Loewy R, Fisher M, Schlosser DA, et al. Intensive auditory cognitive training improves verbal memory in adolescents and young adults at clinical high risk for psychosis. Schizophr Bull. 2016;42(1):118–26.
84. Urben S, Pihet S, Jaugey L, Halfon O, Holzer L. Computer-assisted cognitive remediation in adolescents with psychosis or at risk for psychosis: a 6-month follow-up. Acta Neuropsy. 2012;24(6):328–35.
85. Piskulic D, Barbato M, Liu L, Addington J. Pilot study of cognitive remediation therapy on cognition in young people at clinical high risk of psychosis. Psychiatry Res. 2015;225(1-2):93–8.
86. Choi J, Corcoran CM, Fiszdon JM, et al. Pupillometer-based neurofeedback cognitive training to improve processing speed and social functioning in individuals at clinical high risk for psychosis. Psychiatr Rehabil J. 2017;40(1):33.
87. Bechdolf A, Wagner M, Ruhrmann S, et al. Preventing progression to first-episode psychosis in early initial prodromal states. Br J Psychiatry. 2012;200(1):22–9.
88. Glenthøj LB, Hjorthøj C, Kristensen TD, Davidson CA, Nordentoft M. The effect of cognitive remediation in individuals at ultra-high risk for psychosis: a systematic review. NPJ Schizophr. 2017;3(1):1–8.
89. Devoe DJ, Farris MS, Townes P, Addington J. Interventions and social functioning in youth at risk of psychosis: a systematic review and meta-analysis. Early Interv Psychiatry. 2019;13(2):169–80.
90. Wykes TIL, Brammer M, Mellers J, et al. Effects on the brain of a psychological treatment: cognitive remediation therapy: functional magnetic resonance imaging in schizophrenia. Br J Psychiatry. 2002;181(2):144–52.
91. Penadés R, González-Rodríguez A, Catalán R, Segura B, Bernardo M, Junqué C. Neuroimaging studies of cognitive remediation in schizophrenia: a systematic and critical review. World J Psychiatry. 2017;7(1):34.
92. Morimoto T, Matsuda Y, Matsuoka K, et al. Computer-assisted cognitive remediation therapy increases hippocampal volume in patients with schizophrenia: a randomized controlled trial. BMC Psychiatry. 2018;18(1):83.
93. Cronenwett WJ, Csernansky J. Thalamic pathology in schizophrenia. Behavioral neurobiology of schizophrenia and its treatment. New York: Springer; 2010. p. 509–28.
94. Fuster J. The prefrontal cortex. New York: Academic; 2015.
95. Montagrin A, Saiote C, Schiller D. The social hippocampus. Hippocampus. 2018;28(9):672–9.
96. Bogerts B, Ashtari M, Degreef G, Alvir JMJ, Bilder RM, Lieberman JA. Reduced temporal limbic structure volumes on magnetic resonance images in first episode schizophrenia. Psychiatry Res Neuroimaging. 1990;35(1):1–13.
97. Yildiz M, Borgwardt SJ, Berger GE. Parietal lobes in schizophrenia: do they matter? Schizophr Res Treat. 2011;2011:581686.

Targeting Metabolic Abnormalities in Mental Health Prevention Strategies

Simone Schimmenti, Francesca Maria Camilla Maselli, and Sarah Tosato

People affected by severe mental disorders (SMI) as schizophrenia (SCZ), bipolar disorder (BD), and major depressive disorder (MDD) experience a two to three times higher mortality rate and have a life expectancy shortened of 10–20 years rate compared to the general population [1–3]. The excess mortality observed in SMI is due to physical comorbidities, predominantly cardiovascular diseases (CVD) and type 2 diabetes (T2D) [4, 5]. Specifically, CVD rate is of 11.8%, 8.4%, and 11.7% in SCZ, BD, and MDD, respectively, with only SCZ found significantly associated with the risk of developing coronary heart disease (OR 1.52), cerebrovascular disease (OR 2.05), and congestive heart failure (OR 1.60) [5]. In MDD, a higher risk of stroke (HR 2.04), congestive heart failure (HR 2.02), and coronary heart disease (HR 1.63) has been found compared to the general population [4, 5].

The scandal of "the avoidable mortality" in SMI [6] has made necessary the identification of those patients at high risk of developing physical comorbidities, and it is a clinical imperative [7]. In order to help clinicians to identify these patients, the concept of metabolic syndrome (MetS) may be useful [8]. MetS is a cluster of risk factors consisting of at least three of the following: central obesity, high blood pressure, low high-density lipoprotein cholesterol (HDL-C), elevated triglycerides, and hyperglycemia [9]. These factors significantly increase the risk of CVD, T2D, and all-cause mortality [10].

Simone Schimmenti and Francesca Maria Camilla Maselli contributed equally.

S. Schimmenti · F. M. C. Maselli · S. Tosato (✉)
Department of Neuroscience, Biomedicine and Movement Sciences, Section of Psychiatry, University of Verona, Verona, Italy
e-mail: simone.schimmenti@univr.it; francescamariacamilla.maselli@univr.it; sarah.tosato@univr.it

M. Colizzi, M. Ruggeri (eds.), *Prevention in Mental Health*, https://doi.org/10.1007/978-3-030-97906-5_13

13.1   Metabolic Abnormalities in Psychosis (SCZ and BD)

MetS is highly prevalent in patients with chronic SCZ and BD compared to the general population, with pooled prevalence of 31.7% and 33.4%, respectively [11]. They have almost double probability to develop MetS compared to controls, with body max index (BMI) and age being predictors of MetS [12]. Traditionally, the association between cardio-metabolic abnormalities and psychosis has been attributed to the secondary effects of antipsychotics (APs) [11] or to unhealthy diet or sedentary lifestyle associated with negative symptoms [13]. Interestingly, in the first episode of psychosis (FEP), the overall prevalence rate of MetS and diabetes is 9.8% and 2.1% in drug-naïve patients and 9.9% and 1.3% in medicated ones [14]. Thus, MetS has the same prevalence in FEP patients than in the general population [8].

Waist size, blood pressure, and smoking have been found to be significantly lower in drug-naïve FEP patients compared with those under medication [8], while no differences were found in prevalence of hypertriglyceridemia and HDL-C levels [15]; smoking appears to be elevated early after diagnosis [8, 16]. Indeed, all metabolic components and risk factors are significantly lower in both drug-naïve and medicated FEP patients when compared to those affected by chronic SCZ [8].

A recent meta-review highlights impaired glucose metabolism in drug-naïve FEP patients at the onset compared to controls [17]. Specifically, drug-naïve non-affective FEP patients have higher fasting insulin and insulin resistance levels, while 2-h oral glucose tolerance test (OGTT) results were found to be higher in both affective and non-affective psychosis, compared to controls [18]. Moreover, higher levels of insulin and lower levels of leptin have been found in drug-naïve FEP patients compared to controls and suggest that environmental factors (e.g., unhealthy lifestyle and diet) could explain this association [19].

Total (TC) and LDL cholesterol levels (C-LDL) seem decreased in FEP patients compared to controls, indicating that the hypercholesterolemia found in chronic patients is secondary to unhealthy lifestyle, environmental and genetic factors, and antipsychotics treatment, representing a modifiable risk factor [20]. In contrast, triglycerides are elevated in FEP probably reflecting early glucose dysregulation [20] and insulin resistance [18]. Hypertriglyceridemia is a feature of T2D, conferring about a twofold excess risk for coronary heart disease, stroke, and deaths attributed to other vascular causes [21].

The pooled T2D prevalence is 2.9%, 4.0%, 13.1%, and 9.2% among people with antipsychotic-naïve FEP, FEP, chronic SCZ, and BD, respectively; it is higher in North America (12.5%) than in Europe (7.7%) and in women than in men (RR = 1.43) [22]. The relative risk (RR) of T2D is 2.04 and 1.89 in SCZ and BD, compared to controls [22].

Moreover, obesity and insulin resistance have been associated with non-alcoholic fatty liver disease (NAFLD) that can evolve into non-alcoholic steatohepatitis (NASH), which may lead to liver cirrhosis or hepatocellular carcinoma [23]. Although NAFLD is considered a component of MetS, it has been shown that its presence may itself constitute an independent cardiovascular risk factor [24].

Because of the relationship between cardio-metabolic risk and NAFLD, early detection of NAFLD in clinical practice could be useful in prevention [25].

Finally, young people at ultra-high risk for psychosis (UHR) have increased rates of cardio-metabolic risk factors when compared with controls: they have lower levels of physical activity and higher rates of smoking (33%, pooled OR 2.3) and alcohol abuse, while no differences are found for BMI or blood pressure [26]. Thus, UHR people display cardio-metabolic risk factors which are largely modifiable and, therefore, a possible target for early intervention [26].

Other relevant metabolic abnormalities in FEP are hyperprolactinemia (HPRL) and an increased risk for osteoporosis [27].

HPRL can occur in about one-third of antipsychotic-naïve FEP patients [28] and in nearly three-fourths of the patients treated with first-generation antipsychotics (FGAs) [29].

Finally, over half of people with SCZ have a low bone mineral density (BMD) equating to an almost threefold increased risk compared to the general population [30]. An increased prevalence of osteoporosis was found in patients with SCZ aged 50 or older compared to healthy age-matched controls, and women have twofold higher evidence of osteopenia or osteoporosis compared with men [31]. People with SCZ have also a longer recovery time in case of hip fracture, compared with controls, and they are at a greater risk of adverse events such as postoperative infection and renal failure [32]. Risk factors related to patients' lifestyle (e.g., smoking, sedentariness, alcohol abuse, vitamin D deficiency, diabetes) as well as use of antipsychotics are likely to be involved [33].

Taken together, these data show that cardio-metabolic alterations are present at the onset of psychosis, are probably related to the disease, interact with each other, and worsen with antipsychotics, especially if they are administered for a long time [34]. Indeed, people with psychosis are more likely than the general population to have unhealthy lifestyle behaviors, such as being sedentary [35], smoking [16], and having diets rich in saturated fats while low in fruit and vegetables [36]. These unhealthy lifestyle behaviors could contribute to the worsening of cardio-metabolic alterations.

13.1.1 Pathophysiology

In recent years, the hypothesis that psychosis involves multiple systems at onset has emerged [37] (Fig. 13.1). In fact, dysfunctions in cardio-metabolic [20], immune [38], and hypothalamic-pituitary-adrenal (HPA) systems have been observed at the onset [39]. A recent meta-review confirmed these data, also reporting brain structure and neurophysiology aberrations [37]. Immune abnormalities are those most supported ones both in antipsychotic-naive and FEP patients [37].

Blood **cortisol** level is significantly increased in FEP individuals compared to controls [40]. Increased levels of pro-inflammatory cytokines have been demonstrated in drug-naïve FEP [38] and could cause insulin-like growth factor-1 (IGF-1) resistance and high concentrations of IGF-1, insulin, and C-peptide independently

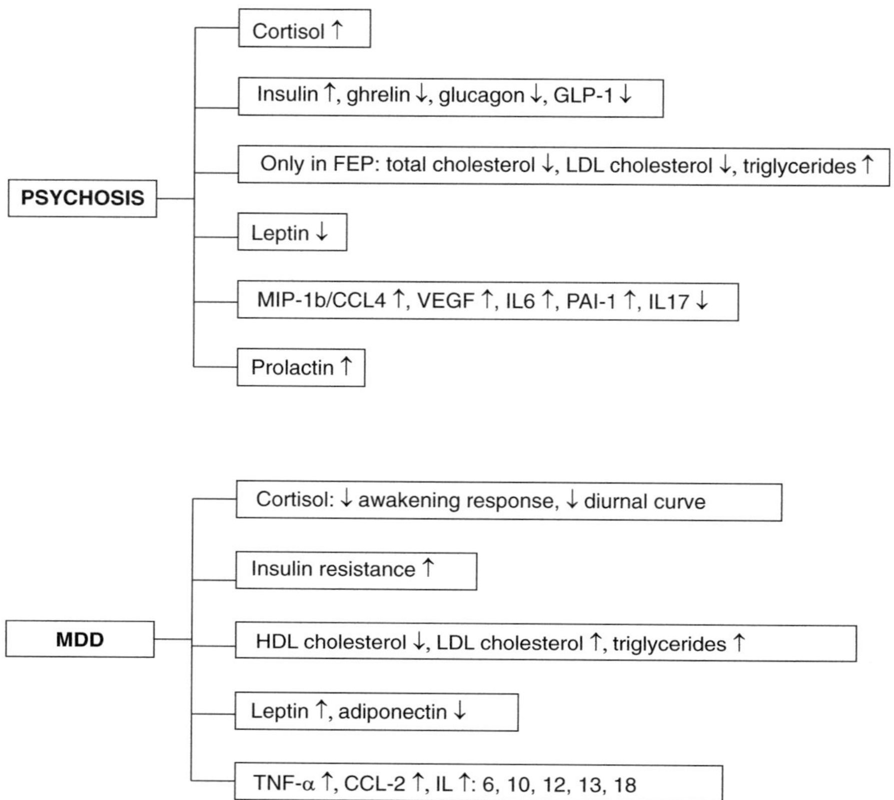

Fig. 13.1 Serum abnormalities in psychosis and major depressive disorders. ↑ increased/increases, ↓ decreased/decreases, *GLP-1* glucagon-like peptide 1, *LDL* low-density lipoprotein, *FEP* first episode of psychosis, *MPI-1b/CCL4* MPI-1b chemokine (C-C motif) ligand 4, *VEGF* vascular endothelial growth factor, *IL* interleukin, *PAI-1* plasminogen activator inhibitor-1, *MDD* major depressive disorder, *HDL* high-density lipoprotein, *TNF-α* tumor necrosis factor-α, *CCL-2* chemokine (C-C motif) ligand 2

of the glucose metabolism and cortisol serum levels. These findings may suggest the presence of insulin resistance in psychosis [41]. These data are in line with analysis of downstream serine-threonine kinases of GSK3β (AKT, mTOR, p70S6K) which revealed lower phosphorylation protein ratios in drug-naive FEP patients, supporting the hypothesis of neuronal insulin resistance which could partially reflect a reduced downstream signal transduction of GABA-R or NMDA-R, D2-R hyperactivity, lower BDNF level, or low-grade inflammation [42].

Other line of evidence suggests specific immune and metabolic signature in FEP: there are reports of an increase of MIP-1b/CCL4, VEGF, IL-6, and PAI-1 in patients compared to controls, while IL-17, ghrelin, glucagon, and GLP-1 have been found decreased [43]. Among these parameters, MIP-1b/CCL4 serum level appears to be the marker that best characterizes FEP. Since MIP-1b/CCL4 is a chemokine linked to neuro-inflammatory processes, it may contribute to the pathogenesis of psychosis [44]. A potential correlation of FEP polygenic risk score [45] with the CCL4 and ghrelin serum concentration was observed, supporting the idea that a genetic liability to inflammatory and metabolic alterations characterizes psychosis onset [46].

Regarding the environmental risk factors of psychosis, it has been demonstrated that FEP patients with a history of childhood trauma (CT) show higher C-peptide and insulin serum concentrations than those without CT, pointing out that hyperinsulinemia could be also the result of environmental exposure [47]. Specifically, patients who had experienced childhood sexual abuse had a higher BMI and C-reactive protein (CRP) compared not only to controls but also to the those without childhood sexual abuse [48]. It is plausible that CT could lead to the development of glucose metabolism dysfunction through HPA axis and the increment of CRP [49], facilitating the progression to TD2 and MetS [50].

Finally, a very important issue to take into account is the regular cannabis use present in one-third of FEP patients [51] that might be crucial in FEP-related metabolic abnormalities. Patients treated with antipsychotics who do not use cannabis show higher serum levels of glucose and triglycerides, lower C-HDL level, and an elevated waist circumference, while cannabis users show no significant changes in metabolic parameters after 1 year of medications [52]. It may be that chronic cannabis use directly suppresses appetite [53], although dietary neglect [54], polysubstance use and smoking [55], and the composition of cannabis [56] could also contribute to these findings. Finally, cannabis consumption may likewise produce a protective effect against liver steatosis in FEP treated patients, probably through the modulation of antipsychotic-induced weight gain [57].

13.1.2 Antipsychotic Treatment

APs play a remarkable role in metabolic abnormalities in FEP, chronic SCZ, and BD [58]. It has been found that after 3 years of APs, 25.1% of FEP individuals show an increase of more than 7% of BMI, increased triglyceride and decreased HDL-C levels, hypertension, increased waist circumference, hyperinsulinemia, and a higher prevalence of MetS [59].

There are marked differences between APs in terms of effects on metabolic parameters (weight, BMI, total cholesterol, C-LDL, triglycerides, and glucose serum levels) in a median treatment duration of 6 weeks: olanzapine and clozapine exhibit the worst profiles, while aripiprazole, brexpiprazole, cariprazine, lurasidone, and ziprasidone show the most benign profiles [60]. Specifically, a weight gain ≥7% compared to baseline was significantly more likely with olanzapine (RR = 3.31) and risperidone (RR = 1.61) than haloperidol and with second-generation antipsychotics (SGAs) than FGAs (RR = 1.45) after 6 months [61]. Interestingly, SGA-FGA effect size differences for weight and lipid outcomes declined with longer follow-up (≥6 months), suggesting that non-medication effects, such as unhealthy lifestyle, the underlying illness, environment, and genetic factors, play a role [62]. Increased baseline weight, male sex, and non-white ethnicity are predictors of susceptibility to AP-induced metabolic change [60].

Antipsychotic-naïve or FEP patients are more vulnerable to weight gain when they start treatment [63]. Generally, weight gain is rapid; then, it slows gradually and often reaches a plateau within 1 year [64]: the first year of AP treatment is a critical period for weight gain and metabolic abnormalities [65], as initial rapid weight gain is a good indicator for long-term obesity [64].

The weight gain risk increases about two times in FEP patients treated with APs compared with placebo, and it is associated with duration of treatment [66]. Except perhaps for ziprasidone, most APs are associated with weight gain and BMI increase. More specifically, over the course of 1 year, increase in BMI ≥ 1 unit occurs with a higher frequency in olanzapine-treated FEP patients compared to those treated with quetiapine or risperidone [67]. An early indicator of an increased risk of weight gain at 1 year during olanzapine therapy may be $\geq 7\%$ weight gain during the first 6 weeks of treatment [68]. There are marked individual variations in weight gain, independently of prescribed AP [69], and this suggests that genetic factors play a role [70]. Specifically, it has been found an association between antipsychotic-induced weight gain [71] and single-nucleotide polymorphisms (SNPs) in HTR2C, the most studied serotonin receptor gene, in FEP patients [61, 72], but not in chronic ones [73].

The mean time to the development of MetS is nearly 12 weeks, and after 1 year of treatment, MetS rate is three times higher compared to baseline and occurs more frequently with olanzapine [67].

The prevalence of diabetes increases rapidly after starting AP [74], and higher AP doses are associated with a higher risk of TD2 [75]. The risk to develop TD2 is higher in FEP patients treated with olanzapine (HR 1.41) and with FGAs (HR 1.60) compared with drug-naïve ones; during longer-term treatment, TD2 risk appears associated with FGAs (OR 1.45), olanzapine (OR 1.57), and clozapine (OR 2.31) [76]. The cumulative risk for TD2 appears to be higher in adolescents and young adults using AP for many different psychiatric disorders when compared with healthy controls (OR 2.58) and with controls affected by psychiatric disorders not treated with AP (OR 2.09) [77]. In addition, TD2 risk is higher in male sex [77].

Finally, olanzapine treatment is associated with higher insulin resistance levels than aripiprazole, ziprasidone, or risperidone [76]. For these reasons, olanzapine should be avoided in FEP [78].

A recent meta-review has investigated metabolic abnormalities in children and adolescents affected by psychiatric disorders treated with APs, finding that lurasidone has the safest profile and olanzapine the worst [79].

Regarding HPRL, it has been established that SGAs cause a minor elevation of the PRL plasma levels than the FGAs [80]. The notable exceptions in this regard are amisulpride, risperidone, and paliperidone [81]. Amisulpride is one of the most pronounced "PRL-raising" AP [58], independently of dosage and duration of administration [82], followed by risperidone and its metabolite paliperidone [83]. On the contrary, aripiprazole, cariprazine, quetiapine, and brexpiprazole have the most favorable profile with respect to PRL elevation toward placebo [58], and aripiprazole at low dose in combination with risperidone or olanzapine significantly reduces the PRL levels induced by these APs [84] probably for its D2R partial agonism [85].

Identifying carriers of the relevant genetic risk factors leading to the greatest increases in PRL levels after AP treatment may help to guide AP choices in FEP patients to avoid adverse effects such as sexual dysfunction and osteoporosis, which are among the most burdensome for patients with psychotic disorders and can compromise the adherence to treatment [86]. To this regard, pharmacogenetic studies have been conducted in FEP patients, showing polymorphisms in NTRK2, DRD2, and ACE genes associated with PRL concentration [87].

Compared with SGAs, a higher fracture risk, in particular of the hip, was found for FGAs in some studies [88, 89], possibly due to extrapyramidal symptoms causing gait disturbances and impairing balance, which are risk factors for falls in older adults [90]. However, other studies found no differences between FGAs and SGAs [91]. No significant differences in BMD between FEP patients and controls before treatment have been found [92]. On the contrary, after 12 months of APs, the decrease in BMD correlated with longer duration of treatment with FGAs, rather than with PRL levels, suggesting that the duration of HPRL may have a greater impact than PRL levels themselves [92].

In conclusion, the choice of AP should be made on an individual basis, considering the clinical circumstances and preferences of patients [60], taking into account that weight gain and HPRL negatively affect adherence rates, especially in younger patients [93] (Fig. 13.2).

13.2 Metabolic Abnormalities in MDD

Patients suffering from MDD are subject to socioeconomic and lifestyle conditions that may influence the development of CVD and MetS [94]. These include poor receipt of physical health care [95], reduced compliance with medical recommendations [96], and adverse medication treatment effects [34], along with modifiable risk factors, such as smoking and physical inactivity [35]. Among medications, APs are the main contributors to increase of MetS risk in MDD compared to controls [7]. A higher BMI is significantly related with lower education, no tobacco use, and male sex [97]. An umbrella review of meta-analyses of cohort studies and randomized controlled trials found that the only risk factor with convincing evidence for obesity in adults is depression [98].

Compared with age- and gender-matched controls, nearly 30% of depressed patients are affected by MetS (RR 1.57), and they also have a heightened risk of hyperglycemia and hypertriglyceridemia [7, 11].

There is a bidirectional relationship between obesity and depression, where the direction depression leading to obesity is stronger than the reverse direction [99]. Adults who were depressed at baseline demonstrated a 37% increase in risk of obesity at follow-up compared with adults who did not experience depression [99]. Conversely, obese adults had an 18% increase in the risk of being depressed over a long-term follow-up [99].

The relationship between MDD and T2D appears also bidirectional [100]. T2D is more common in people with MDD than in age- and gender-matched controls

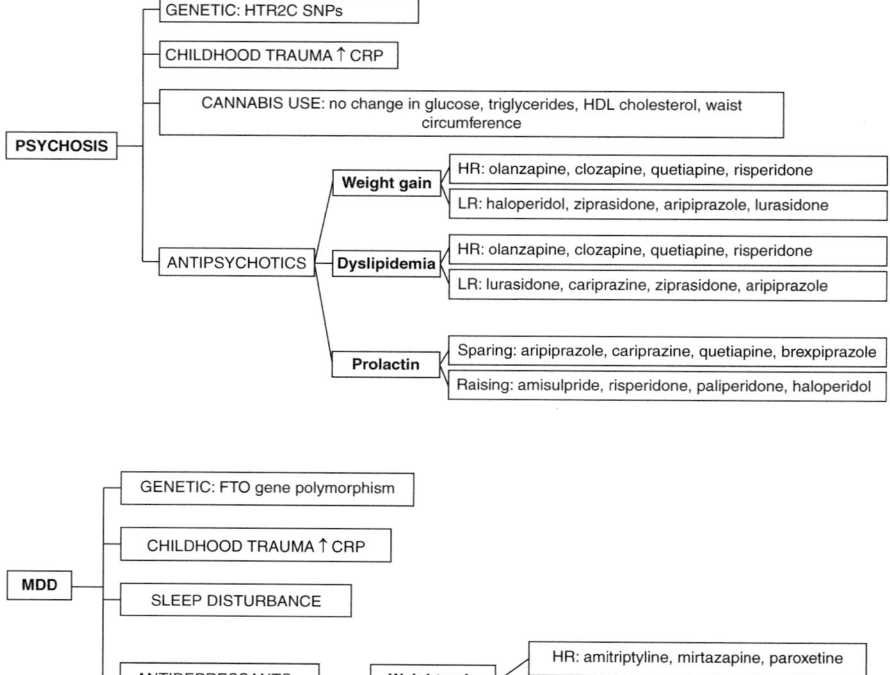

Fig. 13.2 Predictors of obesity in psychosis and major depressive disorder. *HTR2C* 5-hydroxytryptamine receptor 2C, *SNPs* single-nucleotide polymorphisms, ↑ increased/increases, *CRP* C-reactive protein, *HDL* high-density lipoprotein, *MDD* major depressive disorder, *HR* high risk, *LR* low risk, *FTO* FTO alpha-ketoglutarate-dependent dioxygenase

(RR 1.36), whereas there is modest evidence that diabetes is a risk factor for MDD [22, 101]. Treatment duration, antidepressant, and lithium use were significant mediators of T2D prevalence in this population [22].

MDD affects up to 20–25% of adults with T2D [100] and is associated with a nearly twofold risk of all-cause mortality [102]. When combined, depression and diabetes exert an additive effect on all-cause mortality compared with controls without diabetes or MDD (HR 4.59) [103]. Besides, MDD increases the risk of adverse glycemic control: thus, through earlier identification and treatment of long-standing depression, the risk for health complications may be reduced [104].

Depression is prospectively associated with a significant increase in the risk of fracture and bone loss [105]. Hypercortisolemia appears to have a role in decreased bone formation [106]. Higher levels of inflammatory cytokines, such as IL-1β, IL-2, and IL-6, are linked to decreased BMD [107]. Many poor health behaviors associated with MDD, such as smoking, alcohol use, and decreased physical activity, have been found to impact bone metabolism [108]. Specifically, depression has been associated with 39% increase in fracture risk (RR = 1.39) [105]. Due to the high prevalence of MDD and osteoporosis worldwide, the observed relationship has important implications for public health, especially with increased aging of the population worldwide; thus, prevention and treatment of depression might decrease the risk of osteoporotic fracture [105].

Several studies suggest that antidepressants, particularly SSRIs, are associated with decreased BMD and increased fracture risk (RR 1.72), especially in elderly [109]. The risk is higher during the early stages of treatment, reaching a peak within 1 month for tricyclics and 8 months for SSRIs [110].

In summary, these data support the Canadian Network for Mood And Anxiety Treatments (CANMAT) recommendations stating that individuals with MDD, and in particular those taking APs, must be considered a vulnerable group that should be screened proactively for MetS and CVD risk factors [111]. Therefore, psychiatrists and other mental professionals should help individuals with MDD to improve their lifestyle, through smoking cessation, dietary measures, and exercise; if lifestyle interventions do not succeed, preferential use of lower-risk medication should be considered [112].

13.2.1 Pathophysiology

People suffering from MDD have been shown to be at an increased risk for MetS and T2D [7]. Moreover, MetS comorbidity in mood disorders is associated with a more complex affective presentation, lower probability of recovery, more frequent episodes, and suicide attempts [113].

The biological association between MDD and T2D is hypothesized to be due to a dysregulated HPA axis, a shift in sympathetic nervous system tone toward enhanced sympathetic activity, and a proinflammatory state [114]. Depression is associated with a blunted cortisol awakening response and flattening of the diurnal cortisol curve, which is also associated with insulin resistance and T2D [115]. In particular, in melancholic depression hypercortisolemic condition was found, increasing food intake and obesity [116] according to other studies showing that a relatively hyperactive HPA axis leads to melancholy and that a hypoactive stress response leads to atypical depression [117].

Multiple interacting pathways contribute to the comorbidity between MDD and MetS, such as increased levels of pro-inflammatory cytokines and acute-phase proteins, increased lipid peroxidation and oxidized C-LDL, hypernitrosylation, lowered levels of antioxidants, increased atherogenic index of plasma, and reduced levels of C-HDL [118]. Thus, mood disorders are associated with increased atherogenicity, but not with insulin resistance [119].

Patients during acute depressive episodes have higher activity levels of antioxidant enzymes, such as superoxide dismutase and catalase, compared to controls [120]. Immune-oxidative (IO) and nitrosative stress (NS) pathways are activated in people with a sedentary lifestyle, possibly increasing the risk to develop MDD [121]. Oxidative processes, occurring in MetS and MDD, may modify C-LDL and phospholipids leading to a higher risk for atherosclerosis and myocardial infarction [122]. The formation of oxidized LDL and oxidized phospholipids may consequently activate the toll-like receptor 4 (TLR4) complex, a phenomenon described as the TLR radical cycle which may cause chronic inflammation and especially chronic IO and NS, which may further aggravate the immune pathophysiology of mood disorders and MetS [123].

Circulating levels of leptin and TNF-α are elevated both in obesity and MDD [124]. Raised levels of leptin can lead to its resistance, which is evident in MDD with atypical features [125]. By contrast, adiponectin levels, which have anti-inflammatory effect, may be reduced in obesity and MDD [126]. However, controversial findings are reported on this topic in literature: a recent meta-review found no differences in leptin levels in MDD toward healthy controls, apart from subgroup samples with BMI ≥ 25 or age ≥ 40, in which leptin was found increased [127]. In addition, depressed patients with BMI ≥ 25 had lower adiponectin levels compared to controls [127], playing a key role in obesity-related diseases, such as T2D.

Besides the well-known leptin and ghrelin, other biomarkers such as orexin and nesfatin-1 seem to be involved in neurovegetative changes, like sleep and appetite regulation [128]. Sleep disturbance appears a stronger mediator of the relationship between MDD and obesity, compared to stress eating [129]. It is thought that the presence of increased leptin concentrations, despite decreased food intake, could contribute to appetite loss, which is a symptom of typical MDD; on the contrary, in atypical depression higher leptin levels would lead to increased fat body mass [128].

Adiposity-driven inflammation, smoking, and unhealthy lifestyle may contribute to the immune activation in MDD and thus to its relationship with MetS [130]. Levels of IL-6, TNF-α, IL-10, CCL-2, IL-13, IL-18, and IL-12 are significantly elevated in individuals with MDD compared to controls [131].

Regarding genetics, it has been shown that depression enhances the effect of FTO polymorphism on BMI: on average, subjects with MDD carrying the risk allele have a 2.2% higher BMI for each risk allele compared with controls [132]. In addition, cardio-metabolic disease risk genes, associated with mood disorders, have been identified [133]. These risk genes are more than 20 potential pleiotropic genes, and they are implicated in significant pathways: corticotrophin-releasing hormone, AMPK, cAMP-mediated or G-protein coupled receptor, axonal guidance, serotonin or dopamine receptors, circadian rhythm, and leptin signaling [133].

Regarding environmental factors, childhood sexual abuse has been associated with MDD (OR 2.7) and obesity (OR 1.4) in adulthood [134], as previously suggested [135]. Depressed patients with a history of CT show significant elevation in inflammation markers (hsRCP) and are more likely to smoke than those only depressed [136]. Therefore, individuals with CT and MDD are at a greater risk of CVD compared with depressed-only ones [136].

13.2.2 Role of Antidepressants

Antidepressants (ADs) may also be associated with weight gain [137], due to their affinity to H1, M1, and 5-HT2C receptors [138].

AD use is greater in patients with comorbidity, particularly with diagnoses of stroke and diabetes, and co-prescriptions of APs, than in those without [139]. The rate ratio (RR) for weight increase according to AD use is 1.21, indicating that a risk of ≥5% weight gain is 21% higher during AD treatment than during other times [139]. Participants with >1 year of treatment showed an increased risk of weight gain that was maintained at 6 years: RRs were 1.46 at 2 years and 1.48 at 3 years, and then declined, and from year 7 onward, there was no evidence for an increased risk of weight gain [139]. Thus, initiation of AD shows a strong temporal association with weight gain, which is greatest during the second and third years of treatment. During the second year of treatment, the risk of ≥5% weight gain is 46.3%, higher than in the general population (190). In addition, in people who were initially of normal weight, the RR for transition to overweight or obesity was 1.29 [139].

Regarding ADs, amitriptyline, mirtazapine, and paroxetine have been found associated with the greatest risk of weight gain [140]. Interestingly, amitriptyline and mirtazapine were associated with weight gain over both acute (4–12 weeks) and maintenance periods (≥4 months), while paroxetine was associated with weight gain over the medium-long-term period [139]. In contrast, some weight loss occurs with fluoxetine and bupropion, although the effect of fluoxetine appears to be limited to the acute phase of treatment, differently from bupropion [139]. Other ADs have no transient or negligible effect on body weight in the short term; however, the effect of each AD may vary greatly depending on an individual's characteristics and generally became more evident in the long term [139].

Interestingly, lower education status, lower BMI at the onset of AD use, and family history of obesity are independent predictors of weight gain ≥7% compared to the baseline [141].

Noteworthy, an association between ADs and T2D (RR 1.27) has been found, although this finding is still inconclusive [142].

13.3 Treatment and Prevention

Since a range of psychiatric conditions (SCZ, BP, MDD, anxiety, and stress-related disorders) are associated with increased cardio-metabolic disease risk [22] and lower physical fitness [11], the improvement of physical health is both an ethical and clinical priority [6, 143]. The European Psychiatric Association (EPA) stated that maintaining a healthy body weight and shape by healthy eating and regular physical activity is a key component in order to prevent and reduce the risk of developing physical comorbidities, including CVD, and to improve the overall health and well-being of patients [112]. Thus, it is of supreme importance to set up and implement strategies which can prevent and address the problem of physical comorbidity in mental disorders, and it is also crucial to raise the awareness of health professionals regarding these insidious and life-threatening conditions [144]. Two types of interventions can be implemented, pharmacological and non-pharmacological ones, and they can be applied to prevent the onset of cardio-metabolic diseases or to reduce their effects in patients who have already manifested some alterations.

13.3.1 Non-pharmacological Interventions

In the general population, there is consistent evidence that physical activity (PA) and exercise can decrease the risk of developing cardio-metabolic diseases [145, 146] and reduce inflammatory parameters, such as CRP, IL-6, and IL-8 [147, 148], which are commonly raised in SMI. Moreover, there is evidence that PA is equally effective as frontline pharmacological interventions, such as statins and beta-blockers, in preventing CVD mortality [149]. Conversely, high levels of sedentary behavior (SB), which are common in SMI [107], are independently associated with an increased risk of CVD, T2D, and premature mortality [150]. Thus, as increasing PA is a cornerstone of cardio-metabolic prevention in the general population, there is considerable empirical evidence that the same intervention may result useful in several psychiatric disorders. To date, it has been found that the majority of the lifestyle and behavioral interventions produces an increase in PA in SMI [151]. Particularly, it has been recently highlighted that the use of aerobic exercise of moderate-vigorous intensity at a frequency of two to three times a week, ideally supervised by qualified professionals and achieving 150 min of moderate-to-vigorous physical activity (MVPA) per week, could consistently reduce CVD risk markers in people with MDD and SCZ [152]. Moreover, the same PA program is also recommended for reducing the risk of MDD (including postnatal depression) [153]. Similar results seem to be also achieved with a combination of aerobic and resistance training [152]. In order to improve the efficacy of aerobic exercise, higher-intensity training, such as high-intensity interval training (HIIT), has been used in SMI people with cardio-metabolic risk factors and obesity finding that HIIT could significantly improve metabolic parameters, in particular waist circumference, body mass, fasting glucose, HDL-C, and blood pressure [154]. Some studies have found that HIIT intervention has the potentiality to improve parameters of MetS (particularly BMI, body weight, waist circumference, and heart rate), although more research is needed to validate this preliminary data [155, 156].

The EPA guidelines on physical activity [157] state that evidence is sufficient to recommend PA as an effective first-line treatment option for moderate depression and as an adjunctive intervention for improving psychiatric symptoms, cognition, and cardiorespiratory fitness in SMI.

Although to date existing guidelines focus on PA in SCZ and MDD [158], only few interventions have been designed to address the problem of sedentary behavior, with ambiguities on their efficacy [151]. Current findings indicate that isolated exercise interventions are unlikely to induce weight loss in SMI, while adding behavioral interventions or nutritional therapy to exercise programs seems to be a promising approach to reduce body weight [155]. Particularly, the support of qualified professionals who develop motivation results holds great importance in promoting engagement and adherence to PA [159]. The nature of many mental diseases, in particular psychosis, may contribute to physical inactivity due to symptoms such as avolition, blunted affect, and social withdrawal, which could be overcome by implementing exercise routines with support, educational meetings, and motivational counseling [159, 160].

Several studies have evaluated different behavioral interventions (BI) aimed at raising awareness toward healthy behaviors, informing patients about unhealthy lifestyle risk (e.g., smoking) and promoting healthy habits through psychoeducational interventions [161–163]. It has been found that lifestyle counseling is the most effective intervention for body weight and BMI followed by exercise, psychoeducation, and CBT in SCZ [164]. Several psychoeducational approaches have been developed, as far as the format (individual versus group) and the professional characteristics of the staff performing the intervention (psychiatrists versus nurses versus psychologists) are concerned [161]. However, it is still unclear which setup leads to the best result [161]. Particularly, the individual format allows personal advice, to tailor the plan of intervention to the patient's needs and increase motivation to change [161, 165]; on the other hand, the group format gives the possibility to share opinions and reciprocal support and to have imitative behavior [161, 166]. Nevertheless, when the intervention is provided by a multidisciplinary team, its impact on patients' lifestyle behaviors is more effective compared to the ones led by nurses or psychologists alone [161]. Moreover, it has been suggested that medical personnel are important in setting a good example of a healthy lifestyle, which is fundamental for "modeling" the lifestyle of patients [160, 167].

Regarding nutritional therapy (NT), several studies have highlighted that caloric restrictions and healthy diet educational interventions developed by qualified professionals could prevent and reduce weight gain in SMI [160]. Moreover, NT has shown beneficial effects on anthropometric measurements and biochemical variables among patients, with a significant decrease in BMI, body fat percentage, and waist circumference and a slightly improvement in metabolic profiles of fasting blood glucose, triglyceride, and HDL and LDL-C [168]. These beneficial effects have been shown to be achieved even in patients using SGAs such as clozapine and olanzapine, which are known to cause the most significant amount of weight gain and metabolic abnormalities, suggesting that the adverse effects of these medication could be mitigated adopting an adequate NT [160, 169]. However, in SCZ dietary interventions showed a small glucose level reduction and no effect on insulin [164]. Finally, given the paucity of studies, the data do not allow to determine which type of diet (e.g., Mediterranean diet, ketogenic diet) is the more valid to improve cardio-metabolic risk [170].

In conclusion, it can be stated that comprehensive weight and health management programs, including PA, NT, and lifestyle psychoeducation, can be considered more effective than a single-mode approach in preventing and treating cardio-metabolic diseases in SMI [144, 155, 169, 171]. A critical issue is the optimal duration of the intervention. In literature, studies' extent ranges from 3 months to 1–2 years [161]. Although studies do not yet provide clear evidence concerning the optimum length of engagement in these programs [161, 171], experience in the general population suggests that lifestyle change needs to be permanent [172]. Thus, intervention programs should last at least 20 weeks and should provide follow-ups consisting of booster sessions for behavioral, NT, and PA control [171].

13.3.2 Pharmacological Interventions

Psychotropic medications, particularly APs, TCA, and several SSRIs, can cause side effects, including weight gain and metabolic derangements that are often difficult to manage [173]. In this regard, several guidelines have been developed and provide recommendations regarding the monitoring and management for cardio-metabolic risk factors in psychosis [174]. The guidelines recommend several measurements (e.g., weight, glucose, HbA1c, cholesterol/HDL ratio, blood pressure) before starting an antipsychotic and then at the intervals indicated. Tobacco smoking should be inquired, and its cessation should be delivered as part of an overall smoking cessation program [174].

To manage the risk of weight gain and cardio-metabolic disorders associated to APs, some studies have shown that switching antipsychotics to relatively metabolic-neutral agents could lead to an improvement in patients' cardio-metabolic parameters, even if this option is not always feasible (e.g., treatment-resistant patients receiving clozapine) [175]. When non-pharmacological strategies alone are insufficient and switching is not suitable, using concomitant medications to counteract these adversities may be a rational option, although the data concerning this topic are still limited [173]. There is evidence supporting the use of concomitant metformin to mitigate antipsychotic-induced weight gain and other metabolic adversities in SCZ [173, 176]. The use of adjunctive metformin has shown to have a positive effect on different parameters such as body weight, waist circumference, insulin resistance, and serum lipids [173, 176]. Similar but less significant results have also been found for topiramate, sibutramine, and reboxetine [173, 176]. Specifically, topiramate has been found effective in reduction of LDL-C and triglyceride levels, BMI, and weight in SCZ [164]. Pharmacological interventions have shown to be effective in patients affected by psychosis, and FEP patients may derive the most benefit [173]. In fact, FEP patients receiving metformin are less likely to experience clinically relevant weight gain in prevention trials and more likely to achieve clinically relevant weight loss in treatment trials [173, 176]. Specifically, FEP individuals in early treatment lost three times the weight compared with older, more chronic patients [176]. However, given the paucity of studies and the possible onset of side effects related to medications such as metformin, the current evidence is too limited to support the regular clinical use of adjunctive pharmacological treatments, and healthy lifestyle and nutritional interventions should be preferred in the prevention and early treatment of cardio-metabolic alterations [176]. Finally, due to the increased morbidity and mortality among people with SCZ experiencing a fracture, there is a need to develop preventative interventions like more frequent monitoring of serum PRL levels and DEXA scan use in patients with SCZ at high risk of fractures [30, 31]. Importantly, the relatively high prevalence of hypertension, diabetes, smoking, and dyslipidemia is in stark contrast to the lack of related treatment for medical comorbidities in the most patients [95, 177, 178] (Fig. 13.3).

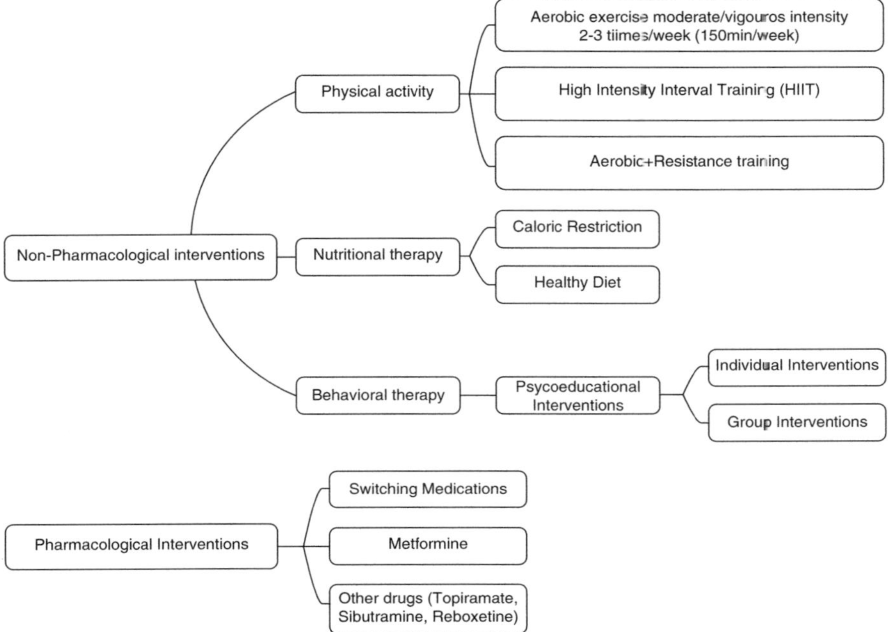

Fig. 13.3 Pharmacological and non-pharmacological interventions to prevent and reduce the risk of developing physical comorbidities in SMI

13.4 Conclusions

Evidence has demonstrated the efficacy of physical activity interventions on cardio-metabolic health and other outcomes as well as psychiatric symptoms in people with SMI [157, 179]. The guidelines have made available to clinicians the adequate tools to monitor metabolic parameters. Despite this and several editorials calling for action [180, 181], "lifestyle interventions" are still limitedly available in clinical routine care [182]. Thus, it is imperative to identify the barriers that make such interventions unavailable in clinical practice, educate professionals to implement them, and monitor their effects.

References

1. Laursen TM. Life expectancy among persons with schizophrenia or bipolar affective disorder. Schizophr Res. 2011;131(1–3):101–4.
2. Reininghaus U, Dutta R, Dazzan P, Doody GA, Fearon P, Lappin J, et al. Mortality in schizophrenia and other psychoses: a 10-year follow-up of the SOP first-episode cohort. Schizophr Bull. 2015;41(3):664–73.

3. Lawrence D, Hancock KJ, Kisely S. The gap in life expectancy from preventable physical illness in psychiatric patients in Western Australia: retrospective analysis of population based registers. BMJ. 2013;346:f2539.

4. Hoang U, Goldacre MJ, Stewart R. Avoidable mortality in people with schizophrenia or bipolar disorder in England. Acta Psychiatr Scand. 2013;127(3):195–201.

5. Correll CU, Solmi M, Veronese N, Bortolato B, Rosson S, Santonastaso P, et al. Prevalence, incidence and mortality from cardiovascular disease in patients with pooled and specific severe mental illness: a large-scale meta-analysis of 3,211,768 patients and 113,383,368 controls. World Psychiatry. 2017;16(2):163–80.

6. Thornicroft G. Physical health disparities and mental illness: the scandal of premature mortality. Br J Psychiatry. 2011;199(6):441–2.

7. Vancampfort D, Correll CU, Wampers M, Sienaert P, Mitchell AJ, De Herdt A, et al. Metabolic syndrome and metabolic abnormalities in patients with major depressive disorder: a meta-analysis of prevalences and moderating variables. Psychol Med. 2014;44(10):2017–28.

8. Mitchell AJ, Vancampfort D, De Herdt A, Yu W, De Hert M. Is the prevalence of metabolic syndrome and metabolic abnormalities increased in early schizophrenia? A comparative meta-analysis of first episode, untreated and treated patients. Schizophr Bull. 2013;39(2):295–305.

9. Grundy SM, Cleeman JI, Daniels SR, Donato KA, Eckel RH, Franklin BA, et al. Diagnosis and management of the metabolic syndrome: an American Heart Association/National Heart, Lung, and Blood Institute Scientific Statement. Circulation. 2005;112(17):2735–52.

10. Mottillo S, Filion KB, Genest J, Joseph L, Pilote L, Poirier P, et al. The metabolic syndrome and cardiovascular risk a systematic review and meta-analysis. J Am Coll Cardiol. 2010;56(14):1113–32.

11. Vancampfort D, Stubbs B, Mitchell AJ, De Hert M, Wampers M, Ward PB, et al. Risk of metabolic syndrome and its components in people with schizophrenia and related psychotic disorders, bipolar disorder and major depressive disorder: a systematic review and meta-analysis. World Psychiatry. 2015;14(3):339–47.

12. Vancampfort D, Vansteelandt K, Correll CU, Mitchell AJ, De Herdt A, Sienaert P, et al. Metabolic syndrome and metabolic abnormalities in bipolar disorder: a meta-analysis of prevalence rates and moderators. Am J Psychiatry. 2013;170(3):265–74.

13. Samele C, Patel M, Boydell J, Leese M, Wessely S, Murray R. Physical illness and lifestyle risk factors in people with their first presentation of psychosis. Soc Psychiatry Psychiatr Epidemiol. 2007;42(2):117–24.

14. Mitchell AJ, Vancampfort D, Sweers K, van Winkel R, Yu W, De Hert M. Prevalence of metabolic syndrome and metabolic abnormalities in schizophrenia and related disorders—a systematic review and meta-analysis. Schizophr Bull. 2013;39(2):306–18.

15. Vancampfort D, Wampers M, Mitchell AJ, Correll CU, De Herdt A, Probst M, et al. A meta-analysis of cardio-metabolic abnormalities in drug naive, first-episode and multi-episode patients with schizophrenia versus general population controls. World Psychiatry. 2013;12(3):240–50.

16. Myles N, Newall HD, Curtis J, Nielssen O, Shiers D, Large M. Tobacco use before, at, and after first-episode psychosis: a systematic meta-analysis. J Clin Psychiatry. 2012;73(4):468–75.

17. Kucukgoncu S, Kosir U, Zhou E, Sullivan E, Srihari VH, Tek C. Glucose metabolism dysregulation at the onset of mental illness is not limited to first episode psychosis: a systematic review and meta-analysis. Early Interv Psychiatry. 2019;13(5):1021–31.

18. Perry BI, McIntosh G, Weich S, Singh S, Rees K. The association between first-episode psychosis and abnormal glycaemic control: systematic review and meta-analysis. Lancet Psychiatry. 2016;3(11):1049–58.

19. Misiak B, Bartoli F, Stramecki F, Samochowiec J, Lis M, Kasznia J, et al. Appetite regulating hormones in first-episode psychosis: a systematic review and meta-analysis. Neurosci Biobehav Rev. 2019;102:362–70.

20. Pillinger T, Beck K, Stubbs B, Howes OD. Cholesterol and triglyceride levels in first-episode psychosis: systematic review and meta-analysis. Br J Psychiatry. 2017;211(6):339–49.

21. Emerging Risk Factors Collaboration, Sarwar N, Gao P, Seshasai SR, Gobin R, Kaptoge S, et al. Diabetes mellitus, fasting blood glucose concentration, and risk of vascular disease: a collaborative meta-analysis of 102 prospective studies. Lancet. 2010;375(9733):2215–22.
22. Vancampfort D, Correll CU, Galling B, Probst M, De Hert M, Ward PB, et al. Diabetes mellitus in people with schizophrenia, bipolar disorder and major depressive disorder: a systematic review and large scale meta-analysis. World Psychiatry. 2016;15(2):166–74.
23. Bugianesi E, Leone N, Vanni E, Marchesini G, Brunello F, Carucci P, et al. Expanding the natural history of nonalcoholic steatohepatitis: from cryptogenic cirrhosis to hepatocellular carcinoma. Gastroenterology. 2002;123(1):134–40.
24. Targher G, Day CP, Bonora E. Risk of cardiovascular disease in patients with nonalcoholic fatty liver disease. N Engl J Med. 2010;363(14):1341–50.
25. Liu H, Lu HY. Nonalcoholic fatty liver disease and cardiovascular disease. World J Gastroenterol. 2014;20(26):8407–15.
26. Carney R, Cotter J, Bradshaw T, Firth J, Yung AR. Cardiometabolic risk factors in young people at ultra-high risk for psychosis: a systematic review and meta-analysis. Schizophr Res. 2016;170(2–3):290–300.
27. Gonzalez-Blanco L, Greenhalgh AMD, Garcia-Rizo C, Fernandez-Egea E, Miller BJ, Kirkpatrick B. Prolactin concentrations in antipsychotic-naive patients with schizophrenia and related disorders: a meta-analysis. Schizophr Res. 2016;174(1–3):156–60.
28. Garcia-Rizo C, Fernandez-Egea E, Oliveira C, Justicia A, Parellada E, Bernardo M, et al. Prolactin concentrations in newly diagnosed, antipsychotic-naive patients with nonaffective psychosis. Schizophr Res. 2012;134(1):16–9.
29. Montgomery J, Winterbottom E, Jessani M, Kohegyi E, Fulmer J, Seamonds B, et al. Prevalence of hyperprolactinemia in schizophrenia: association with typical and atypical antipsychotic treatment. J Clin Psychiatry. 2004;65(11):1491–8.
30. Stubbs B, Gaughran F, Mitchell AJ, De Hert M, Farmer R, Soundy A, et al. Schizophrenia and the risk of fractures: a systematic review and comparative meta-analysis. Gen Hosp Psychiatry. 2015;37(2):126–33.
31. Jung DU, Kelly DL, Oh MK, Kong BG, Kang JW, Lee SJ, et al. Bone mineral density and osteoporosis risk in older patients with schizophrenia. J Clin Psychopharmacol. 2011;31(4):406–10.
32. Menendez ME, Neuhaus V, Bot AG, Vrahas MS, Ring D. Do psychiatric comorbidities influence inpatient death, adverse events, and discharge after lower extremity fractures? Clin Orthop Relat Res. 2013;471(10):3336–48.
33. Crews MP, Howes OD. Is antipsychotic treatment linked to low bone mineral density and osteoporosis? A review of the evidence and the clinical implications. Hum Psychopharmacol. 2012;27(1):15–23.
34. De Hert M, Detraux J, van Winkel R, Yu W, Correll CU. Metabolic and cardiovascular adverse effects associated with antipsychotic drugs. Nat Rev Endocrinol. 2011;8(2):114–26.
35. Vancampfort D, Firth J, Schuch FB, Rosenbaum S, Mugisha J, Hallgren M, et al. Sedentary behavior and physical activity levels in people with schizophrenia, bipolar disorder and major depressive disorder: a global systematic review and meta-analysis. World Psychiatry. 2017;16(3):308–15.
36. Bly MJ, Taylor SF, Dalack G, Pop-Busui R, Burghardt KJ, Evans SJ, et al. Metabolic syndrome in bipolar disorder and schizophrenia: dietary and lifestyle factors compared to the general population. Bipolar Disord. 2014;16(3):277–88.
37. Pillinger T, D'Ambrosio E, McCutcheon R, Howes OD. Is psychosis a multisystem disorder? A meta-review of central nervous system, immune, cardiometabolic, and endocrine alterations in first-episode psychosis and perspective on potential models. Mol Psychiatry. 2019;24(6):776–94.
38. Upthegrove R, Manzanares-Teson N, Barnes NM. Cytokine function in medication-naive first episode psychosis: a systematic review and meta-analysis. Schizophr Res. 2014;155(1–3):101–8.

39. Chaumette B, Kebir O, Mam-Lam-Fook C, Morvan Y, Bourgin J, Godsil BP, et al. Salivary cortisol in early psychosis: new findings and meta-analysis. Psychoneuroendocrinology. 2016;63:262–70.

40. Hubbard DB, Miller BJ. Meta-analysis of blood cortisol levels in individuals with first-episode psychosis. Psychoneuroendocrinology. 2019;104:269–75.

41. Petrikis P, Boumba VA, Tzallas AT, Voulgari PV, Archimandriti DT, Skapinakis P, et al. Elevated levels of Insulin-like Growth Factor-1 (IGF-1) in drug-naive patients with psychosis. Psychiatry Res. 2016;246:348–52.

42. Kapogiannis D, Dobrowolny H, Tran J, Mustapic M, Frodl T, Meyer-Lotz G, et al. Insulin-signaling abnormalities in drug-naive first-episode schizophrenia: transduction protein analyses in extracellular vesicles of putative neuronal origin. Eur Psychiatry. 2019;62:124–9.

43. Bocchio-Chiavetto L, Zanardini R, Tosato S, Ventriglia M, Ferrari C, Bonetto C, et al. Immune and metabolic alterations in first episode psychosis (FEP) patients. Brain Behav Immun. 2018;70:315–24.

44. Hong S, Lee EE, Martin AS, Soontornniyomkij B, Soontornniyomkij V, Achim CL, et al. Abnormalities in chemokine levels in schizophrenia and their clinical correlates. Schizophr Res. 2017;181:63–9.

45. Wang T, Zhang X, Li A, Zhu M, Liu S, Qin W, et al. Polygenic risk for five psychiatric disorders and cross-disorder and disorder-specific neural connectivity in two independent populations. Neuroimage Clin. 2017;14:441–9.

46. Maj C, Tosato S, Zanardini R, Lasalvia A, Favaro A, Leuci E, et al. Correlations between immune and metabolic serum markers and schizophrenia/bipolar disorder polygenic risk score in first-episode psychosis. Early Interv Psychiatry. 2020;14(4):507–11.

47. Tosato S, Bonetto C, Tomassi S, Zanardini R, Faravelli C, Bruschi C, et al. Childhood trauma and glucose metabolism in patients with first-episode psychosis. Psychoneuroendocrinology. 2020;113:104536.

48. Hepgul N, Pariante CM, Dipasquale S, DiForti M, Taylor H, Marques TR, et al. Childhood maltreatment is associated with increased body mass index and increased C-reactive protein levels in first-episode psychosis patients. Psychol Med. 2012;42(9):1893–901.

49. Harris LW, Guest PC, Wayland MT, Umrania Y, Krishnamurthy D, Rahmoune H, et al. Schizophrenia: metabolic aspects of aetiology, diagnosis and future treatment strategies. Psychoneuroendocrinology. 2013;38(6):752–66.

50. Berens AE, Jensen SKG, Nelson CA III. Biological embedding of childhood adversity: from physiological mechanisms to clinical implications. BMC Med. 2017;15(1):135.

51. Myles H, Myles N, Large M. Cannabis use in first episode psychosis: meta-analysis of prevalence, and the time course of initiation and continued use. Aust N Z J Psychiatry. 2016;50(3):208–19.

52. Scheffler F, Kilian S, Chiliza B, Asmal L, Phahladira L, du Plessis S, et al. Effects of cannabis use on body mass, fasting glucose and lipids during the first 12 months of treatment in schizophrenia spectrum disorders. Schizophr Res. 2018;199:90–5.

53. Vidot DC, Prado G, Hlaing WM, Florez HJ, Arheart KL, Messiah SE. Metabolic syndrome among marijuana users in the United States: an analysis of National Health and Nutrition Examination Survey Data. Am J Med. 2016;129(2):173–9.

54. Hahn LA, Galletly CA, Foley DL, Mackinnon A, Watts GF, Castle DJ, et al. Inadequate fruit and vegetable intake in people with psychosis. Aust N Z J Psychiatry. 2014;48(11):1025–35.

55. Dube E, O'Loughlin J, Karp I, Jutras-Aswad D. Cigarette smoking may modify the association between cannabis use and adiposity in males. Pharmacol Biochem Behav. 2015;135:121–7.

56. Thomas A, Baillie GL, Phillips AM, Razdan RK, Ross RA, Pertwee RG. Cannabidiol displays unexpectedly high potency as an antagonist of CB1 and CB2 receptor agonists in vitro. Br J Pharmacol. 2007;150(5):613–23.

57. Vazquez-Bourgon J, Ortiz-Garcia de la Foz V, Suarez-Pereira I, Iruzubieta P, Arias-Loste MT, Setien-Suero E, et al. Cannabis consumption and non-alcoholic fatty liver disease. A three years longitudinal study in first episode non-affective psychosis patients. Prog Neuropsychopharmacol Biol Psychiatry. 2019;95:109677.

58. Huhn M, Nikolakopoulou A, Schneider-Thoma J, Krause M, Samara M, Peter N, et al. Comparative efficacy and tolerability of 32 oral antipsychotics for the acute treatment of adults with multi-episode schizophrenia: a systematic review and network meta-analysis. Lancet. 2019;394(10202):939–51.
59. Morlan-Coarasa MJ, Arias-Loste MT, Ortiz-Garcia de la Foz V, Martinez-Garcia O, Alonso-Martin C, Crespo J, et al. Incidence of non-alcoholic fatty liver disease and metabolic dysfunction in first episode schizophrenia and related psychotic disorders: a 3-year prospective randomized interventional study. Psychopharmacology (Berl). 2016;233(23–24):3947–52.
60. Pillinger T, McCutcheon RA, Vano L, Mizuno Y, Arumuham A, Hindley G, et al. Comparative effects of 18 antipsychotics on metabolic function in patients with schizophrenia, predictors of metabolic dysregulation, and association with psychopathology: a systematic review and network meta-analysis. Lancet Psychiatry. 2020;7(1):64–77.
61. Zhang JP, Lencz T, Zhang RX, Nitta M, Maayan L, John M, et al. Pharmacogenetic associations of antipsychotic drug-related weight gain: a systematic review and meta-analysis. Schizophr Bull. 2016;42(6):1418–37.
62. Zhang JP, Gallego JA, Robinson DG, Malhotra AK, Kane JM, Correll CU. Efficacy and safety of individual second-generation vs. first-generation antipsychotics in first-episode psychosis: a systematic review and meta-analysis. Int J Neuropsychopharmacol. 2013;16(6):1205–18.
63. Bak M, Fransen A, Janssen J, van Os J, Drukker M. Almost all antipsychotics result in weight gain: a meta-analysis. PLoS One. 2014;9(4):e94112.
64. Hasnain M, Vieweg WV, Hollett B. Weight gain and glucose dysregulation with second-generation antipsychotics and antidepressants: a review for primary care physicians. Postgrad Med. 2012;124(4):154–67.
65. Perez-Iglesias R, Martinez-Garcia O, Pardo-Garcia G, Amado JA, Garcia-Unzueta MT, Tabares-Seisdedos R, et al. Course of weight gain and metabolic abnormalities in first treated episode of psychosis: the first year is a critical period for development of cardiovascular risk factors. Int J Neuropsychopharmacol. 2014;17(1):41–51.
66. Tek C, Kucukgoncu S, Guloksuz S, Woods SW, Srihari VH, Annamalai A. Antipsychotic-induced weight gain in first-episode psychosis patients: a meta-analysis of differential effects of antipsychotic medications. Early Interv Psychiatry. 2016;10(3):193–202.
67. Patel JK, Buckley PF, Woolson S, Hamer RM, McEvoy JP, Perkins DO, et al. Metabolic profiles of second-generation antipsychotics in early psychosis: findings from the CAFE study. Schizophr Res. 2009;111(1–3):9–16.
68. Kinon BJ, Kaiser CJ, Ahmed S, Rotelli MD, Kollack-Walker S. Association between early and rapid weight gain and change in weight over one year of olanzapine therapy in patients with schizophrenia and related disorders. J Clin Psychopharmacol. 2005;25(3):255–8.
69. Deng C. Effects of antipsychotic medications on appetite, weight, and insulin resistance. Endocrinol Metab Clin North Am. 2013;42(3):545–63.
70. Reynolds GP. Pharmacogenetic aspects of antipsychotic drug-induced weight gain - a critical review. Clin Psychopharmacol Neurosci. 2012;10(2):71–7.
71. Luo C, Liu J, Wang X, Mao X, Zhou H, Liu Z. Pharmacogenetic correlates of antipsychotic-induced weight gain in the Chinese population. Neurosci Bull. 2019;35(3):561–80.
72. Templeman LA, Reynolds GP, Arranz B, San L. Polymorphisms of the 5-HT2C receptor and leptin genes are associated with antipsychotic drug-induced weight gain in Caucasian subjects with a first-episode psychosis. Pharmacogenet Genomics. 2005;15(4):195–200.
73. Tsai SJ, Hong CJ, Yu YW, Lin CH. 759C/T genetic variation of 5HT(2C) receptor and clozapine-induced weight gain. Lancet. 2002;360(9347):1790.
74. Nielsen J, Skadhede S, Correll CU. Antipsychotics associated with the development of type 2 diabetes in antipsychotic-naive schizophrenia patients. Neuropsychopharmacology. 2010;35(9):1997–2004.
75. Ulcickas Yood M, Delorenze GN, Quesenberry CP Jr, Oliveria SA, Tsai AL, Kim E, et al. Association between second-generation antipsychotics and newly diagnosed treated diabetes mellitus: does the effect differ by dose? BMC Psychiatry. 2011;11:197.

76. Yu L, Wu S, Deng Y, Lei J, Yu L, Li W. Insulin resistance induced by olanzapine and other second-generation antipsychotics in Chinese patients with schizophrenia: a comparative review and meta-analysis. Eur J Clin Pharmacol. 2019;75(12):1621–9.

77. Galling B, Roldan A, Nielsen RE, Nielsen J, Gerhard T, Carbon M, et al. Type 2 diabetes mellitus in youth exposed to antipsychotics: a systematic review and meta-analysis. JAMA Psychiat. 2016;73(3):247–59.

78. Leucht S, Cipriani A, Spineli L, Mavridis D, Orey D, Richter F, et al. Comparative efficacy and tolerability of 15 antipsychotic drugs in schizophrenia: a multiple-treatments meta-analysis. Lancet. 2013;382(9896):951–62.

79. Solmi M, Fornaro M, Ostinelli EG, Zangani C, Croatto G, Monaco F, et al. Safety of 80 antidepressants, antipsychotics, anti-attention-deficit/hyperactivity medications and mood stabilizers in children and adolescents with psychiatric disorders: a large scale systematic meta-review of 78 adverse effects. World Psychiatry. 2020;19(2):214–32.

80. Suzuki Y, Sugai T, Fukui N, Watanabe J, Ono S, Tsuneyama N, et al. Differences in plasma prolactin levels in patients with schizophrenia treated on monotherapy with five second-generation antipsychotics. Schizophr Res. 2013;145(1–3):116–9.

81. Peuskens J, Pani L, Detraux J, De Hert M. The effects of novel and newly approved antipsychotics on serum prolactin levels: a comprehensive review. CNS Drugs. 2014;28(5):421–53.

82. Andrade C. Low-dose amisulpride and elevation in serum prolactin. J Clin Psychiatry. 2013;74(6):e558–60.

83. Bellantuono C, Santone G. [Efficacy, tolerability and safety of paliperidone extended-release in the treatment of schizophrenia and schizoaffective disorder]. Riv Psichiatr. 2012;47(1):5–20.

84. Li X, Tang Y, Wang C. Adjunctive aripiprazole versus placebo for antipsychotic-induced hyperprolactinemia: meta-analysis of randomized controlled trials. PLoS One. 2013;8(8):e70179.

85. Keck PE Jr, McElroy SL. Aripiprazole: a partial dopamine D2 receptor agonist antipsychotic. Expert Opin Investig Drugs. 2003;12(4):655–62.

86. Montejo AL, Arango C, Bernardo M, Carrasco JL, Crespo-Facorro B, Cruz JJ, et al. Spanish consensus on the risks and detection of antipsychotic drug-related hyperprolactinaemia. Rev Psiquiatr Salud Ment. 2016;9(3):158–73.

87. Gasso P, Mas S, Bioque M, Cabrera B, Lobo A, Gonzalez-Pinto A, et al. Impact of NTRK2, DRD2 and ACE polymorphisms on prolactin levels in antipsychotic-treated patients with first-episode psychosis. J Psychopharmacol. 2018;32(6):702–10.

88. Oderda LH, Young JR, Asche CV, Pepper GA. Psychotropic-related hip fractures: meta-analysis of first-generation and second-generation antidepressant and antipsychotic drugs. Ann Pharmacother. 2012;46(7–8):917–28.

89. Wu CS, Chang CM, Tsai YT, Huang YW, Tsai HJ. Antipsychotic treatment and the risk of hip fracture in subjects with schizophrenia: a 10-year population-based case-control study. J Clin Psychiatry. 2015;76(9):1216–23.

90. Jackson JW, Schneeweiss S, VanderWeele TJ, Blacker D. Quantifying the role of adverse events in the mortality difference between first and second-generation antipsychotics in older adults: systematic review and meta-synthesis. PLoS One. 2014;9(8):e105376.

91. Rigler SK, Shireman TI, Cook-Wiens GJ, Ellerbeck EF, Whittle JC, Mehr DR, et al. Fracture risk in nursing home residents initiating antipsychotic medications. J Am Geriatr Soc. 2013;61(5):715–22.

92. Wang M, Hou R, Jian J, Mi G, Qiu H, Cao B, et al. Effects of antipsychotics on bone mineral density and prolactin levels in patients with schizophrenia: a 12-month prospective study. Hum Psychopharmacol. 2014;29(2):183–9.

93. Van Mastrigt S, Addington J, Addington D. Substance misuse at presentation to an early psychosis program. Soc Psychiatry Psychiatr Epidemiol. 2004;39(1):69–72.

94. Atlantis E, Shi Z, Penninx BJ, Wittert GA, Taylor A, Almeida OP. Chronic medical conditions mediate the association between depression and cardiovascular disease mortality. Soc Psychiatry Psychiatr Epidemiol. 2012;47(4):615–25.

95. De Hert M, Cohen D, Bobes J, Cetkovich-Bakmas M, Leucht S, Ndetei DM, et al. Physical illness in patients with severe mental disorders. II. Barriers to care, monitoring and treatment guidelines, plus recommendations at the system and individual level. World Psychiatry. 2011;10(2):138–51.
96. Swardfager W, Herrmann N, Marzolini S, Saleem M, Farber SB, Kiss A, et al. Major depressive disorder predicts completion, adherence, and outcomes in cardiac rehabilitation: a prospective cohort study of 195 patients with coronary artery disease. J Clin Psychiatry. 2011;72(9):1181–8.
97. Lee CJ, Lee LT, Tsai HC, Chang WH, Lee IH, Chen KC, et al. Factors related to metabolic parameters in medicated patients with major depressive disorder—a naturalistic study. Psychiatry Res. 2018;268:28–33.
98. Solmi M, Kohler CA, Stubbs B, Koyanagi A, Bortolato B, Monaco F, et al. Environmental risk factors and nonpharmacological and nonsurgical interventions for obesity: an umbrella review of meta-analyses of cohort studies and randomized controlled trials. Eur J Clin Invest. 2018;48(12):e12982.
99. Mannan M, Mamun A, Doi S, Clavarino A. Is there a bi-directional relationship between depression and obesity among adult men and women? Systematic review and bias-adjusted meta analysis. Asian J Psychiatr. 2016;21:51–66.
100. Khaledi M, Haghighatdoost F, Feizi A, Aminorroaya A. The prevalence of comorbid depression in patients with type 2 diabetes: an updated systematic review and meta-analysis on huge number of observational studies. Acta Diabetol. 2019;56(6):631–50.
101. Mezuk B, Eaton WW, Albrecht S, Golden SH. Depression and type 2 diabetes over the lifespan: a meta-analysis. Diabetes Care. 2008;31(12):2383–90.
102. Sullivan MD, O'Connor P, Feeney P, Hire D, Simmons DL, Raisch DW, et al. Depression predicts all-cause mortality: epidemiological evaluation from the ACCORD HRQL substudy. Diabetes Care. 2012;35(8):1708–15.
103. Black SA, Markides KS, Ray LA. Depression predicts increased incidence of adverse health outcomes in older Mexican Americans with type 2 diabetes. Diabetes Care. 2003;26(10):2822–8.
104. Whitworth SR, Bruce DG, Starkstein SE, Davis WA, Davis TM, Bucks RS. Lifetime depression and anxiety increase prevalent psychological symptoms and worsen glycemic control in type 2 diabetes: the Fremantle Diabetes Study Phase II. Diabetes Res Clin Pract. 2016;122:190–7.
105. Wu Q, Liu B, Tonmoy S. Depression and risk of fracture and bone loss: an updated meta-analysis of prospective studies. Osteoporos Int. 2018;29(6):1303–12.
106. Ganesan K, Teklehaimanot S, Tran TH, Asuncion M, Norris K. Relationship of C-reactive protein and bone mineral density in community-dwelling elderly females. J Natl Med Assoc. 2005;97(3):329–33.
107. van den Berk-Clark C, Secrest S, Walls J, Hallberg E, Lustman PJ, Schneider FD, et al. Association between posttraumatic stress disorder and lack of exercise, poor diet, obesity, and co-occuring smoking: a systematic review and meta-analysis. Health Psychol. 2018;37(5):407–16.
108. Alghadir AH, Gabr SA, Al-Eisa E. Physical activity and lifestyle effects on bone mineral density among young adults: sociodemographic and biochemical analysis. J Phys Ther Sci. 2015;27(7):2261–70.
109. Rabenda V, Nicolet D, Beaudart C, Bruyere O, Reginster JY. Relationship between use of antidepressants and risk of fractures: a meta-analysis. Osteoporos Int. 2013;24(1):121–37.
110. Bruyere O, Reginster JY. Osteoporosis in patients taking selective serotonin reuptake inhibitors: a focus on fracture outcome. Endocrine. 2015;48(1):65–8.
111. Lam RW, McIntosh D, Wang J, Enns MW, Kolivakis T, Michalak EE, et al. Canadian Network for Mood and Anxiety Treatments (CANMAT) 2016 clinical guidelines for the management of adults with major depressive disorder: Section 1. Disease burden and principles of care. Can J Psychiatry. 2016;61(9):510–23.

112. De Hert M, Dekker JM, Wood D, Kahl KG, Holt RI, Moller HJ. Cardiovascular disease and diabetes in people with severe mental illness position statement from the European Psychiatric Association (EPA), supported by the European Association for the Study of Diabetes (EASD) and the European Society of Cardiology (ESC). Eur Psychiatry. 2009;24(6):412–24.
113. Fagiolini A, Frank E, Scott JA, Turkin S, Kupfer DJ. Metabolic syndrome in bipolar disorder: findings from the Bipolar Disorder Center for Pennsylvanians. Bipolar Disord. 2005;7(5):424–30.
114. Champaneri S, Wand GS, Malhotra SS, Casagrande SS, Golden SH. Biological basis of depression in adults with diabetes. Curr Diab Rep. 2010;10(6):396–405.
115. Joseph JJ, Golden SH. Cortisol dysregulation: the bidirectional link between stress, depression, and type 2 diabetes mellitus. Ann N Y Acad Sci. 2017;1391(1):20–34.
116. Bjorntorp P. Do stress reactions cause abdominal obesity and comorbidities? Obes Rev. 2001;2(2):73–86.
117. Juruena MF, Bocharova M, Agustini B, Young AH. Atypical depression and non-atypical depression: is HPA axis function a biomarker? A systematic review. J Affect Disord. 2018;233:45–67.
118. de Melo LGP, Nunes SOV, Anderson G, Vargas HO, Barbosa DS, Galecki P, et al. Shared metabolic and immune-inflammatory, oxidative and nitrosative stress pathways in the metabolic syndrome and mood disorders. Prog Neuropsychopharmacol Biol Psychiatry. 2017;78:34–50.
119. Bortolasci CC, Vargas HO, Vargas Nunes SO, de Melo LG, de Castro MR, Moreira EG, et al. Factors influencing insulin resistance in relation to atherogenicity in mood disorders, the metabolic syndrome and tobacco use disorder. J Affect Disord. 2015;179:148–55.
120. Galecki P, Szemraj J, Bienkiewicz M, Florkowski A, Galecka E. Lipid peroxidation and antioxidant protection in patients during acute depressive episodes and in remission after fluoxetine treatment. Pharmacol Rep. 2009;61(3):436–47.
121. Moylan S, Berk M, Dean OM, Samuni Y, Williams LJ, O'Neil A, et al. Oxidative & nitrosative stress in depression: why so much stress? Neurosci Biobehav Rev. 2014;45:46–62.
122. Bonomini F, Rodella LF, Rezzani R. Metabolic syndrome, aging and involvement of oxidative stress. Aging Dis. 2015;6(2):109–20.
123. Lucas K, Maes M. Role of the Toll Like receptor (TLR) radical cycle in chronic inflammation: possible treatments targeting the TLR4 pathway. Mol Neurobiol. 2013;48(1):190–204.
124. Pasco JA, Jacka FN, Williams LJ, Henry MJ, Nicholson GC, Kotowicz MA, et al. Leptin in depressed women: cross-sectional and longitudinal data from an epidemiologic study. J Affect Disord. 2008;107(1–3):221–5.
125. Milaneschi Y, Lamers F, Bot M, Drent ML, Penninx BW. Leptin dysregulation is specifically associated with major depression with atypical features: evidence for a mechanism connecting obesity and depression. Biol Psychiatry. 2017;81(9):807–14.
126. Leo R, Di Lorenzo G, Tesauro M, Cola C, Fortuna E, Zanasi M, et al. Decreased plasma adiponectin concentration in major depression. Neurosci Lett. 2006;407(3):211–3.
127. Cao B, Chen Y, Brietzke E, Cha D, Shaukat A, Pan Z, et al. Leptin and adiponectin levels in major depressive disorder: a systematic review and meta-analysis. J Affect Disord. 2018;238:101–10.
128. Caroleo M, Carbone EA, Primerano A, Foti D, Brunetti A, Segura-Garcia C. The role of hormonal, metabolic and inflammatory biomarkers on sleep and appetite in drug free patients with major depression: a systematic review. J Affect Disord. 2019;250:249–59.
129. Yu J, Fei K, Fox A, Negron R, Horowitz C. Stress eating and sleep disturbance as mediators in the relationship between depression and obesity in low-income, minority women. Obes Res Clin Pract. 2016;10(3):283–90.
130. Capuron L, Lasselin J, Castanon N. Role of adiposity-driven inflammation in depressive morbidity. Neuropsychopharmacology. 2017;42(1):115–28.
131. Kohler CA, Freitas TH, Maes M, de Andrade NQ, Liu CS, Fernandes BS, et al. Peripheral cytokine and chemokine alterations in depression: a meta-analysis of 82 studies. Acta Psychiatr Scand. 2017;135(5):373–87.

132. Rivera M, Locke AE, Corre T, Czamara D, Wolf C, Ching-Lopez A, et al. Interaction between the FTO gene, body mass index and depression: meta-analysis of 13701 individuals. Br J Psychiatry. 2017;211(2):70–6.
133. Amare AT, Schubert KO, Klingler-Hoffmann M, Cohen-Woods S, Baune BT. The genetic overlap between mood disorders and cardiometabolic diseases: a systematic review of genome wide and candidate gene studies. Transl Psychiatry. 2017;7(1):e1007.
134. Hailes HP, Yu R, Danese A, Fazel S. Long-term outcomes of childhood sexual abuse: an umbrella review. Lancet Psychiatry. 2019;6(10):830–9.
135. Nelson J, Klumparendt A, Doebler P, Ehring T. Childhood maltreatment and characteristics of adult depression: meta-analysis. Br J Psychiatry. 2017;210(2):96–104.
136. Danese A, Moffitt TE, Pariante CM, Ambler A, Poulton R, Caspi A. Elevated inflammation levels in depressed adults with a history of childhood maltreatment. Arch Gen Psychiatry. 2008;65(4):409–15.
137. Arterburn D, Sofer T, Boudreau DM, Bogart A, Westbrook EO, Theis MK, et al. Long-term weight change after initiating second-generation antidepressants. J Clin Med. 2016;5(4):48.
138. Fava M. Weight gain and antidepressants. J Clin Psychiatry. 2000;61(Suppl 11):37–41.
139. Gafoor R, Booth HP, Gulliford MC. Antidepressant utilisation and incidence of weight gain during 10 years' follow-up: population based cohort study. BMJ. 2018;361:k1951.
140. Serretti A, Mandelli L. Antidepressants and body weight: a comprehensive review and meta-analysis. J Clin Psychiatry. 2010;71(10):1259–72.
141. Uguz F, Sahingoz M, Gungor B, Aksoy F, Askin R. Weight gain and associated factors in patients using newer antidepressant drugs. Gen Hosp Psychiatry. 2015;37(1):46–8.
142. Correll CU, Detraux J, De Lepeleire J, De Hert M. Effects of antipsychotics, antidepressants and mood stabilizers on risk for physical diseases in people with schizophrenia, depression and bipolar disorder. World Psychiatry. 2015;14(2):119–36.
143. Rosenbaum S, Stubbs B, Ward PB, Steel Z, Lederman O, Vancampfort D. The prevalence and risk of metabolic syndrome and its components among people with posttraumatic stress disorder: a systematic review and meta-analysis. Metabolism. 2015;64(8):926–33.
144. Gurusamy J, Gandhi S, Damodharan D, Ganesan V, Palaniappan M. Exercise, diet and educational interventions for metabolic syndrome in persons with schizophrenia: a systematic review. Asian J Psychiatr. 2018;36:73–85.
145. Nelson ME, Rejeski WJ, Blair SN, Duncan PW, Judge JO, King AC, et al. Physical activity and public health in older adults: recommendation from the American College of Sports Medicine and the American Heart Association. Med Sci Sports Exerc. 2007;39(8):1435–45.
146. Haskell WL, Lee IM, Pate RR, Powell KE, Blair SN, Franklin BA, et al. Physical activity and public health: updated recommendation for adults from the American College of Sports Medicine and the American Heart Association. Med Sci Sports Exerc. 2007;39(8):1423–34.
147. Hayashino Y, Jackson JL, Hirata T, Fukumori N, Nakamura F, Fukuhara S, et al. Effects of exercise on C-reactive protein, inflammatory cytokine and adipokine in patients with type 2 diabetes: a meta-analysis of randomized controlled trials. Metabolism. 2014;63(3):431–40.
148. Bergstrom G, Behre CJ, Schmidt C. Moderate intensities of leisure-time physical activity are associated with lower levels of high-sensitivity C-reactive protein in healthy middle-aged men. Angiology. 2012;63(6):412–5.
149. Naci H, Ioannidis JP. Comparative effectiveness of exercise and drug interventions on mortality outcomes: metaepidemiological study. BMJ. 2013;347:f5577.
150. Biswas A, Oh PI, Faulkner GE, Bajaj RR, Silver MA, Mitchell MS, et al. Sedentary time and its association with risk for disease incidence, mortality, and hospitalization in adults: a systematic review and meta-analysis. Ann Intern Med. 2015;162(2):123–32.
151. Ashdown-Franks G, Williams J, Vancampfort D, Firth J, Schuch F, Hubbard K, et al. Is it possible for people with severe mental illness to sit less and move more? A systematic review of interventions to increase physical activity or reduce sedentary behaviour. Schizophr Res. 2018;202:3–16.

152. Thivel D, Masurier J, Baquet G, Timmons BW, Pereira B, Berthoin S, et al. High-intensity interval training in overweight and obese children and adolescents: systematic review and meta-analysis. J Sports Med Phys Fitness. 2019;59(2):310–24.
153. Piercy KL, Troiano RP, Ballard RM, Carlson SA, Fulton JE, Galuska DA, et al. The physical activity guidelines for Americans. JAMA. 2018;320(19):2020–8.
154. Ross LM, Porter RR, Durstine JL. High-intensity interval training (HIIT) for patients with chronic diseases. J Sport Health Sci. 2016;5(2):139–44.
155. Schmitt A, Maurus I, Rossner MJ, Roh A, Lembeck M, von Wilmsdorff M, et al. Effects of aerobic exercise on metabolic syndrome, cardiorespiratory fitness, and symptoms in schizophrenia include decreased mortality. Front Psychiatry. 2018;9:690.
156. Abdel-Baki A, Brazzini-Poisson V, Marois F, Letendre E, Karelis AD. Effects of aerobic interval training on metabolic complications and cardiorespiratory fitness in young adults with psychotic disorders: a pilot study. Schizophr Res. 2013;149(1–3):112–5.
157. Stubbs B, Vancampfort D, Hallgren M, Firth J, Veronese N, Solmi M, et al. EPA guidance on physical activity as a treatment for severe mental illness: a meta-review of the evidence and position statement from the European Psychiatric Association (EPA), supported by the International Organization of Physical Therapists in Mental Health (IOPTMH). Eur Psychiatry. 2018;54:124–44.
158. Firth J, Siddiqi N, Koyanagi A, Siskind D, Rosenbaum S, Galletly C, et al. The Lancet Psychiatry Commission: a blueprint for protecting physical health in people with mental illness. Lancet Psychiatry. 2019;6(8):675–712.
159. Mittal VA, Vargas T, Osborne KJ, Dean D, Gupta T, Ristanovic I, et al. Exercise treatments for psychosis: a review. Curr Treat Options Psychiatry. 2017;4(2):152–66.
160. Tumiel E, Wichniak A, Jarema M, Lew-Starowicz M. Nonpharmacological interventions for the treatment of cardiometabolic risk factors in people with schizophrenia-a systematic review. Front Psychiatry. 2019;10:566.
161. De Rosa C, Sampogna G, Luciano M, Del Vecchio V, Pocai B, Borriello G, et al. Improving physical health of patients with severe mental disorders: a critical review of lifestyle psychosocial interventions. Expert Rev Neurother. 2017;17(7):667–81.
162. Bauer IE, Galvez JF, Hamilton JE, Balanza-Martinez V, Zunta-Soares GB, Soares JC, et al. Lifestyle interventions targeting dietary habits and exercise in bipolar disorder: a systematic review. J Psychiatr Res. 2016;74:1–7.
163. Bruins J, Jorg F, Bruggeman R, Slooff C, Corpeleijn E, Pijnenborg M. The effects of lifestyle interventions on (long-term) weight management, cardiometabolic risk and depressive symptoms in people with psychotic disorders: a meta-analysis. PLoS One. 2014;9(12):e112276.
164. Vancampfort D, Firth J, Correll CU, Solmi M, Siskind D, De Hert M, et al. The impact of pharmacological and non-pharmacological interventions to improve physical health outcomes in people with schizophrenia: a meta-review of meta-analyses of randomized controlled trials. World Psychiatry. 2019;18(1):53–66.
165. Reinares M, Sanchez-Moreno J, Fountoulakis KN. Psychosocial interventions in bipolar disorder: what, for whom, and when. J Affect Disord. 2014;156:46–55.
166. Pingani L, Fiorillo A, Luciano M, Catellani S, Vinci V, Ferrari S, et al. Who cares for it? How to provide psychosocial interventions in the community. Int J Soc Psychiatry. 2013;59(7):701–5.
167. Hjorth P, Espensen CH, Madsen NJ, Viuff AG, Munk-Jorgensen P. Reducing the risk of type 2 diabetes in nonselected outpatients with schizophrenia: a 30-month program. J Psychiatr Pract. 2018;24(1):21–31.
168. Amiaz R, Rubinstein K, Czerniak E, Karni Y, Weiser M. A diet and fitness program similarly affects weight reduction in schizophrenia patients treated with typical or atypical medications. Pharmacopsychiatry. 2016;49(3):112–6.
169. Papanastasiou E. Interventions for the metabolic syndrome in schizophrenia: a review. Ther Adv Endocrinol Metab. 2012;3(5):141–62.

170. Joseph J, Depp C, Shih PB, Cadenhead KS, Schmid-Schonbein G. Modified Mediterranean diet for enrichment of short chain fatty acids: potential adjunctive therapeutic to target immune and metabolic dysfunction in schizophrenia? Front Neurosci. 2017;11:155.
171. Bonfioli E, Berti L, Goss C, Muraro F, Burti L. Health promotion lifestyle interventions for weight management in psychosis: a systematic review and meta-analysis of randomised controlled trials. BMC Psychiatry. 2012;12:78.
172. Bushe C, Haddad P, Peveler R, Pendlebury J. The role of lifestyle interventions and weight management in schizophrenia. J Psychopharmacol. 2005;19(6 Suppl):28–35.
173. Mizuno Y, Suzuki T, Nakagawa A, Yoshida K, Mimura M, Fleischhacker WW, et al. Pharmacological strategies to counteract antipsychotic-induced weight gain and metabolic adverse effects in schizophrenia: a systematic review and meta-analysis. Schizophr Bull. 2014;40(6):1385–403.
174. Cooper SJ, Reynolds GP, With expert co-authors (in alphabetical order), Barnes T, England E, Haddad PM, et al. BAP guidelines on the management of weight gain, metabolic disturbances and cardiovascular risk associated with psychosis and antipsychotic drug treatment. J Psychopharmacol. 2016;30(8):717–48.
175. Alptekin K, Hafez J, Brook S, Akkaya C, Tzebelikos E, Ucok A, et al. Efficacy and tolerability of switching to ziprasidone from olanzapine, risperidone or haloperidol: an international, multicenter study. Int Clin Psychopharmacol. 2009;24(5):229–38
176. Maayan L, Vakhrusheva J, Correll CU. Effectiveness of medications used to attenuate antipsychotic-related weight gain and metabolic abnormalities: a systematic review and meta-analysis. Neuropsychopharmacology. 2010;35(7):1520–30.
177. Correll CU, Robinson DG, Schooler NR, Brunette MF, Mueser KT, Rosenheck RA, et al. Cardiometabolic risk in patients with first-episode schizophrenia spectrum disorders: baseline results from the RAISE-ETP study. JAMA Psychiat. 2014;71(12):1350–63.
178. Mitchell AJ, Delaffon V, Vancampfort D, Correll CU, De Hert M. Guideline concordant monitoring of metabolic risk in people treated with antipsychotic medication: systematic review and meta-analysis of screening practices. Psychol Med. 2012;42(1):125–47.
179. Rosenbaum S, Tiedemann A, Sherrington C, Curtis J, Ward PB. Physical activity interventions for people with mental illness: a systematic review and meta-analysis. J Clin Psychiatry. 2014;75(9):964–74.
180. Mitchell AJ, De Hert M. Promotion of physical health in persons with schizophrenia: can we prevent cardiometabolic problems before they begin? Acta Psychiatr Scand. 2015;132(2):83–5.
181. Bartels SJ. Can behavioral health organizations change health behaviors? The STRIDE study and lifestyle interventions for obesity in serious mental illness. Am J Psychiatry. 2015;172(1):9–11.
182. Deenik J, Czosnek L, Teasdale SB, Stubbs B, Firth J, Schuch FB, et al. From impact factors to real impact: translating evidence on lifestyle interventions into routine mental health care. Transl Behav Med. 2020;10(4):1070–3.

Imaging in Psychiatry: A Reappraisal of Preventative Potential

Isabel Valli and Norma Verdolini

14.1 Introduction

The diagnosis of psychiatric disorders is still based on a method available several hundreds of years ago, a clinical interview, associated with significant limitations in terms of accuracy and inter-rater reliability [1]. There has been therefore growing interest in the potential use of biological markers for diagnostic and prognostic purposes [2]. In particular, brain imaging methods, such as structural MRI (sMRI), functional MRI (fMRI) and diffusion tensor imaging (DTI), have provided high-resolution information about the anatomy, the activity and the connections in the brain.

Structural MRI makes it possible to visualise volumetric abnormalities of both cortical and subcortical structures. Functional MRI employs changes in blood oxygenation to detect changes in brain activity and can be used either at rest or in combination with various tasks aimed at activating specific brain circuits. DTI measures the diffusion of water molecules through tissues and is used to assess white matter integrity, often measuring fractional anisotropy (FA), which is an estimate of the net directionality of diffusion and that if decreased can reflect abnormalities in myelination and neural fibre density.

I. Valli (✉)
Department of Psychosis Studies, Institute of Psychiatry Psychology and Neuroscience, King's College London, London, UK

Institut d'Investigacions Biomediques August Pi I Sunyer, University of Barcelona, Barcelona, Spain
e-mail: isabel.valli@kcl.ac.uk

N. Verdolini
Bipolar and Depressive Disorders Unit, Hospital Clinic, University of Barcelona, IDIBAPS, CIBERSAM, Barcelona, Spain
e-mail: NVERDOLINI@clinic.cat

M. Colizzi, M. Ruggeri (eds.), *Prevention in Mental Health*,
https://doi.org/10.1007/978-3-030-97906-5_14

These non-invasive techniques have provided a considerable deal of information about the brain-based abnormalities that underlie psychiatric disorders, both trans-diagnostically and for specific diagnoses [3, 4]. However, these promising findings have thus far brought limited progress in clinical practice. Brain imaging studies have been mostly useful for the characterisation of pathophysiological mechanisms at group level, because mass univariate analyses can only identify differences in terms of group means. For example, when comparing a group of patients with the disorder of interest to a group of healthy participants, univariate analyses can identify differences based on group but cannot inform diagnostic or prognostic reasoning for the single subject. However, imaging findings have been considered to hold significant promise for the development of objective measures, potentially even capable to contribute to the reshaping of nosological criteria and to address a number of diagnostic issues derived from subjectivity [5].

This is why the recent development of multivariate analysis methods, such as machine learning (ML), has sparked a great deal of interest. ML methods are in fact developments of artificial intelligence that can be used to identify complex patterns within data [6]. ML algorithms can be trained to learn a pattern and employ such knowledge to make predictions on new data. They hence offer the advantage of enabling statistical inferences to be made at the level of the individual and thus yield results with high translational potential in clinical practice. Over the past 20 years, they are increasingly being employed to attempt to discriminate individuals with a psychiatric disorder from healthy controls and most importantly with predictive purposes, for example, to identify individuals who will develop a psychiatric disorder among those who show a vulnerability to it [5]. In addition multivariate analysis methods are inherently sensitive to spatially distributed and subtle effects [7]; hence, they appear better suited for the identification of the neural correlates of psychiatric disorders, which are subtle and distributed rather than large abnormalities in a specific region of the brain.

One of the ML learning algorithms most frequently employed is support vector machine (SVM), a technique used for the classification of individual observations into distinct groups or classes, based on the detection of regularities in high-dimensional data [8]. SVM is a supervised multivariate classification method where 'supervised' refers to the way in which the algorithm is trained [9]. The training phase in ML can in fact be developed employing one of two approaches: supervised and unsupervised. In the first case, the algorithm is being provided with group labels, so, for example, it is told which are the patients and which are the controls; hence, it learns to identify the characteristics that define each of the two pre-specified groups. Other approaches use unsupervised training, and in this case the algorithm aims to identify a structure in the data without being given pre-specified groups; hence, it can be employed to group individuals based on the fact that they share a similar structure without a priori given labels [10].

SVM treats each component of the image as a point in a high-dimensional space. To classify participants and discriminate between groups, the algorithm must define a decision boundary or 'hyperplane', which is a plane that splits a high-dimensional space. However many hyperplanes can correctly divide the data. SVM finds the optimal one, in the sense that it is characterised by the largest distance between the closest data points, which are the most difficult to classify and are called support vectors [9]. Once the hyperplane is defined, new subjects are assigned to one group or the other based on their position relative to the hyperplane [9]. Hence, after the training phase comes the testing phase, where the performance of the classifier is assessed based on the proportion of correctly classified new participants [7].

Deep learning (DL) is another type of ML approach that is raising growing interest due to its ability to learn more complex and abstract patterns of brain structure through consecutive nonlinear transformations [10]. The term 'deep' is used in contrast to the more 'shallow' approach used to extract patterns that characterises SVM.

This chapter will focus on the recent developments towards a translational use of brain imaging techniques. Rather than describing the neuroanatomy of brain abnormalities that characterise each of the examined disorders, it will thus focus on the use of ML techniques for clinical purposes.

In particular the chapter will introduce, where possible, psychiatric applications of machine learning that are focusing on a few main areas of clinical interest; it is to say where multivariate techniques have been used to contribute to answer clinically relevant questions.

The majority of studies have sought to discriminate between individuals already experiencing a specific disorder and healthy controls. This was mostly done in order to test the discriminatory potential at the individual level of ML algorithms, and this chapter will initially summarise efforts made in such direction.

To be useful, however, a clinical tool must provide information that is not already available [11]. Then this chapter will move to describe instances when machine learning algorithms have been used to address questions in one of the following areas of clinical utility:

- First, the area of prediction of clinical outcomes in populations who already suffer from an established disorder and prediction of treatment response
- Second, the area of differential diagnosis between different disorders
- Third, the area of disease risk assessment, when machine learning is employed to discriminate which individuals, within a risk group, will go on to develop the disorder of interest

The chapter then will consider the limitations encountered in the development and implementation of machine learning algorithms as clinical tools and why they may have not yet delivered despite the initial promise. Finally, it will offer a glimpse of hope, looking at future directions.

14.2 Psychosis

Schizophrenia (SZ) is characterised by abnormalities in brain structure [12, 13], function [14], connectivity [15] and neurotransmission [16]. However, when analysed at group level, these brain features show considerable overlap between patients and HC [17], so they are valuable descriptors but can't be used for diagnostic purposes in individual patients. Multivariate pattern recognition approaches, on the other hand, appear especially suitable for the identification of neuroimaging-based markers in psychotic disorders [17] as these disorders are characterised by interconnected brain abnormalities that are subtle and distributed rather than localised [18]. Multivariate approaches also offer the additional advantage of providing single subject information. Early analyses of structural MRI data using ML approaches demonstrated their useful potential in discriminating patients with SZ from healthy controls, with a diagnostic accuracy of around 80% [19]. A number of similar studies followed, and a meta-analysis that compared the classification accuracy obtained using different imaging techniques reported diagnostic accuracies ranging from 60 to 100% [17]. Across all studies included in the meta-analysis, the discrimination between SZ and HC was achieved with sensitivity and specificity around 80% [17]. These early studies led to enthusiastic views about the possibility to incorporate neuroimaging to routine diagnostic processes. However, a number of issues became apparent as the field developed and will be discussed in the limitations section in detail.

One of the main limitations of early studies was their reliance on small samples with data collected at one site. More recent studies have therefore employed large multi-site data sets in order to increase sample heterogeneity and assess cross-site generalisability [20]. Rozycki and colleagues trained a ML classifier using multi-centre MRI data from all but one of the available samples and obtained good accuracies, between 70 and 80%, in predicting class membership of the sample left out from the training phase. The authors highlighted that such accuracies offer promising evidence for the future use of brain-based biomarkers and made the classifier publicly available online [20].

Another limitation specifically encountered when examining SZ is the impossibility to discern whether the discrimination is based on abnormalities that are related to the emergence of the illness or rather to the effects of chronicity and antipsychotic treatment on the brain [21]. Both were identified as significant moderators in a meta-analysis of diagnostic biomarkers [17], raising issues about the possibility to employ models developed in chronic SZ to make inferences about first-episode psychosis (FEP). Indeed a model that achieved 74% accuracy in established SZ performed just above chance (54%) in a FEP sample [22]. This suggests that models trained using data from patients with established SZ may not be useful in the early stages of the illness, yet it is in the early stages that ML algorithms could be useful in cases of diagnostic uncertainty and possibly to inform treatment options. However, to date, only a few studies have employed ML to examine neuroanatomical abnormalities in the early phases of psychotic disorders, and results produced inconsistent results [23]. An early study reported 86% accuracy [24], and two others also reported good accuracies, with 86% and 85%, respectively [25, 26]. However other studies reported only fair [27] or even poor accuracies, as low as 51% [28]. Inconsistencies are attributed to the small sample sizes employed [17] and the use of data from a single site, as well as a number of methodological issues related to the way ML algorithms are implemented [29]. A recent study aimed to address some of the aforementioned limitations and clarify whether the analysis of neuro-anatomical data using ML techniques can discriminate between FEP patients and HC at the individual level [23]. The authors employed five different large-sized data sets and employed different classification approaches including both SVM and DL and used methodological precautions aimed at avoiding overoptimistic results. Performance of all methods employed was relatively modest, with the best performance obtained using DL in two of the data sets analysed, reaching accuracies around 70% [23]. However, both of these best-performing classifiers generalised poorly when applied to the other data sets, achieving accuracies around 50%. This is to say that the pattern learnt by the algorithm using one sample was not able to discriminate FEP from HC above chance level when used to classify participants scanned at a different site. The authors interpreted their findings as confirmatory evidence of the likely overoptimistic results secondary to inadequate sample sizes in previous studies. They also acknowledged publication bias, with positive findings more likely to be published. Overall there appears to be a drop in performance from early studies, which were based on small samples and only analysed data from a single site, to more recent ones, which are using larger data sets from multiple sites [20, 23] and are assessing different algorithms and testing their performance on independent samples [23, 30].

14.2.1 Prognosis Prediction and Treatment Response

The discrimination of individuals already experiencing psychosis from healthy controls might not be the most pressing clinical question, as the clinical manifestations are already evident and patients can be distinguished from healthy controls on clinical grounds. However, within those experiencing a psychotic disorder, clinical outcomes are difficult to predict based purely on clinical manifestations [31]. Patients are therefore treated using a similar approach regardless of what will be the clinical trajectory. Brain imaging studies, however, suggest that poorer outcomes are associated with more pronounced grey matter abnormalities at illness onset [32] and longitudinal reductions over time [33]. Poor response to treatment has been associated with elevated glutamate levels together with non-elevated dopamine neurotransmission [34] and has been linked to abnormalities in white matter integrity measured using DTI [35]. These findings, possibly in conjunction with other biomarkers, may be useful for the stratification of patients according to clinical outcome, with a view to optimising treatment using brain-based outcome or response groups [32]. The studies reported above employed a univariate approach and simply described differences between groups. However, a study that examined baseline MRI data applying ML to predict outcome in a first-episode psychosis sample was able to predict a non-remitting clinical course with 72% accuracy [36]. More recently another study compared the performance of six ML algorithms as well as DL in predicting clinical improvement at 1 year follow-up, using fMRI data in a sample of patients comprising both SZ and bipolar disorder (BD) diagnoses [37]. The best discrimination between patients who subsequently improved and those who didn't was 70% and obtained using DL. Multivariate analysis approaches have also been used across different psychosis spectrum diagnoses, for the identification of so-called biotypes [38], aimed at grounding psychiatric nosology in neurobiology and to redefine current diagnostic categories.

One of the key aims of personalised medicine is to be able to tailor treatments to the individual patient based on a prediction of response. This appears to be an especially important issue in SZ, as one third of patients don't respond to antipsychotic treatment and are considered to have a treatment resistant form of the disorder [39]. Yet, based only on the clinical presentation, it is not possible to predict to which treatment the individual patient will respond. The application of ML approaches as support tools for clinical decision-making holds therefore significant promise [40]. This has been attempted using different types of biomarkers; hence, some studies focused on the use of brain imaging data, while others used imaging together with clinical, electrophysiological and cognitive measures. For example, one study examined drug-naïve FEP patients and used hippocampal-whole brain functional connectivity to explore its ability to predict treatment response [41]. The accuracy in predicting class membership of responders versus non-responders was 89%. Another study examined 138 antipsychotic-naïve FEP patients and 151 HC in order to predict short- and long-term treatment response. The model was developed using sMRI data, together with clinical and cognitive information, taking steps to avoid overfitting [42]. The algorithm was able to discriminate FEP patients from HC with about 64% accuracy, with the classification mainly driven by cognitive information, yet it was not able to predict either short- or long-term treatment response. Other studies have employed designs that might improve the predictive power of ML algorithms, for example, by employing a multicentre approach that can grant larger samples and by including more homogenous patient groups in terms of stage of the illness and previous treatment [31]. For example, Koutsouleris and colleagues applied ML to 334 patients from the European First Episode Schizophrenia Trial (EUFEST) and developed a tool to predict good versus poor treatment outcome, yet variables employed were clinical rather than brain-based [43].

14.2.2 Differential Diagnosis

A number of studies sought to use brain imaging data to identify a differential diagnostic signature of SZ, especially attempting to discriminate it from major depressive disorder (MDD) and bipolar disorder (BD). For example, using fMRI in conjunction with a verbal fluency task, Costafreda [44] and colleagues examined 32 patients with SZ, 32 patients with BD and 40 HC individuals. Based on the pattern of neural responses, the authors were able to identify patients with SZ with 92% accuracy and those with BD with 76%. Another study used sMRI data and was able to discriminate patients with SZ from patients with BD with 88% accuracy. Yet, when applying the algorithm to a separate sample, the accuracy dropped to 66% [45].

Using sMRI, Koutsouleris and colleagues [46] examined 158 patients with SZ and 104 patients with MDD and found that the neuroanatomy-based diagnosis was correct for 72% of the patients with schizophrenia and 80% of those with MMD. Ota and colleagues [47] employed a multimodal approach combining measures of grey matter volume and white matter integrity and were able to correctly classify 80% of patients with SZ and 76% of those with MDD. Classification accuracies remained fairly good when the authors applied the model to a second validation sample, yet sizes were modest at each stage.

14.2.3 Risk Assessment and Prediction of Illness

Psychotic disorders are usually preceded by a 1- to 2-year prodromal phase characterised by subtle symptoms, similar yet less severe or less frequent compared to those observed in the full-blown illness [48]. Individuals that present with these sub-threshold manifestations, similar to those observed in the psychosis prodrome, are at a very high risk of developing a psychotic disorder and are defined as having an At Risk Mental State (ARMS) for psychosis [48].

Operationalised criteria for the identification of high-risk individuals hence include the presence of psychotic symptoms that, compared to those observed in psychosis, are less severe or are short-lasting [49]. The criteria also include either the presence of schizotypal personality disorder or a positive family history, indicating increased genetic vulnerability to psychosis, together with functional decline [49]. High psychosis risk is alternatively defined employing the 'basics symptoms approach', which includes the presence of cognitive, perceptual and language abnormalities [50]. The high-risk phase is considered a critical window for the implementation of potential preventative strategies [49]. The identification of vulnerable individuals is therefore at the core of a paradigm shift in psychosis research that, since the 1990s, aims to develop strategies for early intervention that could potentially delay or even prevent psychosis onset [49]. Yet the ARMS is associated with a risk of developing psychosis of 36% at 3 years [51], while the rest of those meeting high-risk criteria will not develop a psychotic disorder and either experience ongoing sub-threshold symptoms, be diagnosed with another psychiatric disorder or recover without treatment [52]. Hence, a key problem at the clinical level is that it is not possible to predict which individuals, of those at high risk, will subsequently go on to develop psychosis. Thus, any intervention for this group would have to be delivered to the entire sample, rather than being targeted at the subgroup that would later develop a psychotic illness. In order to deal with this clinical issue, the incorporation of neurobiological markers into the assessment of risk has received growing interest, due to its potential to increase prognostic precision and support early diagnosis at the individual level [5].

In particular brain imaging data are considered to hold a significant potential due to the fact that psychotic disorders are considered neurodevelopmental in origin. Hence, some of the brain abnormalities make their appearance prior to illness onset, while further changes occur in association with the FEP [53]. As a group, individuals at high risk of psychosis show several abnormalities that are subtler but qualitatively similar to the ones observed in psychosis [5]. However, evidence from cross-sectional volumetric MRI studies also indicates that there are significant differences between high-risk individuals who subsequently transition to psychosis and those who do not [53, 54]. The latter two groups also differ in terms of brain activation [55, 56] and white matter tract integrity [57, 58], as well as dopaminergic [59] and glutamatergic neurotransmission [60].

The results of these univariate analyses have contributed to elucidate the brain mechanisms underlying psychosis risk, but can't be used to make predictions at the individual level. Considerable interest lays therefore in the potential of multivariate approaches to identify individuals at risk of psychosis using different imaging modalities [61] and especially to identify which individuals will develop psychosis among those that show a vulnerability to it [62]. An early study employing this approach found that the structural neuroanatomy of individuals at risk of psychosis provided information that permitted their distinction from controls, irrespective of clinical outcome, and further indicated that structural abnormalities were most pronounced in the individuals that went on to develop psychosis [63]. Other studies, which specifically used ML to predict transition to psychosis in populations at high risk based on neuroanatomical information [64–67], obtained classification accuracies between 80 and 88%. High accuracies suggest that ML learning could be implemented as a clinical tool for psychosis prediction in populations at high risk, yet a number of issues still need addressing, especially in order to achieve generalisability [29]. No study to date has, in fact, externally validated a prediction of transition model in a sample different to the one it was trained with, yet four large multicentre projects are currently underway [62]. The PRONIA consortium, for example, assessed performance and generalisability of a prognostic model that employed clinical and neuroimaging data to predict functioning at 1-year follow-up [68]. The study examined 116 individuals at high risk for psychosis and 120 patients with recent onset depression and found that ML was able to predict social functioning with 82.7% accuracy in psychosis high-risk individuals and 70.3% in recent onset depression. The best accuracy was obtained when combining clinical and imaging information, and the model outperformed expert prognostication, yet not by a great deal. This suggests that precision medicine tools could contribute to provide more accurate risk assessments and hence concur to the potential development of prevention strategies for functional impairment in early depression and psychosis risk.

14.3 Mood Disorders

14.3.1 Major Depressive Disorder

In major depressive disorder (MDD), similarly to other areas of psychiatric research, initial studies using ML approaches assessed the potential of using brain-based abnormalities to discriminate individuals with the disorder from healthy controls [69]. Using sMRI data Costafreda and colleagues [70] were able to discriminate MDD patients from HC based on grey matter volume with 67.6% accuracy. A more recent study, employing a significantly larger sample size, obtained an accuracy of 90% [71]. Other studies employed fMRI, either at rest or while performing a number of different tasks. The latter aimed at activating cognitive- or emotion-based brain circuits considered to be impaired in patients suffering from MDD. For example, a study using a working memory task, obtained an accuracy of 67.5% [72], another using a reinforcement-learning task reported 97% accuracy, while 95% accuracy was obtained using a verbal fluency task [73]. When employing tasks involved in emotion processing, such as the emotional face-processing task, authors reported 84% accuracy [74], while a task examining social and moral values reported 78.3% accuracy [75]. Good results have also been obtained using resting-state fMRI, with accuracies ranging from 84.2 [76] to 95% [77]. A number of studies also employed DTI data and obtained accuracies ranging from 63 to 91% [78–81].

Finally, a number of studies used a multimodal approach in order to assess the potential improvement in discrimination accuracy that could derive from employing different brain-based measures. A large-scale MDD study (total sample size = 307) by Yang and colleagues used structural MRI and DTI data and reported 75% accuracy in discriminating patients from HC [82]. Kambeitz and colleagues [83] did not employ a multimodal approach but rather compared the classificatory success obtained using measures of grey matter structure, white matter integrity and task or resting state fMRI protocols in a meta-analysis including 912 MDD patients and 894 HC. The authors found that both the classification based on resting-state fMRI (85% sensitivity, 83% specificity) and on DTI data (88% sensitivity, 92% specificity) outperformed classifications based on sMRI (70% sensitivity, 71% specificity) and task-based fMRI (74% sensitivity, 77% specificity).

14.3.1.1 Prognosis Prediction and Treatment Response

The course of MDD can vary significantly from one patient to the other, with 20–25% of those experiencing a major depressive episode being at risk for chronic MDD [84]. Hence, there is a significant interest in the potential of different variables for the prediction of clinical outcomes, as the early identification of chronicity markers could have important implications for the development of preventative strategies targeting factors associated with poorer outcomes. A number of clinical variables have been associated with more severe clinical course [84], and several studies have employed structural and functional MRI as well as positron emission tomography to investigate predictors of treatment response [85]. The evidence of brain features associated with a higher likelihood of a poorer clinical course paved the way to the use of brain imaging data as features in ML prediction algorithms. One study used fMRI data to predict disease course in patients with MDD. The study also employed clinical variables, such as depression severity, number of previous episodes and time in remission, which are easy and inexpensive to obtain. However, clinical variables alone did not predict whether patients remained in remission 14 months later, while the accuracy of outcome predictions based on fMRI data reached 75% [86]. Another study employed a multimodal approach, combining clinical, sMRI and fMRI data [87]. The authors were able to discriminate patients with a chronic course of the illness from those with a more favourable clinical trajectory with 73% accuracy using fMRI data in conjunction with an emotion recognition task, while clinical information, sMRI and fMRI of executive function did not permit between-group discrimination. In light of the importance of the clinical question, several MDD studies applied ML techniques to assess their potential to predict antidepressant treatment response [88, 89]. A recent meta-analysis [88] examined the application of ML algorithms for the prediction of therapeutic outcomes in depression, using clinical, genetic and neuroimaging data. The authors reported that the overall pooled estimate for classification accuracy of the 20 studies included was 82%. Studies employing neuroimaging predictors showed greater accuracy (85%) compared to those using clinical (76%) or genetic predictors (68%). Yet models informed by multiple data modalities provided the highest classification accuracy (93%) suggesting that integrating composite information might be the most powerful approach to determine individual patient response to treatment.

14.3.2 Bipolar Disorder

Bipolar disorder (BD) is characterised by abnormalities in brain structure [90], function and neurotransmission [91]. ML studies in BD have therefore assessed the potential of brain imaging data to discriminate patients from controls, as current approaches to diagnosis are considered far from effective, with an average 10-year gap between the first symptoms and diagnosis [92]. Hence, a number of studies attempted to discriminate BD patients from HC, but most of the focus has been towards the possibility to aid the differential diagnosis with other mood disorders, especially unipolar depression, or with schizophrenia [93]. Mangwi and colleagues applied ML to both grey and white matter density in a large cohort of 256 participants in order to assess the discriminatory potential between BD patients and HC. The accuracy obtained using white matter density was 70.3%, and it was 64.9% using grey matter density, while combining the two measures did not improve the accuracy of the algorithm [94]. Interestingly the patients identified with the highest certainty were characterised by the most severe clinical picture in terms of number of lifetime manic episodes and hospitalisations [94]. Another recent study [95] employed a multimodal approach that combined sMRI and fMRI, and even though the accuracy was high (87.5%), the small sample size (44 BD and 36 HC) limited the generalisability of the results. Frangou and colleagues [96] used fMRI in conjunction with a working memory task and assessed its potential to differentiate patients with BD from HC and from patients' relatives who were either diagnosed with MDD or were free of any personal lifetime history of psychopathology. Patients with BD were correctly classified compared to unrelated HC (83.5% accuracy), to their relatives with MDD (73.1% accuracy) and to their healthy relatives (81.8% accuracy).

The ENIGMA Bipolar Disorder Working Group recently applied ML to MRI data from 853 BD and 2167 HC gathered from 13 participating sites [97]. The discrimination accuracies ranged from 45.23 to 81.07% across sites. Despite the significant heterogeneity, there was agreement in terms of the regions that contributed the most to the discrimination of BD participants from HC. The authors thus concluded that the results were promising, although inferior to 80%, which is considered a clinically relevant accuracy threshold.

14.3.2.1 Prognosis Prediction and Treatment Response

In terms of prediction of outcomes, one of the most important clinical aspects is psychosocial functioning. Indeed, in BD, recovery in terms of psychosocial functioning is rarely achieved even after the remission of mood symptoms, and BD is associated with high rates of daily-life disability. One study used ML to analyse MRI volumetric data in BD and HC and identified brain volume changes as predictors of psychosocial functioning [98].

In terms of prediction of treatment, only one study to date used ML techniques to test whether brain-based biological markers can be useful for the prediction of treatment response. The authors employed ML with both fMRI and MRS data and obtained 80% accuracy in predicting lithium response in first-episode mania [99]. The authors acknowledged the very small sample size and considered the study as a proof of concept and a pilot for future work.

14.3.2.2 Differential Diagnosis

An important focus of ML studies has been the discrimination between BD and MDD. Misdiagnosis of BD as MDD may lead to inappropriate treatment and poorer prognosis. Hence, the early discrimination between the two disorders has important implications for clinical management and treatment decisions. This is especially the case when the onset of BD manifests with a depressive episode; hence, the discrimination between unipolar and bipolar depression is an important step towards the prevention of antidepressant use without mood stabilisation. A number of recent studies employed sMRI data to discriminate MDD from BD and obtained accuracies ranging from 54.8 [100] to 88.1% [101]. In particular, Redlich and colleagues were able to discriminate MDD from BD with 79.3% accuracy, yet when they further validated the findings using an independent data set, they obtained an accuracy of 65.5% [102]. Hence, even though the algorithm achieved a good performance, generalisability was poor.

Using resting state fMRI, one study [103] was able to discriminate BD from MDD with 75% accuracy, while another study [104] used resting state fMRI to assess brain connectivity and obtained an accuracy of 86% in the discrimination of unipolar from bipolar depression. Due to the known emotion perception deficits in MDD and BD [105], a number of studies employed fMRI in conjunction with emotion recognition tasks in order to discriminate between the two disorders. One of such studies obtained 72% accuracy in the discrimination between MDD and BD [106], while Grotegerd and colleagues conducted two separate analyses using the same task [107, 108], one considering the whole brain and the other focusing on the amygdala. The whole brain fMRI study reached 90% accuracy [108], while the one focused on amygdala yielded an accuracy of almost 80% [107]. A few studies also employed a multimodal approach [109–111] assessing the ability of sMRI and resting state fMRI data to discriminate MDD from BD, obtaining accuracies ranging from 69.1 [110] to 92.1% [111] Finally, using DTI Deng and colleagues [78] observed that FA measures of the left anterior thalamic radiation could be used to discriminate BD from MDD with 68.3% accuracy.

All of the above-reported studies trained classifiers using data obtained from patients with an established BD diagnosis. However it is in the early stages of a depressive presentation that it is of greatest clinical importance to discriminate between an emergent unipolar or bipolar clinical picture, even before the index manic episode. It is in this phase that a neuroimaging-based tool able to inform the diagnostic process would be most useful. One study used SVM to distinguish between first-episode psychotic mania, first-episode psychotic MDD and HC, but accuracies were modest, with 66.1% when discriminating BD from HC and only 54.7% in BD versus MDD [100]. Another study specifically attempted to discriminate unipolar from bipolar depression before the onset of a manic episode, using resting state fMRI measures of connectivity [112]. The authors were able to discriminate individuals with unipolar depression from individuals who subsequently transitioned to BD from an initial depressive presentation, with 78% accuracy. The study was conducted using data from a single site and lacked external validation yet offered a promising perspective on the potential use of brain-based classifiers for differential diagnosis purposes in the initial stages of affective disorders.

14.3.2.3 Risk Assessment and Prediction of Illness

Children of individuals with BD are at increased risk of developing mood disorders; hence, the study of neurobiological markers in this population is considered of crucial importance for the understanding of vulnerability-related mechanisms. However, there are no strategies, at present, to predict which of the high-risk children will develop a mood disorder. Mourao-Miranda and colleagues examined healthy adolescents at genetic risk of BD and low-risk offspring of healthy parents using fMRI in conjunction with an emotional face recognition task [113]. Using a ML approach, they were able to discriminate the two groups with 75% accuracy and also found that predictive probabilities were significantly higher for the genetic risk adolescents who subsequently went on to develop a psychiatric disorder. The results were hence promising, yet participants were 16 per group. Another study used proton magnetic resonance spectroscopy (H-MRS) data, including measures of glutamate, choline and N-acetyl aspartate obtained from the anterior cingulate and ventrolateral prefrontal cortex [114]. The authors examined 19 high-risk youth who subsequently developed a first mood episode and 19 high-risk participants who did not convert over the follow-up period and were able to discriminate them with 76% accuracy using measures of choline. The authors hence emphasised the possible role of brain metabolites as predictors of future mood episodes in high-risk offspring.

14.4 Anxiety Disorders

Only a few studies employed ML for the analysis of brain imaging data in patients suffering from anxiety disorders. Employing sMRI data to discriminate patients suffering from obsessive-compulsive disorder (OCD) from HC participants, Soriano-Mas and colleagues [115] obtained 76.6% accuracy, while other sMRI studies reported accuracies ranging from 73 to 95.6% [116–119]. Only a small fMRI study in conjunction with an emotional valence task was conducted in OCD, reporting 100% accuracy [120], while the accuracy of studies using resting state fMRI ranged from 72 to 80% [121]. Finally, a multimodal study compared classification results achieved using both resting state and task-related fMRI, while Bu and colleagues [122] assessed the predictive potential of different resting state fMRI parameters, in an effort to identify the most predictive features, and obtained an array of performances, ranging from fairly weak to 95%.

Two ML studies examined social anxiety using different MRI modalities [123, 124]. Both obtained an overall accuracy of around 80% in discriminating patients from HC and highlighted the distributed nature of brain abnormalities associated with social anxiety. One study examined the discrimination potential of sMRI data in *post-traumatic stress disorder* (PTSD). The authors compared 50 earthquake survivors who had developed PTSD with 50 who hadn't and 40 HC who had not been exposed to the earthquake. When survivors with PTSD were compared with HC, measures of grey and white matter provided 91% discrimination accuracy, while the accuracy was only 67% when comparing survivors with and without PTSD [125].

14.5 Neurodevelopmental Disorders

14.5.1 Autism and Autism Spectrum Disorders

Autism and autism spectrum disorders (ASD) have been also studied using ML techniques. These disorders are considered neurodevelopmental in origin and are characterised by impaired social communication and deficits in social-emotional reciprocity. Early studies applied ML to sMRI and examined the discriminatory potential between patients with ASD and HC, obtaining accuracies that ranged from 81 [126] to 90% [127]. In particular, the first study employed whole brain information, while the second one used a region of interest approach. Both studies included only males. Similarly, Uddin and colleagues [128] trained an algorithm based on sMRI features, obtaining a model with 90% accuracy, while Jiao and colleagues [129] sought to compare the accuracy obtained employing whole brain morphometric information versus measurements of cortical thickness. The authors found that thickness-based models (87% accuracy) were superior to those based on volumetric morphometry (74% accuracy). Other MRI techniques were also used for the development of ASD classification models. Task-based fMRI studies obtained accuracies ranging from 69

[130] to 97% [131], while studies employing resting state fMRI reported accuracies ranging from 71.1 [132] to 100% [133]. DTI studies achieved accuracies between 78 and 100% [134]. Finally, a study assessing differences in functional connectivity of large-scale brain networks reached 78 % accuracy [135]. A few studies employed a multimodal approach. The combination of connectivity measures extracted from fMRI and measures of FA from DTI resulted in 95.9% accuracy [136], while a combination of resting state fMRI and sMRI achieved 65% accuracy [137].

In terms of prediction of clinical outcomes, one study successfully predicted future language level in children with ASD on the basis of behavioural and fMRI data, finding that the combination of behavioural and fMRI predictors resulted in the highest accuracy (80%) [138].

These results suggest that different imaging modalities hold potential for the discrimination of clinically diagnosed individuals and appear as an initial step towards the development of algorithms that will be able to answer more complicated clinical questions and possibly inform therapeutic decision-making. Towards these goals future studies should employ larger sample sizes and a prognostic design, for example, in order to dissect the functional heterogeneity of ASD, characterised by different symptom domains and variable levels of psychosocial functioning.

14.5.2 Attention-Deficit/Hyperactivity Disorder

Attention-deficit/hyperactivity disorder (ADHD) has been examined using different MRI modalities. Using sMRI, the classification accuracies for ADHD versus HC ranged between 72 and 93% [139–141]. Studies using task-based fMRI mainly employed tasks assessing attention and impulsiveness and achieved accuracies between 61.1 [142] and 91.2%. Park and colleagues [143] examined connectivity differences between ADHD subtypes, attempting to classify them on the basis of neuroimaging features obtained using six different tasks. ADHD is in fact characterised by different symptom dimensions, manifesting in clinical subtypes such as inattentive, hyperactive/impulsive and combined. The authors found that the classifier was able to distinguish between ADHD subtypes with 91.18% accuracy using both gambling punishment and emotion-related paradigms, which showed a significant correlation with rates of hyperactivity and impulsivity. Studies employing resting state fMRI reported prediction accuracies that ranged between very low (54%) [144] and high (96.06%). No ML study to date has employed DTI-based features for ADHD discrimination, despite previous studies reporting white matter tract abnormalities in ADHD. Finally, several studies employed a multimodal approach for ADHD discrimination including structural and both resting state or task-based fMRI data, with accuracies ranging from very poor (55%) [145] to fairly good (80%) [146].

14.6   Limitations

ML approaches hold considerable clinical promise, yet they are also burdened by significant limitations [29]. The main issue when employing a ML algorithm built using one sample is the possibility for it to generalise to other independent samples, and many factors contribute to render generalisability a difficult process. The first is the issue that arises as a consequence of differences in image acquisition and processing across different centres. An important feature of a real-world tool will therefore be its ability to account for inter-scanner variability. Individuals will be scanned at different locations, and the effects of this variability can be particularly relevant in psychiatry. Such effects can in fact potentially be even larger than the subtle disease-related effects of interest observed in psychiatric disorders [147].

A further issue is the clear definition of the scope of the model, in other words the definition of which individuals the model can make high-quality predictions about [148]. This is fundamentally related to the population used to train the algorithm that needs to be sufficiently representative of the population in which the algorithm itself will be subsequently tested upon [149]. Similarly, training an algorithm in a relatively small sample can lead to overoptimistic results [150]. The use of relatively small sample sizes can in fact lead to inflated estimations due to the relative homogeneity of small samples relative to larger ones, which can make it easier for the algorithm to learn discriminatory patterns [23].

The development and validation of tools that can be employed in clinical practice will thus have to rely on samples that are large enough to reflect the significant heterogeneity that characterises psychiatric disorders, both in clinical and pathophysiological terms, and that makes the development of such tools more challenging [151]. Large data sets may reduce heterogeneity-related problems, as they can represent the whole spectrum of a disorder. Larger samples will also be able to account for gender- and age-specific effects [152].

Other issues are specific to the implementation of ML algorithms themselves. Good accuracies can, for example, reflect overfitting, which occurs when the model describes not only the effects of interest but also the noise in the data. [29]. Overfitting results in very good performance in the training data but generalises very poorly to new data. Models trained using a large number of features and a small number of subjects are more susceptible to overfitting, and this is regularly the case when using brain imaging data [153]. Neuroimaging studies tend in fact to have a relatively small number of subjects and a very large number of features, namely, millions of brain voxels for each subject. This issue, known as the curse of dimensionality, is being dealt with using different strategies for feature selection and will be attenuated by pooling data from large-sized consortia.

The main challenge, once technical difficulties for model development will be addressed, will be the validation of actual tools that can be employed in clinical practice [11, 152]. Models are currently being developed using each time larger data sets, obtained using multicentre study designs. These sets of data are very well characterised in order to obtain the highest discrimination accuracies, yet the transition from models to clinically useful tools will require addressing further problems. The first important issue in the translational process will be the validation of a specific model using real-world data sets. Thus, even for a model showing good performance across different research data sets, there will be additional heterogeneity in clinical practice compared to the relative homogeneity observed in research. This is because the fairly stringent inclusion criteria employed in research settings [11] result in the selection of prototypical patients [2]. Clinical populations will be characterised by a wider range of severities, a higher frequency of comorbidities and a number of other factors likely to reduce the sensitivity, specificity and accuracy of the algorithm, hence the clinical applicability of the method [2].

A further issue towards the development of brain imaging-based clinical tools does not have a technical basis but is rather rooted in taxonomy. Categorical psychiatric diagnoses are not based on biological mechanisms; hence, the search for clinical tools might be complicated by conventional diagnostic boundaries themselves and additionally confounded by frequent comorbidities [2]. It has thus been suggested that a dimensional approach might better reflect clinical reality and permit a stratification of outcomes, due to the unlikely match between DSM-/ICD-defined disorders and biological mechanisms [2]. The research domain criteria (RDoC) approach, for example, is being developed as a different classification framework that might more closely reflect biological mechanisms [154].

14.7   Future Directions

Despite the technical difficulties of this still emerging area of research, a number of encouraging findings have led research teams to implement imaging-based tools aimed at increasing diagnostic and prognostic accuracies compared to those based on clinical data alone [152]. With these tools the clinician can obtain an automatic individual patient report to inform the diagnostic process. However all the tools available at present have been developed to support the diagnosis of specific neurological disorders, in particular Alzheimer's disease and other forms of dementia and multiple sclerosis [152]. All can be used to aid the diagnostic process for a single disorder, but none is validated for the differential diagnosis between multiple disorders. Two can also employ longitudinal data to predict the course of the illness, while none has yet been validated for the prediction of treatment response [152].

No clinical tool is available at the moment for use in psychiatric disorders. This can in part be attributed to the different characteristics of brain abnormalities in psychiatric relative to neurological disorders. The former tend to be subtle and widespread [155], as well as not pathognomonic of a single disorder.

The results of studies employing a ML approach in psychiatry should therefore be interpreted with caution. This is due to the, sometimes, overoptimistic results obtained, especially when employing small samples, and the issues that still prevent their development as clinical tools. They hold however significant potential towards the future development of personalised medicine, and large multicentre studies are warranted to address issues reported above, such as generalisability and reproducibility, which will be fundamental steps towards the clinical implementation of ML algorithms in psychiatry.

References

1. Regier DA, Narrow WE, Clarke DE, Kraemer HC, Kuramoto SJ, Kuhl EA, et al. DSM-5 field trials in the United States and Canada, part II: test-retest reliability of selected categorical diagnoses. Am J Psychiatry. 2013;170(1):59–70.
2. Kapur S, Phillips AG, Insel TR. Why has it taken so long for biological psychiatry to develop clinical tests and what to do about it? Mol Psychiatry. 2012;17(12):1174–9.
3. Goodkind M, Eickhoff SB, Oathes DJ, Jiang Y, Chang A, Jones-Hagata LB, et al. Identification of a common neurobiological substrate for mental illness. JAMA Psychiatry. 2015;72(4):305–15.
4. Mitelman SA. Transdiagnostic neuroimaging in psychiatry: a review. Psychiatry Res. 2019;277:23–38.
5. McGuire P, Sato JR, Mechelli A, Jackowski A, Bressan RA, Zugman A. Can neuroimaging be used to predict the onset of psychosis? Lancet Psychiatry. 2015;2(12):1117–22.
6. Mitchell T. Machine learning. New York: McGraw-Hill; 1998. p. 1998.
7. Orru G, Pettersson-Yeo W, Marquand AF, Sartori G, Mechelli A. Using Support Vector Machine to identify imaging biomarkers of neurological and psychiatric disease: a critical review. Neurosci Biobehav Rev. 2012;36(4):1140–52.
8. Mourao-Miranda J, Bokde AL, Born C, Hampel H, Stetter M. Classifying brain states and determining the discriminating activation patterns: support Vector Machine on functional MRI data. Neuroimage. 2005;28(4):980–95.
9. Vapnik V. The nature of statistical learning theory. New York: Springer; 1995.
10. Vieira S, Pinaya WH, Mechelli A. Using deep learning to investigate the neuroimaging correlates of psychiatric and neurological disorders: methods and applications. Neurosci Biobehav Rev. 2017;74(Pt A):58–75.
11. Mechelli A, Vieira S. From models to tools: clinical translation of machine learning studies in psychosis. NPJ Schizophr. 2020;6(1):4.
12. van Erp TGM, Walton E, Hibar DP, Schmaal L, Jiang W, Glahn DC, et al. Cortical brain abnormalities in 4474 individuals with schizophrenia and 5098 control subjects via the Enhancing Neuro Imaging Genetics Through Meta Analysis (ENIGMA) Consortium. Biol Psychiatry. 2018;84(9):644–54.
13. Kelly S, Jahanshad N, Zalesky A, Kochunov P, Agartz I, Alloza C, et al. Widespread white matter microstructural differences in schizophrenia across 4322 individuals: results from the ENIGMA Schizophrenia DTI Working Group. Mol Psychiatry. 2018;23(5):1261–9.
14. Minzenberg MJ, Laird AR, Thelen S, Carter CS, Glahn DC. Meta-analysis of 41 functional neuroimaging studies of executive function in schizophrenia. Arch Gen Psychiatry. 2009;66(8):811–22.
15. Brandl F, Avram M, Weise B, Shang J, Simoes B, Bertram T, et al. Specific substantial dysconnectivity in schizophrenia: a transdiagnostic multimodal meta-analysis of resting-state functional and structural magnetic resonance imaging studies. Biol Psychiatry. 2019;85(7):573–83.
16. Howes OD, Kapur S. The dopamine hypothesis of schizophrenia: version III--the final common pathway. Schizophr Bull. 2009;35(3):549–62.
17. Kambeitz J, Kambeitz-Ilankovic L, Leucht S, Wood S, Davatzikos C, Malchow B, et al. Detecting neuroimaging biomarkers for schizophrenia: a meta-analysis of multivariate pattern recognition studies. Neuropsychopharmacology. 2015;40(7):1742–51.

18. Chan RC, Di X, McAlonan GM, Gong QY. Brain anatomical abnormalities in high-risk individuals, first-episode, and chronic schizophrenia: an activation likelihood estimation meta-analysis of illness progression. Schizophr Bull. 2011;37(1):177–88.

19. Davatzikos C, Shen D, Gur RC, Wu X, Liu D, Fan Y, et al. Whole-brain morphometric study of schizophrenia revealing a spatially complex set of focal abnormalities. Arch Gen Psychiatry. 2005;62(11):1218–27.

20. Rozycki M, Satterthwaite TD, Koutsouleris N, Erus G, Doshi J, Wolf DH, et al. Multisite machine learning analysis provides a robust structural imaging signature of schizophrenia detectable across diverse patient populations and within individuals. Schizophr Bull. 2018;44(5):1035–44.

21. Vita A, De Peri L, Deste G, Barlati S, Sacchetti E. The effect of antipsychotic treatment on cortical gray matter changes in schizophrenia: does the class matter? A meta-analysis and meta-regression of longitudinal magnetic resonance imaging studies. Biol Psychiatry. 2015;78(6):403–12.

22. Pinaya WH, Gadelha A, Doyle OM, Noto C, Zugman A, Cordeiro Q, et al. Using deep belief network modelling to characterize differences in brain morphometry in schizophrenia. Sci Rep. 2016;6:38897.

23. Vieira S, Gong QY, Pinaya WHL, Scarpazza C, Tognin S, Crespo-Facorro B, et al. Using machine learning and structural neuroimaging to detect first episode psychosis: reconsidering the evidence. Schizophr Bull. 2020;46(1):17–26.

24. Sun D, van Erp TG, Thompson PM, Bearden CE, Daley M, Kushan L, et al. Elucidating a magnetic resonance imaging-based neuroanatomic biomarker for psychosis: classification analysis using probabilistic brain atlas and machine learning algorithms. Biol Psychiatry. 2009;66(11):1055–60.

25. Borgwardt S, Koutsouleris N, Aston J, Studerus E, Smieskova R, Riecher-Rossler A, et al. Distinguishing prodromal from first-episode psychosis using neuroanatomical single-subject pattern recognition. Schizophr Bull. 2013;39(5):1105–14.

26. Xiao Y, Yan Z, Zhao Y, Tao B, Sun H, Li F, et al. Support vector machine-based classification of first episode drug-naive schizophrenia patients and healthy controls using structural MRI. Schizophr Res. 2019;214:11–7.

27. Pettersson-Yeo W, Benetti S, Marquand AF, Dell'acqua F, Williams SC, Allen P, et al. Using genetic, cognitive and multi-modal neuroimaging data to identify ultra-high-risk and first-episode psychosis at the individual level. Psychol Med. 2013;43(12):2547–62.

28. Winterburn JL, Voineskos AN, Devenyi GA, Plitman E, de la Fuente-Sandoval C, Bhagwat N, et al. Can we accurately classify schizophrenia patients from healthy controls using magnetic resonance imaging and machine learning? A multi-method and multi-dataset study. Schizophr Res. 2019;214:3–10.

29. Arbabshirani MR, Plis S, Sui J, Calhoun VD. Single subject prediction of brain disorders in neuroimaging: promises and pitfalls. Neuroimage. 2017;145(Pt B):137–65.

30. Salvador R, Radua J, Canales-Rodriguez EJ, Solanes A, Sarro S, Goikolea JM, et al. Evaluation of machine learning algorithms and structural features for optimal MRI-based diagnostic prediction in psychosis. PLoS One. 2017;12(4):e0175683.

31. McGuire P, Dazzan P. Does neuroimaging have a role in predicting outcomes in psychosis? World Psychiatry. 2017;16(2):209–10.

32. Dazzan P, Arango C, Fleischacker W, Galderisi S, Glenthoj B, Leucht S, et al. Magnetic resonance imaging and the prediction of outcome in first-episode schizophrenia: a review of current evidence and directions for future research. Schizophr Bull. 2015;41(3):574–83.

33. Lappin JM, Morgan C, Chalavi S, Morgan KD, Reinders AA, Fearon P, et al. Bilateral hippocampal increase following first-episode psychosis is associated with good clinical, functional and cognitive outcomes. Psychol Med. 2014;44(6):1279–91.

34. Demjaha A, Egerton A, Murray RM, Kapur S, Howes OD, Stone JM, et al. Antipsychotic treatment resistance in schizophrenia associated with elevated glutamate levels but normal dopamine function. Biol Psychiatry. 2014;75(5):e11–3.

35. Reis Marques T, Taylor H, Chaddock C, Dell'acqua F, Handley R, Reinders AA, et al. White matter integrity as a predictor of response to treatment in first episode psychosis. Brain. 2014;137(Pt 1):172–82.
36. Mourao-Miranda J, Reinders AA, Rocha-Rego V, Lappin J, Rondina J, Morgan C, et al. Individualized prediction of illness course at the first psychotic episode: a support vector machine MRI study. Psychol Med. 2012;42(5):1037–47.
37. Smucny J, Davidson I, Carter CS. Comparing machine and deep learning-based algorithms for prediction of clinical improvement in psychosis with functional magnetic resonance imaging. Hum Brain Mapp. 2021;42:1197–205.
38. Tamminga CA, Clementz BA. Biological fingerprints for psychosis. Neuropsychopharmacology. 2020;45(1):235–7.
39. Meltzer HY. Treatment-resistant schizophrenia--the role of clozapine. Curr Med Res Opin. 1997;14(1):1–20.
40. Korda AI, Andreou C, Borgwardt S. Pattern classification as decision support tool in antipsychotic treatment algorithms. Exp Neurol. 2021;339:113635.
41. Blessing EM, Murty VP, Zeng B, Wang J, Davachi L, Goff DC. Anterior hippocampal-cortical functional connectivity distinguishes antipsychotic naive first-episode psychosis patients from controls and may predict response to second-generation antipsychotic treatment. Schizophr Bull. 2020;46(3):680–9.
42. Ambrosen KS, Skjerbaek MW, Foldager J, Axelsen MC, Bak N, Arvastson L, et al. A machine-learning framework for robust and reliable prediction of short- and long-term treatment response in initially antipsychotic-naive schizophrenia patients based on multimodal neuropsychiatric data. Transl Psychiatry. 2020;10(1):276.
43. Koutsouleris N, Kahn RS, Chekroud AM, Leucht S, Falkai P, Wobrock T, et al. Multisite prediction of 4-week and 52-week treatment outcomes in patients with first-episode psychosis: a machine learning approach. Lancet Psychiatry. 2016;3(10):935–46.
44. Costafreda SG, Fu CH, Picchioni M, Toulopoulou T, McDonald C, Kravariti E, et al. Pattern of neural responses to verbal fluency shows diagnostic specificity for schizophrenia and bipolar disorder. BMC Psychiatry. 2011;11:18.
45. Schnack HG, Nieuwenhuis M, van Haren NE, Abramovic L, Scheewe TW, Brouwer RM, et al. Can structural MRI aid in clinical classification? A machine learning study in two independent samples of patients with schizophrenia, bipolar disorder and healthy subjects. Neuroimage. 2014;84:299–306.
46. Koutsouleris N, Meisenzahl EM, Borgwardt S, Riecher-Rossler A, Frodl T, Kambeitz J, et al. Individualized differential diagnosis of schizophrenia and mood disorders using neuroanatomical biomarkers. Brain. 2015;138(Pt 7):2059–73.
47. Ota M, Ishikawa M, Sato N, Hori H, Sasayama D, Hattori K, et al. Discrimination between schizophrenia and major depressive disorder by magnetic resonance imaging of the female brain. J Psychiatr Res. 2013;47(10):1383–8.
48. Yung AR, McGorry PD. The prodromal phase of first-episode psychosis: past and current conceptualizations. Schizophr Bull. 1996;22(2):353–70.
49. Fusar-Poli P, Borgwardt S, Bechdolf A, Addington J, Riecher-Rossler A, Schultze-Lutter F, et al. The psychosis high-risk state: a comprehensive state-of-the-art review. JAMA Psychiatry. 2013;70(1):107–20.
50. Schultze-Lutter F, Ruhrmann S, Berning J, Maier W, Klosterkotter J. Basic symptoms and ultrahigh risk criteria: symptom development in the initial prodromal state. Schizophr Bull. 2010;36(1):182–91.
51. Fusar-Poli P, Bonoldi I, Yung AR, Borgwardt S, Kempton MJ, Valmaggia L, et al. Predicting psychosis: meta-analysis of transition outcomes in individuals at high clinical risk. Arch Gen Psychiatry. 2012;69(3):220–9.
52. Lin A, Wood SJ, Nelson B, Beavan A, McGorry P, Yung AR. Outcomes of nontransitioned cases in a sample at ultra-high risk for psychosis. Am J Psychiatry. 2015;172(3):249–58.

53. Pantelis C, Velakoulis D, McGorry PD, Wood SJ, Suckling J, Phillips LJ, et al. Neuroanatomical abnormalities before and after onset of psychosis: a cross-sectional and longitudinal MRI comparison. Lancet. 2003;361(9354):281–8.

54. Mechelli A, Riecher-Rossler A, Meisenzahl EM, Tognin S, Wood SJ, Borgwardt SJ, et al. Neuroanatomical abnormalities that predate the onset of psychosis: a multicenter study. Arch Gen Psychiatry. 2011;68(5):489–95.

55. Sabb FW, van Erp TG, Hardt ME, Dapretto M, Caplan R, Cannon TD, et al. Language network dysfunction as a predictor of outcome in youth at clinical high risk for psychosis. Schizophr Res. 2010;116(2-3):173–83.

56. Allen P, Luigjes J, Howes OD, Egerton A, Hirao K, Valli I, et al. Transition to psychosis associated with prefrontal and subcortical dysfunction in ultra high-risk individuals. Schizophr Bull. 2012;38(6):1268–76.

57. Bloemen OJ, de Koning MB, Schmitz N, Nieman DH, Becker HE, de Haan L, et al. White-matter markers for psychosis in a prospective ultra-high-risk cohort. Psychol Med. 2010;40(8):1297–304.

58. Carletti F, Woolley JB, Bhattacharyya S, Perez-Iglesias R, Fusar Poli P, Valmaggia L, et al. Alterations in white matter evident before the onset of psychosis. Schizophr Bull. 2012;38(6):1170–9.

59. Howes OD, Bose SK, Turkheimer F, Valli I, Egerton A, Valmaggia LR, et al. Dopamine synthesis capacity before onset of psychosis: a prospective [18F]-DOPA PET imaging study. Am J Psychiatry. 2011;168(12):1311–7.

60. Bossong MG, Antoniades M, Azis M, Samson C, Quinn B, Bonoldi I, et al. Association of hippocampal glutamate levels with adverse outcomes in individuals at clinical high risk for psychosis. JAMA Psychiatry. 2019;76(2):199–207.

61. Valli I, Marquand AF, Mechelli A, Raffin M, Allen P, Seal ML, et al. Identifying individuals at high risk of psychosis: predictive utility of support vector machine using structural and functional MRI data. Front Psychiatry. 2016;7:52.

62. Andreou C, Borgwardt S. Structural and functional imaging markers for susceptibility to psychosis. Mol Psychiatry. 2020;25(11):2773–85.

63. Koutsouleris N, Gaser C, Bottlender R, Davatzikos C, Decker P, Jager M, et al. Use of neuroanatomical pattern regression to predict the structural brain dynamics of vulnerability and transition to psychosis. Schizophr Res. 2010;123(2-3):175–87.

64. Koutsouleris N, Borgwardt S, Meisenzahl EM, Bottlender R, Moller HJ, Riecher-Rossler A. Disease prediction in the at-risk mental state for psychosis using neuroanatomical biomarkers: results from the FePsy study. Schizophr Bull. 2012;38(6):1234–46.

65. Koutsouleris N, Meisenzahl EM, Davatzikos C, Bottlender R, Frodl T, Scheuerecker J, et al. Use of neuroanatomical pattern classification to identify subjects in at-risk mental states of psychosis and predict disease transition. Arch Gen Psychiatry. 2009;66(7):700–12.

66. Koutsouleris N, Riecher-Rossler A, Meisenzahl EM, Smieskova R, Studerus E, Kambeitz-Ilankovic L, et al. Detecting the psychosis prodrome across high-risk populations using neuroanatomical biomarkers. Schizophr Bull. 2015;41(2):471–82.

67. Zarogianni E, Storkey AJ, Borgwardt S, Smieskova R, Studerus E, Riecher-Rossler A, et al. Individualized prediction of psychosis in subjects with an at-risk mental state. Schizophr Res. 2019;214:18–23.

68. Koutsouleris N, Kambeitz-Ilankovic L, Ruhrmann S, Rosen M, Ruef A, Dwyer DB, et al. Prediction models of functional outcomes for individuals in the clinical high-risk state for psychosis or with recent-onset depression: a multimodal, multisite machine learning analysis. JAMA Psychiatry. 2018;75(11):1156–72.

69. Savitz JB, Rauch SL, Drevets WC. Clinical application of brain imaging for the diagnosis of mood disorders: the current state of play. Mol Psychiatry. 2013;18(5):528–39.

70. Costafreda SG, Chu C, Ashburner J, Fu CH. Prognostic and diagnostic potential of the structural neuroanatomy of depression. PLoS One. 2009;4(7):e6353.

71. Mwangi B, Ebmeier KP, Matthews K, Steele JD. Multi-centre diagnostic classification of individual structural neuroimaging scans from patients with major depressive disorder. Brain. 2012;135(Pt 5):1508–21.
72. Marquand AF, Mourao-Miranda J, Brammer MJ, Cleare AJ, Fu CH. Neuroanatomy of verbal working memory as a diagnostic biomarker for depression. Neuroreport. 2008;19(15):1507–11.
73. Johnston BA, Tolomeo S, Gradin V, Christmas D, Matthews K, Steele JD. Failure of hippocampal deactivation during loss events in treatment-resistant depression. Brain. 2015;138(Pt 9):2766–76.
74. Fu CH, Mourao-Miranda J, Costafreda SG, Khanna A, Marquand AF, Williams SC, et al. Pattern classification of sad facial processing: toward the development of neurobiological markers in depression. Biol Psychiatry. 2008;63(7):656–62.
75. Sato JR, Moll J, Green S, Deakin JF, Thomaz CE, Zahn R. Machine learning algorithm accurately detects fMRI signature of vulnerability to major depression. Psychiatry Res. 2015;233(2):289–91.
76. Yu Y, Shen H, Zeng LL, Ma Q, Hu D. Convergent and divergent functional connectivity patterns in schizophrenia and depression. PLoS One. 2013;8(7):e68250.
77. Craddock RC, Holtzheimer PE III, Hu XP, Mayberg HS. Disease state prediction from resting state functional connectivity. Magn Reson Med. 2009;62(6):1619–28.
78. Deng F, Wang Y, Huang H, Niu M, Zhong S, Zhao L, et al. Abnormal segments of right uncinate fasciculus and left anterior thalamic radiation in major and bipolar depression. Prog Neuropsychopharmacol Biol Psychiatry. 2018;81:340–9.
79. Fang P, Zeng LL, Shen H, Wang L, Li B, Liu L, et al. Increased cortical-limbic anatomical network connectivity in major depression revealed by diffusion tensor imaging. PLoS One. 2012;7(9):e45972.
80. Sacchet MD, Prasad G, Foland-Ross LC, Thompson PM, Gotlib IH. Support vector machine classification of major depressive disorder using diffusion-weighted neuroimaging and graph theory. Front Psychiatry. 2015;6:21.
81. Schnyer DM, Clasen PC, Gonzalez C, Beevers CG. Evaluating the diagnostic utility of applying a machine learning algorithm to diffusion tensor MRI measures in individuals with major depressive disorder. Psychiatry Res Neuroimaging. 2017;264:1–9.
82. Yang J, Zhang M, Ahn H, Zhang Q, Jin TB, Li I, et al. Development and evaluation of a multimodal marker of major depressive disorder. Hum Brain Mapp. 2018;39(11):4420–39.
83. Kambeitz J, Cabral C, Sacchet MD, Gotlib IH, Zahn R, Serpa MH, et al. Detecting neuroimaging biomarkers for depression: a meta-analysis of multivariate pattern recognition studies. Biol Psychiatry. 2017;82(5):330–8.
84. Penninx BW, Nolen WA, Lamers F, Zitman FG, Smit JH, Spinhoven P, et al. Two-year course of depressive and anxiety disorders: results from the Netherlands Study of Depression and Anxiety (NESDA). J Affect Disord. 2011;133(1–2):76–85.
85. Fu CH, Steiner H, Costafreda SG. Predictive neural biomarkers of clinical response in depression: a meta-analysis of functional and structural neuroimaging studies of pharmacological and psychological therapies. Neurobiol Dis. 2013;52:75–83.
86. Lythe KE, Moll J, Gethin JA, Workman CI, Green S, Lambon Ralph MA, et al. Self-blame-selective hyperconnectivity between anterior temporal and subgenual cortices and prediction of recurrent depressive episodes. JAMA Psychiatry. 2015;72(11):1119–26.
87. Schmaal L, Marquand AF, Rhebergen D, van Tol MJ, Ruhe HG, van der Wee NJ, et al. Predicting the naturalistic course of major depressive disorder using clinical and multimodal neuroimaging information: a multivariate pattern recognition study. Biol Psychiatry. 2015;78(4):278–86.
88. Lee Y, Ragguett RM, Mansur RB, Boutilier JJ, Rosenblat JD, Trevizol A, et al. Applications of machine learning algorithms to predict therapeutic outcomes in depression: a meta-analysis and systematic review. J Affect Disord. 2018;241:519–32.
89. Perlman K, Benrimoh D, Israel S, Rollins C, Brown E, Tunteng JF, et al. A systematic meta-review of predictors of antidepressant treatment outcome in major depressive disorder. J Affect Disord. 2019;243:503–15.

90. Hibar DP, Westlye LT, Doan NT, Jahanshad N, Cheung JW, Ching CRK, et al. Cortical abnormalities in bipolar disorder: an MRI analysis of 6503 individuals from the ENIGMA Bipolar Disorder Working Group. Mol Psychiatry. 2018;23(4):932–42.
91. Strakowski SM, Delbello MP, Adler CM. The functional neuroanatomy of bipolar disorder: a review of neuroimaging findings. Mol Psychiatry. 2005;10(1):105–16.
92. Lish JD, Dime-Meenan S, Whybrow PC, Price RA, Hirschfeld RM. The National Depressive and Manic-depressive Association (DMDA) survey of bipolar members. J Affect Disord. 1994;31(4):281–94.
93. Librenza-Garcia D, Kotzian BJ, Yang J, Mwangi B, Cao B, Pereira Lima LN, et al. The impact of machine learning techniques in the study of bipolar disorder: a systematic review. Neurosci Biobehav Rev. 2017;80:538–54.
94. Mwangi B, Wu MJ, Cao B, Passos IC, Lavagnino L, Keser Z, et al. Individualized prediction and clinical staging of bipolar disorders using neuroanatomical biomarkers. Biol Psychiatry Cogn Neurosci Neuroimaging. 2016;1(2):186–94.
95. Li H, Cui L, Cao L, Zhang Y, Liu Y, Deng W, et al. Identification of bipolar disorder using a combination of multimodality magnetic resonance imaging and machine learning techniques. BMC Psychiatry. 2020;20(1):488.
96. Frangou S, Dima D, Jogia J. Towards person-centered neuroimaging markers for resilience and vulnerability in Bipolar Disorder. Neuroimage. 2017;145(Pt B):230–7.
97. Nunes A, Schnack HG, Ching CRK, Agartz I, Akudjedu TN, Alda M, et al. Using structural MRI to identify bipolar disorders - 13 site machine learning study in 3020 individuals from the ENIGMA Bipolar Disorders Working Group. Mol Psychiatry. 2020;25(9):2130–43.
98. Sartori JM, Reckziegel R, Passos IC, Czepielewski LS, Fijtman A, Sodre LA, et al. Volumetric brain magnetic resonance imaging predicts functioning in bipolar disorder: a machine learning approach. J Psychiatr Res. 2018;103:237–43.
99. Fleck DE, Ernest N, Adler CM, Cohen K, Eliassen JC, Norris M, et al. Prediction of lithium response in first-episode mania using the LITHium Intelligent Agent (LITHIA): pilot data and proof-of-concept. Bipolar Disord. 2017;19(4):259–72.
100. Serpa MH, Ou Y, Schaufelberger MS, Doshi J, Ferreira LK, Machado-Vieira R, et al. Neuroanatomical classification in a population-based sample of psychotic major depression and bipolar I disorder with 1 year of diagnostic stability. Biomed Res Int. 2014;2014:706157.
101. Matsuo K, Harada K, Fujita Y, Okamoto Y, Ota M, Narita H, et al. Distinctive neuroanatomical substrates for depression in bipolar disorder versus major depressive disorder. Cereb Cortex. 2019;29(1):202–14.
102. Redlich R, Almeida JJ, Grotegerd D, Opel N, Kugel H, Heindel W, et al. Brain morphometric biomarkers distinguishing unipolar and bipolar depression. A voxel-based morphometry-pattern classification approach. JAMA Psychiatry. 2014;71(11):1222–30.
103. Fan Y, Liu Y, Wu H, Hao Y, Liu H, Liu Z, et al. Discriminant analysis of functional connectivity patterns on Grassmann manifold. Neuroimage. 2011;56(4):2058–67.
104. Li M, Das T, Deng W, Wang Q, Li Y, Zhao L, et al. Clinical utility of a short resting-state MRI scan in differentiating bipolar from unipolar depression. Acta Psychiatr Scand. 2017;136(3):288–99.
105. Kohler CG, Hoffman LJ, Eastman LB, Healey K, Moberg PJ. Facial emotion perception in depression and bipolar disorder: a quantitative review. Psychiatry Res. 2011;188(3):303–9.
106. Burger C, Redlich R, Grotegerd D, Meinert S, Dohm K, Schneider I, et al. Differential abnormal pattern of anterior cingulate gyrus activation in unipolar and bipolar depression: an fMRI and pattern classification approach. Neuropsychopharmacology. 2017;42(7):1399–408.
107. Grotegerd D, Stuhrmann A, Kugel H, Schmidt S, Redlich R, Zwanzger P, et al. Amygdala excitability to subliminally presented emotional faces distinguishes unipolar and bipolar depression: an fMRI and pattern classification study. Hum Brain Mapp. 2014;35(7):2995–3007.
108. Grotegerd D, Suslow T, Bauer J, Ohrmann P, Arolt V, Stuhrmann A, et al. Discriminating unipolar and bipolar depression by means of fMRI and pattern classification: a pilot study. Eur Arch Psychiatry Clin Neurosci. 2013;263(2):119–31.

109. He H, Sui J, Du Y, Yu Q, Lin D, Drevets WC, et al. Co-altered functional networks and brain structure in unmedicated patients with bipolar and major depressive disorders. Brain Struct Funct. 2017;222(9):4051–64.
110. Rive MM, Redlich R, Schmaal L, Marquand AF, Dannlowski U, Grotegerd D, et al. Distinguishing medication-free subjects with unipolar disorder from subjects with bipolar disorder: state matters. Bipolar Disord. 2016;18(7):612–23.
111. Jie NF, Zhu MH, Ma XY, Osuch EA, Wammes M, Theberge J, et al. Discriminating bipolar disorder from major depression based on SVM-FoBa: efficient feature selection with multimodal brain imaging data. IEEE Trans Auton Ment Dev. 2015;7(4):320–31.
112. Shao J, Dai Z, Zhu R, Wang X, Tao S, Bi K, et al. Early identification of bipolar from unipolar depression before manic episode: evidence from dynamic rfMRI. Bipolar Disord. 2019;21(8):774–84.
113. Mourao-Miranda J, Oliveira L, Ladouceur CD, Marquand A, Brammer M, Birmaher B, et al. Pattern recognition and functional neuroimaging help to discriminate healthy adolescents at risk for mood disorders from low risk adolescents. PLoS One. 2012;7(2):e29482.
114. Zhang W, Nery FG, Tallman MJ, Patino LR, Adler CM, Strawn JR, et al. Individual prediction of symptomatic converters in youth offspring of bipolar parents using proton magnetic resonance spectroscopy. Eur Child Adolesc Psychiatry. 2021;30(1):55–64.
115. Soriano-Mas C, Pujol J, Alonso P, Cardoner N, Menchon JM, Harrison BJ, et al. Identifying patients with obsessive-compulsive disorder using whole-brain anatomy. Neuroimage. 2007;35(3):1028–37.
116. Hu X, Liu Q, Li B, Tang W, Sun H, Li F, et al. Multivariate pattern analysis of obsessive-compulsive disorder using structural neuroanatomy. Eur Neuropsychopharmacol. 2016;26(2):246–54.
117. Parrado-Hernandez E, Gomez-Verdejo V, Martinez-Ramon M, Shawe-Taylor J, Alonso P, Pujol J, et al. Discovering brain regions relevant to obsessive-compulsive disorder identification through bagging and transduction. Med Image Anal. 2014;18(3):435–48.
118. Takagi Y, Sakai Y, Lisi G, Yahata N, Abe Y, Nishida S, et al. A neural marker of obsessive-compulsive disorder from whole-brain functional connectivity. Sci Rep. 2017;7(1):7538.
119. Yun JY, Jang JH, Kim SN, Jung WH, Kwon JS. Neural correlates of response to pharmacotherapy in obsessive-compulsive disorder: individualized cortical morphology-based structural covariance. Prog Neuropsychopharmacol Biol Psychiatry. 2015;63:126–33.
120. Weygandt M, Blecker CR, Schafer A, Hackmack K, Haynes JD, Vaitl D, et al. fMRI pattern recognition in obsessive-compulsive disorder. Neuroimage. 2012;60(2):1186–93.
121. Yang X, Hu X, Tang W, Li B, Yang Y, Gong Q, et al. Multivariate classification of drug-naive obsessive-compulsive disorder patients and healthy controls by applying an SVM to resting-state functional MRI data. BMC Psychiatry. 2019;19(1):210.
122. Bu X, Hu X, Zhang L, Li B, Zhou M, Lu L, et al. Investigating the predictive value of different resting-state functional MRI parameters in obsessive-compulsive disorder. Transl Psychiatry. 2019;9(1):17.
123. Frick A, Gingnell M, Marquand AF, Howner K, Fischer H, Kristiansson M, et al. Classifying social anxiety disorder using multivoxel pattern analyses of brain function and structure. Behav Brain Res. 2014;259:330–5.
124. Liu S, Cai W, Liu S, Zhang F, Fulham M, Feng D, et al. Multimodal neuroimaging computing: a review of the applications in neuropsychiatric disorders. Brain Inform. 2015;2(3):167–80.
125. Gong Q, Li L, Tognin S, Wu Q, Pettersson-Yeo W, Lui S, et al. Using structural neuroanatomy to identify trauma survivors with and without post-traumatic stress disorder at the individual level. Psychol Med. 2014;44(1):195–203.
126. Ecker C, Rocha-Rego V, Johnston P, Mourao-Miranda J, Marquand A, Daly EM, et al. Investigating the predictive value of whole-brain structural MR scans in autism: a pattern classification approach. Neuroimage. 2010;49(1):44–56.
127. Ecker C, Marquand A, Mourao-Miranda J, Johnston P, Daly EM, Brammer MJ, et al. Describing the brain in autism in five dimensions--magnetic resonance imaging-assisted

diagnosis of autism spectrum disorder using a multiparameter classification approach. J Neurosci. 2010;30(32):10612–23.

128. Uddin LQ, Menon V, Young CB, Ryali S, Chen T, Khouzam A, et al. Multivariate searchlight classification of structural magnetic resonance imaging in children and adolescents with autism. Biol Psychiatry. 2011;70(9):833–41.

129. Jiao Y, Chen R, Ke X, Chu K, Lu Z, Herskovits EH. Predictive models of autism spectrum disorder based on brain regional cortical thickness. Neuroimage. 2010;50(2):589–99.

130. Chanel G, Pichon S, Conty L, Berthoz S, Chevallier C, Grezes J. Classification of autistic individuals and controls using cross-task characterization of fMRI activity. Neuroimage Clin. 2016;10:78–88.

131. Just MA, Cherkassky VL, Buchweitz A, Keller TA, Mitchell TM. Identifying autism from neural representations of social interactions: neurocognitive markers of autism. PLoS One. 2014;9(12):e113879.

132. Wong E, Anderson JS, Zielinski BA, Fletcher PT. Riemannian regression and classification models of brain networks applied to autism. Connect Neuroimaging. 2018;2018(11083):78–87.

133. Emerson RW, Adams C, Nishino T, Hazlett HC, Wolff JJ, Zwaigenbaum L, et al. Functional neuroimaging of high-risk 6-month-old infants predicts a diagnosis of autism at 24 months of age. Sci Transl Med. 2017;9(393):eaag2882.

134. Ingalhalikar M, Parker D, Bloy L, Roberts TP, Verma R. Diffusion based abnormality markers of pathology: toward learned diagnostic prediction of ASD. Neuroimage. 2011;57(3):918–27.

135. Uddin LQ, Supekar K, Lynch CJ, Khouzam A, Phillips J, Feinstein C, et al. Salience network-based classification and prediction of symptom severity in children with autism. JAMA Psychiatry. 2013;70(8):869–79.

136. Deshpande G, Libero LE, Sreenivasan KR, Deshpande HD, Kana RK. Identification of neural connectivity signatures of autism using machine learning. Front Hum Neurosci. 2013;7:670.

137. Ghiassian S, Greiner R, Jin P, Brown MR. Using functional or structural magnetic resonance images and personal characteristic data to identify ADHD and autism. PLoS One. 2016;11(12):e0166934.

138. Lombardo MV, Pierce K, Eyler LT, Carter Barnes C, Ahrens-Barbeau C, Solso S, et al. Different functional neural substrates for good and poor language outcome in autism. Neuron. 2015;86(2):567–77.

139. Igual L, Soliva JC, Escalera S, Gimeno R, Vilarroya O, Radeva P. Automatic brain caudate nuclei segmentation and classification in diagnostic of attention-deficit/hyperactivity disorder. Comput Med Imaging Graph. 2012;36(8):591–600.

140. Johnston BA, Mwangi B, Matthews K, Coghill D, Konrad K, Steele JD. Brainstem abnormalities in attention deficit hyperactivity disorder support high accuracy individual diagnostic classification. Hum Brain Mapp. 2014;35(10):5179–89.

141. Lim L, Marquand A, Cubillo AA, Smith AB, Chantiluke K, Simmons A, et al. Disorder-specific predictive classification of adolescents with attention deficit hyperactivity disorder (ADHD) relative to autism using structural magnetic resonance imaging. PLoS One. 2013;8(5):e63660.

142. Iannaccone R, Hauser TU, Ball J, Brandeis D, Walitza S, Brem S. Classifying adolescent attention-deficit/hyperactivity disorder (ADHD) based on functional and structural imaging. Eur Child Adolesc Psychiatry. 2015;24(10):1279–89.

143. Park BY, Kim M, Seo J, Lee JM, Park H. Connectivity analysis and feature classification in attention deficit hyperactivity disorder sub-types: a task functional magnetic resonance imaging study. Brain Topogr. 2016;29(3):429–39.

144. Sato JR, Hoexter MQ, Fujita A, Rohde LA. Evaluation of pattern recognition and feature extraction methods in ADHD prediction. Front Syst Neurosci. 2012;6:68.

145. Colby JB, Rudie JD, Brown JA, Douglas PK, Cohen MS, Shehzad Z. Insights into multimodal imaging classification of ADHD. Front Syst Neurosci. 2012;6:59.

146. Bohland JW, Saperstein S, Pereira F, Rapin J, Grady L. Network, anatomical, and non-imaging measures for the prediction of ADHD diagnosis in individual subjects. Front Syst Neurosci. 2012;6:78.
147. Lei D, Pinaya WHL, van Amelsvoort T, Marcelis M, Donohoe G, Mothersill DO, et al. Detecting schizophrenia at the level of the individual: relative diagnostic value of whole-brain images, connectome-wide functional connectivity and graph-based metrics. Psychol Med. 2020;50(11):1852–61.
148. Walter M, Alizadeh S, Jamalabadi H, Lueken U, Dannlowski U, Walter H, et al. Translational machine learning for psychiatric neuroimaging. Prog Neuropsychopharmacol Biol Psychiatry. 2019;91:113–21.
149. Schnack HG. Improving individual predictions: machine learning approaches for detecting and attacking heterogeneity in schizophrenia (and other psychiatric diseases). Schizophr Res. 2019;214:34–42.
150. Bellman RE. Adaptive control processes: a guided tour. Princeton: Princeton University Press; 1961.
151. Janssen RJ, Mourao-Miranda J, Schnack HG. Making individual prognoses in psychiatry using neuroimaging and machine learning. Biol Psychiatry Cogn Neurosci Neuroimaging. 2018;3(9):798–808.
152. Scarpazza C, Ha M, Baecker L, Garcia-Dias R, Pinaya WHL, Vieira S, et al. Translating research findings into clinical practice: a systematic and critical review of neuroimaging-based clinical tools for brain disorders. Transl Psychiatry. 2020;10(1):107.
153. Huys QJ, Maia TV, Frank MJ. Computational psychiatry as a bridge from neuroscience to clinical applications. Nat Neurosci. 2016;19(3):404–13.
154. Insel T, Cuthbert B, Garvey M, Heinssen R, Pine DS, Quinn K, et al. Research Domain Criteria (RDoC): toward a new classification framework for research on mental disorders. Am J Psychiatry. 2010;167(7):748–51.
155. Crossley NA, Scott J, Ellison-Wright I, Mechelli A. Neuroimaging distinction between neurological and psychiatric disorders. Br J Psychiatry. 2015;207(5):429–34.

Functional Neurological Symptoms: A Potential Sentinel of Neurological and Mental Health Disorders

Valeria Sajin and Antonella Macerollo

Abbreviations

BP	Readiness potential (Bereitschaftspotential)
CBT	Cognitive-behavioral therapy
DaTSCAN	Dopamine transporter scintigraphy
DSM-5	*Diagnostic and Statistical Manual of Mental Disorders, 5th Edition*
EEG	Electroencephalography
FMD	Functional movement disorder
FND	Functional neurological disorder
FP	Functional parkinsonism
ICD-10	*International Classification of Diseases, 10th Revision*
ICD-11	*International Classification of Diseases, 11th Revision*
MRI	Magnetic resonance imagery
PNES	Psychogenic non-epileptic seizures
SMA	Supplementary motor area
SPECT	Single-photon emission computed tomography

V. Sajin
Department of Neurology and Clinical Neurophysiology, Schoen Klinik Neustadt, Neustadt in Holstein, Germany
e-mail: vsajin@schoen-klinik.de

A. Macerollo (✉)
Department of Neurology, The Walton Centre for Neurology and Neurosurgery, Liverpool, UK

Institute of Systems, Molecular and Integrative Biology, University of Liverpool, Liverpool, UK
e-mail: a.macerollo@liverpool.ac.uk

M. Colizzi, M. Ruggeri (eds.), *Prevention in Mental Health*,
https://doi.org/10.1007/978-3-030-97906-5_15

15.1 Introduction and Definitions

Functional neurological disorder (FND) is a medical condition defined by the presence of genuine neurological symptoms but lack of compatibility with recognized neurological diseases or organic changes [1–5]. It was also called psychogenic, conversion, somatoform, dissociative, or non-organic disorder. It is believed to be rather the pathology of the nervous "software" than of the "hardware."

FNDs are very common in neurological practice. They are also the most common causes of the neurological disability [6, 7]. Of note, FND is completely distinct from intentionally produced symptoms, as in malingering and factitious disorder. There is a long story of misconceptions and changes of hypotheses and paradigms related to FND. The old assumptions of the pure psychological cause of the functional symptoms ("psychogenic illness") changed nowadays into a complex theory of neurobiological particularities related to this condition.

The term "functional" serves to the better acceptance and understanding of FND by the affected patients [8].

"Psychosomatic" implies the abnormal interaction between body and psychical states but is usually interpreted in the same way as "somatization" [9].

The term "dissociative," a common synonym for FND (used in the *International Classification of Diseases, 11th Revision*, ICD-11), implies the detachment of neurophysiological function from normal awareness [2, 10, 11].

In *Diagnostic and Statistical Manual of Mental Disorders, 5th Edition* (DSM-5), "dissociative disorder" is distinguished from "functional neurological symptom disorder" [1]. Currently there have been changes in classification of FND [12, 13] that serve to an easy diagnosis and a satisfactory management of the disorder.

Misdiagnosis, delayed diagnosis, and inappropriate treatment imply a significant risk of iatrogenic injury, persistence of the morbidity, and high costs to patients and healthcare systems [14, 15].

15.2 General Characteristics

The term "functional" indicates a change of the nervous system function rather than of its structure. It is basically similar to another term used to define FND: "non-organic." The diagnosis of FND as well as its treatment is possible without knowing its exact cause. The knowledge about the etiology makes, however, FND's management much easier.

FNDs manifest with several motor, sensory, visual, and cognitive symptoms causing impairment in the daily activities. However, the most common functional neurological symptoms are non-epileptic seizures ("pseudoseizures") and functional weakness [16]; these symptoms are frequently misdiagnosed with epilepsy or stroke, especially in the emergency situation.

The diagnosis of FND should be based on the criteria of the DSM-5 and of the ICD-11. Clinically, functional neurological symptoms can be undistinguishable from the corresponding non-functional symptoms. Therefore, the differential diagnosis can be only reachable via careful investigations, revealing no abnormalities that would suggest any known disease.

At the same time, there are some positive clinical features that help differentiate an FND (as variability, inconsistency, suggestibility, distractibility, and suppressibility of symptoms) [1, 2]. Psychopathological traits have a supportive value but usually lack of the diagnostic specificity. Electrophysiological brain changes and neuroimaging abnormalities are useful mostly for research purpose and not in clinical practice [4], although they could be helpful for the differential diagnosis.

The treatment of FND should be multidisciplinary and includes psychotherapy. However, the prognosis is usually poor with symptoms unchanged or worse in most patients [4]. A longer duration of symptoms is the predictor of poor outcome [15].

15.3 Etiopathology

Functional neurological symptoms have intrigued neurologists and scientists since the appearance of the first descriptions. Jean-Martin Charcot, Josef Breuer, Sigmund Freud, and Pierre Janet tried to find out the etiology and the pathology of the enigmatic disorders, which seemed to have no organic correlates. Over the last decades, various studies on dissociation and conversion provided data about their physiological and psychopathological mechanisms, and various theories appeared. FNDs were regarded as a personality dissociation due to traumatic experiences [17], as a defense mechanism [18], or as a part of a fragmented self-image [5].

Even if functional neurological symptoms are not anymore considered to be of purely psychogenic origin, scientific data still support the importance of psychological factors and of some personality traits in the development and persistence of these conditions. For instance, patients with psychogenic non-epileptic seizures (PNES) and functional movement disorders (FMDs), two subtypes of FND, have an accentuated neuroticism and lower level of conscientiousness [19].

Patients with PNES also reported significant levels of depressive and anxiety symptoms, overall psychopathology, more frequent history of sexual abuse, higher levels of dissociative symptoms, abnormal levels of alexithymia, and an earlier age at the time of the most traumatic event than FMD patients. Of note, alexithymia is common in all subtypes of FND [20–22].

The FMDs' severity showed a correlation with the fearful attachment style [5, 23].

Other personality traits associated with FNDs are high harm avoidance, low self-directedness, and high novelty seeking [5, 24–26]. A study on 15 patients with mixed sensory-motor FND (PNES excluded) showed severe deficits in personality functioning in all the participants with two distinct subgroups: neurotic and borderline [5, 27].

Childhood and adult life events as well as environmental factors could also predispose to the development of FNDs [28].

A study on FMD patients concluded to a significant childhood emotional abuse and physical neglect, higher levels of fear regarding traumatic experiences, and a larger number of traumatic events in these patients compared to healthy controls and patients with dystonia [29]. Childhood abuse [30–36] and trauma seem to be a predisposing factor for the FND. In this regard, a recent meta-analysis showed that stressful life events during childhood and adulthood were overall more common in patients with FNDs compared to controls [37].

Scientific studies provided a neurophysiological basis to the emotional processing alterations in FND. A limbic hyperactivation with an excessive autonomic arousal and threat-related hypervigilance, an impaired enteroception of visceromotor emotional responses, a suboptimal emotional regulation, and disturbances in subjective interpretations of affective stimuli in FND patients were described [38]. These changes are due to malfunction in the limbic afferences and processed signals as well as to disturbed connections between limbic regions and those involved with awareness of self, body, and behavior (cingulo-insular and temporo-parietal regions).

Notably, the presence of a relevant psychological stressor is not required to establish the diagnosis of FND. Indeed, about one-third of patients with FND have normal scores on psychological measures [39], similarly to patients with organic movement disorders. In addition, a study on pediatric FND patients found no sexual abuse or trauma and no mundane stressors in 25% of patients [40]. These data were supported by another recent study [32]. As a result, the DSM-5 diagnostic criteria for FND have removed preceding stressors as a requirement and instead are currently focused on positive symptoms [1].

Physical trauma has long been considered as the cause of FND, but results of several studies have been inconsistent. Patients with FNDs, especially FMDs, have increased general trauma history [41, 42]. Functional dystonia has frequently an onset after a peripheral trauma [43–49]; the reported incidence of trauma is between 37 and 80% in FMD patients [49–51].

Infections, drug reactions, and pain could also be associated with the development of an FMD [50].

Childhood sexual abuse has been found associated with PNES and some other FNDs [31, 42, 52, 53].

Other predisposing factors for FNDs are stress, comorbid fatigue, chronic pain, irritable bowel syndrome, healthcare profession [54, 55].

Even if stressful events, social influences, and minor trauma may precede the onset of FMDs, their neurobiological basis is still unclear [38]. No single causal mechanism has been found; instead, predisposing factors vary among individual patients. Several cognitive and neurobiological etiological models have been proposed for functional neurological symptoms [54].

Contemporary explanations have moved away from psychodynamic trauma-focused models and nowadays emphasize dysfunction of higher-order cognitive processes. The somatosensory amplification might serve a critical role in somatization [56]. It refers to the tendency of experiencing a wide range of benign bodily sensations as intrusive, intense, noxious, and disruptive. This amplification seems to be associated with a heightened attentional focus on bodily sensations (observed also in FND patients [57, 58]). Somatosensory amplification has been linked to alexithymia, while somatization has been associated with dysphoric-anxious mood and cognitive distortions (particularly pain catastrophizing) [56]. The neurocircuit framework of the somatosensory amplification includes the anterior cingulate cortex, insula, amygdala, hippocampal formation, and striatum. Additionally, there seems to be an altered top-down regulation of motor activities and increased activation of areas implicated in self-awareness, self-monitoring, and active motor inhibition, such as the cingulate and insular cortex [44]. There are some evidences of altered explicit facial emotion processing in people with FNDs [38] with changes in the function of limbic-paralimbic regions.

A hyperactivity of the hypothalamus-pituitary-adrenal axis and autonomous sympathetic system was observed in patients with FNDs [59–66]; however a normal level of salivary cortisol was found in patients with FMDs [67].

Functional and structural brain changes have been found in several studies, including abnormal functional connections in areas associated with cognitive control, behavioral inhibition, and perceptual awareness [68]. Some studies concluded to the strengthened connectivity between limbic and motor networks in patients with FMDs and decreased activation of the supplementary motor area (SMA) and pre-SMA, which are implicated in motor control and preparation [44].

The sensory processing is impaired in patients with FNDs [57, 69–71], even if patients do not manifest functional sensory symptoms. Importantly, there is an impaired feeling of controlling external events in FMD patients with an impaired functional connectivity and hypoactivity of the right temporo-parietal junction [72–75].

Abnormal patterns of cerebral activation and connectivity were shown in FMD patients including hypokinetic (i.e., weakness) [76, 77] and hyperkinetic movements [73, 75, 78–83]. These abnormalities involved the SMA and the pre-SMA (dedicated to the suppression of the motor plans), right temporo-parietal junction and right middle temporal gyrus, cingulate cortex, ventromedial prefrontal cortex and precuneus cortex, paracingulate gyrus and left Heschl's gyrus, right inferior frontal cortex, bilateral cerebellum, bilateral thalamus, left globus pallidus internus (GPi), and right caudate nucleus [72, 73, 75, 80–95].

Some neurophysiological findings are common to both functional and organic disorders. In this regard, organic dystonia and functional dystonia are both characterized by decreased cortical inhibition [44, 94, 96–98], similar local field potentials in the globus pallidus and thalamus, and abnormal activation of the right dorsolateral prefrontal cortex. However, only patients with organic dystonia have increased sensorimotor cortical plasticity [99, 100].

The readiness potential (Bereitschaftspotential, BP), meaning the cortical activation preceding self-initiated movement or volitional muscle relaxation, is an activation pattern of the SMA and premotor cortex [44]. BP usually (but not always) precedes psychogenic jerks [101–104]. Even if BP is recorded prior to the movement, patients with FMDs perceive their movement as "involuntary" [44].

Grey matter is increased in FMD patients in subcortical motor areas (basal ganglia), cerebellum, thalamus, and limbic/paralimbic cortical structures [31, 105–107]. Increased cortical volume of the SMA, superior temporal gyrus, and dorsomedial prefrontal cortex was observed in children and adolescents with FNDs [84, 108]. Volumetric cortical alterations were observed in patients with mobile compared to fixed functional dystonia [109].

Different FNDs constitute a continuum spectrum of functional disorders that share similar etiopathogenic mechanisms [110].

15.4 Comorbidities

FNDs are in comorbidity with some psychiatric disorders. Major depression was reported in 32–58% of cases [33, 111–113], anxiety disorder in 62–79% [22, 33, 111, 114, 115], post-traumatic stress disorder (PTSD) in 23% [116, 117], dissociative disorders in 47% [115], and somatization disorders in 27% [112]. Personality disorder was found in 45–74% FND cases [111, 118, 119]; the borderline personality disorder (BPD) was reported in 34% [120] of FND patients.

There is an association of FNDs with some neurological disorders. Indeed, PNES are common in epilepsy patients [121–124], FMDs are common in Parkinson's disease and dementia with Lewy body cases [125–128], and different FNDs are common in patients with multiple sclerosis [129, 130] or migraine [131, 132].

Twenty-five percent of patients with FMDs have a comorbid organic movement disorder [133]. Functional cognitive disorders (subjective cognitive difficulties causing distress and functional impairment with no underlying structural, neurodegenerative, toxic, or metabolic cause [134]) were reported in patients with depression, bipolar disorder, and anxiety [134–136].

Dissociative symptoms (depersonalization, derealization, dissociative amnesia) could be also comorbid with FNDs [1]. Moreover, FND may overlay with chronic pain conditions such as irritable bowel disease, CRPS, migraine, headaches, or fibromyalgia [137].

Symptoms of lower urinary tract dysfunction were found in 20% of FMD cases; overactive bladder symptoms were the most common [138].

15.5 Epidemiology

The exact prevalence of FNDs is not known, although transient symptoms are common [1]. A prevalence of 5.6% were described in an urban community [139], while the prevalence in neurologic services varies from 6 to 18% of the entire number of patients [1, 140]. The incidence of individual persistent functional symptoms is estimated to be 2–12/100,000 per year [1, 7, 118, 141].

The 1-year prevalence of non-organic disorders in the general community in Florence (673 patients) was reported as 0.3% conversion disorder (equivalent to FND), 0.7% body dysmorphic disorder, 4.5% hypochondriasis, 0.6% somatoform pain disorder, 0.7% somatization disorder, and 13.8% undifferentiated somatoform disorder [142].

In an Australian cohort of FND patients, sensory symptoms were the most common manifestation (48%) followed by limb weakness (37%) and psychogenic non-epileptic seizures (14%). Outcome information was available for 49% of patients at an average of 3 months of follow-up, showing that 45% had some improvement in their symptoms, 43% had static symptoms, and 12% had worsening of symptoms [140].

Around half of FND patients presents with an FMD [143]: 10% (range 1.7–25%) have been categorized as functional parkinsonism (FP) [133].

In two Swiss movement disorders clinics, the prevalence of FP was reported to be 0.64 per 100,000, representing 0.24% of patients with parkinsonism [144]. The majority (87%) of them were women. Six patients had an additional diagnosis of Parkinson's disease (in four of them, the functional symptoms preceded the organic ones), 83% of depression, and 66% of other FNDs.

In a study on 14,568 patients seen in a movement disorders clinic since 1988, 530 patients (3.6%) had FMD [145]. Of them, 17 (3.2%) had parkinsonism, 211 (39.8%) tremor, 215 (40.6%) dystonia, 91 (17.2%) myoclonus, 23 (4.3%) tics, 8 (1.5%) other dyskinesias, and 3 (0.6%) psychogenic chorea [145].

The mean age of onset is 44 years (range 4–73 years) for FMDs [113, 146, 147].

There is a female predominance (mean age 50 years, range 17–83 years) [133] in FNDs including FMDs (61–87%) [113, 145, 148–152].

However, FNDs, especially FMDs, are not uncommon in childhood and in elderly [4]. In a group of 606 pediatric patients with movement disorders, 27 (4%) had FNDs [153]. Child psychiatrists have reported a prevalence of FNDs of 1–3% [154, 155].

The diagnosis of PNES is established in 5 to 10% of outpatients in epilepsy clinics and 20–40% of inpatients in epilepsy monitoring units [156–159]. An incidence of PNES in the general population (from the age of 13 years old and older) in Scotland was estimated as 4.9/100,000/year [160], 1.4/100,000/year in Iceland [140], and 3.03/100,000/year in the USA [161].

The exact prevalence of cognitive functional disorders is unclear. A Dutch study on 2000 healthy patients concluded to a prevalence of functional forgetfulness of 29% in people aged 25–35, rising to 34% in those aged 40–50, 41% in those aged 55–65 years, and 52% in the age group of 70–85 years [162]. In 24% of 418 patients in a memory clinic, no dementia or other organic diagnosis was established. Other studies reported a prevalence of functional cognitive disorders of 24–65% in memory clinic [163–166]. A study on 53 patients with functional retrograde amnesia found a male prevalence (ratio = 3:1) [167].

Functional vision disturbances can be present at any age group [168], and its prevalence is of 1–5% of referrals to ophthalmologists [169, 170].

The prevalence of functional dizziness as a primary cause of vestibular symptoms is of about 10% in neuro-otology centers [171]. It accounts for 19.5% of 17,700 adult outpatients, being the second most common diagnosis after benign paroxysmal positional vertigo in a tertiary referral dizziness unit [172]. It is also very common in childhood with a prevalence of 21%.

15.6 Clinical Diagnosis

The diagnosis of FND requires a careful anamnesis, clinical examination, and usually some investigations in order to exclude the organic causes of neurological symptoms.

FND or conversion disorder is listed in DMS-5 in the section "Somatic Symptom and Related Disorders." While in ICD-10 the dissociative disorders were classified exclusively in the psychiatric section; in ICD-11 the "dissociative neurological symptom disorders" are included in the section "Mental, Behavioral, or Neurodevelopmental Disorders" [2].

The DSM-5 diagnostic criteria of FND include the presence of one or more symptoms of altered voluntary motor or sensory function with clinical findings providing evidence of incompatibility between the symptom and recognized neurological or medical conditions. The symptom or deficit should be not better explained by another medical or mental disorder and should cause clinically significant distress or impairment in social, occupational, or other important areas of functioning or warrant medical evaluation [1].

FNDs in DSM-5 are divided in FND with (1) weakness or paralysis, (2) with abnormal movement (e.g., tremor, dystonic movement, myoclonus, gait disorder), (3) with swallowing symptoms, (4) with speech symptom (e.g., dysphonia, slurred speech), (5) with attacks or seizures, (6) with anesthesia or sensory loss, (7) with special sensory symptom (e.g., visual, olfactory, or hearing disturbance), and (8) with mixed symptoms [1].

In ICD-11 the term "dissociative disorder" is used as the synonym of "functional neurological symptom disorder." It is characterized by paresis or weakness, gait disturbance, movement disturbance, visual disturbance, speech disturbance, other sensory disturbances, non-epileptic seizures, auditory disturbance, vertigo or dizziness, and cognitive symptoms [2].

There can be an acute FND episode (symptoms present for less than 6 months) or persistent FND (symptoms occurring for 6 months or more). Also, FNDs in DSM-5 are divided in those with psychological stressor or without it.

DSM-5 specifies that, although the diagnosis requires that the symptom is not explained by neurological disease, it is not correct to make it simply because results from investigations are normal or because the symptom is "bizarre." There must be specific clinical findings that indicate the incompatibility with neurological disease and an internal inconsistency at examination. The examples of such examination findings supporting FND diagnosis include [1, 4, 10, 14, 28, 173–178]:

1. Hoover's sign (Hoover's test): Weakness of hip extension returns to normal strength with contralateral hip flexion against resistance (Fig. 15.1).
2. Marked weakness of ankle plantar flexion when tested on the bed in an individual who is able to walk on tiptoes.
3. Tremor entrainment test: The unilateral functional tremor changes when the individual is asked to copy the examiner in making a rhythmical movement

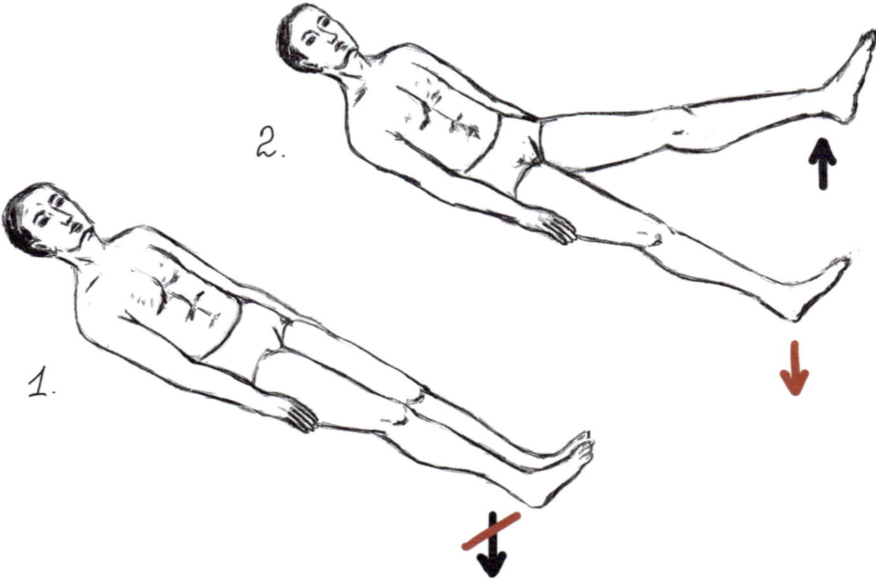

Fig. 15.1 Hoover's test

with their unaffected hand, such that it copies the rhythm of the unaffected hand or the functional tremor is suppressed or no longer makes a simple rhythmical movement.

4. In "psychogenic" non-epileptic attacks (PNES), the occurrence of closed eyes with resistance to opening.
5. For visual symptoms: A tubular visual field (i.e., tunnel vision).
6. Midline splitting and splitting of vibration in functional sensory disorders (Fig. 15.2).
7. Nonanatomic pattern sign and inconsistency for sensory disorders.
8. Dragging gait: Patients with acute functional weakness may drag their whole leg behind them with the hip externally or internally rotated, unlike patients with organic hemiparesis who tend to swing or circumduct their leg.
9. Drift without pronation for upper limb paresis [179].
10. Pelvic thrusting favors PNES, although it can be seen in frontal lobe focal seizures [14].

These signs have good specificity but low sensitivity [173]. Overall, many positive signs have been identified for functional symptoms, although only some of them have been validated [173–175]. Hoover's test has been considered the most useful test for non-organic weakness [129]. The psychogenic gait could be valuably categorized into three patterns—limping of one leg, limping of two legs and truncal imbalance, and the reliability between independent raters was high [173, 180].

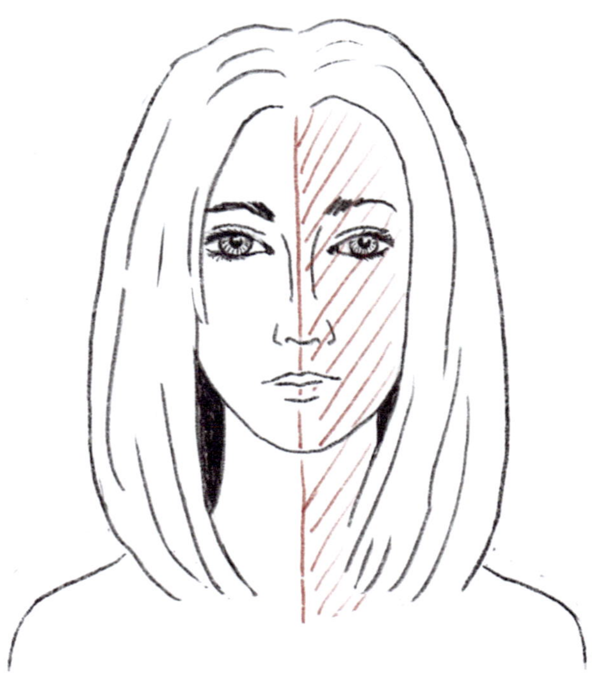

Fig. 15.2 Midline split test

In regard to FMDs, the core clinical features are considered variability of movement frequency, direction, phenomenology, and body location; distractibility (decrease or complete cessation of involuntary movements when engaged in mental tasks or voluntary movements with an unaffected limb); entrainability; and suggestibility [4].

Nonanatomic pattern sign and inconsistency for sensory disorders have demonstrated high sensitivity and specificity [174].

Long duration, fluctuating course, asynchronous movements, pelvic thrusting, side-to-side head or body movement, closed eyes, ictal crying, and memory recall are signs with good evidence from literature specific for PNES [173]. The bringing of an age-inappropriate toy animal to the video-EEG monitoring ("teddy bear sign" [181]) was found in single studies to have a high specificity but low sensitivity, as they are rare.

The phenomenon of "la belle indifference" (i.e., lack of concern about the nature or implications of the symptom) could be present, but it is not specific for FND [28]. A meta-analysis of 11 studies even concluded to a frequency of "la belle indifference" of 21% (range 0–54%) in 356 patients with FND and of 29% (range 0–60%) in 157 patients with organic disease [182].

The anamnesis is a very important part of the FNDs' diagnostical process. It is essential to obtain details regarding onset and evolution of symptoms.

In this regard, FMDs usually begin suddenly (in around 50% cases) and rapidly progress to severe disability [4, 28, 177, 183]. Their course often fluctuates, and transient spontaneous remissions may occur. Frequently, patients associate symptoms with a preceding injury or illness. The movements may be limited to certain situations and not interrupting others (e.g., walking). In addition to the chief complaint, FMD patients often have other transient symptoms. The level of disability in FMDs is often discordant with the physical deficits. Patients may use assistive devices such as canes, walkers, and wheelchairs or become completely dependent on family members for total care. The past medical history in FMDs typically includes a long list of diagnoses and surgical procedures. Childhood traumas may be reported. The typical FNDs' comorbidities (as depression, anxiety) may be present [183]. Family history may reveal other family members with similar disorders or chronic neurologic diseases with similar symptoms [4, 184].

Laboratory tests as well as imaging investigations are important investigations in the diagnostic pathway to exclude organic causes of the diseases.

Magnetic resonance imagery (MRI) can rule out or at least decrease the possibility of an organic brain or spinal cord pathology. Some subtle MRI changes in FNDs are explored in research purpose to understand the FNDs' pathophysiology [185]. The DaTSCAN is used to differentiate FP to idiopathic Parkinson's disease. However, DaTSCAN can be negative in some parkinsonian syndromes.

Electroencephalography (EEG) is useful to differentiate PNES from epileptic seizures. However, some seizures may be missed in the routine EEG. An occurrence from EEG confirmed sleep and postictal confusion supports the diagnosis of epileptic seizure.

Tremor can be investigated by electromyography (EMG).

The Gupta-Lang criteria for FMDs introduced a laboratory-supported, definite diagnostic category based on electrophysiological findings in functional myoclonus (using EMG and EEG back-averaging for the assessment of BP) and functional tremor (surface EMG to document entrainment, which is also termed coherence and coactivation signs) [186].

The differential diagnosis of FNDs should be made with organic neurological (such as epilepsy, stroke, multiple sclerosis, Parkinson's disease) or systemic disorders. Sometimes a supervision of patient and a reassessment of symptoms are required. Differentiation can be difficult, especially in a comorbid of FND and organic neurological disorder. Indeed, it is important to take into account that patients may have a combination of an organic disease with a functional overlay. The differential diagnosis of FNDs is particularly important in the emergency department, when the right decisions and diagnosis can avoid unnecessary investigations and costs [177].

If a mental health syndrome better explains the symptomatic, that diagnosis should be considered. For instance, patients may report general heaviness of their limbs or cognitive changes in depressive disorders. Episodic neurological symptoms (e.g., tremor, paresthesia) can occur in both conversion disorder and panic attacks; however, the panic disorder is usually associated with cardiovascular symptoms.

FNDs should be differentiated from dissociative symptoms, such as depersonalization, derealization, and dissociative amnesia. Patients with malingering or factitious disorder have a "secondary gain" (i.e., when individuals derive external benefits such as money or release from responsibilities) because of their symptoms, which however could also be present in FNDs.

15.7　Special Syndromes

FNDs include a variety of neurological syndromes and symptoms, some of which will be shortly reviewed below.

Functional movement disorders can present with any type of hypokinetic and hyperkinetic, paroxysmal, or continuous movement dysfunction (including tremor, dystonia, gait difficulty, myoclonus, chorea, tics). Patients with FMD are more likely to have ongoing disturbing movement symptoms affecting everyday tasks. The clinical diagnosis of an FMD is based on the presence of movements, which are inconsistent/incongruent with organic movement disorders or sometime on the presence of the psychogenic signs [4, 145]. Distractibility, entrainability, suggestibility, and variability of symptoms are core clinical characteristics of FMDs.

Psychogenic tremor is the most common FMD, accounting for 50% of this group of FNDs [133]. Variability of tremor frequency and direction is common. However, the organic tremor can have variable amplitudes as well, often increasing with stress or anxiety [187]. Several electrophysiological tests to evaluate psychogenic tremor have been validated demonstrating an 89.5% sensitivity and 95.9% specificity with good inter-rater and test-retest reliability [186, 188].

Functional dystonia is characterized by a sudden onset and a rapid progression to a fixed dystonia and early local pain. Patients usually do not have associated sensory tricks and have minimal or no exacerbation with action. Very common is the plantar flexion and inversion of the foot; associated weakness in the dystonic limb might be seen. An active resistance to passive range of motion often occurs. The typical pattern of a functional hand dystonia is a clenched fist with flexion of digits two through five with sparing of the thumb or the index finger, preserving the pincer grasp. When affecting the cervical region, the typical phenotype is a fixed laterocollis with ipsilateral shoulder elevation and contralateral shoulder depression (the latter is not typically seen in organic cervical dystonia) [4]. There is also a controversial entity referred to as peripherally induced dystonia, preceded by a mild injury, and resulting in a fixed dystonia often associated with signs of complex regional pain syndrome [189].

Functional myoclonus often presents as jerking movements of the limbs, head, or trunk. Unlike organic myoclonus, it is often associated with facial grimacing and forceful eyelid closure. Psychogenic myoclonus often occurs in episodes and is typically slower than organic myoclonus. When it is stimulus-induced, it may although occur even before a stimulus is applied, such as before the hammer hits the knee when checking reflexes [4]. It usually does not persist during the sleep. Surface EMG in functional myoclonus typically demonstrates a burst muscle contraction duration greater than 70 ms as opposed to a shorter duration in organic myoclonus [190]. A BP was reported in 63% of functional cases of myoclonus. Variability of muscle recruitment was the most likely parameter to distinguish functional from organic myoclonus [191]. Palatal myoclonus can be functional, as well.

Functional gait disorder frequently occurs in combination with other FMDs. The strength on motor testing is often normal, but patients are unable to bear weight, needing maximal assistance to stand. These patients often exert excessive effort when walking, greater than that seen in organic gait disorders, and might demonstrate the "huffing and puffing sign" characterized by huffing, breath holding, moaning, and facial grimacing [192]. Common manifestations of psychogenic gait are excessive slowness, intermittent buckling at the knees, lurching without falling, and magnet-like attraction to the adjacent walls [192, 193]. Patients may present some dramatic compensatory features such as walking with arms outstretched, referred to as "tightrope walking." Providing minimal support with one finger by the examiner often results in dramatic improvement of the balance. Patients often show an exaggerated response to the pull test. Frequently, the functional gait disorder develops after a fall ("post-fall syndrome"). It is important to distinguish a psychogenic gait disorder from organic disease with a complex gait pattern, such as generalized dystonia, gait affected by dyskinesia in Parkinson's disease, Huntington's disease, spinocerebellar ataxia, or crisscross gait in glucose transporter type 1 deficiency syndrome.

In contrast to Parkinson's disease, patients with *psychogenic parkinsonism* are more commonly female and have a relatively younger age at onset [144]. There is frequently a lack of movements' decrement during the finger-tapping test to investigate the bradykinesia but the presence of hypokinesia and an excessive effort during the movements' performance [194].

Functional facial movements include blepharospasm (involving bilateral contraction of the frontalis and corrugator and resulting in narrowed palpebral fissures without actual contraction of the orbicularis oculi), psychogenic facial spasm (with classic phenotype being ipsilateral platysma contraction with downward deviation of the corner of the mouth), and hemifacial spasm.

Functional paroxysmal dyskinesia has a later onset than the organic dyskinesia [195]. Patients generally do not respond to medications typically used for organic paroxysmal dyskinesias [4].

Psychogenic tics are rare, have an older age of presentation compared to organic tics, have a female predominance, and lack a premonitory urge. However, some organic tics can also present without premonitory sensations. An exaggerated interference with normal movements is common in functional tics and rare in Gilles de la Tourette syndrome [4].

Functional oculomotor disorders usually include oculogyric crises, opsoclonus, and ocular flutter [196].

Functional sensory symptoms represent an alteration or absence of normal sensation in the absence of neurologic disease. There are recognizable clinical patterns, such as hemisensory disturbance ("midline splitting," Fig. 15.1) and sensory disturbance finishing at the groin or shoulder. A nonanatomic sensory loss is also a typical finding. Functional sensory symptoms should be differentiated from unusual organic sensory disturbances, such as synesthesia, cenesthesia, and allochiria [197].

Non-epileptic seizures, also called psychogenic non-epileptic seizures (PNES), consist of paroxysmal changes in responsiveness, movements, or behavior that superficially resemble epileptic seizures, but they are characterized by lack of a neurobiological origin similar to epileptic seizures and are not associated with electrophysiological epileptic changes. PNES are relatively common occurrences in epilepsy centers [198]. Common but not pathognomonic symptoms in PNES are asynchronous limb movements, out-of-phase clonic activity, intermittent shaking movements with episodes of inactivity, side-to-side head movements, pelvic movements, dystonic body posturing, eyes closed during the event, and non-stereotypical seizure patterns [199, 200]. Urinary incontinence and tongue biting do not reliably distinguish between epileptic seizures and PNES [201]. The differential diagnoses of PNES include epilepsy, movement disorders, and other non-epileptic paroxysmal events (e.g., syncope). Frequently, there is a combination of PNES and truly epileptic seizures. Psychiatric comorbidities are also common in PNES [202]. Prolonged video-EEG monitoring with ictal recording is considered as the optimal test for the diagnosis of PNES [202, 203]. However, some seizure types do not present ictal EEG abnormalities (e.g., simple focal seizures), or the ictal EEG changes are obscured by movements (e.g., frontal seizures) [198, 200].

Functional weakness and other stroke mimics are relatively common presenting with limb weakness, numbness, or speech disturbances. Similar to stroke symptoms, the acute functional deficits are usually lateralized (e.g., hemiparesis) [112, 204–206]. Two recent studies from large centers demonstrated rates of functional stroke mimics of 8% [207, 208]. A complete clinical examination, including the clinical bedside tests that point to a functional genesis of the symptoms (as Hoover's test, Fig. 15.2), is not always possible in an emergency department because of lack of time, and only an emergency high-resolution brain imagery (MRI) could rule out the stroke [209].

Functional cognitive disorders usually include functional memory disturbances (inclusive functional retrograde amnesia or so-called dissociative amnesia), decline in attention, and concentration disturbances. Inconsistencies between self-reported symptoms and everyday functioning or neuropsychological test results are one of the core clinical features of functional cognitive disorder. Functional amnesia includes also the psychogenic fugue with a loss of sense of personal identity and a period of wandering from a few days until about 4 weeks, as well as the focal retrograde amnesia [167, 210, 211]. Functional cognitive disorders could be part of anxiety or depression. Overall, psychological distress is considered to be the biggest factor related to the subjective cognitive impairment in younger age group (age 45–64 years old) [212]. Functional cognitive disorders also could occur in association with other functional symptoms or independently. They should be differentiated from dementia and from cognitive dysfunction due to some secondary causes, as drugs, brain injury, encephalitis, stroke, transient global amnesia, vitamin insufficiency, endocrine dysfunction, or other diseases [166].

Functional vison disturbances include the subnormal vision or altered visual fields where no underlying pathology of the visual system can be found. There could be a variety of symptoms including binocular visual loss, monocular visual loss, or monocular decrease in vision. It is not a diagnosis of exclusion but rather the confirmation that the patient has better vision than pretended; hence, the more tests performed showing inconsistencies of symptoms and signs, the more reliable the diagnosis of functional vision disturbances is. Very suggestive is failure to perform tests that actually need no vision but imply the proprioception, such as the fingertip-touching test. The latter is easily performed by a truly blind person (without proprioceptive or coordination pathology) but is frequently failed by patients with functional vision loss. The signing of own name is commonly possible in patient with organic vision loss, but a patient with functional vision disturbance may produce a bizarre signature [213]. Normal pupillary reflexes also may indicate a functional visual problem. However, a thorough differential diagnosis is indispensable as some rare ophthalmic conditions (including Stargardt's disease, cone dystrophies, or other hereditary retinal dystrophies) and paraneoplastic syndromes (i.e., cancer-associated retinopathy or melanoma-associated retinopathy (MAR)) may have very subtle clinical signs [213, 214]. Forty-five to 78% of patients with functional vision loss experience resolution of all visual symptoms under psychotherapeutic treatment [215–219]. Good prognostic indicators include young age and absence of any associated psychiatric disease [215].

Functional auditory symptoms include a non-organic hearing loss and functional auditory hallucinations. They are sometimes difficult to differentiate from an organic auditory dysfunction. Depression and obsessive-compulsive disorder are common in patients with functional musical hallucinations [220].

Functional speech disorders have an inconsistent clinical presentation. Functional aphonia or dysphonia can usually be diagnosed by demonstrating normal sound production on prompted coughing or throat clearing [112].

One of the most common functional speech disorders is stuttering, which can occur in isolation or together with other FNDs [221]. The typical characteristics of a functional stuttering are an excessive variability of presentation, excessive consistency (stuttering on every syllable/word), struggling behaviors such as grimacing and neck extension (though articulatory groping can accompany apraxia of speech), absence of accompanying dysarthria, aphasia or apraxia of speech, and agrammatic or telegraphic speech without aphasia [221].

In functional dysarthria, which rarely occurs in isolation from other FNDs, patients might complain of a globus sensation but will rarely have any other swallowing difficulties [112]. Isolated dysarthria has an 86% likelihood of being a stroke mimic [222].

Functional aphasia is rare and usually presents as non-fluent aphasia with preserved comprehension, and naming and speech patterns are more inconsistent than in truly aphasia [223]. The foreign accent syndrome can be functional, as well [224].

Functional vestibular symptoms are relatively common in adult inpatients and outpatients. A careful anamnesis and clinical examination can help diagnose a functional dizziness. The so-called persistent postural-perceptual dizziness includes core features described over the last 30 years in syndromes like phobic postural vertigo, chronic subjective dizziness, space-motion discomfort, and visual vertigo [225]. Several studies disclosed a number of functional alterations of vestibular and balance mechanisms that distinguished functional vestibular symptoms from primary psychiatric disorders [226–229]. Coexisting anxiety and depressive disorders also are common in patients with functional dizziness, but functional vestibular disorders can occur without psychiatric comorbidity [230].

15.8 Communicating the Diagnosis

When the diagnosis of an FND is established for the physician, the patient should be informed. Not providing the patient with a clear diagnosis can result in a delay in treatment and in additional unnecessary consultations, investigations, as well as emergency department visits [231]. A critical first step in increasing favorable outcomes is the discussion of the diagnosis with the patient, encompassing the critical points: there is an established diagnosis, and the disorder is potentially reversible with treatment [10]. Receiving a diagnosis can be even therapeutic for some patients. The basic communication skills required for patients with FND are similar with those needed for other patients. Communication is more successful if positive and negative factors supporting the diagnosis are listed and the relevance of psychological factors becomes believable to the patients. It is suggested to begin with the patient's particular concerns about this symptom and what may have been told by other doctors, so that specific reassurance can be given [232].

However, it is not helpful simply to inform patients which conditions they do not suffer from. The aims of the conversation should include reducing anxiety and facilitating engagement in further psychological therapy. The etiology of functional symptoms should be explained in a simplified way, linking mood, pathogenesis, and symptoms (e.g., "When people are anxious, the muscles in their neck tend to tense up and that can cause headaches" [233]). The explanation of the diagnosis should make sense to the patient. Clinicians must carefully explain the terms "psychogenic," "conversion," and "functional," so the patient does not misinterpret them to imply that he or she is feigning or malingering. The plan for further management should be presented. Treatment can be described as a form of "brain retraining" [231]. Acute symptoms may improve with an explanation, encouragement, positive suggestion, and physiotherapy. In more chronic cases and to anticipate and prevent relapse, a psychological approach should be offered [232]. If the patient has established healthcare providers, it is important to communicate with them to ensure that they understand the new diagnosis.

Patients in whom PNES is suspected should be referred by the family doctor to an epileptologist for confirmation. If there is no coexisting epilepsy, the patient could be discharged from the neurological care. However, it is important that before discharge patients have accepted their diagnosis and a transition to psychiatry has been established [202]. Possible strategies for communicating the diagnosis of PNES include showing the patient a video-recording of the seizure and presenting the diagnosis as good news (i.e., the absence of epilepsy) [234].

15.9 Treatment

The treatment of the FND patients requires a multidisciplinary approach. The physician who establishes the diagnosis of FND (usually neurologist) should collaborate with psychologists and psychiatrists specialized in the FNDs. The FND's treatment could be outpatient as well as an inpatient one. There are multimodal treatment programs developed specially for FND [235]. In many countries there are also pediatric inpatient and outpatient services specialized on functional symptoms.

Psychotherapeutic interventions have traditionally been considered the treatment of choice of functional disorders. Psychotherapy should be explained in terms of how it will help the patient's symptoms. The patient should understand that "the way the brain processes information" is changed in order to minimize the tendency to express distress through physical symptoms and to create new behaviors that break the established unconscious pattern that leads to those symptoms [235]. The disorder-adapted cognitive-behavioral therapy (CBT) includes education about FND and its pathophysiology and trains patients in stress management techniques and new behavioral responses. It also helps patients identify and change unhelpful thought patterns that reinforce their symptoms [235]. CBT is frequently used for FND [10, 236–242]. Some randomized studies showed a high efficacy of CBT in PNES [243, 244]. In that case it includes components such as education, skills in gaining control of seizures, recognizing triggers, changing cognitions and behaviors associated with seizures, and widening therapy to other aspects of interpersonal functioning [10]. There are also special CBT workbooks which help the patients overcome their functional problems [245, 246]. Hypnosis has also been proven effective for FNDs in randomized controlled trials [238].

There is evidence that physical therapy helps improve FND, especially the one manifested as a movement disorder [247–255]. It has as goal the change in the processing of complex motor programs and the facilitation of engagement in more adaptive patterns of movement or gait. Motor rehabilitation strategies aim to help the patient establish normal control of movement through physiotherapy and occupational or speech therapy. It includes motor retraining that begins with establishing the basic movement patterns (e.g., weight-shifting); the complexity of movement is sequentially increased toward normal movement patterns. Reducing symptom severity by distraction can also be used. Unhelpful cognitions (e.g., thinking "my nerves are damaged") and behaviors (e.g., acting as moving could cause more damage) should be addressed [10, 256]. Outpatient interventions with a physical or neurorehabilitation focus may be beneficial for patients with less severe symptoms.

If the physical therapist is not familiar with FND, he or she should be provided by the referring clinician with the consensus guidelines. The referring clinician should also be available for consultations.

The psychiatric comorbidities in FND (depression, anxiety, post-traumatic stress disorder, etc.) may require a pharmacological treatment. CBT was reported to ameliorate the depression and anxiety in FND patients, as well [237].

Some other non-pharmacological interventions have been proven effective in single cases or small case series of FNDs. These include transcutaneous electrical stimulation, transcranial magnetic stimulation, and therapeutic sedation with propofol [251, 257].

15.10 Outcomes and Prognosis

Data concerning outcome are variable. However, partially because of delayed and poorly delivered diagnoses, the prognosis of FNDs remains generally poor. The largest prospective follow-up study on 716 patients with mixed FNDs followed up over 1 year in Scotland concluded to a poor outcome with 67% of the patients having unchanged symptoms or worse [258]. Even patients with good understanding and acceptance of diagnosis continue to have symptoms over time, which sometimes progress [10]. Consistent negative predictors are long duration of symptoms before diagnosis, receiving a health-related benefit, and comorbid personality disorders, whereas positive predictive factors include young age and early diagnosis [10, 15, 257, 259, 260]. Therefore, the prognosis seems to be better in children than in adolescent and adults [1].

A systematic review on patients with FMD concluded that about 40% have a persistent or worse symptomatic during the follow-up with only 20% showing a complete remission [257]. Only about 40% of patients with PNES achieved the seizure remission during the follow-up period according to other systematic reviews [15, 261]. Sensory symptoms seem to have a similar prognosis with improvement in about 45% [262] (in another study however 83% [205]) of cases.

There are currently no established clinical factors or screening tests to indicate which patients may benefit from specific treatment modalities and over what period [10].

15.11 Prevention of Functional Disorders

Currently there is little knowledge on primary prevention of FMD. However, as emotional and personality disorders are risk factors for FND, an early management of these conditions could result in reduced incidence of functional neurological symptoms. Another point could be reducing the early-life stressors that also seem to be associated with the development of FND.

The presence of other health issues, difficulties in interpersonal relationships, and previous life events such as bereavement are other risk factors for FND. Therefore, their adequate approach can help prevent FNDs. There are sometimes precipitating physical events before the onset of FND [48, 263, 264]; however, preventing all physical injuries is probably not possible. At the same time, an adequate treatment of the traumatic consequences could possibly reduce the occurrence of FND.

The role of the educational background and IQ as risk factors is not clear yet, although it seems that they have little effect on outcome [265]. The news coverage of medical conditions and illnesses portrayed on television and movies seems also to have an important role in the development of neurological functional disorders [54, 58] and could play an important role in education of population in order to prevent or at least early recognize the FND.

15.12 Conclusions

FNDs include several conditions strongly and interdependently associated with mental health. Although their etiopathology per definition includes no organic causes, some underlying minor brain changes were discovered. Early recognition of the FND and their risks, precipitating and perpetuating factors, as well as an adequate management of FND significantly improve the prognosis.

References

1. American Psychiatric Association, DSM-5 Task Force. Diagnostic and statistical manual of mental disorders: DSM-5™. 5th ed. Washington, DC: American Psychiatric Publishing; 2013.
2. World Health Organization. International classification of diseases for mortality and morbidity statistics (11th Revision). 2018. https://icd.who.int/browse11/l-m/en. Accessed 18 Oct 2020.
3. Butler M, Seynaeve M, Nicholson TR, Pick S, Kanaan RA, Lees A, Young AH, Rucker J. Psychedelic treatment of functional neurological disorder: a systematic review. Ther Adv Psychopharmacol. 2020;10:2045125320912125.
4. Thenganatt MA, Jankovic J. Psychogenic (functional) movement disorders. Continuum (Minneap Minn). 2019;25(4):1121–40.
5. Søgaard U, Mathiesen BB, Simonsen E. Personality and psychopathology in patients with mixed sensory-motor functional neurological disorder (conversion disorder): a pilot study. J Nerv Ment Dis. 2019;207(7):546–54.
6. Carson A, Lehn A. Epidemiology. Handb Clin Neurol. 2016;139:47–60.
7. Stone J, Carson A, Duncan R, Roberts R, Warlow C, Hibberd C, Coleman R, Cull R, Murray G, Pelosi A, Cavanagh J, Matthews K, Goldbeck R, Smyth R, Walker J, Sharpe M. Who is referred to neurology clinics?--The diagnoses made in 3781 new patients. Clin Neurol Neurosurg. 2010;112(9):747–51.
8. Ding JM, Kanaan RA. Conversion disorder: a systematic review of current terminology. Gen Hosp Psychiatry. 2017;45:51–5.
9. Stone J. The bare essentials: functional symptoms in neurology. Pract Neurol. 2009;9(3):179–89.
10. Espay AJ, Aybek S, Carson A, Edwards MJ, Goldstein LH, Hallett M, LaFaver K, LaFrance WC Jr, Lang AE, Nicholson T, Nielsen G, Reuber M, Voon V, Stone J, Morgante F. Current concepts in diagnosis and treatment of functional neurological disorders. JAMA Neurol. 2018;75(9):1132–41.
11. Creed F, Guthrie E, Fink P, Henningsen P, Rief W, Sharpe M, White P. Is there a better term than "medically unexplained symptoms"? J Psychosom Res. 2010;68(1):5–8.
12. Stone J, LaFrance WC Jr, Brown R, Spiegel D, Levenson JL, Sharpe M. Conversion disorder: current problems and potential solutions for DSM-5. J Psychosom Res. 2011;71(6):369–76.
13. Stone J, Hallett M, Carson A, Bergen D, Shakir R. Functional disorders in the neurology section of ICD-11: a landmark opportunity. Neurology. 2014;83(24):2299–301.

14. Cock HR, Edwards MJ. Functional neurological disorders: acute presentations and management. Clin Med (Lond). 2018;18(5):414–7.
15. Gelauff J, Stone J. Prognosis of functional neurologic disorders. Handb Clin Neurol. 2016;139:523–41.
16. Stone J. Functional neurological symptoms. J R Coll Physicians Edinb. 2011;41(1):38–42.
17. Nijenhuis E, van der Hart O, Steele K. Trauma-related structural dissociation of the personality. Act Nerv Super. 2010;52:1–23.
18. Howell EF. The dissociative mind. Boca Raton: The Analytic Press/Taylor & Francis Group; 2015.
19. Ekanayake V, Kranick S, LaFaver K, et al. Personality traits in psychogenic nonepileptic seizures (PNES) and psychogenic movement disorder (PMD): neuroticism and perfectionism. J Psychosom Res. 2017;97:23–9.
20. Demartini B, Petrochilos P, Ricciardi L, Price G, Edwards MJ, Joyce E. The role of alexithymia in the development of functional motor symptoms (conversion disorder). J Neurol Neurosurg Psychiatry. 2014;85:1132–7.
21. Koelen JA, Eurelings-Bontekoe EH, Stuke F, Luyten P. Insecure attachment strategies are associated with cognitive alexithymia in patients with severe somatoform disorder. Int J Psychiatry Med. 2015;49:264–78.
22. Martino I, Bruni A, Labate A, Vasta R, Cerasa A, Borzì G, De Fazio P, Gambardella A. Psychopathological constellation in patients with PNES: a new hypothesis. Epilepsy Behav. 2018;78:297–301.
23. Williams B, Ospina JP, Jalilianhasanpour R, Fricchione GL, Perez DL. Fearful attachment linked to childhood abuse, alexithymia, and depression in motor functional neurological disorders. J Neuropsychiatry Clin Neurosci. 2018;31:65–9.
24. Erten E, Yenilmez Y, Fistikci N, Saatcioglu O. The relationship between temperament and character in conversion disorder and comorbid depression. Compr Psychiatry. 2013;54:354–61.
25. Gulec MY, Ynanc L, Yanartathorn O, Uzer A, Gulec H. Predictors of suicide in patients with conversion disorder. Compr Psychiatry. 2014;55:457–62.
26. Sarisoy G, Kaçar ÖF, Öztürk A, Yilman T, Mor S, Özturan DD, Yazici N, Gümüş K. Temperament and character traits in patients with conversion disorder and their relations with dissociation. Psychiatr Danub. 2015;27:390–6.
27. Carson A, Ludwig L, Welch K. Psychologic theories in functional neurologic disorders. In: Hallett M, Stone J, Carson A, editors. Handbook of clinical neurology, vol. 139. Elsevier: Amsterdam; 2016. p. 105–20.
28. Carson A, Hallett M, Stone J. Assessment of patients with functional neurologic disorders. Handb Clin Neurol. 2016;139:169–88.
29. Kranick S, Ekanayake V, Martinez V, Ameli R, Hallett M, Voon V. Psychopathology and psychogenic movement disorders. Mov Disord. 2011;26(10):1844–50.
30. Roelofs K, Keijsers GP, Hoogduin KA, Naring GW, Moene FC. Childhood abuse in patients with conversion disorder. Am J Psychiatry. 2002;159:1908–13.
31. Perez DL, Matin N, Barsky A, Costumero-Ramos V, Makaretz SJ, Young SS, Sepulcre J, LaFrance WC Jr, Keshavan MS, Dickerson BC. Cingulo-insular structural alterations associated with psychogenic symptoms, childhood abuse and PTSD in functional neurological disorders. J Neurol Neurosurg Psychiatry. 2017;88(6):491–7. Erratum in: J Neurol Neurosurg Psychiatry. 2017;88(12):1098.
32. Asadi-Pooya AA, Bahrami Z. Sexual abuse and psychogenic nonepileptic seizures. Neurol Sci. 2019;40(8):1607–10.
33. Pastore A, Pierri G, Fabio G, Ferramosca S, Gigante A, Superbo M, Pellicciari R, Margari F. Differences in psychopathology and behavioral characteristics of patients affected by conversion motor disorder and organic dystonia. Neuropsychiatr Dis Treat. 2018;14:1287–95.
34. Epstein SA, Maurer CW, LaFaver K, Ameli R, Sinclair S, Hallett M. Insights into chronic functional movement disorders: the value of qualitative psychiatric interviews. Psychosomatics. 2016;57(6):566–75.

35. Roelofs K, Pasman J. Stress, childhood trauma, and cognitive functions in functional neurologic disorders. Handb Clin Neurol. 2016;139:139–55.
36. Akyüz F, Gökalp PG, Erdiman S, Oflaz S, Karşidağ Ç. Conversion disorder comorbidity and childhood trauma. Noro Psikiyatr Ars. 2017;54(1):15–20.
37. Ludwig L, Pasman JA, Nicholson T, et al. Stressful life events and maltreatment in conversion (functional neurological) disorder: systematic review and meta-analysis of case-control studies. Lancet Psychiatry. 2018;5(4):307–20.
38. Pick S, Goldstein LH, Perez DL, Nicholson TR. Emotional processing in functional neurological disorder: a review, biopsychosocial model and research agenda. J Neurol Neurosurg Psychiatry. 2019;90(6):704–11.
39. van der Hoeven RM, Broersma M, Pijnenborg GH, Koops EA, van Laar T, Stone J, van Beilen M. Functional (psychogenic) movement disorders associated with normal scores in psychological questionnaires: a case control study. J Psychosom Res. 2015;79:190–4.
40. de Gusmão CM, Guerriero RM, Bernson-Leung ME, Pier D, Ibeziako PI, Bujoreanu S, Maski KP, Urion DK, Waugh JL. Functional neurological symptom disorders in a pediatric emergency room: diagnostic accuracy, features, and outcome. Pediatr Neurol. 2014;51:233–8.
41. Reuber M, Howlett S, Khan A, Grünewald RA. Non-epileptic seizures and other functional neurological symptoms: predisposing, precipitating, and perpetuating factors. Psychosomatics. 2007;48(3):230–8.
42. Sharpe D, Faye C. Non-epileptic seizures and child sexual abuse: a critical review of the literature. Clin Psychol Rev. 2006;26:1020–40.
43. Jankovic J, Van der Linden C. Dystonia and tremor induced by peripheral trauma: predisposing factors. J Neurol Neurosurg Psychiatry. 1988;51(12):1512–9.
44. Baizabal-Carvallo JF, Hallett M, Jankovic J. Pathogenesis and pathophysiology of functional (psychogenic) movement disorders. Neurobiol Dis. 2019;127:32–44.
45. Sankhla C, Lai EC, Jankovic J. Peripherally induced oromandibular dystonia. J Neurol Neurosurg Psychiatry. 1998;65(5):722–8.
46. van Rooijen DE, Geraedts EJ, Marinus J, Jankovic J, van Hilten JJ. Peripheral trauma and movement disorders: a systematic review of reported cases. J Neurol Neurosurg Psychiatry. 2011;82:892–8.
47. Macerollo A, Edwards MJ, Huang HC, Lu MK, Chen HJ, Tsai CH, Chen JC. Peripheral trauma and risk of dystonia: what are the evidences and potential co-risk factors from a population insurance database? PLoS One. 2019;14(5):e0216772.
48. Schrag A, Trimble M, Quinn N, Bhatia K. The syndrome of fixed dystonia: an evaluation of 103 patients. Brain. 2004;127(Pt 10):2360–72.
49. Stone J, Carson A, Aditya H, Prescott R, Zaubi M, Warlow C, Sharpe M. The role of physical injury in motor and sensory conversion symptoms: a systematic and narrative review. J Psychosom Res. 2009;66(5):383–90.
50. Pareés I, Kojovic M, Pires C, Rubio-Agusti I, Saifee TA, Sadnicka A, Kassavetis P, Macerollo A, Bhatia KP, Carson A, Stone J, Edwards MJ. Physical precipitating factors in functional movement disorders. J Neurol Sci. 2014;338(1–2):174–7.
51. Roelofs K, Spinhoven P. Trauma and medically unexplained symptoms: towards an integration of cognitive and neurobiological accounts. Clin Psychol Rev. 2007;27:798–820.
52. Roelofs K, Keijsers GP, Hoogduin KA, Näring GW, Moene FC. Childhood abuse in patients with conversion disorder. Am J Psychiatry. 2002;159(11):1908–13.
53. Selkirk M, Duncan R, Oto M, Pelosi A. Clinical differences between patients with non-epileptic seizures who report antecedent sexual abuse and those who do not. Epilepsia. 2008;49(8):1446–50.
54. Fobian AD, Elliott L. A review of functional neurological symptom disorder etiology and the integrated etiological summary model. J Psychiatry Neurosci. 2019;44(1):8–18.
55. Crimlisk HL, Bhatia K, Cope H, David A, Marsden CD, Ron MA. Slater revisited: 6 year follow up study of patients with medically unexplained motor symptoms. BMJ. 1998;316(7131):582–6.

56. Perez DL, Barsky AJ, Vago DR, Baslet G, Silbersweig DA. A neural circuit framework for somatosensory amplification in somatoform disorders. J Neuropsychiatry Clin Neurosci. 2015;27(1):e40–50.
57. Macerollo A, Chen JC, Pareés I, Kassavetis P, Kilner JM, Edwards MJ. Sensory attenuation assessed by sensory evoked potentials in functional movement disorders. PLoS One. 2015;10(6):e0129507.
58. Edwards MJ, Adams RA, Brown H, Pareés I, Friston KJ. A Bayesian account of 'hysteria'. Brain. 2012;135(Pt 11):3495–512.
59. Apazoglou K, Mazzola V, Wegrzyk J, Frasca Polara G, Aybek S. Biological and perceived stress in motor functional neurological disorders. Psychoneuroendocrinology. 2017;85:142–50.
60. Atmaca M, Baykara S, Mermi O, Yildirim H, Akaslan U. Pituitary volumes are changed in patients with conversion disorder. Brain Imaging Behav. 2016;10(1):92–5.
61. Bakvis P, Spinhoven P, Giltay EJ, Kuyk J, Edelbroek PM, Zitman FG, Roelofs K. Basal hypercortisolism and trauma in patients with psychogenic nonepileptic seizures. Epilepsia. 2010;51(5):752–9.
62. Bakvis P, Spinhoven P, Roelofs K. Basal cortisol is positively correlated to threat vigilance in patients with psychogenic nonepileptic seizures. Epilepsy Behav. 2009;16(3):558–60.
63. Bakvis P, Roelofs K, Kuyk J, Edelbroek PM, Swinkels WA, Spinhoven P. Trauma, stress, and preconscious threat processing in patients with psychogenic nonepileptic seizures. Epilepsia. 2009;50(5):1001–11.
64. Bakvis P, Spinhoven P, Putman P, Zitman FG, Roelofs K. The effect of stress induction on working memory in patients with psychogenic nonepileptic seizures. Epilepsy Behav. 2010;19(3):448–54.
65. Simeon D, Knutelska M, Yehuda R, Putnam F, Schmeidler J, Smith LM. Hypothalamic-pituitary-adrenal axis function in dissociative disorders, post-traumatic stress disorder, and healthy volunteers. Biol Psychiatry. 2007;61(8):966–73.
66. Tak LM, Bakker SJ, Rosmalen JG. Dysfunction of the hypothalamic-pituitary-adrenal axis and functional somatic symptoms: a longitudinal cohort study in the general population. Psychoneuroendocrinology. 2009;34(6):869–77.
67. Maurer CW, LaFaver K, Ameli R, Toledo R, Hallett M. A biological measure of stress levels in patients with functional movement disorders. Parkinsonism Relat Disord. 2015;21(9):1072–5.
68. Perez DL, Dworetzky BA, Dickerson BC, Leung L, Cohn R, Baslet G, Silbersweig DA. An integrative neurocircuit perspective on psychogenic nonepileptic seizures and functional movement disorders: neural functional unawareness. Clin EEG Neurosci. 2015;46(1):4–15.
69. Pareés I, Brown H, Nuruki A, Adams RA, Davare M, Bhatia KP, Friston K, Edwards MJ. Loss of sensory attenuation in patients with functional (psychogenic) movement disorders. Brain. 2014;137(Pt 11):2916–21.
70. Bryant RA, Das P. The neural circuitry of conversion disorder and its recovery. J Abnorm Psychol. 2012;121(1):289–96.
71. Ghaffar O, Staines WR, Feinstein A. Unexplained neurologic symptoms: an fMRI study of sensory conversion disorder. Neurology. 2006;67(11):2036–8.
72. Maurer CW, LaFaver K, Ameli R, Epstein SA, Hallett M, Horovitz SG. Impaired self-agency in functional movement disorders: a resting-state fMRI study. Neurology. 2016;87(6):564–70.
73. Voon V, Gallea C, Hattori N, Bruno M, Ekanayake V, Hallett M. The involuntary nature of conversion disorder. Neurology. 2010;74(3):223–8.
74. Nahab FB, Kundu P, Maurer C, Shen Q, Hallett M. Impaired sense of agency in functional movement disorders: an fMRI study. PLoS One. 2017;12(4):e0172502.
75. Roelofs JJ, Teodoro T, Edwards MJ. Neuroimaging in functional movement disorders. Curr Neurol Neurosci Rep. 2019;19(3):12.
76. Marshall JC, Halligan PW, Fink GR, Wade DT, Frackowiak RS. The functional anatomy of a hysterical paralysis. Cognition. 1997;64(1):B1–8.
77. Halligan PW, Athwal BS, Oakley DA, Frackowiak RS. Imaging hypnotic paralysis: implications for conversion hysteria. Lancet. 2000;355(9208):986–7.

78. Hedera P. Metabolic hyperactivity of the medial posterior parietal lobes in psychogenic tremor. Tremor Other Hyperkinet Mov (NY). 2012;2:tre-02-50-441-1.
79. Blakemore RL, Sinanaj I, Galli S, Aybek S, Vuilleumier P. Aversive stimuli exacerbate defensive motor behaviour in motor conversion disorder. Neuropsychologia. 2016;93(Pt A):229–41.
80. Schrag AE, Mehta AR, Bhatia KP, Brown RJ, Frackowiak RS, Trimble MR, Ward NS, Rowe JB. The functional neuroimaging correlates of psychogenic versus organic dystonia. Brain. 2013;136(Pt 3):770–81.
81. Espay AJ, Maloney T, Vannest J, Norris MM, Eliassen JC, Neefus E, Allendorfer JB, Lang AE, Szaflarski JP. Impaired emotion processing in functional (psychogenic) tremor: a functional magnetic resonance imaging study. Neuroimage Clin. 2018;17:179–87.
82. Bègue I, Adams C, Stone J, Perez DL. Structural alterations in functional neurological disorder and related conditions: a software and hardware problem? Neuroimage Clin. 2019;22:101798.
83. Voon V, Brezing C, Gallea C, Hallett M. Aberrant supplementary motor complex and limbic activity during motor preparation in motor conversion disorder. Mov Disord. 2011;26(13):2396–403.
84. Aybek S, Nicholson TR, Draganski B, Daly E, Murphy DG, David AS, Kanaan RA. Grey matter changes in motor conversion disorder. J Neurol Neurosurg Psychiatry. 2014;85(2):236–8.
85. Aybek S, Vuilleumier P. Imaging studies of functional neurologic disorders. Handb Clin Neurol. 2016;139:73–84.
86. Xue G, Aron AR, Poldrack RA. Common neural substrates for inhibition of spoken and manual responses. Cereb Cortex. 2008;18(8):1923–32.
87. Vuilleumier P. Brain circuits implicated in psychogenic paralysis in conversion disorders and hypnosis. Neurophysiol Clin. 2014;44:323–37.
88. Vuilleumier P, Chicherio C, Assal F, Schwartz S, Slosman D, Landis T. Functional neuro-anatomical correlates of hysterical sensorimotor loss [published correction appears in Brain. 2016 May;139(Pt 5):e29]. Brain. 2001;124(Pt 6):1077–90.
89. Kanaan RA, Craig TK, Wessely SC, David AS. Imaging repressed memories in motor conversion disorder. Psychosom. Med. 2007;69:202–5.
90. Boy F, Husain M, Singh KD, Sumner P. Supplementary motor area activations in unconscious inhibition of voluntary action. Exp Brain Res. 2010;206(4):441–8.
91. Nachev P, Kennard C, Husain M. Functional role of the supplementary and pre-supplementary motor areas. Nat Rev Neurosci. 2008;9(11):856–69.
92. de Lange FP, Toni I, Roelofs K. Altered connectivity between prefrontal and sensorimotor cortex in conversion paralysis. Neuropsychologia. 2010;48:1782–8.
93. van Beilen M, Vogt BA, Leenders KL. Increased activation in cingulate cortex in conversion disorder: what does it mean? J Neurol Sci. 2010;289(1–2):155–8.
94. Avanzino L, Martino D, van de Warrenburg BP, Schneider SA, Abbruzzese G, Defazio G, Schrag A, Bhatia KP, Rothwell JC. Cortical excitability is abnormal in patients with the "fixed dystonia" syndrome. Mov Disord. 2008;23(5):646–52.
95. Cojan Y, Waber L, Carruzzo A, Vuilleumier P. Motor inhibition in hysterical conversion paralysis. Neuroimage. 2009;47:1026–37.
96. Meunier S, Russmann H, Shamim E, Lamy JC, Hallett M. Plasticity of cortical inhibition in dystonia is impaired after motor learning and paired-associative stimulation. Eur J Neurosci. 2012;35(6):975–86.
97. Espay AJ, Morgante F, Purzner J, Gunraj CA, Lang AE, Chen R. Cortical and spinal abnormalities in psychogenic dystonia. Ann Neurol. 2006;59(5):825–34.
98. Tisch S. Recent advances in understanding and managing dystonia. F1000Res. 2018;7:F1000 Faculty Rev-1124.
99. Quartarone A, Rizzo V, Terranova C, et al. Abnormal sensorimotor plasticity in organic but not in psychogenic dystonia. Brain. 2009;132(Pt 10):2871–7.

100. Conte A, Defazio G, Mascia M, Belvisi D, Pantano P, Berardelli A. Advances in the pathophysiology of adult-onset focal dystonias: recent neurophysiological and neuroimaging evidence. F1000Res. 2020;9:F1000 Faculty Rev-67.
101. Hallett M. Physiology of psychogenic movement disorders. J Clin Neurosci. 2010;17(8):959–65.
102. Voon V, Cavanna AE, Coburn K, et al. Functional neuroanatomy and neurophysiology of functional neurological disorders (conversion disorder). J Neuropsychiatry Clin Neurosci. 2016;28(3):168–90.
103. Scott RL, Anson JG. Neural correlates of motor conversion disorder. Motor Control. 2009;13(2):161–84.
104. Spence SA. Hysteria: a new look. Psychiatry. 2006;5(2):56–60.
105. Maurer CW, LaFaver K, Limachia GS, et al. Gray matter differences in patients with functional movement disorders. Neurology. 2018;91(20):e1870–9.
106. Perez DL, Williams B, Matin N, et al. Corticolimbic structural alterations linked to health status and trait anxiety in functional neurological disorder. J Neurol Neurosurg Psychiatry. 2017;88(12):1052–9.
107. Atmaca M, Aydin A, Tezcan E, Poyraz AK, Kara B. Volumetric investigation of brain regions in patients with conversion disorder. Prog Neuropsychopharmacol Biol Psychiatry. 2006;30(4):708–13.
108. Kozlowska K, Griffiths KR, Foster SL, Linton J, Williams LM, Korgaonkar MS. Grey matter abnormalities in children and adolescents with functional neurological symptom disorder. Neuroimage Clin. 2017;15:306–14.
109. Tomic A, Agosta F, Sarasso E, Petrovic I, Basaia S, Pesic D, Kostic M, Fontana A, Kostic VS, Filippi M. Are there two different forms of functional dystonia? A multimodal brain structural MRI study. Mol Psychiatry. 2020;25:3350.
110. Erro R, Brigo F, Trinka E, Turri G, Edwards MJ, Tinazzi M. Psychogenic nonepileptic seizures and movement disorders. Neurol Clin Pract. 2016;6(2):138–49.
111. Feinstein A, Stergiopoulos V, Fine J, Lang AE. Psychiatric outcome in patients with a psychogenic movement disorder: a prospective study. Neuropsychiatry Neuropsychol Behav Neurol. 2001;14:169–76.
112. Stone J, Warlow CF, Sharpe M. The symptom of functional weakness: a controlled study of 107 patients. Brain. 2010;133:1537–51.
113. Lempert T, Dieterich M, Huppert D, Brandt T. Psychogenic disorders in neurology: frequency and clinical spectrum. Acta Neurol Scand. 1990;82(5):335–40.
114. Dimaro LV, Dawson DL, Roberts NA, et al. Anxiety and avoidance in psychogenic nonepileptic seizures: the role of implicit and explicit anxiety. Epilepsy Behav. 2014;33:77–86.
115. Sar V, Akyuz G, Kundakci T, Kiziltan E, Dogan O. Childhood trauma, dissociation, and psychiatric comorbidity in patients with conversion disorder. Am J Psychiatry. 2004;161:2271–6.
116. Scevola L, Teitelbaum J, Oddo S, Centurion E, Loidl CF, Kochen S, Alessio D, L. Psychiatric disorders in patients with psychogenic nonepileptic seizures and drug-resistant epilepsy: a study of an Argentine population. Epilepsy Behav. 2013;29:155–60.
117. Plioplys S, Doss J, Siddarth P, Bursch B, Falcone T, Forgey M, Hinman K, LaFrance WC Jr, Laptook R, Shaw RJ, Weisbrot DM, Willis MD, Caplan R. Risk factors for comorbid psychopathology in youth with psychogenic nonepileptic seizures. Seizure. 2016;38:32–7.
118. Binzer M, Andersen PM, Kullgren G. Clinical characteristics of patients with motor disability due to conversion disorder: a prospective control group study. J Neurol Neurosurg Psychiatry. 1997;63:83–8.
119. Direk N, Kulaksizoglu IB, Alpay K, Gurses C. Using personality disorders to distinguish between patients with psychogenic nonepileptic seizures and those with epileptic seizures. Epilepsy Behav. 2012;23:138–41.
120. Sar V, Islam S, Ozturk E. Childhood emotional abuse and dissociation in patients with conversion symptoms. Psychiatry Clin Neurosci. 2009;63:670–7.

121. Labudda K, Frauenheim M, Illies D, Miller I, Schrecke M, Vietmeier N, Brandt C, Bien CG. Psychiatric disorders and trauma history in patients with pure PNES and patients with PNES and coexisting epilepsy. Epilepsy Behav. 2018;88:41–8.
122. Baroni G, Martins WA, Piccinini V, da Rosa MP, de Paola L, Paglioli E, Margis R, Palmini A. Neuropsychiatric features of the coexistence of epilepsy and psychogenic nonepileptic seizures. J Psychosom Res. 2018;111:83–8.
123. Reuber M, Qurishi A, Bauer J, Helmstaedter C, Fernandez G, Widman G, Elger CE. Are there physical risk factors for psychogenic non-epileptic seizures in patients with epilepsy? Seizure. 2003;12(8):561–7.
124. Bautista RE, Gonzales-Salazar W, Ochoa JG. Expanding the theory of symptom modeling in patents with psychogenic nonepileptic seizures. Epilepsy Behav. 2008;13:407–9.
125. Onofrj M, Bonanni L, Manzoli L, Thomas. Cohort study on somatoform disorders in Parkinson disease and dementia with Lewy bodies. Neurology. 2010;74:1598–606.
126. Ebmeier KP, O'Brien JT, Taylor J-P, editors. Psychiatry of Parkinson's disease. Advances in biological psychiatry, vol. 27. Basel: Karger; 2012. p. 125–32.
127. Paulus KS, Meloni M, Carpentras G, Sassu C, De Natale E, Deriu F, Galistu P, Agnetti V. 4 Parkinson's disease and conversion disorder: case report and literature review. Basal Ganglia. 2012;2(4):258.
128. Wissel BD, Dwivedi AK, Merola A, Chin D, Jacob C, Duker AP, Vaughan JE, Lovera L, LaFaver K, Levy A, Lang AE, Morgante F, Nirenberg MJ, Stephen C, Sharma N, Romagnolo A, Lopiano L, Balint B, Yu XX, Bhatia KP, Espay AJ. Functional neurological disorders in Parkinson disease. J Neurol Neurosurg Psychiatry. 2018;89(6):566–71.
129. Stone J, Carson A, Duncan R, Roberts R, Coleman R, Warlow C, Murray G, Pelosi A, Cavanagh J, Matthews K, Goldbeck R, Sharpe M. Which neurological diseases are most likely to be associated with "symptoms unexplained by organic disease". J Neurol. 2012;259(1):33–8.
130. Krashin D, Murinova N. Association of conversion disorder and migraine. Neurology. 2019;92(15S):P3.10-022.
131. García-Albea E. Jaqueca asociada a trastorno de conversión (jaqueca de Babinski). Análisis de una serie de 43 casos [Migraine associated with conversion symptoms (Babinski's migraine): evaluation of a series of 43 cases]. Neurologia. 2012;27(3):125–35.
132. Factor SA, Podskalny GD, Molho ES. Psychogenic movement disorders: frequency, clinical profile, and characteristics. J Neurol Neurosurg Psychiatry. 1995;59:406–12.
133. Pennington C, Newson M, Hayre A, Coulthard E. Functional cognitive disorder: what is it and what to do about it? Pract Neurol. 2015;15(6):436–44.
134. Stone J, Carson A. Functional neurologic symptoms: assessment and management. Neurol Clin. 2011;29:1–18.
135. Austin MP, Mitchell P, Goodwin GM. Cognitive deficits in depression: possible implications for functional neuropathology. Br J Psychiatry. 2001;178:200–6.
136. Tsui P, Deptula A, Yuan DY. Conversion disorder, functional neurological symptom disorder, and chronic pain: comorbidity, assessment, and treatment. Curr Pain Headache Rep. 2017;21(6):29.
137. Batla A, Pareés I, Edwards MJ, et al. Lower urinary tract dysfunction in patients with functional movement disorders. J Neurol Sci. 2016;361:192–4.
138. Deveci A, Taskin O, Dinc G, Yilmaz H, Demet MM, Erbay-Dundar P, Kaya E, Ozmen E. Prevalence of pseudoneurologic conversion disorder in an urban community in Manisa, Turkey. Soc Psychiatry Psychiatr Epidemiol. 2007;42(11):857–64.
139. Ahmad O, Ahmad KE. Functional neurological disorders in outpatient practice: an Australian cohort. J Clin Neurosci. 2016;28:93–6.
140. Szaflarski JP, Ficker DM, Cahill WT, Privitera MD. Four-year incidence of psychogenic non-epileptic seizures in adults in Hamilton County, OH. Neurology. 2000;55(10):1561–3.
141. Faravelli C, Salvatori S, Galassi F, Aiazzi L, Drei C, Cabras P. Epidemiology of somatoform disorders: a community survey in Florence. Soc Psychiatry Psychiatr Epidemiol. 1997;32(1):24–9.

142. Morgante F, Edwards MJ, Espay AJ. Psychogenic movement disorders. Continuum. 2013;19(5 Movement Disorders):1383–96.
143. Frasca Polara G, Fleury V, Stone J, et al. Prevalence of functional (psychogenic) parkinsonism in two Swiss movement disorders clinics and review of the literature. J Neurol Sci. 2018;387:37–45.
144. Thomas M, Jankovic J. Psychogenic movement disorders: diagnosis and management. CNS Drugs. 2004;18(7):437–52.
145. Williams DT, Ford B, Fahn S. Phenomenology and psychopathsion related to psychogenic movement disorders. Adv Neurol. 1995;65:231–57.
146. Zeigler FJ, Imboden JB, Meyer E. Contemporary conversion al. reactions: a clinical study. Am J Psychiatry. 1960;116:901–10.
147. Lempert T, Diettrich M, Huppert D, et al. Psychogenic disorders in neurology: frequency and clinical spectrum. Acta Neurol Scand. 1990;82:335–40.
148. Marsden CD. Hysteria - a neurologist's view. Psychol Med. 1986;16:277–88.
149. Trimble MR. Neuropsychiatry. Chichester: Wiley; 1981. p. 79–87.
150. Cubo E, Hinson VK, Goetz CG, Garcia Ruiz P, Garcia de Yebenes J, Marti MJ, Rodriguez Oroz MC, Linazasoro G, Chacón J, Vázquez A, López del Val J, Leurgans S, Wuu J. Transcultural comparison of psychogenic movement disorders. Mov Disord. 2005;20(10):1343–5.
151. Williams DT, Ford B, Fahn S. Phenomenology and psychopathsion related to psy chogenic movement disorders. Adv Neurol. 1995;65:231–57.
152. Bäumer T, Sajin V, Münchau A. Childhood-onset movement disorders: a clinical series of 606 cases. Mov Disord Clin Pract. 2016;4(3):437–40.
153. Gelder M, Gath D, Mayou R, Cowen P, editors. Oxford Textbook of Psychiatry. Oxford: Oxford University Press; 1996. p. 353.
154. Goodyer I. Hysterical conversion reactions in childhood. J Child Psychol Psychiatry. 1981;22(2):179–88.
155. Asadi-Pooya AA, Emami Y, Emami M. Psychogenic non-epileptic seizures in Iran. Seizure. 2014;23(3):175–7.
156. Alsaadi TM, Marquez AV. Psychogenic non-epileptic seizures. Am Fam Physician. 2005;72:849–56.
157. Martin R, Burneo JG, Prasad A, et al. Frequency of epilepsy in patients with psychogenic seizures monitored by video-EEG. Neurology. 2003;61:1791–2.
158. Asadi-Pooya AA, Sperling MR. Epidemiology of psychogenic nonepileptic seizures. Epilepsy Behav. 2015;46:60–5.
159. Duncan R, Razvi S, Mulhern S. Newly presenting psychogenic nonepileptic seizures: incidence, population characteristics, and early outcome from a prospective audit of a first seizure clinic. Epilepsy Behav. 2011;20:308–11.
160. Sigurdardottir KR, Olafsson E. Incidence of psychogenic seizures in adults: a population-based study in Iceland. Epilepsia. 1998;39:749–52.
161. Commissaris CJ, Ponds RW, Jolles J. Subjective forgetfulness in a normal Dutch population: possibilities for health education and other interventions. Patient Educ Couns. 1998;34:25–32.
162. Almeida OP, Hill K, Howard R, O'Brien J, Levy R. Demographic and clinical features of patients attending a memory clinic. Int J Geriatr Psychiatry. 1993;8:497–501.
163. Menon R, Larner AJ. Use of cognitive screening instruments in primary care: the impact of national dementia directives (NICE/SCIE, National dementia strategy). Fam Pract. 2011;28:272–6.
164. Blackburn DJ, Shanks MF, Harkness KA, Reuber M, Venneri A. Political drive to screen for pre-dementia: not evidence based and ignores the harms of diagnosis. BMJ. 2013;347:f5125.
165. Stone J, Pal S, Blackburn D, Reuber M, Thekkumpurath P, Carson A. Functional (psychogenic) cognitive disorders: a perspective from the neurology clinic. J Alzheimers Dis. 2015;48(Suppl 1):S5–S17.
166. Harrison NA, Johnston K, Corno F, Casey SJ, Friedner K, Humphreys K, Jaldow EJ, Pitkanen M, Kopelman MD. Psychogenic amnesia: syndromes, outcome, and patterns of retrograde amnesia. Brain. 2017;140(9):2498–510.

167. Egan RA. Functional visual loss. Ophthalmol Clin N Am. 2004;17:321–8.
168. Bose S, Kupersmith MJ. Neuro-ophthalmologic presentations of functional visual disorders. Neurol Clin. 1995;13:321–39.
169. Dieterich M, Staab JP. Functional dizziness: from phobic postu ral vertigo and chronic subjective dizziness to persistent postural-perceptual dizziness. Curr Opin Neurol. 2017;30(1):107–13.
170. Schlaegel TF, Quilala FV, Hysterical amblyopia. Statistical analysis of forth-two cases found in survey of eight hundred unselected eye patients at a state medical centre. Arch Ophthalmol. 1955;54:875–84.
171. Brandt T, Dieterich M, Strupp M. Vertigo and dizziness: common complaints. 2nd ed. London: Springer; 2013.
172. Batu ED, Anlar B, Topcu M, Turanli G. Vertigo in childhood: a retrospective series of 100 children. Eur J Paediatr Neurol. 2015;19:226–32.
173. Daum C, Gheorghita F, Spatola M, et al. Interobserver agreement and validity of bedside 'positive signs' for functional weakness, sensory and gait disorders in conversion disorder: a pilot study. J Neurol Neurosurg Psychiatry. 2015;86(4):425–30.
174. Daum C, Hubschmid M, Aybek S. The value of 'positive' clinical signs for weakness, sensory and gait disorders in conversion disorder: a systematic and narrative review. J Neurol Neurosurg Psychiatry. 2014;85(2):180–90.
175. Hoeritzauer I, Doherty CM, Thomson S, et al. 'Scan-negative' cauda equina syndrome: evidence of functional disorder from a prospective case series. Br J Neurosurg. 2015;29:178–80.
176. Anderson JR, Nakhate V, Stephen CD, Perez DL. Functional (psychogenic) neurological disorders: assessment and acute management in the Emergency Department. Semin Neurol. 2019;39(1):102–14.
177. Tremolizzo L, Susani E, Riva MA, Cesana G, Ferrarese C, Appollonio I. Positive signs of functional weakness. J Neurol Sci. 2014;340(1–2):13–8.
178. Daum C, Aybek S. Validity of the "Drift without pronation" sign in conversion disorder. BMC Neurol. 2013;13:31.
179. Jordbru AA, Smedstad LM, Moen VP, Martinsen EW. Identifying patterns of psychogenic gait by video-recording. J Rehabil Med. 2012;44(1):31–5.
180. Burneo JG, Martin R, Powell T, Greenlee S, Knowlton RC, Faught RE, Prasad A, Mendez M, Kuzniecky RI. Teddy bears: an observational finding in patients with non-epileptic events. Neurology. 2003;61(5):714–5.
181. Stone J, Smyth R, Carson A, Warlow C, Sharpe M. La belle indifférence in conversion symptoms and hysteria: systematic review. Br J Psychiatry. 2006;188:204–9.
182. Park JE. Clinical characteristics of functional movement disorders: a clinic-based study. Tremor Other Hyperkinet Mov (NY). 2018;8:504.
183. Stamelou M, Cossu G, Edwards MJ, et al. Familial psychogenic movement disorders. Mov Disord. 2013;28(9):1295–8.
184. de Abreu LPF, Teodoro T, Edwards MJ. Neuroimaging applications in functional movement disorders. Int Rev Neurobiol. 2018;143:163–77.
185. Gupta A, Lang AE. Psychogenic movement disorders. Curr Opin Neurol. 2009;22(4):430–6.
186. Mostile G, Fekete R, Giuffrida JP, et al. Amplitude fluctuations in essential tremor. Parkinsonism Relat Disord. 2012;18(7):859–63.
187. Schwingenschuh P, Saifee TA, Katschnig-Winter P, et al. Validation of "laboratory-supported" criteria for functional (psychogenic) tremor. Mov Disord. 2016;31(4):555–62.
188. Schmerler DA, Espay AJ. Functional dystonia. Handb Clin Neurol. 2016;139:235–45.
189. Kamble NL, Pal PK. Electrophysiological evaluation of psychogenic movement disorders. Parkinsonism Relat Disord. 2016;22(Suppl 1):S153–8.
190. van der Salm SM, Erro R, Cordivari C, et al. Propriospinal myoclonus: clinical reappraisal and review of literature. Neurology. 2014;83(20):1862–70.
191. Laub HN, Dwivedi AK, Revilla FJ, et al. Diagnostic performance of the "huffing and puffing" sign in psychogenic (functional) movement disorders Mov Disord Clin Pract. 2015;2(1):29–32.

192. Sudarsky L. Psychogenic gait disorders. Semin Neurol. 2006;26(3):351–6.
193. Peckham EL, Hallett M. Psychogenic movement disorders. Neurol Clin. 2009;27(3):801–vii.
194. Ganos C, Aguirregomozcorta M, Batla A, et al. Psychogenic paroxysmal movement disorders—clinical features and diagnostic clues. Parkinsonism Relat Disord. 2014;20(1):41–6.
195. Baizabal-Carvallo JF, Jankovic J. Psychogenic ophthalmologic movement disorders. J Neuropsychiatry Clin Neurosci. 2016;28(3):195–8.
196. Stone J, Vermeulen M. Functional sensory symptoms. Handb Clin Neurol. 2016;139:271–81.
197. Asadi-Pooya AA. Psychogenic nonepileptic seizures: a concise review. Neurol Sci. 2017;38(6):935–40.
198. Avbersek A, Sisodiya S. Does the primary literature provide support for clinical signs used to distinguish psychogenic nonepileptic seizures from epileptic seizures? J Neurol Neurosurg Psychiatry. 2010;81(7):719–25.
199. Perez DL, LaFrance WC Jr. Nonepileptic seizures: an updated review. CNS Spectr. 2016;21(3):239–46.
200. Brigo F, Nardone R, Ausserer H, et al. The diagnostic value of urinary incontinence in the differential diagnosis of seizures. Seizure. 2013;22:85–90.
201. Milán-Tomás Á, Persyko M, Del Campo M, Shapiro CM, Farcnik K. An overview of psychogenic non-epileptic seizures: etiology, diagnosis and management. Can J Neurol Sci. 2018;45(2):130–6.
202. LaFrance WC Jr, Baker GA, Duncan R, Goldstein LH, Reuber M. Minimum requirements for the diagnosis of psychogenic nonepileptic seizures: a staged approach: a report from the International League Against Epilepsy Nonepileptic Seizures Task Force. Epilepsia. 2013;54(11):2005–18.
203. Popkirov S, Stone J, Buchan AM. Functional neurological disorder: a common and treatable stroke mimic. Stroke. 2020;51(5):1629–35.
204. Toth C. Hemisensory syndrome is associated with a low diagnostic yield and a nearly uniform benign prognosis. J Neurol Neurosurg Psychiatry. 2003;74:1113–6.
205. Jones A, Smakowski A, O'Connell N, Chalder T, David AS. Functional stroke symptoms: a prospective observational case series. J Psychosom Res. 2020;132:109972.
206. Gargalas S, Weeks R, Khan-Bourne N, Shotbolt P, Simblett S, Ashraf L, et al. Incidence and outcome of functional stroke mimics admitted to a hyperacute stroke unit. J Neurol Neurosurg Psychiatry. 2017;88:2–6.
207. Wilkins SS, Bourke P, Salam A, Akhtar N, D'Souza A, Kamran S, et al. Functional stroke mimics: incidence and characteristics at a primary stroke center in the Middle East. Psychosom Med. 2018;80:416–21.
208. Behrouz R, Benbadis SR. Psychogenic pseudostroke. J Stroke Cerebrovasc Dis. 2014;23(4):e243–8.
209. Staniloiu A, Markowitsch HJ. Dissociative amnesia. Lancet Psychiatry. 2014;1(3):226–41.
210. Markowitsch HJ, Staniloiu A. Functional (dissociative) retrograde amnesia. Handb Clin Neurol. 2016;139:419–45.
211. Paradise MB, Glozier NS, Naismith SL, Davenport TA, Hickie IB. Subjective memory complaints, vascular risk factors and psychological distress in the middle-aged: a cross-sectional study. BMC Psychiatry. 2011;11:108.
212. Chen CS, Lee AW, Karagiannis A, Crompton JL, Selva D. Practical clinical approaches to functional visual loss. J Clin Neurosci. 2007;14(1):1–7.
213. Greenstein VC, Holopigian K, Seiple W, Carr RE, Hood DC. Atypical multifocal ERG responses in patients with diseases affecting the photoreceptors. Vision Res. 2004;44:2867–74.
214. Beatty S. Psychogenic medicine: non-organic visual loss. Postgrad Med J. 1999;75:201–7.
215. Kathol RG, Cox TA, Corbett JJ, Thompson HS, Clancy J. Functional visual loss: I. A true psychiatric disorder? Psychol Med. 1983;13:307–14.
216. Kathol RG, Cox TA, Corbett JJ, Thompson HS, Clancy J. Functional visual loss: II. Psychiatric aspects in 42 patients followed for 4 years. Psychol Med. 1983;13:315–24.
217. Sletteberg O, Bertelsen T, Hovding G. The prognosis of patients with hysterical visual impairment. Acta Ophthalmol. 1989;67:159–63.

218. Catalano RA, Simon JW, Krohel GB, Rosenber PN. Functional visual loss in children. Ophthalmology. 1986;93:385–90.
219. Baguley DM, Cope TE, McFerran DJ. Functional auditory disorders. Handb Clin Neurol. 2016;139:367–78.
220. Duffy JR. Functional speech disorders: clinical manifestations, diagnosis, and management. Handb Clin Neurol. 2016;139:379–88.
221. Casella G, Llinas RH, Marsh EB. Isolated aphasia in the emergency department: the likelihood of ischemia is low. Clin Neurol Neurosurg. 2017;163:24–6.
222. Mendez MF. Non-neurogenic language disorders: a preliminary classification. Psychosomatics. 2018;59:28–35.
223. Lee O, Ludwig L, Davenport R, Stone J. Functional foreign accent syndrome. Pract Neurol. 2016;16(5):409–11.
224. Staab JP, Eckhardt-Henn A, Horii A, et al. Diagnostic criteria for persistent postural-perceptual dizziness (PPPD): consensus document of the committee for the Classification of Vestibular Disorders of the Bárány Society. J Vestib Res. 2017;27(4):191–208.
225. Querner V, Krafczyk S, Dieterich M, Brandt T. Somatoform phobic postural vertigo: body sway during optokinetically induced roll vection. Exp Brain Res. 2002;143:269–75.
226. Querner V, Krafczyk S, Dieterich M, Brandt T. Patients with somatoform phobic postural vertigo: the more difficult the balance task, the better the balance performance. Neurosci Lett. 2000;285:21–4.
227. Holmberg J, Tjernström F, Karlberg M, et al. Reduced postural differences between phobic postural vertigo patients and healthy subjects during postural threat. J Neurol. 2009;256:1258–62.
228. Ödman M, Maire R. Chronic subjective dizziness. Acta Otolaryngol. 2008;128:1085–8.
229. Staab JP. Chronic subjective dizziness. Continuum (Minneap Minn). 2012;18:1118–41.
230. Brandt T, Huppert D, Strupp M, Dieterich M. Functional dizziness: diagnostic keys and differential diagnosis. J Neurol. 2015;262(8):1977–80.
231. O'Neal MA, Baslet G. Treatment for patients with a functional neurological disorder (conversion disorder): an integrated approach. Am J Psychiatry. 2018;175(4):307–14.
232. Reuber M, Mitchell AJ, Howlett SJ, Crimlisk HL, Grünewald RA. Functional symptoms in neurology: questions and answers. J Neurol Neurosurg Psychiatry. 2005;76(3):307–14.
233. Goldberg D, Gask L, O'Dowd T. The treatment of somatization: teaching techniques of reattribution. J Psychosom Res. 1989;33:689–95.
234. Marie GP. Psychogenic nonepileptic seizures. Innov Clin Neurosci. 2013;10(11-12):15–8.
235. Williams DT, Lafaver K, Carson A, Fahn S. Inpatient treatment for functional neurologic disorders. Handb Clin Neurol. 2016;139:631–41.
236. Tazaki M, Landlaw K. Behavioural mechanisms and cognitive-behavioural interventions of somatoform disorders. Int Rev Psychiatry. 2006;18(1):67–73.
237. Dallocchio C, Tinazzi M, Bombieri F, Arnó N, Erro R. Cognitive behavioural therapy and adjunctive physical activity for functional movement disorders (conversion disorder): a pilot, single-blinded, randomized study. Psychother Psychosom. 2016;85(6):381–3.
238. Moene FC, Spinhoven P, Hoogduin KAL, van Dyck R. A randomised controlled clinical trial on the additional effect of hypnosis in a comprehensive treatment programme for in-patients with conversion disorder of the motor type. Psychother Psychosom. 2002;71(2):66–76.
239. Moene FC, Spinhoven P, Hoogduin KAL, van Dyck R. A randomized controlled clinical trial of a hypnosis-based treatment for patients with conversion disorder, motor type. Int J Clin Exp Hypn. 2003;51(1):29–50.
240. Sharpe M, Walker J, Williams C, Stone J, Cavanagh J, Murray G, Butcher I, Duncan R, Smith S, Carson A. Guided self-help for functional (psychogenic) symptoms: a randomized controlled efficacy trial. Neurology. 2011;77(6):564–72.
241. Hubschmid M, Aybek S, Maccaferri GE, Chocron O, Gholamrezaee MM, Rossetti AO, Vingerhoets F, Berney A. Efficacy of brief interdisciplinary psychotherapeutic intervention for motor conversion disorder and nonepileptic attacks. Gen Hosp Psychiatry. 2015;37(5):448–55.

242. Ricciardi L, Edwards MJ. Treatment of functional (psychogenic) movement disorders. Neurotherapeutics. 2014;11:201–7.
243. LaFrance WC Jr, Baird GL, Barry JJ, Blum AS, Frank Webb A, Keitner GI, Machan JT, Miller I, Szaflarski JP, NES Treatment Trial (NEST-T) Consortium. Multicenter pilot treatment trial for psychogenic nonepileptic seizures: a randomized clinical trial. JAMA Psychiatry. 2014;71(9):997–1005.
244. Goldstein LH, Chalder T, Chigwedere C, Khondoker MR, Moriarty J, Toone BK, Mellers JD. Cognitive-behavioral therapy for psychogenic nonepileptic seizures: a pilot RCT. Neurology. 2010;74(24):1986–94.
245. Williams C, Carson A, Smith S, Sharpe M. Overcoming functional neurological symptoms: a five areas approach. London: Hodder Arnold; 2011.
246. Reiter JM, Andrews D, Reiter C, LaFrance WC. Taking control of your seizures: workbook. New York: Oxford University Press; 2015.
247. Kaur J, Garnawat D, Ghimiray D, Sachdev M. Conversion disorder and physical therapy. Delphi Psychiatry J. 2012;15:394–7.
248. Ness D. Physical therapy management for conversion disorder: case series. J Neurol Phys Ther. 2007;31:30–9.
249. Jordbru AA, Smedstad LM, Klungsøyr O, Martinsen EW. Psychogenic gait disorder: a randomized controlled trial of physical rehabilitation with one-year follow-up. J Rehabil Med. 2014;46(2):181–7.
250. Nielsen G, Ricciardi L, Demartini B, Hunter R, Joyce E, Edwards MJ. Outcomes of a 5-day physiotherapy programme for functional (psychogenic) motor disorders. J Neurol. 2015;262(3):674–81.
251. Lehn A, Gelauff J, Hoeritzauer I, Ludwig L, McWhirter L, Williams S, Gardiner P, Carson A, Stone J. Functional neurological disorders: mechanisms and treatment. J Neurol. 2016;263(3):611–20. https://doi.org/10.1007/s00415-015-7893-2.
252. Nielsen G, Buszewicz M, Stevenson F, et al. Randomised feasibility study of physiotherapy for patients with functional motor symptoms. J Neurol Neurosurg Psychiatry. 2017;88(6):484–90.
253. Czarnecki K, Thompson JM, Seime R, Geda YE, Duffy JR, Ahlskog JE. Functional movement disorders: successful treatment with a physical therapy rehabilitation protocol. Parkinsonism Relat Disord. 2012;18(3):247–51.
254. McCormack R, Moriarty J, Mellers JD, Shotbolt P, Pastena R, Landes N, Goldstein L, Fleminger S, David AS. Specialist inpatient treatment for severe motor conversion disorder: a retrospective comparative study. J Neurol Neurosurg Psychiatry. 2014;85(8):895–900.
255. Nielsen G, Stone J, Edwards MJ. Physiotherapy for functional (psychogenic) motor symptoms: a systematic review. J Psychosom Res. 2013;75(2):93–102.
256. Nielsen G, Stone J, Matthews A, et al. Physiotherapy for functional motor disorders: a consensus recommendation. J Neurol Neurosurg Psychiatry. 2015;86(10):1113–9.
257. Gelauff J, Stone J, Edwards M, Carson A. The prognosis of functional (psychogenic) motor symptoms: a systematic review. J Neurol Neurosurg Psychiatry. 2014;85(2):220–6.
258. Sharpe M, Stone J, Hibberd C, et al. Neurology out-patients with symptoms unexplained by disease: illness beliefs and financial benefits predict 1-year outcome. Psychol Med. 2010;40:689–98.
259. Barbey A, Aybek S. Functional movement disorders. Curr Opin Neurol. 2017;30(4):427–34.
260. Jankovic J, Vuong KD, Thomas M. Psychogenic tremor: long-term outcome. CNS Spectr. 2006;11:501–8.
261. Durrant J, Rickards H, Cavanna AE. Prognosis and outcome predictors in psychogenic nonepileptic seizures. Epilepsy Res Treat. 2011;2011:274736.
262. Stone J, Sharpe M, Rothwell PM, Warlow CP. The 12 year prognosis of unilateral functional weakness and sensory disturbance. J Neurol Neurosurg Psychiatry. 2003;74(5):591–6.
263. Wilshire CE, Ward T. Psychogenic explanations of physical illness: time to examine the evidence. Perspect Psychol Sci. 2016;11:606–31.

264. Stone J, Warlow C, Sharpe M. Functional weakness: clues to mechanism from the nature of onset. J Neurol Neurosurg Psychiatry. 2012;83:67–9.
265. Carson A, Lehn A. Epidemiology. Funct Neurol Disord. 2016;5:47–60.

Part III

Future Perspectives

Unmet Therapeutic Needs in Psychotic Illness: The Gut Microbiome-Endocannabinoid Axis as a Target for the Development of New Preventative Strategies

Amedeo Minichino

In this chapter I will present a series of findings aimed at shedding light on the relationship between two recently discovered biological systems (the gut microbiome and the endocannabinoid system) and anhedonia and amotivation, debilitating symptoms that characterise psychotic illness since its earliest stages [1–3].

The rationale of investigating new potential biological pathways underlying anhedonia and amotivation is to facilitate treatment breakthroughs [4], as current therapies aimed at palliating these symptoms lack in efficacy [5].

A growing body of literature shows that modifications in the diversity and composition of the gut microbiota occur in psychotic illness [6], even before the onset of the disorder [7]. These modifications have been related to more severe illness outcomes, including poor response to treatment [8]. While most of the evidence on the relationship between psychotic illness and the gut microbiome is associational, new studies using novel methodological approaches suggest causality [9, 10]. With the gut microbiome being modifiable, these new findings strongly encourage the search for novel therapeutics that could improve illness trajectories in psychotic illness by targeting the gut microbiome ("psychobiotics") [11].

Most of the currently available psychobiotics have broad effects on the gut microbiome [12]. This results in downstream aspecific effects on the gut-brain axis, which might explain the mixed nature of current literature on the efficacy of psychobiotics in psychotic illness [12]. To unveil the real potential of psychobiotics as therapeutic aids for treating psychotic illness, it is important to first clarify the mechanisms through which changes in gut microbiome taxonomy and functionality translate into specific mental health phenotypes [11]. The endocannabinoid system modulates key central (glutamatergic, GABAergic and dopaminergic

A. Minichino (✉)
Department of Psychiatry, St John's College, University of Oxford, Oxford, UK
e-mail: amedeo.minichino@psych.ox.ac.uk

© The Author(s), under exclusive license to Springer Nature Switzerland AG 2022
M. Colizzi, M. Ruggeri (eds.), *Prevention in Mental Health*,
https://doi.org/10.1007/978-3-030-97906-5_16

neurotransmission) and peripheral (inflammation, metabolism) mechanisms of key relevance for pathophysiological models of psychotic illness [13]. A consistent body of evidence suggests a specific involvement of the endocannabinoid system in anhedonia and amotivation [14, 15], a view that is in line with large-scale initiatives such as the Research Domain Criteria (RDoC—endocannabinoids are among the molecular targets of positive valence system) [16]. Evidence from other fields of medicine, such as cardiology, neurology and immunology, suggests that the gut microbiome is a key modulator of the endocannabinoid system [17].

Based on these and other considerations presented later in the chapter, I will discuss the evidence on the existence of a gut microbiome-endocannabinoid axis that might represent a novel target of intervention for anhedonia and amotivation. This evidence could provide a theoretical background for the development of therapeutics in an area of unmet need, with potential implications for the field of early intervention.

The chapter is structured as follows:

1. A brief introduction to anhedonia and amotivation and their relevance in psychotic illness.
2. An introduction to the gut microbiome and its relevance for psychotic illness, anhedonia/amotivation and implications for treatment.
3. A synthesis of the evidence on the involvement of the endocannabinoid system in psychotic illness and the relevance for anhedonia/amotivation.
4. New data suggesting the existence of a gut microbiome-endocannabinoid axis in psychotic illness.
5. Final considerations.

16.1 Anhedonia and Amotivation: The Search for Novel Therapeutic Targets

Anhedonia and amotivation are highly debilitating symptoms, traditionally considered a unique feature of schizophrenia, where they manifest in 60–90% of patients [18]. More recently, it has become clear that these symptoms manifest across the whole psychosis spectrum [19, 20], where they represent key predictors of poor illness trajectories.

In the context of schizophrenia and related psychoses, anhedonia and amotivation are often referred to as "experiential negative symptoms" [4, 18]. The term "experiential" is used to underlie the experiential nature of these symptoms, which is in contrast with the expressive features of other frequently observed negative symptoms (blunted/flat affect and alogia, referred to as "expressive negative symptoms") (see also Table 16.1).

This differentiation has clinical relevance as experiential, but not expressive, negative symptoms are tightly related to poor illness trajectories, loss in functioning and reduced response to treatment (for a more detailed description, including primary vs. secondary, please see ref. [4]). Anhedonia and amotivation, and related

Table 16.1 Anhedonia and amotivation as experiential negative symptoms

		Definition
Experiential	*Avolition*	Reduction in the initiation of and persistence in activities
	Anhedonia	Impairments in the intensity of pleasure (anticipated and/or experienced during the act) from activities usually perceived as pleasurable. This might be associated with reduced engagement in activities
	Asociality	Reduced interaction with others and diminished will to form social bonds
Expressive	*Blunted or flat affect*	Decrease in the outward expression of emotion
	Alogia	Reduction in the quantity of speech and amount of spontaneous elaboration

social withdrawal, manifest as early as in the prodromal phase of psychosis, years before the appearance of delusions and hallucinations [4, 18, 21]. Therefore, these symptoms represent an important target for preventative interventions [2, 3]. Antipsychotics, the cornerstone of psychotic illness treatment, have limited, if any, efficacy on anhedonia/amotivation [5]. This has made the research on novel effective therapeutic targets for these symptoms an utmost priority. In schizophrenia, anhedonia and amotivation are traditionally related to a complex combination of dysfunctional dopaminergic, glutamatergic and cholinergic neurotransmission [18]. Based on this knowledge, a number of clinical trials used compounds (NMDA receptor enhancers, mGluR2-/mGluR3-positive allosteric modulators, muscarinic acetylcholine agonists, amphetamine-based compounds) aimed at targeting these neurotransmitter systems in patients with psychosis, with limited success [22]. More recently, the inflammatory system has received increasing attention from the clinical and scientific community as follows: (1) genome-wide association studies pointed out an association between the genes of the major histocompatibility complex and schizophrenia [23]; (2) meta-analytic evidence showed increased circulating pro-inflammatory cytokines in patients with psychotic illness compared to controls [24]; and (3) population studies suggested high comorbidity rates between autoimmune disorders and psychosis [25].

Several authors advocate for a specific involvement of peripheral and central inflammation in the genesis of anhedonia and amotivation in psychosis [26]. However, the specificity of this association has been often questioned as pro-inflammatory mechanisms have been related to other key symptoms of the psychotic spectrum, such as delusions, hallucination, cognitive deficits [27, 28] as well as other psychiatric syndromes [29]. Furthermore, the exact mechanisms underlying the association between altered peripheral and central inflammation and anhedonia/amotivation are unclear. Molecules such as C-reactive proteins and cytokines, on which the majority of studies are focused, are relatively large and do not cross the blood-brain barrier, raising the question of how they could influence brain functions [26]. More recent complementary hypotheses, such as a hyperactive complement system (involved in altered synaptic pruning) and microglia dysfunctions, did not find confirmation in large prospective studies in clinical cohorts [30]. These considerations might explain why the large majority of trials using anti-inflammatory compounds (inhibitor of cyclooxygenase type 2 [31], non-steroidal anti-inflammatory drugs [31], minocycline [12], methotrexate [32]) in psychotic illness were ineffective for the treatment of anhedonia/amotivation.

The search for new targets for the treatment of anhedonia/amotivation has continued and expanded beyond inflammation.

## 16.2	The Gut Microbiome: Relevance for Psychosis and Anhedonia/Amotivation

The gut microbiome is a highly dynamic and complex ecosystem of bacteria, viruses and fungi located in the human intestinal tract [33]. A consistent body of evidence suggests that the gut microbiome contributes to the regulation of many physiological processes of key relevance for the host's health [34], such as the maturation and modulation of the activity of the immune system; the regulation of appetite and body weight; and relevant for psychotic illness, neurodevelopment and neurodegeneration [35]. Many different gut microbiome-to-brain paths have been identified (summarised in Table 16.2), and each of them has potential relevance for psychotic illness.

### 16.2.1	The Gut Microbiome in Psychotic Illness

The gut microbiome is part of the interface between environmental risk factors and pathophysiological pathways of key relevance for psychotic disorders [39, 40]. Urbanicity, migration/ethnicity, diet and substance misuse, well-known risk factors for psychosis [41], have all been shown to modify the gut microbiome.

Significant differences in the taxonomy of gut microbes have emerged in all studies that have investigated the gut microbiome in patients with psychotic disorder vs. control [6, 7, 9, 42–44]. One key study showed that a specific panel of bacteria (*Aerococcaceae*, *Bifidobacteriaceae*, *Brucellaceae*, *Pasteurellaceae* and *Rikenellaceae*) can be used to distinguish patients with schizophrenia from controls [10]. Another longitudinal study identified certain taxonomic features (a lower abundance of *Lachnospiraceae*, *Ruminococcaceae* and some *Bacteroides* spp.) within psychotic patients that could be used to predict their poor outcomes [45]. Two recent studies showed that the transplantation of gut microbes from unmedicated patients with schizophrenia to germ-free mice can induce schizophrenia-like behaviours in recipient animals [9, 10]. These two latter studies provided the first evidence suggesting a causal link between abnormalities of the gut microbiome and schizophrenia.

The evidence from these early studies coherently showed that abnormalities of the gut microbiome, in particular a reduced microbial diversity ("gut dysbiosis") in patients with psychotic disorders, could be clinically informative as diagnostic and prognostic biomarkers.

Table 16.2 Interplay between the gut microbiome and biological systems of known relevance for psychotic disorders

Biological system	Metabolites/molecules	Relevance for psychotic disorder
Immune system [36]	Cytokines, antibodies against neural surface antigens (e.g. anti-NMDAR), C4	Altered gut microbiome composition can affect immune development by enhancing the sensitivity to both internal and external antigens, a common finding in psychotic disorder. In the host, this translates in the activation of a pro-inflammatory response that includes the release of pro-inflammatory cytokines (IL-6, IFN-γ and TNF-α), the activation of the complement system and molecular mimicry mechanisms that underlie more specific autoimmunity phenomena (antibodies against antigens of the neural surface) Meta-analytic evidence and GWAS analyses advocate for a key role of the immune system in psychotic disorder. Both direct (C4 and synaptic pruning, NMDAR antagonism) and indirect (increased blood-brain barrier permeability) mechanisms might be at play
Indole and tryptophan metabolism [37]	Kynurenate/tryptophan ratio	Production of kynurenate, a N-methyl-D-aspartate receptor (NMDAR) antagonist, is influenced by certain bacterial species, and the activity of indoleamine-pyrrole-2,3-dioxygenase (IDO, a key enzyme on the conversion pathway from tryptophan to kynurenate) is upregulated by cytokines such as IFN-γ and TNF-α NMDA hypofunction in cortical and hippocampal areas is central for pathophysiological models of psychotic disorder
Biological barriers [38]	Short-chain fatty acid (SCFA)	SCFA (acetate, butyrate, propionate) is a primary product of the breakdown of non-digestible carbohydrates by gut bacteria. SCFA facilitates the tight-junction assembly in intestinal (gut barrier) and endothelial (blood-brain barrier) cells In pathophysiological models of psychosis, increased permeability of biological barriers is believed to facilitate the leakage of neuroactive material (e.g. kynurenate, antibodies, cytokines) in the brain
Endocannabinoid system [15, 17]	Anandamide (AEA) and 2-arachidonoylglycerol (2-AG)	In the gastrointestinal tract, the engagement of the endocannabinoid is modulated by the gut microbiome. The main endocannabinoid mediators which are anandamide (AEA) and 2-arachydonoilglycerol (2-AG) are protective towards psychotic disorder. The relevance of endocannabinoids for psychosis lies in the modulation of key neurotransmitter systems (glutamate, dopamine, GABA) and NMDAR expression

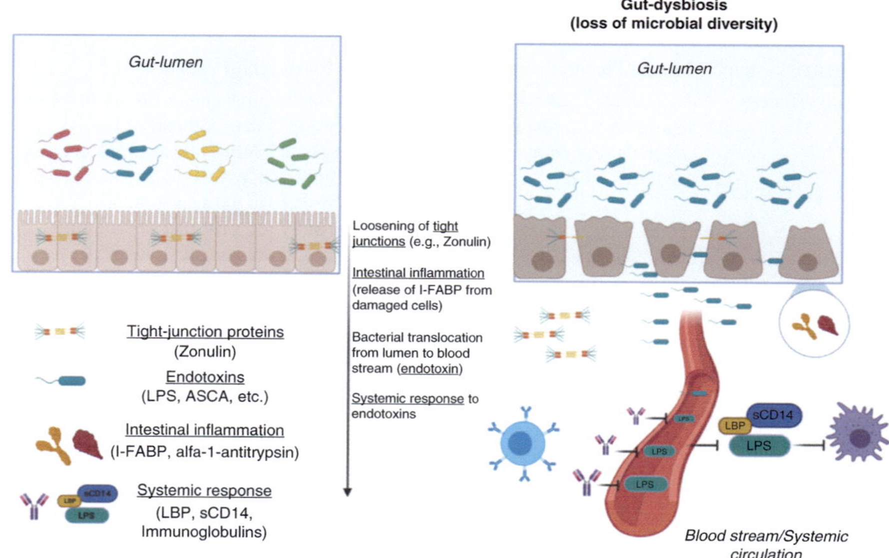

Fig. 16.1 Gut dysbiosis. Reduced microbial diversity ("gut dysbiosis") triggers a cascade of events, including loosening of gut barrier permeability, intestinal inflammation, translocation of bacterial antigens from the gut lumen to the bloodstream and a systemic response to endotoxins. Each of these events can be measured with specific biomarkers. In order: tight junction proteins, intestinal fatty acid-binding protein (I-FABP), alfa-1-antitripsin, endotoxins (*LPS* lipopolysaccharide, ASCA Saccharomyces cerevisiae antigens), lipopolysaccharide-binding protein (LBP), soluble CD14 (sCD14) and immunoglobulins against bacterial endotoxins. (Taken from Safadi et al. (2021). Gut dysbiosis in severe mental illness and chronic fatigue: a novel trans-diagnostic construct? A systematic review and meta-analysis. Mol Psychiatry)

16.2.2 Gut Dysbiosis and Anhedonia/Amotivation

Microbial diversity is considered by many as the hallmark of a "healthy" gut microbiome [36, 46]. Gut dysbiosis can trigger a cascade of events that are detrimental for the host's health (Fig. 16.1).

These events include the loosing of gut barrier integrity and the leakage of bacterial endotoxin (e.g. lipopolysaccharide—LPS) and false neurotransmitters from the gut lumen to the bloodstream ("endotoxemia") [40]. These events can affect brain functions through both direct (e.g. neurotoxic triggers) and indirect (vagal system modulation) mechanisms [40]. Experimental animal and human models showed that gut dysbiosis and the consequent endotoxemia can induce in the host a series of symptoms that are often referred to as "sickness behaviour" [47].

Sickness behaviour is commonly used as a pathophysiological model of anhedonia and amotivation [47]. A recent meta-analysis from our research group showed that gut dysbiosis occurs in severe mental illness (schizophrenia, bipolar disorder, depression) and is associated with the severity of anhedonia and amotivation across diagnostic boundaries [40]. Similar findings were obtained when chronic fatigue was investigated [40]. This is relevant as the only symptoms of chronic fatigue that overlap with those of severe mental illness are anhedonia/amotivation, suggesting that gut dysbiosis might specifically contribute to these symptoms.

16.2.3 Therapeutic Implications

As accumulating evidence advocates for a key role for the gut microbiome in psychotic illness, a few clinical trials have used compounds that target the gut microbiome as add-on to treatment as usual (TAU) [12]. Currently available compounds with psychobiotic potential belong to four main categories: antibiotics/antimicrobials, probiotics (live microorganisms), prebiotics (nutrients for putatively beneficial bacteria) and symbiotics (a combination of probiotics and prebiotics) [11]. A recent meta-analysis from our research group summarised the evidence from 28 randomised placebo-controlled trials investigating the efficacy of add-on psychobiotics for the treatment of negative symptoms in psychotic illness [12]. The pooled estimates showed no difference between add-on psychobiotics and placebo for the treatment of negative symptoms of psychotic illness. However, most of the included studies used add-on antibiotics, with paucity of evidence (only three studies) on pre–/probiotics [12]. Antibiotics have extensive effects on the composition and functionality of gut microbes [48]. These broad effects lack specificity and could explain why their use as add-on treatment to TAU in psychotic illness is not supported by evidence. These considerations highlight the need to clarify which mechanisms underlie the observed association between gut dysbiosis and anhedonia/amotivation before engaging in further trials.

16.3 The Endocannabinoid System: Relevance for Psychotic Illness and Anhedonia/Amotivation

The endocannabinoid system is a ubiquitous endogenous modulatory system. It encompasses two main agonists (anandamide—AEA; 2-acylglycerol—2-AG), two main receptors (CB1R and CB2R), two synthesising and two degrading enzymes (see Fig. 16.2) [49]. In the brain, endocannabinoid agonists provide inhibitory regulatory feedback at the synaptic level and modulate the release of neurotransmitters, such as dopamine, glutamate and gamma-aminobutyric acid (GABA) [49]. Endocannabinoid agonists and their receptors are also involved in the modulation on brain rhythms, including gamma-oscillations (more details in Fig. 16.2).

In the periphery, endocannabinoid agonists modulate several physiological processes, including inflammation, gut permeability and metabolism [49].

A recent meta-analysis from our research group showed that the endocannabinoid system is altered in psychotic illness [49]. Pooled data from 18 studies showed that patients with psychosis have higher levels of endocannabinoid agonists and receptors in the cerebrospinal fluid and blood compared to controls. We also found that this increase occurred at any stage of illness (including the prodrome), and it

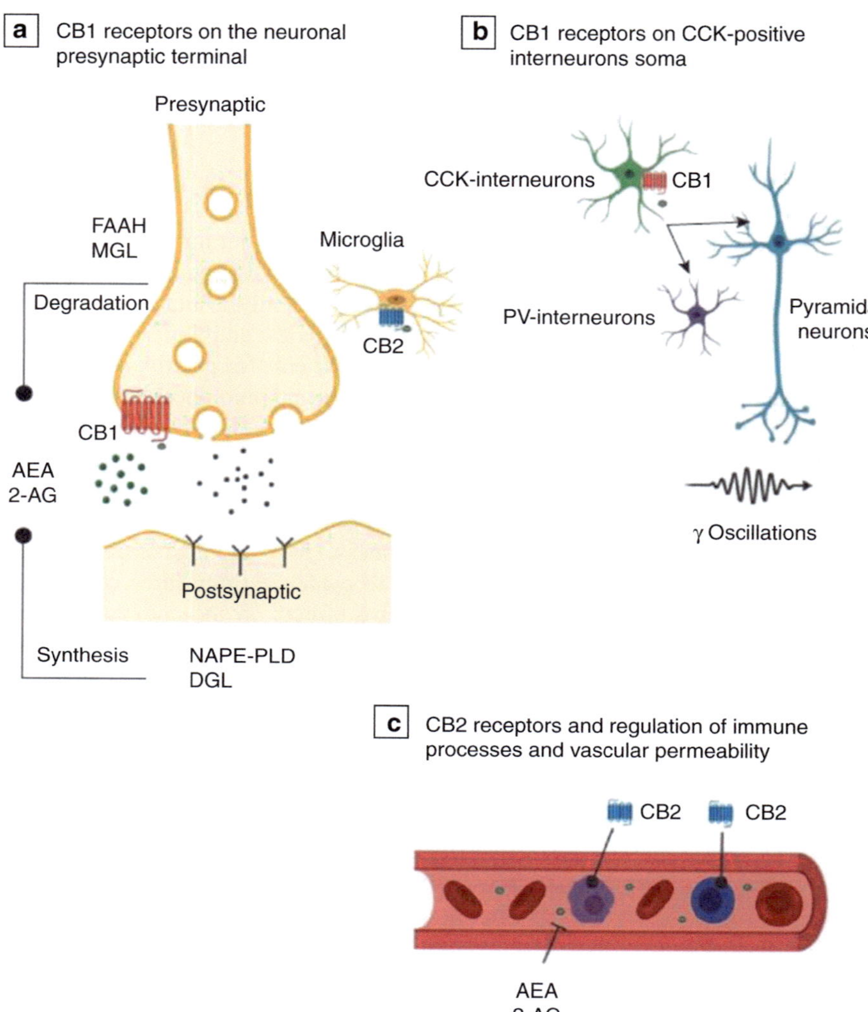

Fig. 16.2 The endocannabinoid system. (From: Minichino et al., Measuring Disturbance of the Endocannabinoid System in Psychosis: A Systematic Review and Meta-analysis. JAMA Psychiatry. 2019 Jun 5:76(9):914–23.) (**a**) Type 1 cannabinoid (CB1) receptors are mainly localised on the neuronal presynaptic terminal, possibly mediating retrograde inhibitory feedback and neurotransmitter release. (**b**) CB1 receptors are also localised on the soma of cholecystokinin (CCK)-positive interneurons, contributing to the synchronisation of pyramidal cell cortical firing, which is involved in the genesis of γ oscillations. (**c**) Given their high expression on immune cells, type 2 cannabinoid (CB2) receptors are mainly associated with the peripheral functions of the endocannabinoid system, particularly the regulation of immune processes and vascular permeability. However, CB2 receptors are expressed in the human brain (microglia and blood vessels). *AEA* anandamide, *2-AG* 2-arachidonoylglicerol, *DGL* diacylglycerol lipase, *FAAH* fatty acid amide hydrolase, *MGL* monoacylglycerol lipase, *NAPE-PLD* N-acyl-phosphatidylethanolamine phospholipase D, *PV* parvalbumin

was independent of cannabis use and medications. Furthermore, in patients with lower levels of endocannabinoid agonists, negative symptoms were manifesting in a more severe manner [49].

As other authors previously hypothesised [50], these findings suggest that the endocannabinoid system is involved in the pathophysiology of psychotic illness (and in the genesis of negative symptoms) and that its activation might be protective towards illness mechanisms.

This might occur through two main mechanisms: (1) endocannabinoid agonists prevent the depletion of dopamine in the ventral striatum, a key brain area involved in the processing of rewarding cues [51], and (2) endocannabinoid agonists help in stabilising the communication between parvalbumin interneurons and pyramidal cells and the resulting brain rhythm coordination [52]. Dysfunctions in either one or both of these two mechanisms, as it might occur when the endocannabinoid system is dysfunctional, are responsible for hedonic and cognitive impairments, respectively, and underlie anhedonic/amotivational behaviours [4, 22].

16.4 The Gut Microbiome-Endocannabinoid Axis

In the previous two subheadings, we presented some evidence suggesting that the gut microbiome and the endocannabinoid system might independently contribute to the pathophysiology of anhedonia/amotivation. Here, we will bring these two biological systems together and report data from some key studies showing how their interplay might be relevant for anhedonia/amotivation.

Reduced gut microbiome diversity ("gut dysbiosis") has been shown to be a strong trigger for the activation of the endocannabinoid system [17]. Gut dysbiosis can induce the transcription of *cnr1* and *cnr2*, which codify for the cannabinoid receptors 1 (CB1R) and 2 (CB2R), respectively [17]. The endocannabinoid system, activated upon the dysbiosis stimuli and the resulting gut leakage, exerts "gatekeeper" function by providing regulatory feedback and increasing the synthesis of tight junction proteins [17]. A recent study showed that the effect of gut dysbiosis on the endocannabinoid system goes beyond the gut and extend to the brain [15]. The authors showed that the transplant of gut microbes from an animal model of depression to recipient germ-free mice caused central modifications in the expression of cannabinoid receptors (in particular, reduced levels of endocannabinoid signalling) and anhedonia/amotivation [15]. These symptoms and the related endocannabinoid abnormalities were reversed by complementation with a strain of the *Lactobacilli* genus (a probiotic) [15].

These findings, albeit obtained in mice, represent the first evidence showing a causal link between gut dysbiosis, endocannabinoid system abnormalities and anhedonia/amotivation. They also suggest that these abnormalities are reversible and that interventions aimed at improving the diversity of gut microbes might have the potential to palliate highly debilitating symptoms.

Our research group recently replicated these findings in a general population cohort. We used longitudinal data collected over 5 years from 786 twins from the

TwinsUK registry [53]. In this cohort, reduced gut microbiome diversity was associated with the severity of anhedonia and amotivation. This association was mediated by the peripheral levels of endocannabinoids.

16.4.1 Future Directions

In this chapter, we presented a series of evidence aimed at highlighting the potential role of the gut microbiome-endocannabinoid axis for the pathophysiology of anhedonia/amotivation, two debilitating symptoms that often manifest in the earliest stages of psychotic illness and are current unmet therapeutic needs. The data presented in support of the existence of this biological axis needs to be validated in adequately powered prospective longitudinal studies on clinical samples. Ideally, gut microbiome data will need to be collected at multiple time points to take into account the high intra- and inter-individual variability of this biomarker. Furthermore, taxonomic analysis of the gut microbiome should be complemented with other "omics" data to provide a complete readout of the functional contribution of the gut microbes to the host's health.

References

1. Minichino A, Francesconi M, Carrión RE, Delle Chiaie R, Bevilacqua A, Parisi M, et al. From neurological soft signs to functional outcome in young individuals in treatment with secondary services for non-psychotic disorders: a path analysis. Psychol Med. 2017;47:1192.
2. Minichino A, Francesconi M, Carrión RE, Bevilacqua A, Parisi M, Rullo S, et al. Prediction of functional outcome in young patients with a recent-onset psychiatric disorder: beyond the traditional diagnostic classification system. Schizophr Res. 2017;185:114.
3. Francesconi M, Minichino A, Carrión RE, Delle Chiaie R, Bevilacqua A, Parisi M, et al. Psychosis prediction in secondary mental health services. A broad, comprehensive approach to the "at risk mental state" syndrome. Eur Psychiatry. 2017;40:96.
4. Galderisi S, Mucci A, Buchanan RW, Arango C. Negative symptoms of schizophrenia: new developments and unanswered research questions. Lancet Psychiatry. 2018;5:664–77.
5. Fusar-Poli P, Papanastasiou E, Stahl D, Rocchetti M, Carpenter W, Shergill S, et al. Treatments of negative symptoms in schizophrenia: meta-analysis of 168 randomized placebo-controlled trials. Schizophr Bull. 2015;41:892–9.
6. Kelly JR, Minuto C, Cryan JF, Clarke G, Dinan TG. The role of the gut microbiome in the development of schizophrenia. Schizophr Res. 2020; https://doi.org/10.1016/j.schres.2020.02.010.
7. He Y, Kosciolek T, Tang J, Zhou Y, Li Z, Ma X, et al. Gut microbiome and magnetic resonance spectroscopy study of subjects at ultra-high risk for psychosis may support the membrane hypothesis. Eur Psychiatry. 2018;53:37–45.
8. Schwarz E, Maukonen J, Hyytiäinen T, Kieseppä T, Orešič M, Sabunciyan S, et al. Analysis of microbiota in first episode psychosis identifies preliminary associations with symptom severity and treatment response. Schizophr Res. 2018;192:398–403.
9. Zheng P, Zeng B, Liu M, Chen J, Pan J, Han Y, et al. The gut microbiome from patients with schizophrenia modulates the glutamate-glutamine-GABA cycle and schizophrenia-relevant behaviors in mice. Sci Adv. 2019;5:eaau8317.
10. Zheng P, Zeng B, Zhou C, Liu M, Fang Z, Xu X, et al. Gut microbiome remodeling induces depressive-like behaviors through a pathway mediated by the host's metabolism. Mol Psychiatry. 2016;21:786–96.

11. Dinan TG, Stanton C, Cryan JF. Psychobiotics: a novel class of psychotropic. Biol Psychiatry. 2013;74:720–6.
12. Minichino A, Brondino N, Solmi M, del Giovane C, Fusar-Poli P, Burnet P, et al. The gut-microbiome as a target for the treatment of schizophrenia: a systematic review and meta-analysis of randomised controlled trials of add-on strategies. Schizophr Res. 2020; https://doi.org/10.1016/j.schres.2020.02.012.
13. Minichino A, Senior M, Brondino N, Zhang SH, Godwlewska BR, Burnet PWJ, et al. Measuring disturbance of the endocannabinoid system in psychosis: a systematic review and meta-analysis. JAMA Psychiatry. 2019;76:914.
14. Hill MN, Carrier EJ, McLaughlin RJ, Morrish AC, Meier SE, Hillard CJ, et al. Regional alterations in the endocannabinoid system in an animal model of depression: effects of concurrent antidepressant treatment. J Neurochem. 2008;106:2322–36.
15. Chevalier G, Siopi E, Guenin-Macé L, Pascal M, Laval T, Rifflet A, et al. Effect of gut microbiota on depressive-like behaviors in mice is mediated by the endocannabinoid system. Nat Commun. 2020;11:1–15.
16. Karhson DS, Hardan AY, Parker KJ. Endocannabinoid signaling in social functioning: an RDoC perspective. Transl Psychiatry. 2016;6:e905.
17. Cani PD, Plovier H, van Hul M, Geurts L, Delzenne NM, Druart C, et al. Endocannabinoids-at the crossroads between the gut microbiota and host metabolism. Nat Rev Endocrinol. 2016;12:133–43.
18. Millan MJ, Fone K, Steckler T, Horan WP. Negative symptoms of schizophrenia: clinical characteristics, pathophysiological substrates, experimental models and prospects for improved treatment. Eur Neuropsychopharmacol. 2014;24:645–92.
19. Winograd-Gurvich C, Fitzgerald PB, Georgiou-Karistianis N, Bradshaw JL, White OB. Negative symptoms: a review of schizophrenia, melancholic depression and Parkinson's disease. Brain Res Bull. 2006;70:312–21.
20. Moritz S, Fritzsche A, Engel M, Meiseberg J, Klingberg S, Hesse K. A plea for a transdiagnostic conceptualization of negative symptoms and for consistent psychiatric vocabulary. Schizophr Res. 2019;204:427–9.
21. Fusar-Poli P, Salazar De Pablo G, Correll CU, Meyer-Lindenberg A, Millan MJ, Borgwardt S, et al. Prevention of psychosis: advances in detection, prognosis, and intervention. JAMA Psychiatry. 2020;77:755–65.
22. Davis MC, Horan WP, Marder SR. Psychopharmacology of the negative symptoms: current status and prospects for progress. Eur Neuropsychopharmacol. 2014;24:788–99.
23. Sekar A, Bialas AR, de Rivera H, Davis A, Hammond TR, Kamitaki N, et al. Schizophrenia risk from complex variation of complement component 4. Nature. 2016;530:177–83.
24. Pillinger T, Osimo EF, Brugger S, Mondelli V, McCutcheon RA, Howes OD. A meta-analysis of immune parameters, variability, and assessment of modal distribution in psychosis and test of the immune subgroup hypothesis. Schizophr Bull. 2019;45:1120–33.
25. Cullen AE, Holmes S, Pollak TA, Blackman G, Joyce DW, Kempton MJ, et al. Associations between non-neurological autoimmune disorders and psychosis: a meta-analysis. Biol Psychiatry. 2019;85:35–48.
26. Goldsmith DR, Rapaport MH. Inflammation and negative symptoms of schizophrenia: implications for reward processing and motivational deficits. Front Psychiatry. 2020;11:46.
27. Bergink V, Gibney SM, Drexhage HA. Autoimmunity, inflammation, and psychosis: a search for peripheral markers. Biol Psychiatry. 2014;75:324–31.
28. Suárez-Pinilla P, López-Gil J, Crespo-Facorro B. Immune system: a possible nexus between cannabinoids and psychosis. Brain Behav Immun. 2014;40:269–82.
29. Jeon SW, Kyoung YH, Kim YK. Role of inflammation in psychiatric disorders. In: Advances in experimental medicine and biology, vol. 1192. New York: Springer; 2019. p. 491–501.
30. Inta D, Lang UE, Borgwardt S, Meyer-Lindenberg A, Gass P. Microglia activation and schizophrenia: lessons from the effects of minocycline on postnatal neurogenesis, neuronal survival and synaptic pruning. Schizophr Bull. 2017;43:493–6.

31. Nitta M, Kishimoto T, Müller N, Weiser M, Davidson M, Kane JM, et al. Adjunctive use of nonsteroidal anti-inflammatory drugs for schizophrenia: a meta-analytic investigation of randomized controlled trials. Schizophr Bull. 2013;39:1230–41.
32. Chaudhry IB, Husain MO, Khoso AB, Husain MI, Buch MH, Kiran T, et al. A randomised clinical trial of methotrexate points to possible efficacy and adaptive immune dysfunction in psychosis. Transl Psychiatry. 2020;10:415.
33. Goodrich JK, Waters JL, Poole AC, Sutter JL, Koren O, Blekhman R, et al. Human genetics shape the gut microbiome. Cell. 2014;159:789–99.
34. Wang WL, Xu SY, Ren ZG, Tao L, Jiang JW, Zheng S, sen. Application of metagenomics in the human gut microbiome. World J Gastroenterol. 2015;21:803–14.
35. Sarkar A, Harty S, Johnson KVA, Moeller AH, Carmody RN, Lehto SM, et al. The role of the microbiome in the neurobiology of social behaviour. Biol Rev. 2020;95:1131–66.
36. Gilbert JA, Blaser MJ, Caporaso JG, Jansson JK, Lynch S, v., Knight R. Current understanding of the human microbiome. Nat Med. 2018;24:392–400.
37. Kennedy PJ, Cryan JF, Dinan TG, Clarke G. Kynurenine pathway metabolism and the microbiota-gut-brain axis. Neuropharmacology. 2017;112:399–412.
38. Peng L, Li ZR, Green RS, Holzman IR, Lin J. Butyrate enhances the intestinal barrier by facilitating tight junction assembly via activation of AMP-activated protein kinase in Caco-2 cell monolayers. J Nutr. 2009;139:1619–25.
39. Minichino A, Ando A, Francesconi M, Salatino A, Delle Chiaie R, Cadenhead K. Investigating the link between drug-naive first episode psychoses (FEPs), weight gain abnormalities and brain structural damages: relevance and implications for therapy. Prog Neuropsychopharmacol Biol Psychiatry. 2017;77:9.
40. Safadi JM, Quinton AMG, Lennox BR, Burnet PWJ, Minichino A. Gut dysbiosis in severe mental illness and chronic fatigue: a novel trans-diagnostic construct? A systematic review and meta-analysis. Mol Psychiatry. 2021; https://doi.org/10.1038/s41380-021-01032-1.
41. Fusar-Poli P, Tantardini M, de Simone S, Ramella-Cravaro V, Oliver D, Kingdon J, et al. Deconstructing vulnerability for psychosis: meta-analysis of environmental risk factors for psychosis in subjects at ultra high-risk. Eur Psychiatry. 2017;40:65–75.
42. Nguyen TT, Kosciolek T, Eyler LT, Knight R, Jeste DV. Overview and systematic review of studies of microbiome in schizophrenia and bipolar disorder. J Psychiatr Res. 2018;99:50–61.
43. Castro-Nallar E, Bendall ML, Pérez-Losada M, Sabuncyan S, Severance EG, Dickerson FB, et al. Composition, taxonomy and functional diversity of the oropharynx microbiome in individuals with schizophrenia and controls. PeerJ. 2015;2015:e1140.
44. He Y, Kosciolek T, Tang J, Zhou Y, Li Z, Ma X, et al. Gut microbiome and magnetic resonance spectroscopy study of subjects at ultra-high risk for psychosis may support the membrane hypothesis. Eur Psychiatry. 2018;53:37–45.
45. Schwarz E, Maukonen J, Hyytiäinen T, Kieseppä T, Orešič M, Sabunciyan S, et al. Analysis of microbiota in first episode psychosis identifies preliminary associations with symptom severity and treatment response. Schizophr Res. 2018;192:398–403.
46. Zierer J, Jackson MA, Kastenmüller G, Mangino M, Long T, Telenti A, et al. The fecal metabolome as a functional readout of the gut microbiome. Nat Genet. 2018;50:790–5.
47. Grigoleit J-S, Engler H, Schedlowski M. Experimental human endotoxemia, sickness behavior, and neuropsychiatric diseases. Cham: Springer; 2015. p. 63–82.
48. Willing BP, Russell SL, Finlay BB. Shifting the balance: antibiotic effects on host-microbiota mutualism. Nat Rev Microbiol. 2011;9:233–43.
49. Minichino A, Senior M, Brondino N, Zhang SH, Godwlewska BR, Burnet PWJ, et al. Measuring disturbance of the endocannabinoid system in psychosis: a systematic review and meta-analysis. JAMA Psychiatry. 2019;76:914–23.
50. Koethe D, Hoyer C, Leweke FM. The endocannabinoid system as a target for modelling psychosis. Psychopharmacology (Berl). 2009;206:551–61.

51. Solinas M, Goldberg SR, Piomelli D. The endocannabinoid system in brain reward processes. Br J Pharmacol. 2008;154:369–83.
52. Berghuis P, Dobszay MB, Wang X, Spano S, Ledda F, Sousa KM, et al. Endocannabinoids regulate interneuron migration and morphogenesis by transactivating the TrkB receptor. Proc Natl Acad Sci U S A. 2005;102:19115–20.
53. Minichino A, Jackson M, Francesconi M, Steves C, Menni C, Burnet P, et al. Endocannabinoid system mediates the association between gut microbial diversity and anhedonia/amotivation in a general population cohort. Mol Psychiatry. Accepted/In press.

Prodromal Dementias with Lewy Bodies: A Paradigm for Identifying People at Ultra-High Risk

17

Gennaro Pagano

17.1 Introduction

Dementia with Lewy bodies (DLB) is not only the most common dementia after Alzheimer's disease (AD) and vascular dementia, affecting 7–15% of all individuals with dementia [1], but also the dementia with the highest likelihood of having an onset with pure psychiatric symptoms. Individuals with DLB have high frequency of visual hallucinations (clinical cohort, 72%; neuropathological cohort, 65%), auditory hallucinations (clinical cohort, 38%; neuropathological cohort, 35%), delusions (clinical cohort, 57%; neuropathological cohort, 60%), and depression (clinical cohort, 19%; neuropathological cohort, 32.5%) at presentation to clinical services in patients with dementia with Lewy bodies. Visual and auditory hallucinations, delusions, and depression all occurred at significantly higher rates in patients with dementia with Lewy bodies than in people with Alzheimer's disease [2].

DLB is also the most recently described at the pathological level (only in 1987 [3]), with the first operational criteria only in 1992 [4], and the first International Consensus Diagnostic Criteria on Dementia with Lewy Bodies published in 1996 [5], refined in 2006 [6] and later in 2017 [7].

The pathognomonic characteristics of DLB are the presence of Lewy bodies (mostly composed of alpha-synuclein) in postmortem brain and the impairment of noradrenergic and dopaminergic systems, which can be measured in vivo by using metaiodobenzylguanidine (MIBG) single-photon emission computed tomography (SPECT) for the myocardial norepinephrine transporter (NET) [8, 9] and by using ioflupane SPECT for the brain dopamine transporter (DAT) [10]. Ioflupane SPECT

G. Pagano (✉)
University of Exeter Medical School, London, UK

Roche Pharma Research and Early Development (pRED), Neuroscience and Rare Diseases, Roche Innovation Center Basel, Basel, Switzerland
e-mail: gennaro.pagano@roche.com

is used in clinical practice for the differential diagnosis between DLB and AD [11]. On the clinical side, DLB is characterized by dementia together with varying combinations of the core clinical features of parkinsonism, REM sleep behavior disorder (RBD), fluctuating cognition/alertness, and visual hallucinations [7]. Despite substantial advances have been made in understanding the genetics and pathology of DLB, the causes and the pathophysiological mechanisms preceding the dementia onset remain unknown.

The main theory on the development of DLB suggests a progressive neurodegeneration of the limbic system induced by the presence of aggregated toxic alpha-synuclein species. To date, however, there are no reliable measures of aggregated toxic alpha-synuclein species in vivo neither of brain damage. Moreover, the neurodegenerative process may start decades before the full DLB syndrome develops and likely determines the pattern of early clinical changes. These changes include cognitive and non-cognitive features, such as delirium and psychiatric symptoms (e.g., delusions, hallucinations, depression, and anxiety), but also parkinsonism and rapid eye movement (REM) sleep behavior disorder (RBD) [12]. The diagnosis of prodromal DLB is particularly challenging because of the long duration of this phase (even 20 years), the lack of clear in vivo biomarkers of disease, and the relatively non-specificity of the symptoms, overlapping with other psychiatric or neurodegenerative conditions such as late-onset psychosis, Parkinson's disease (PD), or AD.

Cognitive and non-cognitive symptoms are not only non-specific but also often overlapping with each other. However, a higher number and greater severity of symptoms is associated with increased risk of developing the full DLB phenotype. For example, in individuals with MCI, both parkinsonism and RBD strongly predict a later transition to DLB rather than to AD or other dementia types [13, 14]. Delirium can occur during the MCI stage of DLB (or even earlier) [15] as can fluctuations of cognition and arousal that may give rise to a diagnosis of delirium [12]. Psychiatric symptoms such as visual hallucinations (either spontaneous or provoked by illness or medication) are more likely to occur compared with normal controls or prodromal AD [16, 17], and prodromal DLB often experience also delusions, depression, and anxiety [18].

In the following sections, we will describe the three most common phenotypes of prodromal DLB [19], MCI-DLB, delirium-DLB, and psychiatric-DLB, and which evidence should be generated to propose formal criteria for these types of prodromal DLB moving in the direction of a unique framework for ultra-high risk for DLB.

17.2 MCI-DLB

MCI-DLB phenotype is the most common and characterized prodromal type of DLB, with clear clinical criteria and supportive biomarker features. The National Institute on Aging and Alzheimer's Association criteria [20] include the presence of cognitive complaint from the patient or from an informant or clinician who knows them and has observed a decline, with deficits in one or more cognitive domains that are greater than would be expected from normal aging. These deficits should not be associated with acute conditions nor linked to lifelong patterns of lower cognitive function (e.g., neurodevelopmental disorders). MCI-DLB usually have an overall preservation of their prior level of independence with minimal interference in day-to-day functional abilities, which, by definition, does not constitute a dementia.

Subjective cognitive impairment represents as step 1 of the diagnosis that is always followed by using standardized neuropsychological assessment to confirm an objective cognitive impairment. The main issues in all objective measures are (1) the lack of proper individualized cut-off (typically 1.5 standard deviation below the mean for their age and education-matched peers on culturally appropriate normative data is used, but often the data are lacking, especially in a multicultural environment); (2) the fluctuating nature of the symptoms, which requires serial testing to be accurate (but it is hard to reduce the effect of learning on serial measures); and (3) the difficulty in measuring longitudinal changes versus cross-sectional time-points. MCI and dementia are defined by deterioration or loss of cognitive function from the baseline of each individual person, which is often impossible to get considering that, when people seek doctors' opinion, it is when the symptoms and the decline have already started. In clinical practice, several categorizations are used to define the type of MCI including single- or multiple-domain deficits and amnestic or non-amnestic status. These categorizations aid in the identification of biomarkers and in the differentiation in rate of decline and progression to dementia, each of which may be important in the conduct of clinical trials.

Prodromal MCI-DLB have a very heterogeneous clinical pattern, but on the cognitive side, they often show a disproportionate attention/executive and visual processing deficits with a relatively well-preserved memory and object naming [21]. In particular, people with MCI-DLB show low attention, processing speed, and verbal fluency and difficulty in visual discrimination, assembly, and figure drawing [13, 22–24].

Another key aspect to consider is the presence of co-pathology. For example, people with MCI-DLB with impaired memory often show an extended coexisting AD-related pathology, characterized by greater hippocampal atrophy on imaging and greater CA1 hippocampal subfield pathology on autopsy. Moreover, similar to other subtypes of MCI, a proportion of people with MCI-DLB may revert to being cognitively normal, although they remain at a greater risk of the eventual development of dementia. Some instability of an MCI-DLB diagnosis is to be expected given inherent fluctuating cognition, worsening with neuroleptics or anticholinergics, or improvement with levodopa-carbidopa or cholinesterase inhibitors. In the differential diagnosis between MCI-DLB and MCI-AD, one of the aspects to consider is whether or not it is multi-domain and if is amnestic or nonamnestic. Nonamnestic single-domain MCI seldom develops into AD but is associated with a greater risk of transition to DLB [16, 25] with a tenfold risk compared with amnestic MCI [12]. However, considering that a high number of people with DLB have coexisting AD-related pathology (that may influence their cognitive profile), MCI-DLB still should be considered an important part of the differential diagnosis in amnestic subjects.

17.3 Delirium-DLB

An acute confusional state in people with no history of cognitive impairment is common in the years preceding MCI-DLB or full DLB syndrome [26]. One of the key diagnostic challenges is to identify if these acute confusional states are real delirium episodes or misdiagnosed severe cognitive fluctuations associated with clouding of consciousness (or a combination of both). Fluctuations in DLB are usually detectable by observation or informant report but also measurable using sensitive cognitive and electrophysiologic measures. Approximately half of the caregivers of DLB patients reports at least one episode of delirium before the full DLB diagnosis [27], and previous episodes of delirium were much more frequent in patients with DLB compared with patients with AD (25% vs. 7%), with a quarter of those with DLB having repeated delirium [17].

Beyond the academic exercise to identify prodromal delirium-DLB to potentially include them in clinical trials testing disease-modifying drugs, recognition that DLB may first present as delirium is important because most guidelines for behavioral disturbances in delirium recommend antipsychotics as first-line pharmacologic treatment. In people with DLB, typical antipsychotics can induce severe drug-induced parkinsonism. One biomarker available to identify whether a person with delirium is at high risk of DLB is the FDG-PET imaging. A study in people with prolonged delirium showed that 32% of subjects had a DLB-like pattern at FDG-PET imaging scan, which is a high proportion in regard both to the known prevalence of the disease and to that of their matched cognitively impaired control group (4%). Despite very few pathologic studies showed a link between delirium and pathology at autopsy, a significantly increased risk of postoperative delirium in those with peripheral alpha-synuclein pathology has been described [28]. Delirium has been suggested to be more common in those subjects with DLB with later age at onset, but further evidence is needed. In general, MCI-DLB are more susceptible to delirium than MCI-AD, and this delirium may occur as their presenting complaint before MCI develops. Delirium may be provoked by multiple factors including surgery, infections/sepsis, fever, or other system illnesses or secondary to use or sudden withdrawal of alcohol or psycho-active drugs. Prodromal delirium-DLB should be suspected in people in whom adequate provoking factors for delirium are not found, and delirium is prolonged or recurrent and later develops progressive cognitive decline and dementia. Moreover, the core clinical features of DLB might not be really helpful in this situation because, for example, cognitive fluctuation and clouding of consciousness and visual hallucinations can also occur in non-DLB delirium, motor parkinsonism could be related to the use of antipsychotics and not linked to DLB itself, and the diagnostic significance of a history of RBD in a person with delirium is not yet established.

17.4 Psychiatric-DLB

First episodes of major depression or psychosis in older adults are the most frequently reported presentations of prodromal psychiatric-DLB, which differs markedly from the construct of MCI-DLB and is sometimes sufficiently severe to require hospitalization. However, based on primary psychiatric features alone, psychiatric-DLB cases are not easily differentiated from non-neurodegenerative late-onset psychosis cases [29]. To date, only few centers were able to describe prodromal psychiatric-DLB with clinicopathologic correlations with the presence of Lewy bodies, but in these studies, DLB may present as a primary psychiatric disorder [30–32].

Visual hallucination is the most common symptom of prodromal psychiatric-DLB and is often associated with Capgras syndrome [33–36], apathy, anxiety, and depression [18]. Psychomotor retardation such as slowed speech, thinking, and body movements can resemble the bradykinesia of parkinsonism. The occurrence of rest tremor or rigidity is more helpful than bradykinesia to suspect prodromal DLB in patients with depressive disorder [37], but psychotropic-induced parkinsonism may complicate diagnosis. Atypical clinical features may prove valuable pointers to underlying DLB pathology, particularly the presence of recurrent visual hallucinations [18] when these occur before cognitive impairment becomes evident. As with all alpha-synucleinopathies, RBD may be a useful indicator, although a relationship between antidepressant usage and subsequent RBD onset is a potential confounder. Although the primary psychiatric manifestations are often accompanied by mild cognitive deficits [29], cognitive evaluation and interpretation of performance can be difficult when psychiatric symptoms are prominent. The frequency of cognitive fluctuations in psychiatric-DLB cases has not been determined.

Initial reports suggest that ^{123}I-MIBG scintigraphy may be helpful in psychiatric-onset DLB [32, 37, 38]. Eighteen of 35 patients with a first onset of major depressive disorder >50 years and with bradykinesia developed a clinical diagnosis of DLB after 6 years of follow-up. All 18 had an abnormal ventilatory response to hypercapnia, indicative of severe autonomic dysfunction, whereas none of the 17 patients with a normal response converted to DLB within the study period. For the converters, the most common presentation was with psychotic and melancholic features simultaneously. The frequency of hypersensitivity to antipsychotics, antidepressants, and antianxiety drugs was higher in converters than in nonconverters [37]. Further studies need to confirm these findings and to determine the value of other DLB biomarkers in psychiatric-onset cases [32, 38].

17.5 Moving to a Unified Framework of Ultra-High Risk of DLB

Considering the clear link between DLB and delirium, in people diagnosed with delirium, a careful search for other DLB features should be made with a low threshold for undertaking DLB biomarker examinations, especially in those with recurrent, unexplained, or prolonged delirium. The extent to which delirium presentations of DLB have the biomarker abnormalities associated with established DLB or other prodromal DLB presentations is unclear, although the FDG-PET imaging or DaTSPECT, showing reduced DAT uptake, has shown promising results [39]. However, the link between delirium and DLB is an important area for future research, to clarify the relationship between the two and to establish which factors associated with delirium should raise the index of suspicion for underlying prodromal DLB.

For psychiatric-DLB, it is not yet clear how to identify patients with prominent late-onset psychiatric symptoms who may have underlying Lewy body pathology disease and subsequently progress to DLB. It is premature to try to construct formal criteria for psychiatric-onset DLB, but clinicians in mental health and other settings need to be aware that this possibility exists, not least because of the risk of severe antipsychotic sensitivity reactions with increased morbidity and mortality.

Another approach could be using available biomarkers to create a score of risk of developing DLB that is incorporating the clinical phenotype (MCI-DLB, delirium-DLB, or psychiatric-DLB) but take also into account the presence of alpha-synuclein pathology in the brain. The latter can be measured with seeding assay in the CSF [40]; the presence of genetic mutations as a proxy for pronounced α-Syn pathology, e.g., GBA [40]; and the presence of neurodegeneration of noradrenergic, dopaminergic, and limbic systems measurable with SPECT and MRI, in which probable DLB is followed by the typical FDG-PET imaging pattern.

Clinical studies are needed to develop and validate a score for ultra-high risk for DLB, which should be then integrated with deeper biomarker assessment. This will allow clearer definition of prodromal DLB and facilitate the initiation of disease modification trials targeting the earliest stages of the disease. These criteria for prodromal DLB may be helpful for psychiatrists working with older adults with late onset of psychiatric symptoms. Psychiatrists could have a key role in the early stages/prevention of DLB. A flowchart has been proposed here as potential call for action (Fig. 17.1).

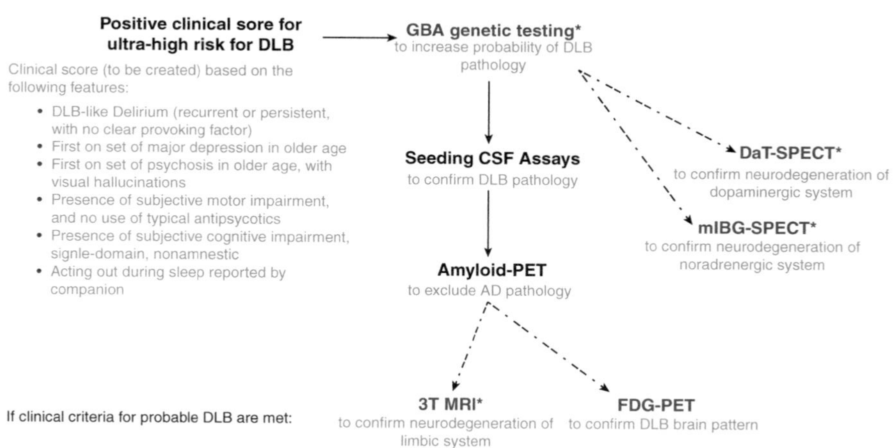

Fig. 17.1 Flowchart for ultra-high risk for DLB

17.6 Conclusions

MCI-DLB, delirium-DLB, and psychiatric-DLB are the three prodromal types of DLB characterized on the basis of the symptoms that precede the dementia. The clinicopathologic heterogeneity of these phenotypes highlights the need for a diagnosis based on in vivo pathology-driven biomarkers. A series of studies are necessary to move toward a unique framework for ultra-high risk for DLB.

References

1. Walker Z, Possin KL, Boeve BF, Aarsland D. Lewy body dementias. Lancet. 2015;386(10004):1683–97.
2. Ballard C, Holmes C, McKeith I, Neill D, O'Brien J, Cairns N, et al. Psychiatric morbidity in dementia with Lewy bodies: a prospective clinical and neuropathological comparative study with Alzheimer's disease. Am J Psychiatry. 1999;156(7):1039–45.
3. Gibb WR, Esiri MM, Lees AJ. Clinical and pathological features of diffuse cortical Lewy body disease (Lewy body dementia). Brain. 1987;110(Pt 5):1131–53.
4. McKeith IG, Perry RH, Fairbairn AF, Jabeen S, Perry EK. Operational criteria for senile dementia of Lewy body type (SDLT). Psychol Med. 1992;22(4):911–22.
5. McKeith IG, Galasko D, Kosaka K, Perry EK, Dickson DW, Hansen LA, et al. Consensus guidelines for the clinical and pathologic diagnosis of dementia with Lewy bodies (DLB): report of the consortium on DLB international workshop. Neurology. 1996;47(5):1113–24.
6. McKeith IG. Consensus guidelines for the clinical and pathologic diagnosis of dementia with Lewy bodies (DLB): report of the consortium on DLB international workshop. J Alzheimers Dis. 2006;9(3 Suppl):417–23.
7. McKeith IG, Boeve BF, Dickson DW, Halliday G, Taylor JP, Weintraub D, et al. Diagnosis and management of dementia with Lewy bodies: fourth consensus report of the DLB consortium. Neurology. 2017;89(1):88–100.
8. Suzuki M, Kurita A, Hashimoto M, Fukumitsu N, Abo M, Ito Y, et al. Impaired myocardial 123I-metaiodobenzylguanidine uptake in Lewy body disease: comparison between dementia with Lewy bodies and Parkinson's disease. J Neurol Sci. 2006;240(1–2):15–9.
9. Watanabe H, Ieda T, Katayama T, Takeda A, Aiba I, Doyu M, et al. Cardiac (123)I-meta-iodobenzylguanidine (MIBG) uptake in dementia with Lewy bodies: comparison with Alzheimer's disease. J Neurol Neurosurg Psychiatry. 2001;70(6):781–3.
10. Walker Z, Costa DC, Ince P, McKeith IG, Katona CL. In-vivo demonstration of dopaminergic degeneration in dementia with Lewy bodies. Lancet. 1999;354(9179):646–7.
11. McKeith I, O'Brien J, Walker Z, Tatsch K, Booij J, Darcourt J, et al. Sensitivity and specificity of dopamine transporter imaging with 123I-FP-CIT SPECT in dementia with Lewy bodies: a phase III, multicentre study. Lancet Neurol. 2007;6(4):305–13.
12. Ferman TJ, Smith GE, Kantarci K, Boeve BF, Pankratz VS, Dickson DW, et al. Nonamnestic mild cognitive impairment progresses to dementia with Lewy bodies. Neurology. 2013;81(23):2032–8.
13. Cagnin A, Busse C, Gardini S, Jelcic N, Guzzo C, Gnoato F, et al. Clinical and cognitive phenotype of mild cognitive impairment evolving to dementia with Lewy bodies. Dement Geriatr Cogn Dis Extra. 2015;5(3):442–9.
14. Sadiq D, Whitfield T, Lee L, Stevens T, Costafreda S, Walker Z. Prodromal dementia with Lewy bodies and prodromal Alzheimer's disease: a comparison of the cognitive and clinical profiles. J Alzheimers Dis. 2017;58(2):463–70.

15. FitzGerald JM, Perera G, Chang-Tave A, Price A, Rajkumar AP, Bhattarai M, et al. The incidence of recorded delirium episodes before and after dementia diagnosis: differences between dementia with Lewy bodies and Alzheimer's disease. J Am Med Dir Assoc. 2019;20(5):604–9.

16. Jicha GA, Schmitt FA, Abner E, Nelson PT, Cooper GE, Smith CD, et al. Prodromal clinical manifestations of neuropathologically confirmed Lewy body disease. Neurobiol Aging. 2010;31(10):1805–13.

17. Vardy E, Holt R, Gerhard A, Richardson A, Snowden J, Neary D. History of a suspected delirium is more common in dementia with Lewy bodies than Alzheimer's disease: a retrospective study. Int J Geriatr Psychiatry. 2014;29(2):178–81.

18. Fujishiro H, Nakamura S, Sato K, Iseki E. Prodromal dementia with Lewy bodies. Geriatr Gerontol Int. 2015;15(7):817–26.

19. McKeith I, Taylor JP, Thomas A, Donaghy P, Kane J. Revisiting DLB diagnosis: a consideration of prodromal DLB and of the diagnostic overlap with Alzheimer disease. J Geriatr Psychiatry Neurol. 2016;29(5):249–53.

20. Albert MS, DeKosky ST, Dickson D, Dubois B, Feldman HH, Fox NC, et al. The diagnosis of mild cognitive impairment due to Alzheimer's disease: recommendations from the National Institute on Aging-Alzheimer's Association workgroups on diagnostic guidelines for Alzheimer's disease. Alzheimers Dement. 2011;7(3):270–9.

21. Ferman TJ, Smith GE, Boeve BF, Graff-Radford NR, Lucas JA, Knopman DS, et al. Neuropsychological differentiation of dementia with Lewy bodies from normal aging and Alzheimer's disease. Clin Neuropsychol. 2006;20(4):623–36.

22. Donaghy PC, Taylor JP, O'Brien JT, Barnett N, Olsen K, Colloby SJ, et al. Neuropsychiatric symptoms and cognitive profile in mild cognitive impairment with Lewy bodies. Psychol Med. 2018;48(14):2384–90.

23. Cagnin A, Busse C, Jelcic N, Gnoato F, Mitolo M, Caffarra P. High specificity of MMSE pentagon scoring for diagnosis of prodromal dementia with Lewy bodies. Parkinsonism Relat Disord. 2015;21(3):303–5.

24. Yoon JH, Kim M, Moon SY, Yong SW, Hong JM. Olfactory function and neuropsychological profile to differentiate dementia with Lewy bodies from Alzheimer's disease in patients with mild cognitive impairment: a 5-year follow-up study. J Neurol Sci. 2015;355(1–2):174–9.

25. Kondo D, Ota K, Kasanuki K, Fujishiro H, Chiba Y, Murayama N, et al. Characteristics of mild cognitive impairment tending to convert into Alzheimer's disease or dementia with Lewy bodies: a follow-up study in a memory clinic. J Neurol Sci. 2016;369:102–8.

26. Gore RL, Vardy ER, O'Brien JT. Delirium and dementia with Lewy bodies: distinct diagnoses or part of the same spectrum? J Neurol Neurosurg Psychiatry. 2015;86(1):50–9.

27. Auning E, Rongve A, Fladby T, Booij J, Hortobagyi T, Siepel FJ, et al. Early and presenting symptoms of dementia with Lewy bodies. Dement Geriatr Cogn Disord. 2011;32(3):202–8.

28. Sunwoo MK, Hong JY, Choi J, Park HJ, Kim SH, Lee PH. Alpha-Synuclein pathology is related to postoperative delirium in patients undergoing gastrectomy. Neurology. 2013;80(9):810–3.

29. Van Assche L, Van Aubel E, Van de Ven L, Bouckaert F, Luyten P, Vandenbulcke M. The neuropsychological profile and phenomenology of late onset psychosis: a cross-sectional study on the differential diagnosis of very-late-onset schizophrenia-like psychosis, dementia with Lewy bodies and Alzheimer's type dementia with psychosis. Arch Clin Neuropsychol. 2019;34(2):183–99.

30. Ballard CG, Jacoby R, Del Ser T, Khan MN, Munoz DG, Holmes C, et al. Neuropathological substrates of psychiatric symptoms in prospectively studied patients with autopsy-confirmed dementia with Lewy bodies. Am J Psychiatry. 2004;161(5):843–9.

31. Iseki E, Marui W, Nihashi N, Kosaka K. Psychiatric symptoms typical of patients with dementia with Lewy bodies—similarity to those of levodopa-induced psychosis. Acta Neuropsychiatr. 2002;14(5):237–41.

32. Kobayashi K, Nakano H, Akiyama N, Maeda T, Yamamori S. Pure psychiatric presentation of the Lewy body disease is depression—an analysis of 60 cases verified with myocardial meta-iodobenzylguanidine study. Int J Geriatr Psychiatry. 2015;30(6):663–8.

33. Koga S, Dickson DW, Wszolek ZK. Capgras syndrome in dementia with Lewy bodies: a possible association of severe cortical Lewy body pathology. Neurol Neurochir Pol. 2021;55(6):592–4.
34. Thaipisuttikul P, Lobach I, Zweig Y, Gurnani A, Galvin JE. Capgras syndrome in dementia with Lewy bodies. Int Psychogeriatr. 2013;25(5):843–9.
35. Ohara K, Morita Y. Case with probable dementia with Lewy bodies, who shows reduplicative paramnesia and Capgras syndrome. Seishin Shinkeigaku Zasshi. 2006;108(7):705–14.
36. Marantz AG, Verghese J. Capgras' syndrome in dementia with Lewy bodies. J Geriatr Psychiatry Neurol. 2002;15(4):239–41.
37. Takahashi S, Mizukami K, Arai T, Ogawa R, Kikuchi N, Hattori S, et al. Ventilatory response to hypercapnia predicts dementia with Lewy bodies in late-onset major depressive disorder. J Alzheimers Dis. 2016;50(3):751–8.
38. Fujishiro H, Iseki E, Nakamura S, Kasanuki K, Chiba Y, Ota K, et al. Dementia with Lewy bodies: early diagnostic challenges. Psychogeriatrics. 2013;13(2):128–38.
39. Akintade O, Pierres F. Acute presentation of dementia with Lewy bodies. Clin Med (Lond). 2019;19(4):327–30.
40. Brockmann K, Quadalti C, Lerche S, Rossi M, Wurster I, Baiardi S, et al. Association between CSF alpha-synuclein seeding activity and genetic status in Parkinson's disease and dementia with Lewy bodies. Acta Neuropathol Commun. 2021;9(1):175.

Neglected Vulnerabilities in Mental Health: Where Do We Need to Do More?

Pasquale Pezzella, Giulia Maria Giordano, and Silvana Galderisi

18.1 Introduction

"Mental health is a dynamic state of internal equilibrium which enables individuals to use their abilities in harmony with universal values of society. Basic cognitive and social skills; the ability to recognize, express, and modulate one's own emotions, as well as empathize with others; flexibility and the ability to cope with adverse life events and function in social roles; and harmonious relationship between body and mind represent important components of mental health which contribute, to varying degrees, to the state of internal equilibrium." This definition was elaborated by Galderisi et al. in 2015 [1]. According to it, mental and psychological well-being is influenced not only by individual characteristics but also by the socioeconomic circumstances in which people find themselves and the environment in which they live; these determinants interact with each other dynamically and may threaten (risk factors) or protect (protective factors) an individual's mental health state [2]. This "internal equilibrium" is disrupted in one of every three individuals, or more, during their lifetimes [3, 4].

Mental illnesses constitute a substantial economic burden worldwide, and there is between-disorder variation in societal cost per patient; in particular, disorders such as schizophrenia and intellectual disabilities are generally associated with higher societal cost compared to "neurotic" disorders and eating disorders [5]. Mental illnesses have a considerable impact on the healthcare system that is heavily oriented toward treatment and disability management, with minimal resources devoted to prevention [6]. However, strategies focused on treatment of mental illnesses exclusively will not be sufficient to meet the challenge of the growing burden of mental disorders, and it is critical that countries invest in their prevention and early recognition and treatment, as well as in promotion of mental health at the

P. Pezzella · G. M. Giordano · S. Galderisi (✉)
University of Campania "Luigi Vanvitelli", Naples, Italy

© The Author(s), under exclusive license to Springer Nature Switzerland AG 2022
M. Colizzi, M. Ruggeri (eds.), *Prevention in Mental Health*,
https://doi.org/10.1007/978-3-030-97906-5_18

population level [7, 8]. Indeed, although for the most common major mental illnesses we now have medical and psychosocial interventions of proven efficacy, the available treatments appear still insufficient. For instance, in schizophrenia current treatments target mainly positive symptoms, but cognitive or negative symptoms remain, so far an unmet therapeutic need [9–11], and for autism spectrum disorders, effective treatments for the core symptoms are not available [12]. To improve this picture, we need a more effective bridge between basic research discoveries and the development of novel therapeutic strategies for preventing mental illnesses and for treating and rehabilitating people with mental disorders [13, 14].

The identification of vulnerability factors, in particular the most neglected ones, as well as novel diagnostic markers or pharmacological targets, could be exploited for the development of innovative preventive approaches, psychosocial interventions, and treatment strategies. Many potential risk factors early in life (ages 0–25 years), including parental mental and physical illnesses; child abuse and neglect; exposure to domestic violence; perinatal and obstetric insults; bullying; as well as mental, emotional, and behavioral problems in childhood or adolescence, and being a member of ethnic minority, have been addressed in previous chapters. In the present chapter, starting from the definition of mental health reported above [1], we will focus on vulnerability factors, in particular the most neglected ones (Tables 18.1 and 18.2), for which an in-depth knowledge might foster the promotion of mental health and prevention of mental disorders.

Table 18.1 Normative life events addressed in the chapter

Normative life events	Effects on mental health	What do we need to do?
	Several studies on the relationship between life events or life changes and various measures of morbidity, including psychiatric illnesses, found that morbidity tends to increase with higher exposure to these events and changes. The normative life events we focused on are listed below: 1. Adolescence 2. Marriage 3. Becoming parent 4. Retirement	It would be necessary to: 1. Increase public awareness that important life changes and events are often associated with stress increase 2. Identify factors that might increase stress of the target population and their key health needs 3. Promote sustainable and evidence-based interventions that may target psychological distress related to life changes/events 4. Coordinate and support efforts for the prevention of stress associated with life changes/events and for health promotion at the national and international level 5. Focus research on effective methods for prevention and health promotion

Table 18.1 (continued)

Normative life events	Effects on mental health	What do we need to do?
Adolescence	Critical life epoch characterized by many changes in which new physical, social, and emotional habits or important skills for a person's well-being are developed and maintained. Adolescents and young adults are at a key stage in establishing an independent identity, making educational and professional decisions and life choices, as well as establishing interpersonal relationships. Mental health issues in adolescents represent an important public health challenge worldwide. Globally, an estimated 10–20% of adolescents experience mental health conditions, yet these remain underdiagnosed and undertreated	It would be necessary to: 1. Identify the main factors and vulnerabilities that might influence mental well-being of young people 2. Promote healthy and supportive environments (home, school etc.) 3. Involve family, teachers, and relevant community agencies to promote supportive environments and social networks 4. Provide school programs and interventions, aimed to improve life or social skills of adolescents, to cope with stress, to deal with different emotional states, and to improve personal relationships 5. Implement prevention and health promotion strategies, taking into account the biopsychosocial and cultural characteristics and needs of adolescents 6. Strengthen an individual's capacity to regulate emotions, provide alternatives to risk-taking behaviors, and build resilience for difficult situations and adversities
Marriage	The association between marriage and mental health may depend on different social, family, and friend contexts of the person and consequently may not hold up in different contexts or groups of people, although marriage on average seems to improve mental health. However, early, non-normative marriage or even forced marriage is more likely to have a negative impact on mental health and is linked to higher lifetime prevalence and higher punctual prevalence of mental disorders than adult marriage	It would be necessary to: 1. Adopt and implement laws, policies, and strategies to address factors contributing to early, non-normative marriage and to prevent forced marriage for women 2. Adopt comprehensive social protection measures for children and women that are forced to marry 3. Safeguard children's and adolescents' access to education 4. Create a protective legal and political framework for more vulnerable people 5. Provide health and social services for women, in particular in low-income countries

(continued)

Table 18.1 (continued)

Normative life events	Effects on mental health	What do we need to do?
Becoming parent	Becoming a parent could be associated with psychological distress and with anxiety and, to a lesser extent, depression. It often reduces social networks, partly due to less available free time, different daily routines, an increased focus on the child and romantic partner, as well as diverging interests with childless affiliates. Sleep deprivation due to the child could also contribute to the development of mental health problems and could lead parents to experience anger toward the child	It would be necessary to: 1. Identify aspects that can influence the parents' relationship and their psychological distress 2. Identify parents at high risk of psychological distress 3. Direct interventions in the context of family therapy for high-risk parents that might need help 4. Implement projects targeting the general population to provide education on mental health during this period and to reduce parents' psychological burden 5. Assess whether specific social or psychoeducational interventions enhance resilience and reduce mental health sequelae among parents at higher risk of psychological distress 6. Provide home assistance for parents, especially early in a marriage, for the first child, and for unplanned children, situations in which parents might be unprepared and susceptible to psychological distress
Retirement	Retirement does not necessarily harm or benefit health. Its health consequences vary across individuals. A negative impact might be due to the eventual difficulty for the person to decide about the time of retirement or to psychological factors, such as fear of retirement and self-efficacy. Workers who perceive retirement as involuntary show a worsening in self-perceived health	It would be necessary to: 1. Consider retirement as a life change that might affect many aspects of life, including physical, psychological, and financial ones, and whose consequences can vary from person to person 2. Identify factors that might mostly influence the psychological well-being of the elderly people before and after retirement 3. Provide early interventions to support workers who perceive retirement as involuntary 4. Provide early retirement support interventions that focus on: (a) Emotional difficulties posed by anticipating the end of work (b) Gradual implementation of alternative activities after retirement

Table 18.2 Other neglected vulnerabilities addressed in the chapter

Vulnerabilities	Effects on mental health	What do we need to do?
Transition from CAMHS to AMHS	The transition from CAMHS to AMHS is poorly planned, executed, and experienced. Nearly one in four young people transit from CAMHS to AMHS after reaching the age limit. Some of them may be lost during the transition and develop severe and long-lasting mental health problems because of: 1. Resistance to transfer 2. Inadequate training of adult care providers on adolescents' disorders 3. Different models of care in child and adult services 4. Desire of young people to solve their problems by themselves 5. Unwillingness to repeat their story to a new clinician	It would be necessary to: 1. Provide a service in which the young patient continues the treatment path with the health workers from mental health services for both adults and children/adolescents, so that they can be accompanied in a gradual process of transition and can be helped establish a relationship with the new therapist while accompanied by the previous therapist with whom she/he is already familiar 2. Supply adequate funding and resources to effectively establish and manage these services
Basic cognition	Basic cognition is a determining factor in managing and carrying out daily activities. Cognitive impairment and consequent poor functioning in real life represent a major burden for patients (especially patients with psychosis, in particular schizophrenia) and contribute to their disability	It would be necessary to: 1. Identify cognitive impairment, particularly in patients at high risk to show these deficits 2. Provide assessment of cognitive impairment in line with current conceptualization and up-to-date assessment instruments, not only in research but also in clinical settings 3. Provide and use available integrative approach (pharmacological and psychosocial), as even minimal improvement in cognitive deficits can be associated with better functioning and quality of life 4. Provide cognitive remediation interventions, associated with family psychoeducation, cognitive behavior therapy, social skills training, physical exercise, and supported education or work interventions 5. Focus on the research of new innovative treatments effective for cognition

(continued)

Table 18.2 (continued)

Vulnerabilities	Effects on mental health	What do we need to do?
Emotional regulation	Poor emotional regulation is a common mechanism across many mental disorders (such as depression, bipolar disorder, anxiety disorders, attention-deficit/hyperactivity disorder, eating disorders, borderline personality disorder, autism spectrum disorders, insomnia, substance use disorders, and gambling disorder)	It would be necessary to: 1. Implement school-based and media-based programs to promote adaptative emotional regulation, focusing on emotions 2. Provide interventions targeting at emotional regulation, such as cognitive therapy, emotional regulation therapy, dialectical behavior therapy, and mindfulness-based interventions 3. Focus future research on interventions aimed to improve emotional regulations
Negative symptoms	Negative symptoms represent a key aspect of schizophrenia. They have a huge impact on patient outcome. Unfortunately, these symptoms are poorly recognized, and they do not respond satisfactorily to current available treatment. Therefore, they represent to date an unmet need in the care of people suffering from schizophrenia	It would be necessary to: 1. Recognize and carefully assess negative symptoms to achieve better patient outcomes 2. Provide assessment of negative symptoms in line with current conceptualization and up-to-date assessment instruments, not only in research but also in clinical settings 3. Train clinicians in recognition and assessment of negative symptoms 4. Educate patients and family members about the importance of negative symptoms, and increase their ability to recognize them, especially in FEP and prodromal subjects (CHR, UHR) 5. Use available interventions for treatment of negative symptoms, as even minimal improvement can be associated with better functioning and quality of life 6. Focus on research of innovative treatments effective for negative symptoms

Table 18.2 (continued)

Vulnerabilities	Effects on mental health	What do we need to do?
Body image	Concerns about body image are associated with maladaptive body change and weight loss strategies, such as dieting, low self-esteem, depression, and eating disorders. The populations most at risk are young people, especially women and those with pre-existing mental disorders. Body image is not only associated with eating disorders but also may occur simultaneously and exacerbate other psychopathological symptoms, such as depression, suicidal ideation, and social anxiety	It would be necessary to: 1. Develop psychoeducational interventions that provide parents with appropriate guidance and skills, in order to create a home environment that favors healthy weight-related behaviors and limits dissatisfaction with own body 2. Implement school-based screening programs for high-risk adolescents, providing information about eating disorders and teaching students to analyze and deconstruct social body image ideals and media messages 3. Implement media-based campaigns to promote positive body image and address body image issues 4. Use available interventions, such as cognitive behavioral therapy, to target cognitive, emotional, and behavioral factors that might influence body image
Humanitarian emergencies	Stress-related mental health disorders are associated with large-scale human disasters, such as natural disasters, pandemics, armed conflicts, large population displacements, food shortages, social disruption, and collapse of public health infrastructure. Complex humanitarian emergencies can negatively affect mental health of involved individuals, especially women and children and minorities in general, in low- and middle-income and conflict-affected countries. During humanitarian emergencies people are exposed to many stressful factors and have numerous and significant mental health needs. However, mental health care is often not provided in these contexts	It would be necessary to: 1. Develop national guidelines, standards, and support tools for the provision of mental health care and psychosocial support during emergencies, offering psychological first aid in all complex humanitarian emergencies 2. Strengthen the capacity of health professionals to identify and manage mental disorders during emergencies 3. Identify vulnerable groups, and evaluate what mental health support and clinical care are available 4. Train and educate individuals at the forefront of health care 5. Develop shared decision-making processes 6. Prevent negative mental health consequences in mental health providers 7. Develop sustainable mental health services 8. Adapt the humanitarian response system to local, national, and regional requirements

CAMHS Child and Adolescent Mental Health Services, *AMHS* Adult Mental Health Services, *FEP* first episode of psychosis, *CHR* clinical high risk, *UHR* ultra-high risk

18.2 Vulnerabilities

18.2.1 Life Epochs

Taking into account the concept of "dynamic state of internal equilibrium," different life events or changes could bring modifications in the achieved equilibrium. There have been many studies on the relationship between life events or life changes and various measures of morbidity, including psychiatric illnesses, and it has been found that morbidity tends to increase with increasing levels of exposure to life events [15–17]. Life events can be classified as normative (i.e., of high probability for most people at a certain age, such as marriage or job entry) or non-normative (i.e., often unexpected and occurring at any time during the lifespan) [17]. Normative life events, such as adolescent crises and puberty, transition to adulthood, job entry, marriage, pregnancy, becoming a parent, or retirement (Table 18.1), are good examples of life events requiring an active search for a new internal equilibrium. Non-normative events have been addressed in the relevant chapter. In this chapter, the focus is on neglected vulnerabilities that deserve attention and might be targeted by psychosocial interventions.

As to normative events, *adolescence* is a crucial period of transition from childhood to adulthood, during which the person develops and maintains physical, social, and emotional habits or skills important for her/his well-being. Adopting healthy sleep patterns; taking regular exercise; developing coping, problem-solving, and interpersonal skills; and learning to manage emotions are just examples of those habits/skills. Mental health issues in adolescents represent an important public health challenge worldwide. Globally, an estimated 10–20% of adolescents experience mental health conditions, yet these remain underdiagnosed and undertreated [18, 19]. Adolescence is also the period of *puberty*, a life event involving major biological and social changes [20]. Puberty itself is associated with increased behavioral problems in boys and increased social anxiety, depression, and self-harm in girls and is also associated with a lower sense of well-being and increased reports of fatigue, irritability, and somatic complaints in both boys and girls [21]. It is also possible that early puberty and mental health problems during adolescence share a range of common risk factors. These may include stressful family environment, early childhood adversity, bullying, emotional and/or physical abuse, and lack of parental warmth [22–25]. Furthermore, bad communication within the family can interfere with psychological development causing low self-esteem, poor self-determination, and resilience and lead to anxiety and depression symptoms [26–28]. Preventive measures that can help avoid the development and progression of mental health issues in adolescents include strengthening individual's capacity to regulate emotions, enhancing alternatives to risk-taking behaviors, building resilience for difficult situations and adversities, and promoting supportive social environments and social networks. Protection of mental health in adolescents requires a multilevel approach involving the family, schoolteachers, and relevant community agencies, to create healthy and supportive environments and implement preventive and health-promoting strategies that take into account adolescents' biopsychosocial and cultural characteristics and needs [18, 26].

Marriage is often regarded as a mean to increase psychological, social, and economic resources [29, 30] and to help individuals avoid the stress of relationship dissolution [29–31]. Married individuals enjoy better mental health than never married and previously married individuals [32–38]. Marriage has been linked with mental health outcomes such as self-worth, a sense of connectedness, and subjective well-being [39]. However, these associations can either suggest that marriage leads to improvements in health or that healthy individuals are more likely to "be selected" for marriage and stay married compared with their unhealthy counterparts [39, 40]. Uecker [40] showed that married young adults have lower psychological distress than single young adults, but they do not have a clear advantage over young adults in other types of romantic relationship. Actually, young adults who are engaged and not cohabiting have lower levels of distress than married young adults. However, these findings are controversial, and discrepant data have also been reported [34, 40]. Some studies found that men and women who get and stay married are less depressed than those who remain single [35, 41–43] or divorce [31, 41, 44–46]. Most individuals divorcing after a long-term marriage adapt successfully over time, and it depends primarily on intrapersonal resources, although a minority of divorcees exhibit enduring difficulties [47]. However, studies evaluating the association between marriage and mental health tend to observe the average effects of marriage on mental health, and few studies have attempted to identify potential moderators of this relationship [48]. In other words, the association between marriage and mental health may depend on different social, family, and friend contexts of the person and consequently may not hold up in different contexts or groups of people, although marriage on average seems to improve mental health. For instance, if we consider some particular contexts, not only marriage could be unrelated to a better mental health but may even make it worse. In particular, marriage at an early, non-normative age or even forced marriage, still occurring in some contexts, is more likely to have a negative impact on mental health [30, 49]. A cross-sectional study conducted in 2011 evaluated the sociodemographic characteristics and psychiatric comorbidities of a large sample of women married at an early, non-normative age [50]. According to this study, the majority of women who married before 18 years had a higher lifetime prevalence and a higher point prevalence of mental disorders compared to women married as adults. Disorders with the highest lifetime prevalence were major depressive disorder, nicotine dependence, and, after controlling for sociodemographic characteristic, antisocial personality disorder, while disorders with the highest point prevalence were specific phobias, nicotine dependence, and, after controlling for sociodemographic characteristic, dysthymia. If we consider the COVID-19 pandemic, according to a UNICEF report, the risk of early and forced marriages could increase, due to worsening economic conditions of families and communities, school closures, and service interruptions. Though it is still unclear what effect the pandemic will have on this problem, adopting comprehensive social protection measures, safeguarding children's and adolescents' access to education, creating a protective legal and political framework, and providing social guidance and the guarantee that health and social services for girls are adequately resourced and available are some of the measures that UNICEF has suggested to end early and forced marriages by 2030 [51].

Becoming parents, that is, the *transition to parenthood*, could be associated, in both men and women, with psychological distress [52] and adverse effects on parental mental health, such as anxiety and, to a lesser extent, depression [53–58], although many parents adapt well to the demands of parenthood. According to an epidemiological community survey, parenthood is associated with a better mental health, especially for men [57]. Perinatal psychiatry is the focus of another chapter. Our goal here is to emphasize that parenthood is a normative life change, which needs to be mentioned and generally considered as a possible time of stress, and poorly addressed as a risk factor for mental disorders. Parental mental disorders are also associated with an increased risk of developmental problems in children [59]. It must be said that parenthood often reduces social networks [60], partly due to logistic reasons, such as less available free time and different daily routines, and partly due to psychological processes, such as an increased focus on the child and romantic partner, as well as diverging interests with childless affiliates [61]. Moreover, sleep deprivation, both in pregnancy and postpartum, also could contribute to the development of mental health problems [62, 63] and could lead parents to experience anger toward the child [64]. It is not yet entirely clear, up to now, which diagnostic categories are most associated with this life change, what is the direction, and which are the mediators of these associations. The most studied diagnostic category is depression. Manic episodes, suicide risk, and social phobia are also often reported [65]. Some studies have evaluated unintended pregnancy as a risk factor for maternal mental health, and an association has been found between unintended pregnancy and an increased risk of perinatal maternal depression and parental stress, as well as low levels of psychological well-being and life satisfaction [66–68], although such an association may be a result of confounding factors such as socioeconomic status [69]. In case of offspring with physical defects, low birth weight, abnormal fetal activity and development, and behavioral/emotional problems, anxiety was the most prevalent disturbance in parents [70–73].

The transition to parenthood is an important period of stressful and sometimes maladaptive change for a significant proportion of new parents that are at risk of a range of mental health adjustments and relationship problems. It is important to highlight the central role that the quality of the relationship within the couple could play in aiding the mental health of new parents and the importance of focusing interventions on strengthening this relationship, as well as avoiding postnatal sleep deprivation, to avoid long-term unfavorable outcomes.

Retirement, i.e., the transition from an active working life to relatively inactive life, is a significant social life event. It has repercussions on many aspects of life including physical, psychological, and financial domains and could be a major trigger for developing mental health problems and threatening psychological well-being of the elderly [74–76]. However, some studies reported advantages, after retirement, such as decrease in the work-related stress, a reduction in mental and physical fatigue, and, in general, an improvement in mental health [77–79].

According to a longitudinal study, retirement does not categorically harm or benefit health, but its health consequences vary across individuals. A negative impact might be due to the eventual difficulty for the person to decide about the time of retirement or due to psychological factors such as fear of retirement and self-efficacy. It has been reported that older workers who perceived retirement as involuntary showed decreases in perceived health [80, 81]. Anyway, the findings point to the desirability of supportive pre-retirement interventions that focus on emotional difficulties posed by the anticipation of ending work and gradual implementation of alternative activities.

18.2.2 Transition from Child to Adult Mental Health Services

In spite of the high frequency of mental disorders before adulthood, and of the likelihood that they persist and even worsen during adulthood [82–84], most young people experience a clear discontinuity of care due to the so-called transition gap. Transition from child and adolescent mental health services (CAMHS) to adult mental health services (AMHS) is a common experience for young people with enduring health problems who reach the age boundary between services. For most patients, the transition from CAMHS to AMHS is poorly planned, executed, and experienced [85]. A recent review on this topic shows a gap in the care at the end of CAMHS: nearly one in four young people transit from CAMHS to AMHS after reaching the age limit [86]. Young people with a severe and enduring mental illness, such as psychosis, and those who have been hospitalized or are on medication with psychotropic drugs are more likely to move to adult services due to the severity of their condition; instead, those with neurodevelopmental, emotional/neurotic, and personality disorders most likely fall through the CAMHS–AMHS gap and have more pronounced transition difficulties [86–91]. Additionally, those patients who moved to AMHS were less likely to live with their parents, had more psychiatric hospital admissions, and were treated with psychotropic medications in the last 2 years before moving to AMHS [92]. Some of them may be lost during the transition and develop severe and long-lasting mental health problems because of resistance to transfer or inadequate training of adult care providers on adolescents' disorders, different models of care in child and adult services, young people who desire to solve their problems themselves, or unwillingness to repeat their story to a new clinician [93–95]. The TRACK study identified a cohort of young people, aged between 16 and 21, who had received mental health care within the UK National Health Services, and assessed their transitions from young to adult mental health services. Of the total sample, 85% were considered "suitable" for adult services by children mental health providers. However, only 49% actually transferred to AMHS [93]. The results are consistent with other national studies conducted in countries other than the UK [90, 92, 96].

One of the problems related to the transition is the abovementioned lack of or inadequate training for care providers and variations in the content of training programs. Transition is more often addressed in child and adolescent psychiatry training only [97]. While for child and adolescent psychiatric trainees the mean number of months spent working in services for minors and adults is about the same, adult psychiatric trainees spend most part of their working time in adult services [98]. The current inadequate knowledge could contribute to the suboptimal transition process and to young people falling through the care gap between services.

There is a problem even at the service level, that is, in the different approaches of CAMHS and AMHS [99]. Patients and parents are not always fully satisfied with the transition to adult mental health services, and this might lead to the abandonment of care programs. Some studies have defined the transition from youth to adult services as sharp, as it might cause relapses and discontinuation of access to mental health services [100]. Healthcare providers have also shown awareness of this gap and attempts at collaborative work between services [101]. As emerges from a systematic review, one of the main obstacles to a successful transition process is the lack of two-way communication between young people, parents, and doctors and between doctors from young and adult mental health services, which suggests the need for joint work between these care providers [102].

Overall, the available results show that there are two main approaches to transition problems: one is to improve the liaison between services for children and adults by keeping services as they currently exist [85, 91, 103, 104], and the other one is to develop new service models such as integrated mental health services for young people [105–110]. Both keeping existing services separate and developing new services can have advantages and limitations. Maintaining existing services requires models to enhance close collaboration between services, including transition coordinators [111]. Instead, the implementation of specific transition clinics, often seen as a solution, can result in a double transition, a temporary solution before accessing adult services [102, 112]. In our opinion, regardless of the two approaches mentioned above, young individuals, upon reaching the age limit at which they should leave such services, should continue the treatment path, for a defined period, with health workers from both adult and childhood/adolescence mental health services, so that they can be accompanied in a gradual transition process. Such a process would help the young person establish a therapeutic relationship with the new therapist while accompanied by the previous therapist with whom she/he is already familiar. However, adequate funding and resources would be needed to establish and effectively operate these services.

Although transition from CAMHS to AMHS should be a planned and efficient process, to date, there is no consensus about this decision-making process, and the management of the young patients depends on the clinical judgment. The 5-year (2014–19) European Union-funded "Managing the Link and Strengthening Transition from Child to Adult Mental Health Care" (MILESTONE) project aims to improve transition from CAMHS to AMHS in 28 European countries [113, 114]. The MILESTONE project developed and validated [115] a 64-item instrument for assessing transition, the Transition Readiness and Appropriateness Measure (TRAM), which guides clinicians' actions by identifying areas in which clinicians on both sides can work to ease the transition of the young person and by training them about good transition practices. Hopefully, this and other research projects will result in evidence-based guidelines that clinicians can follow to support their decision-making and direct their actions.

Future research should record the long-term outcomes of CAMHS leavers, to document whether they continue to receive mental health care and assess the level of functioning after transition. Finally, to help bridge the gap between CAMHS and AMHS, it would be advisable to involve young people more in research and service design by creating more youth-centered transitions [116, 117].

18.2.3 Basic Cognition, Social Skills, and Emotional Regulation

Basic cognitive and social skills are considered an important component of mental health due to the impact they have on every aspect of daily life [118–124]. Cognitive domains encompass a wide range of functions, such as the ability to pay attention, remember and organize information, solve problems, and make decisions, as well as social cognition skills, such as emotion processing, the ability to perceive and use emotional information; theory of mind, the ability to infer the intentions, dispositions, emotions, and beliefs of others and to use one's own repertoire of verbal/non-verbal abilities to communicate and interact with others; social perception, the ability to decode and interpret social cues; and attribution style/bias, the tendency to attribute hostile intentions to others and infer the causes of particular positive and negative social situations [125, 126]. All of these skills are interdependent and allow people to function in their environment. While mild degrees of impairment are compatible with mental health, moderate to severe degrees of impairment, especially if not balanced by other aspects, may require the support of others. Cognition is a determining factor in managing and carrying out daily activities. Only if a person can remember, concentrate, communicate, plan, and reason. she/he is able to cope with the requirements of life [127]. The link between cognition and functioning has been demonstrated not only in people with cognitive impairments [122] or mental health issues [128] but also in healthy individuals [129]. There is accumulating evidence that approximately one third of patients with mild cognitive impairment have difficulties in instrumental activities of daily living that require and rely heavily on memory and complex reasoning, especially in managing their finances, making medical decisions, and leading to finish daily activities [130–136]. In subjects with psychosis, particularly with schizophrenia, cognitive domains predict daily functioning, work skills, and interpersonal relationship [137–139]. Cognitive impairment and consequent poor functioning in real life represent a major burden for patients and contribute to their disability [140, 141]. Therefore, the identification of cognitive deficits represents an essential part of effective management of people with schizophrenia or other mental disorders to achieve recovery and psychosocial reintegration [142]. In fact, cognitive remediation interventions can improve the deficits of individuals with schizophrenia or other schizophrenia spectrum disorders, as demonstrated by several meta-analyses [143, 144]. Furthermore. it has been shown that cognitive remediation interventions associated with psychosocial interventions, such as social skills training or job support, have positive repercussions on functioning in real life and improve the outcome of psychosocial interventions [143–148].

Emotional regulation is a component of emotional processing domain and is generally defined as the ability to recognize, express, and modulate one's own emotional state that promotes adaptive and goal-directed behavior [149]. It is also regarded as an important component of mental health. Indeed, individuals show a quite large degree of variability in emotional abilities [150, 151]. In particular, the ability to regulate emotions reflects variation in how well people adjust emotional responses to meet current situational demands [152, 153]. An individual with this ability can aptly modify the intensity of the emotional experience and expression [154]. Furthermore, it has been shown that individuals who can best modulate their emotional expressive behavior have the highest well-being, disposable income, and socioeconomic status [155]. Unfortunately, in a society in which the accent is always on rational thinking and the expression of emotions is often regarded as negative feature, it is not surprising that alexithymia, i.e., the difficulty of distinguishing and describing emotions, is rather common in the population. Maladaptive emotional regulation and psychiatric disorders are closely related [156]. In particular, poor emotional regulation is a common mechanism across many mental disorders, such as depression [157–159], bipolar disorder [159–161], anxiety disorders [162–164], attention-deficit/hyperactivity disorder [165–167], eating disorders [168, 169], borderline personality disorder [170–173], autism spectrum disorders [174–176], insomnia [162, 177], substance use disorders [178, 179], and gambling disorder [180–182]. Poor emotional regulation can act as a maintenance factor of addiction [183, 184] and contribute to alcohol consumption and poor outcomes of alcohol use disorder [185, 186]. Research on the topic suggests that depression can be regarded as a consequence of dysfunctional emotional regulation; it is associated with a more frequent use of maladaptive strategies (rumination, suppression) and less frequent use of adaptive emotion regulation strategies (distraction, re-evaluation) [187–190]. Individuals with generalized anxiety disorder (GAD) have significantly more difficulty identifying and describing emotions; greater negative reactivity to their emotions as they fear the negative consequences of these experiences; and difficulty experiencing other emotions including depressed mood, anger, and even positive emotions such as euphoria; they also report less confidence than controls in their own ability to calm down following a negative emotional state [191–193]. Individuals affected by eating disorders have difficulties to cope with certain emotional states, such as adverse mood states, anger, anxiety, or depression, the so-called mood intolerance. Due to a reduced awareness of the triggering mood (and the associated cognitions), these patients tend to regulate or suppress negative emotions through dysfunctional behaviors, such as binging, purging, and/or restricting food intake [194–199]. In fact, negative mood predicts binging and purging in bulimia nervosa [200, 201], as well as binge episodes in binge eating disorder (BED) [202–204]. In subjects with bulimia nervosa, binge eating disorders, and anorexia nervosa, research studies showed emotion-processing deficits with alexithymia, difficulties with emotional awareness [205–207], tendency to avoid emotions, and less ability to accept and manage emotions [208]. The goal of improving emotional regulation strategies has become an important target for many psychological interventions, such as cognitive behavioral therapy, emotional regulation therapy, and dialectical behavior therapy, among others [209]. Even treatments that do not have emotional regulation as their main target may have positive effects on this transdiagnostic construct [178]. Mindfulness-based interventions have been proposed to involve cognitive reappraisal and facilitate the expression of emotions [210, 211]. Since emotion regulation is associated with various mental disorders, future research should investigate causal relationships and clarify which patients or individuals are at risk of or already have difficulties in the regulation of emotions and, finally, which interventions are most effective.

18.2.4 Negative Symptoms

One of the goals of DSM-5 was a shift from a categorical approach, in which diagnosis is based on defined criteria that can be met or not, to a dimensional approach, defining disorders based on psychopathological dimensions along a continuum of severity or intensity [212]. The Research Domain Criteria (RDoC) project was promoted by the National Institute of Mental Health (NIMH) in 2008, with the aim to "develop, for research purposes, new ways of classifying mental disorders based on dimensions of observable behavior and neurobiological measures" [213]. A dimensional assessment is also recommended for psychoses by identifying the severity and clinical heterogeneity of the main symptom domains: positive, negative, depressive, manic, psychomotor, and cognitive symptoms [214]. However, while some of these psychopathological dimensions are well understood, recognized, and often adequately treated, the same does not apply to the negative and cognitive dimensions. For instance, although negative and cognitive symptoms have long been recognized as a core component of schizophrenia, limited treatment options are available for negative and cognitive dimensions, and despite advances in understanding the epidemiology, etiology, biology, and psychopharmacology of schizophrenia, they remain so far an unmet therapeutic need [10, 11, 215–217]. Cognition, in general, has been briefly analyzed in the previous paragraph and addressed in another chapter of this book; therefore, hereafter, we will focus on negative symptoms.

First, negative symptoms in schizophrenia may be classified as primary or secondary. Primary negative symptoms represent the phenomenological expression of the disorder, while secondary negative symptoms may be caused by other psychopathological dimensions (i.e., positive symptoms, depression), as well as by treatment-related (i.e., parkinsonism due to treatment) or environmental factors [218–220]. Both primary and secondary negative symptoms cluster in two domains: a motivational one, consisting of avolition, anhedonia, and asociality, and an expressive deficit domain, consisting of blunted affect and alogia [10, 221, 222]. The distinction between primary and secondary negative symptoms has significant therapeutic implications. For instance, in some cases, it is possible to obtain an improvement in secondary negative symptoms by removing the underlying causes; instead, the primary negative symptoms tend to persist despite pharmacological intervention with both first- and second-generation antipsychotics [223]. Primary and secondary negative symptoms can be difficult to differentiate although this distinction is important for researchers and for clinical trial design.

Negative symptoms are present since the onset of schizophrenia and probably long before it [224, 225]; in 73% of cases, they first appear before the onset of positive symptoms [226]. Depending on how negative symptoms are defined, 50–90% of patients at the first admission present them [227, 228]. Negative symptoms have an elevated stability in the course of the illness, mostly in the presence of poor premorbid outcome [229, 230]. The presence of persistent negative symptoms has also been related to prolonged duration of untreated psychosis, which is a very robust predictor of poor treatment response [231].

Negative symptoms should be recognized, carefully assessed, and managed to achieve better patient outcomes. Especially when primary and persistent, they are closely related to poor patient functioning, worse quality of life, and lowered productivity, more than positive symptoms, which can be better addressed by available treatment options; however, often they are not recognized by clinicians. Limited evidence-based treatment is available, and, to date, effective treatment of persistent negative symptoms remains an unmet medical need in schizophrenia. However, some pharmacological and non-pharmacological treatment methods have been shown to be effective in treating the negative symptoms of schizophrenia, and some psychosocial interventions have shown promise although few studies have yet been conducted [10, 11]. Every effort should be made to use available interventions for their treatment, as even minimal improvement in negative symptoms can be associated with better functioning and quality of life. Treatment should be personalized and guided by the preferences of the individual patient as much as possible.

18.2.5 Body Image

Body image is the perception that individuals have of their physical appearance (weight, size, and body shape); it is related to satisfaction or concern about the appearance and can be associated with avoidance of exposure, as well as anxiety and discomfort [232, 233]. Adolescents are often targeted by messages related to their body and how it should be, not only from the media but also from their family and friends [234], and this may negatively influence the image they have of their own body [235, 236]. We are surrounded by advice on how to improve our physical appearance, from how to lose weight to how to surgically alter appearance, and from the importance of being thin to the techniques for developing muscles. All these messages may contribute to the greater focus on appearance in young people today, as compared to previous generation [237]; they regard ideal appearance as the standard for their own body, and when their appearance does not match the internalized ideal body, dissatisfaction arises, i.e., a negative attitude toward own physical appearance [232]. Social media may amplify dissatisfaction: adolescents post photographs of themselves and view photos of others [238], and, in these activities, physical appearance plays an important role [239]. Adolescents report a pressure to "look perfect" on social media, and, due to that, they tend to carefully select and edit their posts to get close to the ideal [240]. Several factors can moderate the associations between the use of social media and body dissatisfaction, from individual to environmental and social factors, such as the relationship with parents and in particular mother-adolescent relationship [241, 242]. Sociocultural influences (peers, parents, media) and mediational factors (internalization of the thin-ideal, appearance comparison) seem to predict body dissatisfaction and eating disorders [243]. Actually, multiple factors may be in place: (a) pubertal changes that may induce the development of body image problems, for instance, girls' physical changes during puberty may involve weight gain [244]; (b) family environment and the perception of family, friends, and romantic relationship experiences [245–249]; and (c) parents' behaviors such as suggesting going on a diet, making comments on adolescent's weight/appearance, and excessive physical exercise [250]. Romantic partners also have a role in both men's and women's body image experiences and could also influence individual's vulnerability to disordered eating and, in general, their psychological health [251–253]. In both girls [254–256] and boys [257, 258], body dissatisfaction consistently predicts disordered and maladaptive eating behaviors, as well as other psychological problems. In particular, concerns about body image are associated with weight loss strategies, such as dieting, with low self-esteem, depression, eating disorders, and adoption of maladaptive body change strategies. However, as mentioned, body image is not only associated with eating disorders but also may occur simultaneously and exacerbate other psychopathological symptoms, such as depression [259–264], suicidal ideation [265–267], and social anxiety [268–271]. Several strategies can be used by researchers, educators, and mental health professionals to address body image problems; among them, psycho-education, cognitive behavioral psychotherapy, and ecological/activist approaches are the most frequent. In order to create a home environment that favors healthy weight-related behaviors and limits dissatisfaction with one's body, it would be necessary to develop psycho-educational interventions that provide parents with appropriate guidance and skills [272]. Cognitive behavioral therapy (CBT) is also an important tool. CBT for body image targets cognitive, emotional, and behavioral factors and generally includes psycho-education, cognitive intervention, exposure to avoided situations, and prevention of rituals and perceptual retraining [273, 274].

18.2.6 Humanitarian Emergencies and Mental Health

The United Nations (UN) defines a complex humanitarian emergency as "a humanitarian crisis in a country, region or society where there is a total or considerable breakdown of authority resulting from internal or external conflict, and which requires an international response that goes beyond the mandate or capacity of any single agency and/or the ongoing UN country programme" [275]. Stress-related mental health disorders are associated with large-scale human disasters, such as natural disasters, like pandemics, armed conflict, large population displacements, food shortages, social disruption, and collapse of public health infrastructure [276–279]. Complex humanitarian emergencies can negatively affect the mental health of the involved individuals [280–282]. A meta-analysis of epidemiological surveys of refugees and other conflict-affected persons from 40 countries showed average rates of 15–20% for depression and post-traumatic stress disorder [283]. The UNESCO EFA Global Monitoring Report shows that almost all (about 95%) unschooled children live in low- and middle-income countries and half of them live in countries caught up by conflicts [284]. In addition to the educational consequences, children and adolescents living in conflict-afflicted countries, exposed to violence and trauma, face a number of consequences for their mental health and emotional, cognitive, and social development, which result in problems in social relationships, including a difficulty in trusting others, poor quality relationships, and a high risk of re-victimization and of developing several physical health problems [285]. Women and adolescent girls are more involved in humanitarian emergency situations, since these categories, following displacement, are particularly vulnerable to high-risk and unintended pregnancies, spontaneous abortions, perinatal complications, unsafe abortions, unsafe births, and deaths; despite this, problems related to gender-based violence and reproductive and sexual health are less and insufficiently addressed [286]. When we talk about violence against women and violence against children, the emphasis is often on some forms of violence, those related to the emergency situation, in particular physical and sexual violence and abuse by armed groups. Domestic violence, in particular by close partners or caregivers, is often neglected, although it is clear that the family seems to be the place in which most of the acts of violence take place [287]. Women in low- and middle-income and conflict-affected countries who reported being victims of sexual violence and other social stressors were significantly more likely to have suicidal thoughts and experience depression, anxiety, and PTSD symptoms [288]. In the chaos of an emergency, not only it is possible that due to stressful factors, some individuals may experience psychiatric symptoms, as we have said, but individuals with pre-existing mental disorders may also experience a relapse or exacerbation of existing symptoms; people with pre-existing chronic psychosis, bipolar disorder, intellectual disability, and epilepsy are particularly at risk of neglect, abandonment, abuse, discontinuation of maintenance medications, and lack of access to health services [289].

While there is evidence of the influence that humanitarian emergencies have on mental health, mental health care is often not provided, particularly in low- and middle-income countries, which are often affected by conflicts. During humanitarian emergencies people are exposed to a large number of stressful factors, so they have numerous and significant mental health needs, which are often neglected by health professionals. Some plans aimed to improve mental health in humanitarian emergencies are based on early support to public health activities aimed at reducing mortality and morbidity, offering psychological first aid, identifying vulnerable groups, evaluating what mental health support and clinical care are available, training and educating individuals at the forefront of health care, sharing decision-making processes, and preventing negative mental health consequences in mental health providers [290]. Other plans rely on the development of national guidelines, standards, and support tools for the provision of actions for mental health and psychosocial support (MHPSS) during emergencies, on strengthening the capacity of health professionals to identify and manage mental disorders during emergencies and on the development of sustainable mental health services [291]. During the World Humanitarian Summit on challenges and opportunities for humanitarian assistance in 2015, the text adopted by the European Parliament "emphasizes the need to adapt the humanitarian response system to local, national and regional requirements, and to empower and engage regularly affected populations, including women of all ages, children, persons with disabilities, minorities and indigenous people recognizing their role as change agents by ensuring, whenever possible, feedback from and prior consultation with these populations in the programming and implementation of humanitarian action."

There are different approaches to address mental health problems and support people in complex humanitarian emergencies: (1) the "traumatic approach" which emphasizes trauma-centered interventions (e.g., narrative exposure therapy, trauma-focused cognitive behavioral therapy, and Eye Movement Desensitization and Reprocessing—EMDR); (2) the "psychosocial approach," which is based on the close relationship between individual emotional well-being and the social context and therefore concrete relationships with others within the family and community; (3) "the global mental health approach" which provides appropriate health interventions for a range of mental health problems, regardless of the humanitarian context, and is based on the idea that the provision of health care in any setting must include mental health care, as there is "no health without mental health" [292].

Nowadays, the pandemic due to Sars-Cov-2 has created emergencies everywhere, and its effects on the health of the general population and of those with pre-existing mental disorders are still to be fully acknowledged and far from being adequately managed.

Due to quarantine and its effects, as well as the economic impact and increased unemployment, mental health disorders (such as PTSD, anxiety disorders, depression) will increase and have a strong societal impact. Furthermore, most likely, the pandemic will have a negative influence on risk factors for mental disorders, for example, by contributing to an increase in risk behaviors (e.g., use of alcohol and tobacco, social isolation) and stress-related reactions (insomnia, anger, fear) [293]. The psychosocial responses of the general population to the most recent epidemics of infectious disease of the past two decades (such as the severe acute respiratory syndrome epidemic (SARS), the H1N1 pandemic, Middle East Respiratory Syndrome (MERS), or Ebola virus outbreaks) have been variable and have included feelings of anxiety and shame, experiences of individual and societal failure or weakness, an underestimation of the probability of survival, an overestimation of the probability of infection, the adoption of excessive and inappropriate precautionary measures, as well as an increased demand for health services at a time of shortage [294, 295]. The pandemic can be particularly serious for those who have been directly or indirectly in contact with the virus, who are already biologically vulnerable or subject to psychosocial stressors (including people with physical illnesses, mental or substance use disorders), health workers (due to the high level of exposure and stress associated with the increase in working hours), and those who follow news through numerous media channels [296]. As a result of the COVID-19 pandemic, 33% of the global population started experiencing symptoms related to depression, anxiety, insomnia, or suicidal ideas, especially individuals with a history of mental illnesses [297], and subjects with pre-existing mental disorders were even more at risk of relapses or aggravation of their symptomatology [298]. In particular, subjects with schizophrenia [299, 300], bipolar disorder [301, 302], obsessive-compulsive disorder [303–305], eating disorders [306, 307], gambling disorder, and substance use disorder [308, 309]. ADHD [310, 311], intellectual disability [312], and autism [313] showed an increased vulnerability to a worsening of symptoms. Therefore, it is important to consider that the mental health consequences may be present for longer and peak later than the actual pandemic. The involvement of psychiatrists and mental health professionals in the COVID-19 Task Force appears essential to guide policies aimed at preventing consequences on mental health and to guide the implementation of adequate therapeutic interventions where prevention fails. At the beginning of the pandemic, healthcare workers were particularly vulnerable to emotional distress, given the risk of exposure to the virus, before the vaccine, concern for infection and care of loved ones, shortage of personal protective equipment (PPE), more working hours, and involvement in emotionally and ethically demanding decisions on resource allocation. Healthcare professionals, particularly frontline workers during the first lockdown, have reported negative consequences as a result of exposure to stress and the fear of infecting loved ones [314–316]. In order to prepare for the immediate and near future, it would seem essential to invest in the training of healthcare professionals who are unexpectedly at the forefront of responding to disastrous events such as pandemics, as well as in the implementation of adequate and advanced therapeutic and rehabilitation programs [317]. It would be necessary to improve and adapt existing mental health services to current needs and facilitate access of individuals who suffer from mental disorders or those who de novo develop a psychiatric disorder [295]. We need to learn more about the psychiatric and psychological aspects of COVID-19 and about effective initiatives from a public and global mental health perspective [295]. In conclusion, the COVID-19 pandemic could represent an opportunity to improve the care of people with mental disorders, increase the quality of monitoring of needs and the efficiency of services of mental health, and accelerate the implementation of remote interventions with the use of digital platforms, helping reduce inequalities and improve mental health globally [318].

18.3   Final Remarks

Findings reported in this chapter confirm that several vulnerability factors, which are often neglected, are involved in establishing dysfunctional mechanisms that can lead to the development of mental disorders. The overview provided in the chapter is far from covering all neglected factors and is focused on those factors deemed as relevant to the definition of mental health proposed by Galderisi et al. [1] and not always clearly addressed as part of mental health care.

It is clear from the presented overview that much is needed to address risks for and vulnerabilities to mental health issues that may appear in different life epochs and involve different spheres of life. Knowledge of vulnerabilities and risk factors for mental disorders is the basis for successful prevention of mental disorders and promotion of mental health.

References

1. Galderisi S, Heinz A, Kastrup M, Beezhold J, Sartorius N. Toward a new definition of mental health. World Psychiatry. 2015;14(2):231–3.
2. Organization WH. Risks to mental health: an overview of vulnerabilities and risk factors. Geneva: World Health Organization; 2012.
3. Steel Z, Marnane C, Iranpour C, Chey T, Jackson JW, Patel V, et al. The global prevalence of common mental disorders: a systematic review and meta-analysis 1980–2013. Int J Epidemiol. 2014;43(2):476–93.
4. Vigo D, Thornicroft G, Atun R. Estimating the true global burden of mental illness. Lancet Psychiatry. 2016;3(2):171–8.
5. Christensen MK, Lim CCW, Saha S, Plana-Ripoll O, Cannon D, Presley F, et al. The cost of mental disorders: a systematic review. Epidemiol Psychiatr Sci. 2020;29:e161.
6. Furber G, Leach M, Guy S, Segal L. Developing a broad categorisation scheme to describe risk factors for mental illness, for use in prevention policy and planning. Aust NZ J Psychiat. 2017;51(3):230–40.
7. Organization WH. Mental Health Action Plan 2013–2020. Geneva: World Health Organization; 2013.
8. Barry MM, Clarke AM, Petersen I. Promotion of mental health and prevention of mental disorders: priorities for implementation. East Mediterr Health J. 2015;21(7):503–11.
9. Stepnicki P, Kondej M, Kaczor AA. Current concepts and treatments of Schizophrenia. Molecules. 2018;23(8):2087.
10. Galderisi S, Mucci A, Dollfus S, Nordentoft M, Falkai P, Kaiser S, et al. EPA guidance on assessment of negative symptoms in schizophrenia. Eur Psychiatry. 2021;64(1):e23.
11. Galderisi S, Kaiser S, Bitter I, Nordentoft M, Mucci A, Sabe M, et al. EPA guidance on treatment of negative symptoms in schizophrenia. Eur Psychiatry. 2021;64(1):e21.
12. Pandina G, Ring RH, Bangerter A, Ness S. Current approaches to the pharmacologic treatment of core symptoms across the lifespan of Autism Spectrum disorder. Child Adolesc Psychiatr Clin N Am. 2020;29(2):301.
13. Insel TR, Scolnick EM. Cure therapeutics and strategic prevention: raising the bar for mental health research. Mol Psychiatry. 2006;11(1):11–7.
14. Cirulli F, Francia N, Berry A, Aloe L, Alleva E, Suomi SJ. Early life stress as a risk factor for mental health: role of neurotrophins from rodents to non-human primates. Neurosci Biobehav Rev. 2009;33(4):573–85.
15. Fergusson DM, Horwood LJ. Vulnerability to life events exposure. Psychol Med. 1987;17(3):739–49.
16. Tibubos AN, Burghardt J, Klein EM, Brahler E, Junger C, Michal M, et al. Frequency of stressful life events and associations with mental health and general subjective health in the general population. J Public Health. 2020;29:1071–80.
17. Wrzus C, Hanel M, Wagner J, Neyer FJ. Social network changes and life events across the life span: a meta-analysis. Psychol Bull. 2013;139(1):53–80.
18. Organization WH. Adolescent mental health. Geneva: WHO; 2019.

19. Kessler RC, Angermeyer M, Anthony JC, De Graaf R, Demyttenaere K, Gasquet I, et al. Lifetime prevalence and age-of-onset distributions of mental disorders in the World Health Organization's World Mental Health Survey Initiative. World Psychiatry. 2007;6(3):168–76.
20. Brim OGJ, Ryff CD. On the properties of life events. In: Baltes Jr PB, Brim OG, editors. Life-span development and behavior. 3rd ed. New York: Academic Press; 1980. p. 367–88.
21. R. V. Puberty, The Brain and Mental Health in Adolescence. In: Bourguignon JP, Carel JC, Christen Y, editors. Brain crosstalk in puberty and adolescence research and perspectives in endocrine interactions, vol. 13. Cham: Springer; 2015.
22. Basu S, Banerjee B. Impact of environmental factors on mental health of children and adolescents: a systematic review. Child Youth Serv Rev. 2020;119:105515.
23. Butterfield RD, Silk JS, Lee KH, Siegle GS, Dahl RE, Forbes EE, et al. Parents still matter! Parental warmth predicts adolescent brain function and anxiety and depressive symptoms 2 years later. Dev Psychopathol. 2021;33(1):226–39.
24. Nelson CA, Scott RD, Bhutta ZA, Harris NB, Danese A, Samara M. Adversity in childhood is linked to mental and physical health throughout life. Br Med J. 2020;371:m3048.
25. McKay MT, Cannon M, Chambers D, Conroy RM, Coughlan H, Dodd P, et al. Childhood trauma and adult mental disorder: a systematic review and meta-analysis of longitudinal cohort studies. Acta Psychiatr Scand. 2021;143(3):189–205.
26. Zarnaghash M, Zarnaghash M, Zarnaghash N. The relationship between family communication patterns and mental health. Procedia Soc Behav Sci. 2013;84:405–10.
27. Pinto ACS, Luna IT, Silva ADA, Pinheiro PND, Braga VAB, Souza AMAE. Risk factors associated with mental health issues in adolescents: a integrative review. Rev Esc Enferm USP. 2014;48(3):552–61.
28. Ioffe M, Pittman LD, Kochanova K, Pabis JM. Parent–adolescent communication influences on anxious and depressive symptoms in early adolescence. J Youth Adolesc. 2020;49(8):1716–30.
29. Liu H, Elliott S, Umberson D. Marriage in young adulthood. In: Grant JE, Potenza MN, editors. Young adult mental health. New York: Oxford University Press; 2010. p. 169–80.
30. Williams K, Umberson D. Marital status, marital transitions, and health: a gendered life course perspective. J Health Soc Behav. 2004;45(1):81–98.
31. Simon RW, Barrett AE. Nonmarital romantic relationships and mental health in early adulthood: does the association differ for women and men? J Health Soc Behav. 2010;51(2):168–82.
32. Brown SL. The effect of union type on psychological well-being: depression among cohabitors versus marrieds. J Health Soc Behav. 2000;41(3):241–55.
33. Gove WR, Style CB, Hughes M. The effect of marriage on the well-being of adults: a theoretical analysis. J Fam Issues. 1990;11(1):4–35.
34. Horwitz AV, White HR. Becoming married, depression, and alcohol problems among young adults. J Health Soc Behav. 1991;32(3):221–37.
35. Lamb KA, Lee GR, DeMaris A. Union formation and depression: selection and relationship effects. J Marriage Fam. 2003;65(4):953–62.
36. Marcussen K. Explaining differences in mental health between married and cohabiting individuals. Soc Psychol Q. 2005;68(3):239–57.
37. Ross CE. Reconceptualizing marital status as a continuum of social attachment. J Marriage Fam. 1995;57(1):129–40.
38. Simon RW. Revisiting the relationships among gender, marital status, and mental health. Am J Sociol. 2002;107(4):1065–96.
39. Koball HL, Moiduddin E, Henderson J, Goesling B, Besculides M. What do we know about the link between marriage and health? J Fam Issues. 2010;31(8):1019–40.
40. Uecker JE. Marriage and mental health among young adults. J Health Soc Behav. 2012;53(1):67–83.
41. Horwitz AV, White HR, Howell-White S. Becoming married and mental health: a longitudinal study of a cohort of young adults. J Marriage Fam. 1996;58(4):895–907.
42. Kim HK, McKenry PC. The relationship between marriage and psychological well-being: a longitudinal analysis. J Fam Issues. 2002;23(8):885–911.

43. Meadows SO, McLanahan SS, Brooks-Gunn J. Stability and change in family structure and maternal health trajectories. Am Sociol Rev. 2008;73(2):314–34.
44. Aseltine RH, Kessler RC. Marital disruption and depression in a community sample. J Health Soc Behav. 1993;34(3):237–51.
45. Johnson DR, Wu J. An empirical test of crisis, social selection, and role explanations of the relationship between marital disruption and psychological distress: a pooled time-series analysis of four-wave panel data. J Marriage Fam. 2002;64(1):211–24.
46. Marks NF, Lambert JD. Marital status continuity and change among young and midlife adults: longitudinal effects on psychological well-being. J Fam Issues. 1998;19(6):652–86.
47. Knöpfli B, Morselli D, Perrig-Chiello P. Trajectories of psychological adaptation to marital breakup after a long-term marriage. Gerontology. 2016;62(5):541–52.
48. Frech A, Williams K. Depression and the psychological benefits of entering marriage. J Health Soc Behav. 2007;48(2):149–63.
49. Rauf B, Saleem N, Clawson R, Sanghera M, Marston G. Forced marriage: implications for mental health and intellectual disability services. Adv Psychiatr Treat. 2013;19(2):135–43.
50. Le Strat Y, Dubertret C, Le Foll B. Child marriage in the United States and its association with mental health in women. Pediatrics. 2011;128(3):524–30.
51. (UNICEF) UNICsEF. COVID-19: A threat to progress against child marriage. 2021.
52. McKenzie SK, Carter K. Does transition into parenthood lead to changes in mental health? Findings from three waves of a population based panel study. J Epidemiol Community Health. 2013;67(4):339.
53. Heron J, O'Connor TG, Evans J, Golding J, Glover V. The course of anxiety and depression through pregnancy and the postpartum in a community sample. J Affect Disord. 2004;80(1):65–73.
54. Matthey S, Barnett B, Howie P, Kavanagh DJ. Diagnosing postpartum depression in mothers and fathers: whatever happened to anxiety? J Affect Disord. 2003;74(2):139–47.
55. Wenzel A, Haugen EN, Jackson LC, Brendle JR. Anxiety symptoms and disorders at eight weeks postpartum. J Anxiety Disord. 2005;19(3):295–311.
56. Umberson D, Pudrovska T, Reczek C. Parenthood, childlessness, and well-being: a life course perspective. J Marriage Fam. 2010;72(3):612–29.
57. Helbig S, Lampert T, Klose M, Jacobi F. Is parenthood associated with mental health? Findings from an epidemiological community survey. Soc Psychiatry Psychiatr Epidemiol. 2006;41(11):889–96.
58. Parfitt Y, Ayers S. Transition to parenthood and mental health in first-time parents. Infant Ment Health J. 2014;35(3):263–73.
59. Stein A, Pearson RM, Goodman SH, Rapa E, Rahman A, McCallum M, et al. Effects of perinatal mental disorders on the fetus and child. Lancet. 2014;384(9956):1800–19.
60. Bost KK, Cox MJ, Burchinal MR, Payne C. Structural and supportive changes in couples' family and friendship networks across the transition to parenthood. J Marriage Fam. 2002;64(2):517–31.
61. Bernardi L. Channels of social influence on reproduction. Popul Res Policy Rev. 2003;22(5):427–555.
62. Hiscock H, Bayer JK, Hampton A, Ukoumunne OC, Wake M. Long-term mother and child mental health effects of a population-based infant sleep intervention: cluster-randomized, controlled trial. Pediatrics. 2008;122(3):e621–7.
63. Skouteris H, Wertheim EH, Germano C, Paxton SJ, Milgrom J. Assessing sleep during pregnancy: a study across two time points examining the Pittsburgh Sleep Quality Index and associations with depressive symptoms. Womens Health Issues. 2009;19(1):45–51.
64. Cummings EM, Davies PT. Maternal depression and child development. J Child Psychol Psychiatry. 1994;35(1):73–122.
65. Pearson RM, Culpin I, Loret de Mola C, Quevedo L, Murray J, Matijasevich A, et al. Transition to parenthood and mental health at 30 years: a prospective comparison of mothers and fathers in a large Brazilian birth cohort. Arch Womens Ment Health. 2019;22(5):621–9.

66. Orr ST, Arden MC. Unintended pregnancy and the psychosocial well-being of pregnant women. Womens Health Issues. 1997;7(1):38–46.
67. Yanikkerem E, Ay S, Piro N. Planned and unplanned pregnancy: effects on health practice and depression during pregnancy. J Obstet Gynaecol Res. 2013;39(1):180–7.
68. McCrory C, McNally S. The effect of pregnancy intention on maternal prenatal behaviours and parent and child health: results of an irish cohort study. Paediatr Perinat Epidemiol. 2013;27(2):208–15.
69. Gipson JD, Koenig MA, Hindin MJ. The effects of unintended pregnancy on infant, child, and parental health: a review of the literature. Stud Fam Plann. 2008;39(1):18–38.
70. Hansen D, Lou HC, Olsen J. Serious life events and congenital malformations: a national study with complete follow-up. Lancet. 2000;356(9233):875–80.
71. Hedegaard M, Henriksen TB, Sabroe S, Secher NJ. Psychological distress in pregnancy and preterm delivery. BMJ. 1993;307(6898):234–9.
72. DiPietro JA, Hilton SC, Hawkins M, Costigan KA, Pressman EK. Maternal stress and affect influence fetal neurobehavioral development. Dev Psychol. 2002;38(5):659–68.
73. O'Connor TG, Heron J, Glover V. Antenatal anxiety predicts child behavioral/emotional problems independently of postnatal depression. J Am Acad Child Adolesc Psychiatry. 2002;41(12):1470–7.
74. Kim JE, Moen P. Retirement transitions, gender, and psychological well-being: a life-course, ecological model. J Gerontol Ser B. 2002;57(3):P212–P22.
75. Osborne JW. Psychological effects of the transition to retirement. Can J Couns Psychother. 2011;46(1):45–58.
76. Szinovacz ME, DeViney S. The retiree identity: gender and race differences. J Gerontol Ser B. 1999;54B(4):S207–S18.
77. Westerlund H, Vahtera J, Ferrie JE, Singh-Manoux A, Pentti J, Melchior M, et al. Effect of retirement on major chronic conditions and fatigue: French GAZEL occupational cohort study. BMJ. 2010;341:c6149.
78. Oksanen T, Vahtera J, Westerlund H, Pentti J, Sjösten N, Virtanen M, et al. Is retirement beneficial for mental health?: antidepressant use before and after retirement. Epidemiology. 2011;22(4):553–9.
79. Mein G, Martikainen P, Hemingway H, Stansfeld S, Marmot M. Is retirement good or bad for mental and physical health functioning? Whitehall II longitudinal study of civil servants. J Epidemiol Community Health. 2003;57(1):46–9.
80. van Solinge H. Health change in retirement: a longitudinal study among older workers in the Netherlands. Res Aging. 2007;29(3):225–56.
81. Jokela M, Ferrie JE, Gimeno D, Chandola T, Shipley MJ, Head J, et al. From midlife to early old age: health trajectories associated with retirement. Epidemiology. 2010;21(3):284–90.
82. Kessler RC, Berglund P, Demler O, Jin R, Merikangas KR, Walters EE. Lifetime prevalence and age-of-onset distributions of DSM-IV disorders in the National Comorbidity Survey Replication. Arch Gen Psychiatry. 2005;62(6):593–602.
83. McGorry PD, Purcell R, Goldstone S, Amminger GP. Age of onset and timing of treatment for mental and substance use disorders: implications for preventive intervention strategies and models of care. Curr Opin Psychiatry. 2011;24(4):301–6.
84. Gibb SJ, Fergusson DM, Horwood LJ. Burden of psychiatric disorder in young adulthood and life outcomes at age 30. Br J Psychiatry. 2010;197(2):122–7.
85. Pottick KJ, Bilder S, Vander Stoep A, Warner LA, Alvarez MF. US patterns of mental health service utilization for transition-age youth and young adults. J Behav Health Serv Res. 2008;35(4):373–89.
86. Appleton R, Connell C, Fairclough E, Tuomainen H, Singh SP. Outcomes of young people who reach the transition boundary of child and adolescent mental health services: a systematic review. Eur Child Adolesc Psychiatry. 2019;28(11):1431–46.
87. McNicholas F, Adamson M, McNamara N, Gavin B, Paul M, Ford T, et al. Who is in the transition gap? Transition from CAMHS to AMHS in the Republic of Ireland. Irish J Psychol Med. 2015;32(1):61–9.

88. Perera RH, Rogers SL, Edwards S, Hudman P, Malone C. Determinants of transition from child and adolescent to adult mental health services: a Western Australian Pilot Study. Aust Psychol. 2017;52(3):184–90.
89. Leavey G, McGrellis S, Forbes T, Thampi A, Davidson G, Rosato M, et al. Improving mental health pathways and care for adolescents in transition to adult services (IMPACT): a retrospective case note review of social and clinical determinants of transition. Soc Psychiatry Psychiatr Epidemiol. 2019;54(8):955–63.
90. Pontoni G, Di Pietro E, Neri T, Mattei G, Longo F, Neviani V, et al. Factors associated with the transition of adolescent inpatients from an intensive residential ward to adult mental health services. Eur Child Adolesc Psychiatry. 2021.
91. Singh SP, Paul M, Ford T, Kramer T, Weaver T, McLaren S, et al. Process, outcome and experience of transition from child to adult mental healthcare: multiperspective study. Br J Psychiatry. 2010;197(4):305–12.
92. Stagi P, Galeotti S, Mimmi S, Starace F, Castagnini AC. Continuity of care from child and adolescent to adult mental health services: evidence from a regional survey in Northern Italy. Eur Child Adolesc Psychiatry. 2015;24(12):1535–41.
93. Singh SP, Paul M, Ford T, Kramer T, Weaver T. Transitions of care from child and adolescent mental health services to adult mental health services (TRACK Study): a study of protocols in Greater London. BMC Health Serv Res. 2008;8:135.
94. Davis M, Butler M. Service system supports during the transition from adolescence to adulthood: parent perspectives. Shrewsbury, MA: Implementation Science and Practice Advances Research Center Publications; 2002.
95. McNamara N, Coyne I, Ford T, Paul M, Singh S, McNicholas F. Exploring social identity change during mental healthcare transition. Eur J Soc Psychol. 2017;47(7):889–903.
96. Cappelli M, Davidson S, Racek J, Leon S, Vloet M, Tataryn K, et al. Transitioning youth into adult mental health and addiction services: an outcomes evaluation of the youth transition project. J Behav Health Serv Res. 2016;43(4):597–610.
97. Singh S, Tuomainen H, Madan J, Warwick J, Street C, Wolke D, et al. Training of adult psychiatrists and child and adolescent psychiatrists in Europe: a systematic review of training characteristics and transition from child/adolescent to adult mental health services. BMC Med Educ. 2019;19(1):204.
98. Hendrickx G, De Roeck V, Russet F, Dieleman G, Franic T, Maras A, et al. Transition as a topic in psychiatry training throughout Europe: trainees' perspectives. Eur Child Adolesc Psychiatry. 2020;29(1):41–9.
99. Birchwood M, Singh SP. Mental health services for young people: matching the service to the need. Br J Psychiatry. 2013;202(s54):s1–2.
100. Youth Select Committee. Young people's mental health. London: British Youth Council; 2015.
101. McLaren S, Belling R, Paul M, Ford T, Kramer T, Weaver T, et al. 'Talking a different language': an exploration of the influence of organizational cultures and working practices on transition from child to adult mental health services. BMC Health Serv Res. 2013;13:254.
102. Reale L, Bonati M. Mental disorders and transition to adult mental health services: a scoping review. Eur Psychiatry. 2015;30(8):932–42.
103. Manteuffel B, Stephens RL, Sondheimer DL, Fisher SK. Characteristics, service experiences, and outcomes of transition-aged youth in systems of care: programmatic and policy implications. J Behav Health Serv Res. 2008;35(4):469–87.
104. Davis M, Sondheimer DL. State child mental health efforts to support youth in transition to adulthood. J Behav Health Serv Res. 2005;32(1):27–42.
105. Curtis SV, Wodarski JS. The East Tennessee Assertive Adolescent Family Treatment Program: a three-year evaluation. Soc Work Public Health. 2015;30(3):225–35.
106. Gilmer TP, Ojeda VD, Fawley-King K, Larson B, Garcia P. Change in mental health service use after offering youth-specific versus adult programs to transition-age youths. Psychiatr Serv. 2012;63(6):592–6.

107. Heflinger CA, Hoffman C. Transition age youth in publicly funded systems: identifying high-risk youth for policy planning and improved service delivery. J Behav Health Serv Res. 2008;35(4):390–401.
108. Scal P, Evans T, Blozis S, Okinow N, Blum R. Trends in transition from pediatric to adult health care services for young adults with chronic conditions. J Adolesc Health. 1999;24(4):259–64.
109. Purcell R, Jorm AF, Hickie IB, Yung AR, Pantelis C, Amminger GP, et al. Transitions Study of predictors of illness progression in young people with mental ill health: study methodology. Early Interv Psychiatry. 2015;9(1):38–47.
110. Wilson J, Clarke T, Lower R, Ugochukwu U, Maxwell S, Hodgekins J, et al. Creating an innovative youth mental health service in the United Kingdom: The Norfolk Youth Service. Early Interv Psychiatry. 2018;12(4):740–6.
111. Hendrickx G, De Roeck V, Maras A, Dieleman G, Gerritsen S, Purper-Ouakil D, et al. Challenges during the transition from child and adolescent mental health services to adult mental health services. BJPsych Bull. 2020;44(4):163–8.
112. Crowley R, Wolfe I, Lock K, McKee M. Improving the transition between paediatric and adult healthcare: a systematic review. Arch Dis Child. 2011;96(6):548–53.
113. Singh SP, Tuomainen H, Girolamo G, Maras A, Santosh P, McNicholas F, et al. Protocol for a cohort study of adolescent mental health service users with a nested cluster randomised controlled trial to assess the clinical and cost-effectiveness of managed transition in improving transitions from child to adult mental health services (the MILESTONE study). BMJ Open. 2017;7(10):e016055.
114. Tuomainen H, Schulze U, Warwick J, Paul M, Dieleman GC, Franić T, et al. Managing the link and strengthening transition from Child to Adult Mental Health Care in Europe (MILESTONE): background, rationale and methodology. BMC Psychiatry. 2018;18(1):167.
115. Santosh P, Singh J, Adams L, Mastroianni M, Heaney N, Lievesley K, et al. Validation of the transition readiness and appropriateness measure (TRAM) for the managing the link and strengthening transition from child to adult mental healthcare in Europe (MILESTONE) study. BMJ Open. 2020;10(6):e033324.
116. Singh SP, Tuomainen H. Transition from child to adult mental health services: needs, barriers, experiences and new models of care. World Psychiatry. 2015;14(3):358–61.
117. Broad KL, Sandhu VK, Sunderji N, Charach A. Youth experiences of transition from child mental health services to adult mental health services: a qualitative thematic synthesis. BMC Psychiatry. 2017;17(1):380.
118. Artero S, Touchon J, Ritchie K. Disability and mild cognitive impairment: a longitudinal population-based study. Int J Geriatr Psychiatry. 2001;16(11):1092–7.
119. Gigi K, Werbeloff N, Goldberg S, Portuguese S, Reichenberg A, Fruchter E, et al. Borderline intellectual functioning is associated with poor social functioning, increased rates of psychiatric diagnosis and drug use—a cross sectional population based study. Eur Neuropsychopharmacol. 2014;24(11):1793–7.
120. Moritz DJ, Kasl SV, Berkman LF. Cognitive functioning and the incidence of limitations in activities of daily living in an elderly community sample. Am J Epidemiol. 1995;141(1):41–9.
121. Warren EJ, Grek A, Conn D, Herrmann N, Icyk E, Kohl J, et al. A correlation between cognitive performance and daily functioning in elderly people. J Geriatr Psychiatry Neurol. 1989;2(2):96–100.
122. Aretouli E, Brandt J. Everyday functioning in mild cognitive impairment and its relationship with executive cognition. Int J Geriatr Psychiatry. 2010;25(3):224–33.
123. Wadley VG, Okonkwo O, Crowe M, Ross-Meadows LA. Mild cognitive impairment and everyday function: evidence of reduced speed in performing instrumental activities of daily living. Am J Geriatr Psychiatry. 2008;16(5):416–24.
124. Lee MT, Jang Y, Chang WY. How do impairments in cognitive functions affect activities of daily living functions in older adults? PLoS One. 2019;14(6):e0218112.
125. Green MF, Nuechterlein KH. The MATRICS initiative: developing a consensus cognitive battery for clinical trials. Schizophr Res. 2004;72(1):1–3.

126. Harvey PD. Domains of cognition and their assessment. Dialogues Clin Neurosci. 2019;21(3):227–37.
127. Daniëls NEM, Bartels SL, Verhagen SJW, Van Knippenberg RJM, De Vugt ME, Delespaul P. Digital assessment of working memory and processing speed in everyday life: feasibility, validation, and lessons-learned. Internet Interv. 2020;19:100300.
128. Mansueto G, van Nierop M, Schruers K, Alizadeh BZ, Bartels-Velthuis AA, van Beveren NJ, et al. The role of cognitive functioning in the relationship between childhood trauma and a mixed phenotype of affective-anxious-psychotic symptoms in psychotic disorders. Schizophr Res. 2018;192:262–8.
129. Shimada H, Makizako H, Lee S, Doi T, Lee S, Tsutsumimoto K, et al. Impact of cognitive frailty on daily activities in older persons. J Nutr Health Aging. 2016;20(7):729–35.
130. Albert SM, Tabert MH, Dienstag A, Pelton G, Devanand D. The impact of mild cognitive impairment on functional abilities in the elderly. Curr Psychiatry Rep. 2002;4(1):64–8.
131. Tuokko H, Morris C, Ebert P. Mild cognitive impairment and everyday functioning in older adults. Neurocase. 2005;11(1):40–7.
132. Farias ST, Mungas D, Reed BR, Harvey D, Cahn-Weiner D, Decarli C. MCI is associated with deficits in everyday functioning. Alzheimer Dis Assoc Disord. 2006;20(4):217–23.
133. Pérès K, Chrysostome V, Fabrigoule C, Orgogozo JM, Dartigues JF, Barberger-Gateau P. Restriction in complex activities of daily living in MCI: impact on outcome. Neurology. 2006;67(3):461–6.
134. Perneczky R, Pohl C, Sorg C, Hartmann J, Tosic N, Grimmer T, et al. Impairment of activities of daily living requiring memory or complex reasoning as part of the MCI syndrome. Int J Geriatr Psychiatry. 2006;21(2):158–62.
135. Okonkwo OC, Wadley VG, Griffith HR, Ball K, Marson DC. Cognitive correlates of financial abilities in mild cognitive impairment. J Am Geriatr Soc. 2006;54(11):1745–50.
136. Allaire JC, Gamaldo A, Ayotte BJ, Sims R, Whitfield K. Mild cognitive impairment and objective instrumental everyday functioning: the everyday cognition battery memory test. J Am Geriatr Soc. 2009;57(1):120–5.
137. Shamsi S, Lau A, Lencz T, Burdick KE, DeRosse P, Brenner R, et al. Cognitive and symptomatic predictors of functional disability in schizophrenia. Schizophr Res. 2011;126(1-3):257–64.
138. Galderisi S, Rucci P, Mucci A, Rossi A, Rocca P, Bertolino A, et al. The interplay among psychopathology, personal resources, context-related factors and real-life functioning in schizophrenia: stability in relationships after 4 years and differences in network structure between recovered and non-recovered patients. World Psychiatry. 2020;19(1):81–91.
139. Mucci A, Galderisi S, Gibertoni D, Rossi A, Rocca P, Bertolino A, et al. Factors associated with real-life functioning in persons with Schizophrenia in a 4-year follow-up study of the Italian Network for Research on Psychoses. JAMA Psychiat. 2021;78(5):550–9.
140. Bellack AS, Green MF, Cook JA, Fenton W, Harvey PD, Heaton RK, et al. Assessment of community functioning in people with schizophrenia and other severe mental illnesses: a white paper based on an NIMH-sponsored workshop. Schizophr Bull. 2007;33(3):805–22.
141. Green MF, Horan WP, Lee J. Nonsocial and social cognition in schizophrenia: current evidence and future directions. World Psychiatry. 2019;18(2):146–61.
142. Kerns JG, Berenbaum H. Cognitive impairments associated with formal thought disorder in people with schizophrenia. J Abnorm Psychol. 2002;111(2):211–24.
143. Wykes T, Huddy V, Cellard C, McGurk SR, Czobor P. A meta-analysis of cognitive remediation for schizophrenia: methodology and effect sizes. Am J Psychiatry. 2011;168(5):472–85.
144. Vita A, Barlati S, Ceraso A, Nibbio G, Ariu C, Deste G, et al. Effectiveness, core elements, and moderators of response of cognitive remediation for schizophrenia: a systematic review and meta-analysis of randomized clinical trials. JAMA Psychiat. 2021;78:848–58.
145. Barlati S, Deste G, De Peri L, Ariu C, Vita A. Cognitive remediation in schizophrenia: current status and future perspectives. Schizophr Res Treat. 2013;2013:156084.
146. Barlati S, Deste G, Galluzzo A, Perin AP, Valsecchi P, Turrina C, et al. Factors associated with response and resistance to cognitive remediation in schizophrenia: a critical review. Front Pharmacol. 2018;9:1542.

147. Galderisi S, Davidson M, Kahn RS, Mucci A, Boter H, Gheorghe MD, et al. Correlates of cognitive impairment in first episode schizophrenia: the EUFEST study. Schizophr Res. 2009;115(2–3):104–14.
148. McGurk SR, Mueser KT, Xie H, Welsh J, Kaiser S, Drake RE, et al. Cognitive enhancement treatment for people with mental illness who do not respond to supported employment: a randomized controlled trial. Am J Psychiatry. 2015;172(9):852–61.
149. Thompson RA. Emotion regulation: a theme in search of definition. Monogr Soc Res Child Dev. 1994;59(2–3):25–52.
150. Mayer JD, Roberts RD, Barsade SG. Human abilities: emotional intelligence. Annu Rev Psychol. 2008;59:507–36.
151. Mayer JD, Salovey P, Caruso DR. Emotional intelligence: new ability or eclectic traits? Am Psychol. 2008;63(6):503–17.
152. Gross JJ, Thompson RA. Emotion regulation: conceptual foundations. In: Gross JJ, editor. Handbook of emotion regulation. New York: Guilford Press; 2007. p. 3–24.
153. Mayer JD, Salovey P. Emotional intelligence, imagination, cognition, and personality. Cognit Pers. 1990;9:185–211.
154. Gross JJ. The emerging field of emotion regulation: an integrative review. Rev Gen Psychol. 1998;2(3):271–99.
155. Côté S, Gyurak A, Levenson RW. The ability to regulate emotion is associated with greater well-being, income, and socioeconomic status. Emotion. 2010;10(6):923–33.
156. Berking M, Wupperman P. Emotion regulation and mental health: recent findings, current challenges, and future directions. Curr Opin Psychiatry. 2012;25(2):128–34.
157. Schäfer J, Naumann E, Holmes EA, Tuschen-Caffier B, Samson AC. Emotion regulation strategies in depressive and anxiety symptoms in youth: a meta-analytic review. J Youth Adolesc. 2017;46(2):261–76.
158. Diedrich A, Burger J, Kirchner M, Berking M. Adaptive emotion regulation mediates the relationship between self-compassion and depression in individuals with unipolar depression. Psychol Psychother. 2017;90(3):247–63.
159. Musket CW, Hansen NS, Welker KM, Gilbert KE, Gruber J. A pilot investigation of emotional regulation difficulties and mindfulness-based strategies in manic and remitted bipolar I disorder and major depressive disorder. Int J Bipolar Disord. 2021;9(1):2.
160. Townsend J, Altshuler LL. Emotion processing and regulation in bipolar disorder: a review. Bipolar Disord. 2012;14(4):326–39.
161. Dodd A, Lockwood E, Mansell W, Palmier-Claus J. Emotion regulation strategies in bipolar disorder: a systematic and critical review. J Affect Disord. 2019;246:262–84.
162. Kirwan M, Pickett SM, Jarrett NL. Emotion regulation as a moderator between anxiety symptoms and insomnia symptom severity. Psychiatry Res. 2017;254:40–7.
163. O'Toole MS, Zachariae R, Mennin DS. Social anxiety and emotion regulation flexibility: considering emotion intensity and type as contextual factors. Anxiety Stress Coping. 2017;30(6):716–24.
164. Picó-Pérez M, Radua J, Steward T, Menchón JM, Soriano-Mas C. Emotion regulation in mood and anxiety disorders: a meta-analysis of fMRI cognitive reappraisal studies. Prog Neuropsychopharmacol Biol Psychiatry. 2017;79(Pt B):96–104.
165. Lugo-Candelas C, Flegenheimer C, McDermott JM, Harvey E. Emotional understanding, reactivity, and regulation in young children with ADHD symptoms. J Abnorm Child Psychol. 2017;45(7):1297–310.
166. Shaw P, Stringaris A, Nigg J, Leibenluft E. Emotion dysregulation in attention deficit hyperactivity disorder. Am J Psychiatry. 2014;171(3):276–93.
167. Shenaar-Golan V, Wald N, Yatzkar U. Patterns of emotion regulation and emotion-related behaviors among parents of children with and without ADHD. Psychiatry Res. 2017;258:494–500.
168. Dingemans A, Danner U, Parks M. Emotion regulation in binge eating disorder: a review. Nutrients. 2017;9(11):1274.

169. Mallorquí-Bagué N, Vintró-Alcaraz C, Sánchez I, Riesco N, Agüera Z, Granero R, et al. Emotion regulation as a transdiagnostic feature among eating disorders: cross-sectional and longitudinal approach. Eur Eat Disord Rev. 2018;26(1):53–61.
170. Gratz KL, Rosenthal MZ, Tull MT, Lejuez CW, Gunderson JG. An experimental investigation of emotion dysregulation in borderline personality disorder. J Abnorm Psychol. 2006;115(4):850–5.
171. Schulze L, Domes G, Krüger A, Berger C, Fleischer M, Prehn K, et al. Neuronal correlates of cognitive reappraisal in borderline patients with affective instability. Biol Psychiatry. 2011;69(6):564–73.
172. Dixon-Gordon KL, Turner BJ, Zachary Rosenthal M, Chapman AL. Emotion regulation in borderline personality disorder: an experimental investigation of the effects of instructed acceptance and suppression. Behav Ther. 2017;48(6):750–64.
173. Metcalfe RK, Fitzpatrick S, Kuo JR. A laboratory examination of emotion regulation skill strengthening in borderline personality disorder. J Pers Disord. 2017;8(3):237–46.
174. Zantinge G, van Rijn S, Stockmann L, Swaab H. Physiological arousal and emotion regulation strategies in young children with autism spectrum disorders. J Autism Dev Disord. 2017;47(9):2648–57.
175. Mazefsky CA, Herrington J, Siegel M, Scarpa A, Maddox BB, Scahill L, et al. The role of emotion regulation in autism spectrum disorder. J Am Acad Child Adolesc Psychiatry. 2013;52(7):679–88.
176. Cai RY, Richdale AL, Uljarević M, Dissanayake C, Samson AC. Emotion regulation in autism spectrum disorder: where we are and where we need to go. Autism Res. 2018;11(7):962–78.
177. Vanek J, Prasko J, Genzor S, Ociskova M, Holubova M, Sova M, et al. Insomnia and emotion regulation. Neuro Endocrinol Lett. 2020;41(5):255–69.
178. Sloan E, Hall K, Moulding R, Bryce S, Mildred H, Staiger PK. Emotion regulation as a transdiagnostic treatment construct across anxiety, depression, substance, eating and borderline personality disorders: a systematic review. Clin Psychol Rev. 2017;57:141–63.
179. Evren B, Evren C, Dalbudak E, Topcu M, Kutlu N. Relationship of internet addiction severity with probable ADHD and difficulties in emotion regulation among young adults. Psychiatry Res. 2018;269:494–500.
180. Mestre-Bach G, Fernández-Aranda F, Jiménez-Murcia S, Potenza MN. Emotional regulation in gambling disorder. Curr Opin Behav Sci. 2020;31:102–8.
181. Munguía L, Jiménez-Murcia S, Granero R, Baenas I, Agüera Z, Sánchez I, et al. Emotional regulation in eating disorders and gambling disorder: a transdiagnostic approach. J Behav Addict. 2021;10:508–23.
182. Navas JF, Contreras-Rodríguez O, Verdejo-Román J, Perandrés-Gómez A, Albein-Urios N, Verdejo-García A, et al. Trait and neurobiological underpinnings of negative emotion regulation in gambling disorder. Addiction. 2017;112(6):1086–94.
183. Dingle GA, Neves DDC, Alhadad SSJ, Hides L. Individual and interpersonal emotion regulation among adults with substance use disorders and matched controls. Br J Clin Psychol. 2018;57(2):186–202.
184. Zimmermann K, Walz C, Derckx RT, Kendrick KM, Weber B, Dore B, et al. Emotion regulation deficits in regular marijuana users. Hum Brain Mapp. 2017;38(8):4270–9.
185. Herman AM, Duka T. Facets of impulsivity and alcohol use: what role do emotions play? Neurosci Biobehav Rev. 2019;106:202–16.
186. Jakubczyk A, Trucco EM, Kopera M, Kobyliński P, Suszek H, Fudalej S, et al. The association between impulsivity, emotion regulation, and symptoms of alcohol use disorder. J Subst Abuse Treat. 2018;91:49–56.
187. Gross JJ, Muñoz RF. Emotion regulation and mental health. Clin Psychol Sci Pract. 1995;2(2):151–64.
188. Kring AM, Werner KH. Emotion regulation and psychopathology. In: Philippot Pierre FRS, editor. The regulation of emotion. Mahwah, NJ: Lawrence Erlbaum Associates; 2004. p. 359–85.

189. Hollon SD, Muñoz RF, Barlow DH, Beardslee WR, Bell CC, Bernal G, et al. Psychosocial intervention development for the prevention and treatment of depression: promoting innovation and increasing access. Biol Psychiatry. 2002;52(6):610–30.
190. Joormann J, Stanton CH. Examining emotion regulation in depression: a review and future directions. Behav Res Ther. 2016;86:35–49.
191. Mennin DS, Heimberg RG, Turk CL, Fresco DM. Preliminary evidence for an emotion dysregulation model of generalized anxiety disorder. Behav Res Ther. 2005;43(10):1281–310.
192. Tull MT, Stipelman BA, Salters-Pedneault K, Gratz KL. An examination of recent nonclinical panic attacks, panic disorder, anxiety sensitivity, and emotion regulation difficulties in the prediction of generalized anxiety disorder in an analogue sample. J Anxiety Disord. 2009;23(2):275–82.
193. Novick-Kline P, Turk CL, Mennin DS, Hoyt EA, Gallagher CL. Level of emotional awareness as a differentiating variable between individuals with and without generalized anxiety disorder. J Anxiety Disord. 2005;19(5):557–72.
194. Markland D, Ingledew DK. The measurement of exercise motives: factorial validity and invariance across gender of a revised Exercise Motivations Inventory. Br J Health Psychol. 1997;2(4):361–76.
195. Geller J, Cockell SJ, Hewitt PL, Goldner EM, Flett GL. Inhibited expression of negative emotions and interpersonal orientation in anorexia nervosa. Int J Eat Disord. 2000;28(1):8–19.
196. Fairburn CG, Cooper Z, Shafran R. Cognitive behaviour therapy for eating disorders: a "transdiagnostic" theory and treatment. Behav Res Ther. 2003;41(5):509–28.
197. Peñas-Lledó E, Vaz Leal FJ, Waller G. Excessive exercise in anorexia nervosa and bulimia nervosa: relation to eating characteristics and general psychopathology. Int J Eat Disord. 2002;31(4):370–5.
198. Smyth JM, Wonderlich SA, Heron KE, Sliwinski MJ, Crosby RD, Mitchell JE, et al. Daily and momentary mood and stress are associated with binge eating and vomiting in bulimia nervosa patients in the natural environment. J Consult Clin Psychol. 2007;75(4):629–38.
199. Wild B, Eichler M, Feiler S, Friederich HC, Hartmann M, Herzog W, et al. Dynamic analysis of electronic diary data of obese patients with and without binge eating disorder. Psychother Psychosom. 2007;76(4):250–2.
200. Crosby RD, Wonderlich SA, Engel SG, Simonich H, Smyth J, Mitchell JE. Daily mood patterns and bulimic behaviors in the natural environment. Behav Res Ther. 2009;47(3):181–8.
201. Smyth JM, Wonderlich SA, Sliwinski MJ, Crosby RD, Engel SG, Mitchell JE, et al. Ecological momentary assessment of affect, stress, and binge-purge behaviors: day of week and time of day effects in the natural environment. Int J Eat Disord. 2009;42(5):429–36.
202. Chua JL, Touyz S, Hill AJ. Negative mood-induced overeating in obese binge eaters: an experimental study. Int J Obes Relat Metab Disord. 2004;28(4):606–10.
203. Hilbert A, Tuschen-Caffier B. Maintenance of binge eating through negative mood: a naturalistic comparison of binge eating disorder and bulimia nervosa. Int J Eat Disord. 2007;40(6):521–30.
204. Stein RI, Kenardy J, Wiseman CV, Dounchis JZ, Arnow BA, Wilfley DE. What's driving the binge in binge eating disorder?: a prospective examination of precursors and consequences. Int J Eat Disord. 2007;40(3):195–203.
205. Bydlowski S, Corcos M, Jeammet P, Paterniti S, Berthoz S, Laurier C, et al. Emotion-processing deficits in eating disorders. Int J Eat Disord. 2005;37(4):321–9.
206. Carano A, De Berardis D, Gambi F, Di Paolo C, Campanella D, Pelusi L, et al. Alexithymia and body image in adult outpatients with binge eating disorder. Int J Eat Disord. 2006;39(4):332–40.
207. Svaldi J, Caffier D, Tuschen-Caffier B. Emotion suppression but not reappraisal increases desire to binge in women with binge eating disorder. Psychother Psychosom. 2010;79(3):188–90.
208. Corstorphine E, Mountford V, Tomlinson S, Waller G, Meyer C. Distress tolerance in the eating disorders. Eat Behav. 2007;8(1):91–7.
209. Naragon-Gainey K, McMahon TP, Chacko TP. The structure of common emotion regulation strategies: a meta-analytic examination. Psychol Bull. 2017;143(4):384–427.

210. Brockman R, Ciarrochi J, Parker P, Kashdan T. Emotion regulation strategies in daily life: mindfulness, cognitive reappraisal and emotion suppression. Cogn Behav Ther. 2017;46(2):91–113.
211. Passanisi A, D'Urso G, Pace U. The interplay between maladaptive personality traits and mindfulness deficits among adolescent regular gamblers: a mediation model. J Gambl Stud. 2019;35(1):93–105.
212. Kupfer DJ, Kuhl EA, Regier DA. DSM-5—the future arrived. JAMA. 2013;309(16):1691–2.
213. Cuthbert BN. The RDoC framework: facilitating transition from ICD/DSM to dimensional approaches that integrate neuroscience and psychopathology. World Psychiatry. 2014;13(1):28–35.
214. Keeley JW, Gaebel W. Symptom rating scales for schizophrenia and other primary psychotic disorders in ICD-11. Epidemiol Psychiatr Sci. 2018;27(3):219–24.
215. Citrome L. Unmet needs in the treatment of schizophrenia: new targets to help different symptom domains. J Clin Psychiatry. 2014;75(Suppl 1):21–6.
216. Foussias G, Siddiqui I, Fervaha G, Agid O, Remington G. Dissecting negative symptoms in schizophrenia: opportunities for translation into new treatments. J Psychopharmacol. 2015;29(2):116–26.
217. Marder SR, Galderisi S. The current conceptualization of negative symptoms in schizophrenia. World Psychiatry. 2017;16(1):14–24.
218. Kirkpatrick B, Buchanan RW, Ross DE, Carpenter WT Jr. A separate disease within the syndrome of schizophrenia. Arch Gen Psychiatry. 2001;58(2):165–71.
219. Kirkpatrick B, Galderisi S. Deficit schizophrenia: an update. World Psychiatry. 2008;7(3):143–7.
220. Kirkpatrick B, Mucci A, Galderisi S. Primary, enduring negative symptoms: an update on research. Schizophr Bull. 2017;43(4):730–6.
221. Strauss GP, Horan WP, Kirkpatrick B, Fischer BA, Keller WR, Miski P, et al. Deconstructing negative symptoms of schizophrenia: avolition-apathy and diminished expression clusters predict clinical presentation and functional outcome. J Psychiatr Res. 2013;47(6):783–90.
222. Kaiser S, Lyne J, Agartz I, Clarke M, Mørch-Johnsen L, Faerden A. Individual negative symptoms and domains—relevance for assessment, pathomechanisms and treatment. Schizophr Res. 2017;186:39–45.
223. Mucci A, Merlotti E, Üçok A, Aleman A, Galderisi S. Primary and persistent negative symptoms: concepts, assessments and neurobiological bases. Schizophr Res. 2017;186:19–28.
224. Lyne J, O'Donoghue B, Roche E, Renwick L, Cannon M, Clarke M. Negative symptoms of psychosis: a life course approach and implications for prevention and treatment. Early Interv Psychiatry. 2018;12(4):561–71.
225. an der Heiden W, Häfner H. The epidemiology of onset and course of schizophrenia. Eur Arch Psychiatry Clin Neurosci. 2000;250(6):292–303.
226. An der Heiden W, Leber A, Häfner H. Negative symptoms and their association with depressive symptoms in the long-term course of schizophrenia. Eur Arch Psychiatry Clin Neurosci. 2016;266(5):387–96.
227. Mäkinen J, Miettunen J, Isohanni M, Koponen H. Negative symptoms in schizophrenia: a review. Nord J Psychiatry. 2008;62(5):334–41.
228. Malla AK, Norman RM, Takhar J, Manchanda R, Townsend L, Scholten D, et al. Can patients at risk for persistent negative symptoms be identified during their first episode of psychosis? J Nerv Ment Dis. 2004;192(7):455–63.
229. Galderisi S, Mucci A, Bitter I, Libiger J, Bucci P, Fleischhacker WW, et al. Persistent negative symptoms in first episode patients with schizophrenia: results from the European First Episode Schizophrenia Trial. Eur Neuropsychopharmacol. 2013;23(3):196–204.
230. Austin SF, Mors O, Budtz-Jørgensen E, Secher RG, Hjorthøj CR, Bertelsen M, et al. Long-term trajectories of positive and negative symptoms in first episode psychosis: a 10year follow-up study in the OPUS cohort. Schizophr Res. 2015;168(1-2):84–91.
231. Carbon M, Correll CU. Thinking and acting beyond the positive: the role of the cognitive and negative symptoms in schizophrenia. CNS Spectr. 2014;19(Suppl 1):38–52; quiz 35-7, 53.

232. Heider N, Spruyt A, De Houwer J. Body dissatisfaction revisited: on the importance of implicit beliefs about actual and ideal body image. Psychol Belg. 2018;57(4):158–73.
233. Ferreira C, Pinto-Gouveia J, Duarte C. Physical appearance as a measure of social ranking: the role of a new scale to understand the relationship between weight and dieting. Clin Psychol Psychother. 2013;20(1):55–66.
234. Thompson JK, Heinberg LJ, Altabe M, Tantleff-Dunn S. Exacting beauty: theory, assessment, and treatment of body image disturbance, vol. 12. Washington, DC: American Psychological Association; 1999. p. 396.
235. Barlett CP, Vowels C, Saucier DA. Meta-analyses of the effects of media images on men's body-image concerns. J Soc Clin Psychol. 2008;27:279–310.
236. Grabe S, Ward LM, Hyde JS. The role of the media in body image concerns among women: a meta-analysis of experimental and correlational studies. Psychol Bull. 2008;134(3):460–76.
237. Markey CH, Gillen MM. Body Image. In: Levesque RJR, editor. Encyclopedia of Adolescence. Cham: Springer International; 2016. p. 1–14.
238. Espinoza G, Juvonen J. The pervasiveness, connectedness, and intrusiveness of social network site use among young adolescents. Cyberpsychol Behav Soc Netw. 2011;14(12):705–9.
239. Chua THH, Chang L. Follow me and like my beautiful selfies: Singapore teenage girls' engagement in self-presentation and peer comparison on social media. Comput Hum Behav. 2016;55:190–7.
240. Siibak A. Constructing the self through the photo selection—visual impression management on social networking websites. Cyberpsychology. 2009;3:1.
241. Valkenburg PM, Peter J. The Differential susceptibility to media effects model. J Commun. 2013;63(2):221–43.
242. de Vries DA, Vossen HGM, van der Boom PVK. Social media and body dissatisfaction: investigating the attenuating role of positive parent-adolescent relationships. J Youth Adolesc. 2019;48(3):527–36.
243. Keery H, van den Berg P, Thompson JK. An evaluation of the tripartite influence model of body dissatisfaction and eating disturbance with adolescent girls. Body Image. 2004;1(3):237–51.
244. Warren MP. Physical and biological aspects of puberty. In: Brooks-Gunn J, Petersen AC, editors. Girls at puberty: biological and psychosocial perspectives. Boston, MA: Springer US; 1983. p. 3–28.
245. Babio N, Arija V, Sancho C, Canals J. Factors associated with body dissatisfaction in non-clinical adolescents at risk of eating disorders. J Public Health. 2008;16(2):107–15.
246. Bearman SK, Stice E. Testing a gender additive model: the role of body image in adolescent depression. J Abnorm Child Psychol. 2008;36(8):1251–63.
247. Benedikt R, Wertheim EH, Love A. Eating attitudes and weight-loss attempts in female adolescents and their mothers. J Youth Adolesc. 1998;27(1):43–57.
248. Davison KK, Markey CN, Birch LL. Etiology of body dissatisfaction and weight concerns among 5-year-old girls. Appetite. 2000;35(2):143–51.
249. Wertheim EH, Mee V, Paxton SJ. Relationships among adolescent girls' eating behaviors and their parents' weight-related attitudes and behaviors. Sex Roles. 1999;41(3):169–87.
250. Haines J, Neumark-Sztainer D, Hannan P, Robinson-O'Brien R. Child versus parent report of parental influences on children's weight-related attitudes and behaviors. J Pediatr Psychol. 2008;33(7):783–8.
251. Markey CN, Markey PM. romantic relationships and body satisfaction among young women. J Youth Adolesc. 2006;35(2):256–64.
252. Goins LB, Markey CN, Gillen MM. Understanding men's body image in the context of their romantic relationships. Am J Mens Health. 2012;6(3):240–8.
253. Tantleff-Dunn S, Thompson JK. Romantic partners and body image disturbance: further evidence for the role of perceived—actual disparities. Sex Roles. 1995;33(9):589–605.
254. Smolak L. Body image in children and adolescents: where do we go from here? Body Image. 2004;1(1):15–28.
255. Stice E, Bearman SK. Body-image and eating disturbances prospectively predict increases in depressive symptoms in adolescent girls: a growth curve analysis. Dev Psychol. 2001;37(5):597–607.

256. Stice E, Shaw HE. Role of body dissatisfaction in the onset and maintenance of eating pathology: a synthesis of research findings. J Psychosom Res. 2002;53(5):985–93.
257. McCabe MP, Ricciardelli LA. Body image dissatisfaction among males across the lifespan: a review of past literature. J Psychosom Res. 2004;56(6):675–85.
258. Cafri G, Thompson JK, Ricciardelli L, McCabe M, Smolak L, Yesalis C. Pursuit of the muscular ideal: physical and psychological consequences and putative risk factors. Clin Psychol Rev. 2005;25(2):215–39.
259. Paxton SJ, Neumark-Sztainer D, Hannan PJ, Eisenberg ME. Body dissatisfaction prospectively predicts depressive mood and low self-esteem in adolescent girls and boys. J Clin Child Adolesc Psychol. 2006;35(4):539–49.
260. Shin NY, Shin MS. Body dissatisfaction, self-esteem, and depression in obese Korean children. J Pediatr. 2008;152(4):502–6.
261. Satghare P, Mahesh MV, Abdin E, Chong SA, Subramaniam M. The relative associations of body image dissatisfaction among psychiatric out-patients in Singapore. Int J Environ Res Public Health. 2019;16(24):5162.
262. Balta S, Emirtekin E, Kircaburun K, Griffiths MD. The mediating role of depression in the relationship between body image dissatisfaction and cyberbullying perpetration. Int J Ment Health Addict. 2020;18(6):1482–92.
263. Barnes M, Abhyankar P, Dimova E, Best C. Associations between body dissatisfaction and self-reported anxiety and depression in otherwise healthy men: a systematic review and meta-analysis. PLoS One. 2020;15(2):e0229268.
264. You S, Shin K. Body dissatisfaction and mental health outcomes among Korean college students. Psychol Rep. 2016;118(3):714–24.
265. Rodríguez-Cano T, Beato-Fernández L, Llario AB. Body dissatisfaction as a predictor of self-reported suicide attempts in adolescents: a Spanish community prospective study. J Adolesc Health. 2006;38(6):684–8.
266. Perkins NM, Brausch AM. Body dissatisfaction and symptoms of bulimia nervosa prospectively predict suicide ideation in adolescents. Int J Eat Disord. 2019;52(8):941–9.
267. Brausch AM, Muehlenkamp JJ. Body image and suicidal ideation in adolescents. Body Image. 2007;4(2):207–12.
268. Archibald K. The role of body image and social anxiety in problematic drinking behavior. Undergrad Rev. 2010;6:15–20.
269. Simbar M, Nazarpour S, Alavi Majd H, Dodel Andarvar K, Jafari Torkamani Z, Alsadat RF. Is body image a predictor of women's depression and anxiety in postmenopausal women? BMC Psychiatry. 2020;20(1):202.
270. Pawijit Y, Likhitsuwan W, Ludington J, Pisitsungkagarn K. Looks can be deceiving: body image dissatisfaction relates to social anxiety through fear of negative evaluation. Int J Adolesc Med Health. 2017;31(4).
271. Davison TE, McCabe MP. Relationships between men's and women's body image and their psychological, social, and sexual functioning. Sex Roles. 2005;52(7):463–75.
272. Gillen MM, Markey CN. Body image and mental health. In: Friedman HS, editor. Encyclopedia of mental health. New York: Elsevier; 2016. p. 187–92.
273. Deckersbach T, Otto MW, Savage CR, Baer L, Jenike MA. The relationship between semantic organization and memory in obsessive-compulsive disorder. Psychother Psychosom. 2000;69(2):101–7.
274. Ayub N, Kimong P, Ee G. A distorted body image: cognitive behavioral therapy for body dysmorphic disorder. London: IntechOpen; 2018.
275. (UNHCR) UNHCfR. Coordination in Complex Emergencies. 2001. https://www.unhcr.org/partners/partners/3ba88e7c6/coordination-complex-emergencies.html.
276. Brennan RJ, Nandy R. Complex humanitarian emergencies: a major global health challenge. Emerg Med (Fremantle). 2001;13(2):147–56.
277. Ćosić K, Popović S, Šarlija M, Kesedžić I. Impact of human disasters and COVID-19 pandemic on mental health: potential of digital psychiatry. Psychiatr Danub. 2020;32(1):25–31.

278. Mental health and psychosocial consequences of armed conflict and natural disasters. Int J Soc Psychiatry. 2011;57(1_suppl):57–78.
279. Organization WH. Mental health and psychosocial well–being among children in severe food shortage situations. Geneva: WHO; 2006.
280. Hussain A, Nygaard E, Siqveland J, Heir T. The relationship between psychiatric morbidity and quality of life: interview study of Norwegian tsunami survivors 2 and 6 years post-disaster. BMC Psychiatry. 2016;16:173.
281. Mollica RF, McInnes K, Sarajlić N, Lavelle J, Sarajlić I, Massagli MP. Disability associated with psychiatric comorbidity and health status in Bosnian refugees living in Croatia. JAMA. 1999;282(5):433–9.
282. Weiss DS, Marmar CR, Schlenger WE, Fairbank JA, Jordan BK, Hough RL, et al. The prevalence of lifetime and partial post-traumatic stress disorder in Vietnam theater veterans. J Trauma Stress. 1992;5(3):365–76.
283. Steel Z, Chey T, Silove D, Marnane C, Bryant RA, van Ommeren M. Association of torture and other potentially traumatic events with mental health outcomes among populations exposed to mass conflict and displacement: a systematic review and meta-analysis. JAMA. 2009;302(5):537–49.
284. United nations educational, scientific and cultural organization (UNESCO). Global education monitoring report team. The hidden crisis: armed conflict and education; EFA global monitoring report. 2011.
285. de Jong JT, Berckmoes LH, Kohrt BA, Song SJ, Tol WA, Reis R. A public health approach to address the mental health burden of youth in situations of political violence and humanitarian emergencies. Curr Psychiatry Rep. 2015;17(7):60.
286. Activities UNFfP. Women and girls in humanitarian emergencies in Eastern Europe and Central Asia. 2016.
287. Asghar K, Rubenstein B, Stark L. Preventing household violence: promising strategies for humanitarian settings. CPC Learning Network. 2017. http://www.cpcnetwork.org/wp-content/uploads/2017/02/Landscaping-review-Final-Jan-2017.pdf.
288. Jaung M, Jani S, Banu S, Mackey JM. International emergency psychiatry challenges: disaster medicine, war, human trafficking, displaced persons. Psychiatr Clin North Am. 2017;40(3):565–74.
289. Ventevogel P, van Ommeren M, Schilperoord M, Saxena S. Improving mental health care in humanitarian emergencies. Bull World Health Organ. 2015;93(10):666.
290. Mollica RF, Cardozo BL, Osofsky HJ, Raphael B, Ager A, Salama P. Mental health in complex emergencies. Lancet. 2004;364(9450):2058–67.
291. van Ommeren M, Hanna F, Weissbecker I, Ventevogel P. Mental health and psychosocial support in humanitarian emergencies. East Mediterr Health J. 2015;21(7):498–502.
292. Ventevogel P. Interventions for mental health and psychosocial support in complex humanitarian emergencies: moving towards consensus in policy and action? In: Morina N, Nickerson A, editors. Mental health of refugee and conflict-affected populations: theory, research and clinical practice. Cham: Springer International; 2018. p. 155–80.
293. Shigemura J, Ursano RJ, Morganstein JC, Kurosawa M, Benedek DM. Public responses to the novel 2019 coronavirus (2019-nCoV) in Japan: mental health consequences and target populations. Psychiatry Clin Neurosci. 2020;74(4):281–2.
294. Sim K, Huak Chan Y, Chong PN, Chua HC, Wen SS. Psychosocial and coping responses within the community health care setting towards a national outbreak of an infectious disease. J Psychosom Res. 2010;68(2):195–202.
295. Moreno C, Wykes T, Galderisi S, Nordentoft M, Crossley N, Jones N, et al. How mental health care should change as a consequence of the COVID-19 pandemic. Lancet Psychiatry. 2020;7(9):813–24.
296. Fiorillo A, Gorwood P. The consequences of the COVID-19 pandemic on mental health and implications for clinical practice. Eur Psychiatry. 2020;63(1):e32.
297. McCracken LM, Badinlou F, Buhrman M, Brocki KC. Psychological impact of COVID-19 in the Swedish population: depression, anxiety, and insomnia and their associations to risk and vulnerability factors. Eur Psychiatry. 2020;63(1):e81.

298. Fiorillo A, Sampogna G, Giallonardo V, Del Vecchio V, Luciano M, Albert U, et al. Effects of the lockdown on the mental health of the general population during the COVID-19 pandemic in Italy: results from the COMET collaborative network. Eur Psychiatry. 2020;63(1):e87.
299. Fonseca L, Diniz E, Mendonça G, Malinowski F, Mari J, Gadelha A. Schizophrenia and COVID-19: risks and recommendations. Rev Bras Psiquiatr. 2020;42(3):236–8.
300. Kozloff N, Mulsant BH, Stergiopoulos V, Voineskos AN. The COVID-19 global pandemic: implications for people with Schizophrenia and related disorders. Schizophr Bull. 2020;46(4):752–7.
301. Hernández-Gómez A, Andrade-González N, Lahera G, Vieta E. Recommendations for the care of patients with bipolar disorder during the COVID-19 pandemic. J Affect Disord. 2021;279:117–21.
302. Stefana A, Youngstrom EA, Chen J, Hinshaw S, Maxwell V, Michalak E, et al. The COVID-19 pandemic is a crisis and opportunity for bipolar disorder. Bipolar Disord. 2020;22(6):641–3.
303. Banerjee DD. The other side of COVID-19: Impact on obsessive compulsive disorder (OCD) and hoarding. Psychiatry Res. 2020;288:112966.
304. Sulaimani MF, Bagadood NH. Implication of coronavirus pandemic on obsessive-compulsive-disorder symptoms. Rev Environ Health. 2021;36(1):1–8.
305. Kumar A, Somani A. Dealing with Corona virus anxiety and OCD. Asian J Psychiatr. 2020;51:102053.
306. Fernández-Aranda F, Casas M, Claes L, Bryan DC, Favaro A, Granero R, et al. COVID-19 and implications for eating disorders. Eur Eat Disord Rev. 2020;28(3):239–45.
307. Cooper M, Reilly EE, Siegel JA, Coniglio K, Sadeh-Sharvit S, Pisetsky EM, et al. Eating disorders during the COVID-19 pandemic and quarantine: an overview of risks and recommendations for treatment and early intervention. Eat Disord. 2020:1–23.
308. Ko CH, Yen JY. Impact of COVID-19 on gaming disorder: monitoring and prevention. J Behav Addict. 2020;9(2):187–9.
309. King D, Delfabbro P, Billieux J, Potenza M. Problematic online gaming and the COVID-19 pandemic. J Behav Addict. 2020;9:184–6.
310. Cortese S, Asherson P, Sonuga-Barke E, Banaschewski T, Brandeis D, Buitelaar J, et al. ADHD management during the COVID-19 pandemic: guidance from the European ADHD Guidelines Group. Lancet Child Adolesc Health. 2020;4(6):412–4.
311. McGrath J. ADHD and Covid-19: current roadblocks and future opportunities. Irish J Psychol Med. 2020;37(3):204–11.
312. Courtenay K, Perera B. COVID-19 and people with intellectual disability: impacts of a pandemic. Irish J Psychol Med. 2020;37(3):231–6.
313. Narzisi A. Handle the Autism Spectrum condition during Coronavirus (COVID-19) stay at home period: ten tips for helping parents and caregivers of young children. Brain Sci. 2020;10(4):207.
314. Pfefferbaum B, North CS. Mental health and the Covid-19 pandemic. N Engl J Med. 2020;383(6):510–2.
315. Du J, Dong L, Wang T, Yuan C, Fu R, Zhang L, et al. Psychological symptoms among frontline healthcare workers during COVID-19 outbreak in Wuhan. Gen Hosp Psychiatry. 2020;67:144–5.
316. Zhang WR, Wang K, Yin L, Zhao WF, Xue Q, Peng M, et al. Mental health and psychosocial problems of medical health workers during the COVID-19 epidemic in China. Psychother Psychosom. 2020;89(4):242–50.
317. Kang L, Ma S, Chen M, Yang J, Wang Y, Li R, et al. Impact on mental health and perceptions of psychological care among medical and nursing staff in Wuhan during the 2019 novel coronavirus disease outbreak: a cross-sectional study. Brain Behav Immun. 2020;87:11–7.
318. Pezzella P, Galderisi S. L'impatto della pandemia di COVID-19 sulla salute mentale. Noos Aggiornamenti in Psichiatria. 2020;26(3):171–82.

Afterword: Prevention of the Risk of Mental Suffering, A General and Specific Objective at Every Stage of Life

Matteo Balestrieri

> *Budding psychiatric rehabilitator, referring to patients*
> *"Why can't they have a slightly more normal life?"*
> *Psychiatrist*
> *"Because normal life for them is a risk".*
> *Rehabilitator*
> *"It is for everyone!".*
>
> *"Si può fare (You can do it)", a film by Giulio Manfredonia*

Prevention in mental health is aimed in a general sense at achieving good mental health and in a more specific sense at reducing the risk of mental disorders. Mental health has been defined as "a state of well-being in which the individual realises his or her abilities, can cope with the normal stresses of life, can work productively and fruitfully, and is able to make a contribution to his or her community" [1]. As far as mental disorders are concerned, they should be understood broadly as "a behavioural or mental pattern that causes significant distress or impairment in personal functioning" [2].

As is well illustrated in this volume, the quantity and quality of factors involved in prevention are extremely vast. We know that mental disorders are dynamic and heterogeneous phenomena whose pathogenesis is necessarily multi-causal, which entails an extreme expansion of the objectives of prevention. In order to systematise them, the concepts of primary, secondary and tertiary prevention have been used for a long time, although they are not always clearly differentiated. As pointed out by Lasalvia in one of the chapters of this volume, a framework of reference perhaps

M. Balestrieri
University of Udine, Udine, Italy

Psychiatric Clinic, Integrated University Health Authority, Udine, Italy

Psychiatry Residency Training Program, Udine, Italy

Degree Course in Professional Education, University of Udine, Udine, Italy more useful is instead that described by Mrazek and Haggerty, who list three types of prevention [3]: (a) universal (aimed at the general population); (b) selective (aimed at high-risk groups); (c) indicated (aimed at high-risk subjects who already present some symptoms without coming to meet all the diagnostic criteria of a disorder). This type of classification, in my opinion, allows to define the different approaches that must be proper to these three types of prevention. And each approach is defined by the characteristics of the following constituent elements: the actor (the expert who carries out the prevention), the user, the type of intervention, the place where the prevention takes place and the timing of the prevention.

If we consider *universal prevention*, the users could be families, teachers, and students. The approach to families is less codifiable, as they are less easily reached and are exposed to information from many sources, from television (more generalist) or the web in all its forms (with the risks of fake and confirmation bias). Schools therefore remain the preferred place for universal prevention. A recent meta-analysis of randomised controlled trials evaluating school-based programmes to prevent depression and anxiety in children and adolescents suggests that school-based depression and anxiety prevention programmes produce moderate positive effects, but these tend to fade over time [4]. Universal interventions tend to be less effective than selective or indicated prevention interventions. This is not surprising, as change effects are more likely to be achieved in young people who are at risk or already symptomatic. In addition, very large sample sizes are needed to achieve significant universal prevention effects: by exporting the data obtained on a large scale, estimates suggest that existing programmes can prevent 21% of new cases of depression, with about 22 individuals who need to be treated to prevent one case of depression. Another aspect that emerges in the meta-analysis, which answers the question of who should be the actor of prevention, is that there is a certain greater effectiveness, only in the short term, of prevention programmes carried out by external staff (more experienced in mental health) than those carried out by teachers. Obviously, there are practical limitations associated with hiring external staff, as they can be expensive and difficult to sustain in the medium and long term.

With regard to *selective prevention*, the identification of cases at risk and the quantification of the risk itself are fundamental. The latter estimation is often complex, since it can refer to biological as well as behavioural parameters and varies greatly in relation to the type of psychopathology studied. In this regard, the subject of endophenotypes, biological and psychological phenomena that link genetic contributions to the symptoms of a disorder, has been much studied. Their early recognition, often in a specialist context, can pave the way for selective prevention, but quantifying the risk is never easy in individual patients. When only the behavioural aspect is taken into account, suicidal ideation can be considered a risk factor for suicide, but it is much more widespread than the latter. The gradation of risk therefore depends on the frequency with which the ideation manifests itself and interferes with daily life. Similarly, hopelessness in an adolescent is a risk for depressive disorder, but may dissipate completely with increasing age. High risk can be defined here by a combination of unfavourable factors, in which hopelessness is aggravated by an unsupportive environment, easy access to substances, economic poverty and lack of social and health services.

In this volume, there are many chapters dealing with the definition of risk from a selective prevention perspective. Within the systematisation of clinical staging for mental health, analysed by Rutigliano and Del Grande, risk states should correspond precisely to stage 0. On the contrary, the definition of at-risk mental states (ARMS) used in the literature coincides with stage 1 of clinical staging (i.e., high-risk individuals seeking help). This distinction underlines the difficulty of identifying at-risk individuals before the onset of symptoms or personal suffering. Who is the actor of recognition in this case? Once again, the school, or the paediatrician or any educator involved in the growth of the child or adolescent. On the contrary, it is very important to recognise cognitive neurodevelopmental assets in the premorbid phase (see Bellani et al. and Zoccante et al. in this volume), which are instead observed by mental health specialists from a perspective of selective prevention of psychiatric disorders. A broad overview of the mental health risk factors to be considered is contained in a document published by the World Health Organisation a few years ago, in which individual, social and environmental factors related to the risk of psychiatric disorders are systematically analysed [5]. I refer to it for a more detailed discussion of this issue.

Finally, *indicated prevention* refers to those individuals at risk who have the first manifestations of illness or who come in for observation due to a state of distress. The quality of indicated prevention depends both on factors relating to the individual and on the organisational characteristics of healthcare. As far as the individual is concerned, a central aspect is illness behaviour, i.e. the behaviour that each individual engages in at the onset of a state of mental suffering. The variables that modulate illness behaviour range from personal beliefs about illness (the reference to no-vax is inevitable in this historical moment) to the degree of medical culture, the subjective threshold of suffering, the level of fear of illness and treatment and the attitudes of family members and acquaintances. All these contribute not only to the failure to detect the disorder but also to the degree of adherence to the prescribed treatments.

The other aspect to consider is the organisation of healthcare. Healthcare that is proximal to the citizen will be able to recognise and intervene earlier. General practitioners and paediatricians must be able to recognise the first symptoms of illness, but they must also have easier access to mental health services. Clinical skills and organisational opportunities must go hand in hand to avoid long months, or sometimes years, before treatment starts. This means that we need to have an effective and efficient healthcare system, which is not split between services that are poorly communicating with each other. In this sense, it is important to recall the chapter by Pezzella et al. on the importance of the delicate transition from mental health services for minors to those for adults.

A large body of literature has long told us that the longer the period of untreated illness, the worse the prognosis of the disorder. A recent meta-analysis on the duration of untreated psychosis (DUP), for example, found highly suggestive evidence of a relationship between a longer DUP and more severe positive and negative symptoms and global psychopathology in general, a greater likelihood of self-harm before first contact, as well as a lower likelihood of remission at follow-up [6].

Even in the case of indicated prevention, this volume provides numerous insights that I do not mention for the sake of brevity and the variety of topics addressed, with the exception of Lemon and Thompson's chapter on pharmacological treatments in at-risk individuals, which attempts to take stock of a rather critical and criticised subject by highlighting the potential neuroprotective role of a number of psychotropic drugs that are on the market or may soon be introduced.

Finally, a careful reflection on the costs of prevention is needed. It has been said many times that prevention costs less than treatment, even in the case of mental health. A recent systematic review by Le et al. [7] took stock by selecting 65 studies published from 2008 to 2020 which assessed the cost-effectiveness of preventing mental disorders (especially depression and anxiety disorders) and promoting mental well-being, compared to usual care or no intervention. Most studies showed that interventions for prevention and mental health promotion were cost-effective. Screening plus school psychological interventions were the most cost-effective interventions for prevention in children and adolescents, while parental and workplace interventions were more effective for mental health promotion in children and adults, respectively. Overall, therefore, prevention appears to be cost-effective, which contrasts with the fact that it very often attracts little attention and resources.

In conclusion, the points of reflection offered by this volume are many, and I have tried to highlight how many of them open up to further considerations, in particular by highlighting the practical feasibility of prevention interventions. I believe that reading various chapters will provide younger and more attentive psychiatrists, in particular with many stimuli for their profession, the aim of which is to promote a healthy life free from the condition of illness.

References

1. Galderisi S, Heinz A, Kastrup M, Beezhold J, Sartorius N. Toward a new definition of mental health. World Psychiatry. 2015;14(2):231–3. https://doi.org/10.1002/wps.20231.
2. Bolton D. What is mental disorder? An essay in philosophy, science, and values. Oxford: Oxford University Press; 2008. p. 6. https://books.google.it/books?id=Ohzt1HBilXcC&pg=PA6&redir_esc=y#v=onepage&q&f=false
3. Institute of Medicine (US) Committee on Prevention of Mental Disorders. In: Mrazek PJ, Haggerty RJ, editors. Reducing risks for mental disorders: frontiers for preventive intervention research. New directions in definitions. Washington, DC: National Academies Press (US); 1994. https://doi.org/10.17226/2139. https://www.ncbi.nlm.nih.gov/books/NBK236318/.
4. Werner-Seidler A, Spanos S, Calear AL, Perry Y, Torok M, O'Dea B, Christensen H, Newby JM. School-based depression and anxiety prevention programs: an updated systematic review and meta-analysis. Clin Psychol Rev. 2021;89:102079. https://doi.org/10.1016/j.cpr.2021.102079.
5. WHO. Risks to mental health: an overview of vulnerabilities and risk factors. In: Background paper by WHO secretariat for the development of a comprehensive mental health action plan. Geneva: World Health Organization; 2012. https://www.who.int/mental_health/mhgap/risks_to_mental_health_EN_27_08_12.pdf.
6. Howes OD, Whitehurst T, Shatalina E, et al. The clinical significance of duration of untreated psychosis: an umbrella review and random-effects meta-analysis. World Psychiatry. 2021;20(1):75–95. https://doi.org/10.1002/wps.20822.
7. Le LK-D, Esturas AC, Mihalopoulos C, Chiotelis O, Bucholc J, Chatterton ML, et al. Cost-effectiveness evidence of mental health prevention and promotion interventions: a systematic review of economic evaluations. PLoS Med. 2021;18(5):e1003606. https://doi.org/10.1371/journal.pmed.1003606.